Novel Approaches for Overcoming Biological Barriers

Novel Approaches for Overcoming Biological Barriers

Editors

Vibhuti Agrahari
Prashant Kumar

MDPI • Basel • Beijing • Wuhan • Barcelona • Belgrade • Manchester • Tokyo • Cluj • Tianjin

Editors
Vibhuti Agrahari
Department of
Pharmaceutical Sciences
University of Oklahoma
Health Sciences Center
Oklahoma City
United States

Prashant Kumar
Vaccine Analytics and
Formulation Center (VAFC)
University of Kansas
Lawrence
United States

Editorial Office
MDPI
St. Alban-Anlage 66
4052 Basel, Switzerland

This is a reprint of articles from the Special Issue published online in the open access journal *Pharmaceutics* (ISSN 1999-4923) (available at: www.mdpi.com/journal/pharmaceutics/special_issues/novel_approaches_biological_barriers).

For citation purposes, cite each article independently as indicated on the article page online and as indicated below:

LastName, A.A.; LastName, B.B.; LastName, C.C. Article Title. *Journal Name* **Year**, *Volume Number*, Page Range.

ISBN 978-3-0365-7699-2 (Hbk)
ISBN 978-3-0365-7698-5 (PDF)

Contents

About the Editors . . . . **vii**

Vibhuti Agrahari and Prashant Kumar
Novel Approaches for Overcoming Biological Barriers
Reprinted from: *Pharmaceutics* **2022**, *14*, 1851, doi:10.3390/pharmaceutics14091851 . . . . **1**

Sahar Jafari, Ittai S. Baum, Oleg G. Udalov, Yichien Lee, Olga Rodriguez and Stanley T. Fricke et al.
Opening the Blood Brain Barrier with an Electropermanent Magnet System
Reprinted from: *Pharmaceutics* **2022**, *14*, 1503, doi:10.3390/pharmaceutics14071503 . . . . **5**

Rehab A. Alshammari, Fadilah S. Aleanizy, Amal Aldarwesh, Fulwah Y. Alqahtani, Wael A. Mahdi and Bushra Alquadeib et al.
Retinal Delivery of the Protein Kinase C-β Inhibitor Ruboxistaurin Using Non-Invasive Nanoparticles of Polyamidoamine Dendrimers
Reprinted from: *Pharmaceutics* **2022**, *14*, 1444, doi:10.3390/pharmaceutics14071444 . . . . **17**

Angelo Corti, Teresa Calimeri, Flavio Curnis and Andres J. M. Ferreri
Targeting the Blood–Brain Tumor Barrier with Tumor Necrosis Factor-α
Reprinted from: *Pharmaceutics* **2022**, *14*, 1414, doi:10.3390/pharmaceutics14071414 . . . . **39**

Ramesh Nimma, Anil Kumar Kalvala, Nilkumar Patel, Sunil Kumar Surapaneni, Li Sun and Rakesh Singh et al.
Combined Transcriptomic and Proteomic Profiling to Unravel Osimertinib, CARP-1 Functional Mimetic (CFM 4.17) Formulation and Telmisartan Combo Treatment in NSCLC Tumor Xenografts
Reprinted from: *Pharmaceutics* **2022**, *14*, 1156, doi:10.3390/pharmaceutics14061156 . . . . **55**

Toni Todorovski, Diogo A. Mendonça, Lorena O. Fernandes-Siqueira, Christine Cruz-Oliveira, Giuseppina Guida and Javier Valle et al.
Targeting Zika Virus with New Brain- and Placenta-Crossing Peptide–Porphyrin Conjugates
Reprinted from: *Pharmaceutics* **2022**, *14*, 738, doi:10.3390/pharmaceutics14040738 . . . . **75**

Hojun Choi, Kyungsun Choi, Dae-Hwan Kim, Byung-Koo Oh, Hwayoung Yim and Soojin Jo et al.
Strategies for Targeted Delivery of Exosomes to the Brain: Advantages and Challenges
Reprinted from: *Pharmaceutics* **2022**, *14*, 672, doi:10.3390/pharmaceutics14030672 . . . . **89**

Puneet Tyagi, Mika Koskinen, Jari Mikkola, Sanjay Sarkhel, Lasse Leino and Asha Seth et al.
Injectable Biodegradable Silica Depot: Two Months of Sustained Release of the Blood Glucose Lowering Peptide, Pramlintide
Reprinted from: *Pharmaceutics* **2022**, *14*, 553, doi:10.3390/pharmaceutics14030553 . . . . **103**

Ameeduzzafar Zafar, Nabil K Alruwaili, Syed Sarim Imam, Mohd Yasir, Omar Awad Alsaidan and Ali Alquraini et al.
Development and Optimization of Nanolipid-Based Formulation of Diclofenac Sodium: In Vitro Characterization and Preclinical Evaluation
Reprinted from: *Pharmaceutics* **2022**, *14*, 507, doi:10.3390/pharmaceutics14030507 . . . . **115**

Yongchao Chu, Tao Sun, Zichen Xie, Keyu Sun and Chen Jiang
Physicochemical Characterization and Pharmacological Evaluation of Novel Propofol Micelles with Low-Lipid and Low-Free Propofol
Reprinted from: *Pharmaceutics* **2022**, *14*, 414, doi:10.3390/pharmaceutics14020414 . . . . **131**

Adam J. Plaunt, Tam L. Nguyen, Michel R. Corboz, Vladimir S. Malinin and David C. Cipolla
Strategies to Overcome Biological Barriers Associated with Pulmonary Drug Delivery
Reprinted from: *Pharmaceutics* **2022**, *14*, 302, doi:10.3390/pharmaceutics14020302 . . . . **145**

Zhuxian Wang, Yaqi Xue, Zhaoming Zhu, Yi Hu, Quanfu Zeng and Yufan Wu et al.
Quantitative Structure-Activity Relationship of Enhancers of Licochalcone A and Glabridin Release and Permeation Enhancement from Carbomer Hydrogel
Reprinted from: *Pharmaceutics* **2022**, *14*, 262, doi:10.3390/pharmaceutics14020262 . . . . **167**

Thomas C. Chen, Clovis O. da Fonseca, Daniel Levin and Axel H. Schönthal
The Monoterpenoid Perillyl Alcohol: Anticancer Agent and Medium to Overcome Biological Barriers
Reprinted from: *Pharmaceutics* **2021**, *13*, 2167, doi:10.3390/pharmaceutics13122167 . . . . **189**

Mai M. El Taweel, Mona H. Aboul-Einien, Mohammed A. Kassem and Nermeen A. Elkasabgy
Intranasal Zolmitriptan-Loaded Bilosomes with Extended Nasal Mucociliary Transit Time for Direct Nose to Brain Delivery
Reprinted from: *Pharmaceutics* **2021**, *13*, 1828, doi:10.3390/pharmaceutics13111828 . . . . **217**

Gaëlle Hugon, Sébastien Goutal, Ambre Dauba, Louise Breuil, Benoit Larrat and Alexandra Winkeler et al.
[^{18}F]2-Fluoro-2-deoxy-sorbitol PET Imaging for Quantitative Monitoring of Enhanced Blood-Brain Barrier Permeability Induced by Focused Ultrasound
Reprinted from: *Pharmaceutics* **2021**, *13*, 1752, doi:10.3390/pharmaceutics13111752 . . . . **245**

About the Editors

Vibhuti Agrahari

Vibhuti Agrahari, Ph.D. is an assistant professor at the University of Oklahoma Health Sciences Center. Her laboratory focuses on therapeutic biomaterials and long-term drug delivery, and currently focused on nanoformulations development for ocular/otic diseases, supported by foundational and organizational grants. Her research work has been credited with two US patents, co-authored more than 35 peer-reviewed articles, 7 book chapters, and over 20 conference presentations. Dr. Agrahari's work was recognized with numerous research awards and honors, such as BJD Faculty Research Award (2018), SU Faculty Development Grant (2017), AAPS-NBC Biotechnology Graduate Student Symposium Award (2016 and 2015), Ronald MacQuarrie Fellowship (2015), Judith Hemberger Graduate Scholarship (2014), Scholar of Preparing Future Faculty Program of School of Graduate Studies (2014–2016), meritorious scholar of UMKC GAF Women's Council (2014–2017), and Research Fellowship by Ministry of Human Resource Development, Government of India (2005). She strongly believes in promoting academic excellence in learning environments that are inclusive of teaching, scholarship, community services, and leadership roles. She is an active member of professional organizations and served in various leadership roles, including Co-Chair and Scientific Committee Chair of 2016 Pharmaceutics Graduate Student Research Meeting; Council of Faculty—Junior Faculty Community Leadership Group, American Association of Colleges of Pharmacy (2018); Ambassador, Controlled Release Society—Young Scientists Committee (2018–2020); Member of AAPS Nomination Committee (2019), AAPS Strategic Planning Task Force (2020–2021) AAPS Horizon Planning Committee (2021–2022), and UMKC Women's Council Board of Directors (2022–2025).

Prashant Kumar

Dr. Prashant Kumar is a Scientific Assistant Director working on the development of low-cost and stable vaccine formulations to extend global access to the vaccines. He is currently working on AAV-based COVID-19, sIPV and combination vaccine, Measles and Rubella, and Shigella vaccine projects at Vaccine Analytics and Formulation Center (VAFC) at KU. Dr. Kumar's past projects include the development of live attenuated RV3-BB rotavirus, non-replicating rotavirus vaccine (NRRV), HPV, Salmonella, and Shigella vaccines. Most of his current/past projects are in phase 1 to 3 of clinical trials. Dr. Kumar's multidisciplinary background in bioprocessing, formulation development, analytical and biophysical characterization coupled with statistical design of experiments (DOE) has helped him in efficient process development, and cost minimization needed to make these projects a success. Dr. Kumar serves on the editorial board of several scientific journals and has a number of scientific papers and book chapters to his credit.

pharmaceutics

MDPI

Editorial

Novel Approaches for Overcoming Biological Barriers

Vibhuti Agrahari [1,*] and Prashant Kumar [2,*]

[1] Department of Pharmaceutical Sciences, University of Oklahoma Health Sciences Center, 1110 N. Stonewall Avenue, Oklahoma City, OK 73117, USA
[2] Vaccine Analytics and Formulation Center, Department of Pharmaceutical Chemistry, University of Kansas, Lawrence, KS 66047, USA
* Correspondence: vibhuti-agrahari@ouhsc.edu (V.A.); prashant.kumar@ku.edu (P.K.)

Citation: Agrahari, V.; Kumar, P. Novel Approaches for Overcoming Biological Barriers. *Pharmaceutics* **2022**, *14*, 1851. https://doi.org/10.3390/pharmaceutics14091851

Received: 26 August 2022
Accepted: 30 August 2022
Published: 2 September 2022

Publisher's Note: MDPI stays neutral with regard to jurisdictional claims in published maps and institutional affiliations.

The human body poses a spectrum of biological mechanisms operating at different levels that are important for its normal functioning and development. Due to the complex nature and varying properties of the body's biological barriers, the development of novel drug delivery systems to specific targets represents both a challenge as well as an opportunity. Extensive attempts have been made to overcome the barriers that prevent entry of therapeutic drugs and vaccines necessary for the treatment of several diseases, impaired conditions or use as prophylaxis. Novel technologies or approaches focusing on overcoming the specific barriers have been studied by investigators in this field to address specific needs. The delivery of a wide range of therapeutic molecules across a variety of barriers is now possible, as experimentally demonstrated by various in vivo and in vitro systems. This Special Issue on the novel approaches for overcoming biological barriers is a collection of efforts led by the several investigators and their groups to address the unmet need and development of the advanced drug delivery systems.

Among all the barriers in the human body, the blood–brain barrier (BBB) has always been challenging, despite several efforts made over the decades to breach it. The first article of this Special Issue by Hugon et al. corroborates the application of a [^{18}F] 2-fluoro-2-deoxy-sorbitol ([^{18}F]FDS) PET imaging technique as a translational and quantitative marker of BBB permeability to probe the impact of spatially controlled focused ultrasound (FUS) together with microbubbles on the integrity of the BBB in mice for the first time [1]. [^{18}F] FDS PET imaging presents a sensitive, quantitative, and noninvasive marker of BBB permeability. Other advantages of [^{18}F] FDS PET include its safety, low MW, low distribution across the intact BBB, and low diffusion from the sonicated volume to the non-sonicated brain with an intact BBB over time scales of minutes [1]. In another study, Taweel et al. demonstrated the direct delivery of intranasal zolmitriptan to rat brain using zolmitriptan-loaded bilosomes in a mucoadhesive in situ gel [2]. This technique involving an in-situ gelling system has high viscosity and therefore extends nasal mucociliary transit time by resisting mucociliary clearance. This system is a promising intranasal substitute with boosted therapeutic effect for treating patients suffering from migraines [2]. In the next article, Chen et al. summarized several clinical and preclinical investigations of monoterpenoid Perillyl alcohol (POH), a naturally available anti-cancer agent for overcoming biological barriers [3]. The application of POH for intranasal, nose-to-brain, intra-arterial BBB delivery and permeation-enhancing functions are noteworthy. The authors also described the use of POH in combination with other therapeutic agents for the creation of new entities with enhanced transport across biological barriers. Thus, POH underlies its ability to overcome the obstacles placed by different types of biological barriers and accordingly shape its multifaceted promise in the drug development for cancer therapy [3]. In a novel approach, Jafari et al. demonstrated proof-of-principle of a hybrid electropermanent magnets (EPM)-based device for temporarily opening the BBB using both an in vitro cell culture and an in vivo mice model [4]. This technique is useful for safe and effective drug transport across the BBB and can selectively target different parts of the brain by tailoring electrical waveforms [4].

Corti et al. compiled the development and application of a derivative of tumor necrosis factor-α (TNF) to target the blood–brain–tumor barrier (BBTB) [5]. A peptide–cytokine fusion (NGR-TNF) was prepared by combining TNF to Cys-Asn-Gly-Arg-Cys-Gly peptide (NGR), a ligand of aminopeptidase N (CD13)-positive tumor blood vessels. NGR-TNF demonstrated effective TNF delivery to tumor vessels by overcoming the biological barriers restricting drug penetration in cancer lesions [5]. In comparison to other TNF-related drugs, extremely low-doses of NGR-TNF or its derivativities were able to successfully overcome the BBTB. Choi et al. discussed the recent advances in the targeted delivery of exosomes to the brain [6]. Exosomes carry various membrane proteins (e.g., CD9, CD63, PTGFRN, and Lamp2b) and lipids (e.g., phosphatidylserine) that can serve as the targeting moieties. Thus, gaining attention for their potential for natural BBB crossing, broad surface-engineering capability, promising results for CNS delivery, and potential as next-generation therapeutics for treating CNS diseases. This comprehensive review also highlights receptor-mediated transcytosis (RMT) as one of the widely investigated methods to cross the BBB for drug delivery to the central nervous system (CNS). Drugs can hijack RMT by expressing specific molecules that bind to RMT, such as the transferrin receptor (TfR), low-density lipoprotein receptor (LDLR), and insulin receptor (INSR). Cell-penetrating peptides and components of neurotropic viruses have also demonstrated efficient drug delivery across the BBB [6]. The next article is focused on the Zika virus (ZIKV). It is a global concern because it invades the brains of adults and fetuses. The investigations by Todorovski et al. described that Placenta-Crossing Peptide-Porphyrin Conjugates (PPCs) exhibited BBB translocation capacity in a mouse model that could potentially fill the Zika virus (ZIKV) treatment gap [7]. This group recently evaluated the in vitro BBB and blood–placental barrier (BPB) crossing ability and anti-ZIKV activity of eight new PPCs. They identified PP-P1 as the most promising candidate, with elevated trans-BBB and -BPB scores and the highest antiviral potency and high serum stability, with a $t_{1/2} > 22$ h, which bodes well for in vivo application [7]. Thus, peptide–porphyrin conjugation is a promising strategy to tackle brain-resident viruses. Alshammari et al. developed a non-invasive therapy using Ruboxistaurin (RBX) nanoparticles incorporated into the polyamidoamine (PAMAM) dendrimer generation 5 for the treatment of diabetic retinopathy [8]. This nanoformulation possesses high drug loading capacity and is safe on the human retinal macroglial Müller cells (MIO-M1). Thus, the nanoformulation developed in this study holds promise to improve the therapeutic outcomes of anti-VEGF therapy and the bioavailability of RBX to prevent vision loss, overcome ocular barriers, and increase patient adherence [8]. Wang et al. provide insight into the drug–enhancers–Carbomer Hydrogel (CP) and drug–enhancers–skin interactions and the structural characteristics of enhancers to ground the drug-specific molecular mechanisms of enhancers and pharmaceutical hydrogel design [9]. A systematic approach was established to evaluate the enhanced release and retention of whitening agents from CP hydrogel in the presence of enhancers based on interactions between drugs, enhancers, and CP or skin. In conclusion, this study provides a strategy for the reasonable utilization of enhancers and formulation optimization in topical hydrogel whitening. [9]. Zafar et al. rationally designed the nanolipid-based formulation of diclofenac (DC) for the treatment of inflammation to be administered by the oral route [10]. The bilosomes (BC) nanoformulation showed a prolonged DC release with high permeation flux in the in vitro release and ex vivo permeation study. The pharmacokinetic and pharmacodynamics studies revealed the enhanced bioavailability and anti-inflammatory activity of BC-DC compared to pure DC and DC-Liposomes (LP) [10]. Therefore, the developed nanoformulation improves the therapeutic efficacy and overcomes complications of gastric irritation and ulcers. In another study, Chu et al. developed a novel propofol-mixed micelle as a clinical alternative for anesthetics [11]. This novel micellar formulation reduces injection-site pain and the risk of hyperlipidemia due to the low content of free propofol and low-lipid constituent. In addition, the developed formulation overcomes the biological barrier of the reticuloendothelial system and complications of the marketed propofol formulation [11]. The rat paw-lick study showed a significant reduction in pain compared to Diprivan.

Thus, overcoming the major problem of the commercial formulation. Notably, the novel propofol formulation had a non-hemolytic reaction and exhibited a good safety profile, displayed similar anesthetic actions, absorption, and clearance effects after a single dose in comparison with the marketed formulation [11]. In a novel approach, Tyagi et al. developed a pramlintide–silica microparticle hydrogel depot which offers a significant advantage for the formulation (in near-native conditions) and delivery (degraded products do not destabilize protein structure) of biologicals [12]. The sustained delivery of Pramlintide from the silica depot was investigated in a rat model for two-months after subcutaneous administration [12]. In conclusion, the injectable, scalable, and biodegradable silica-based delivery system has great potential for therapeutic applications and can mitigate risk factors and compliance issues related to multiple dosing of different drugs. Nimma et al. findings revealed that a Telmisartan–(CARP-1) functional mimetic–Osimertinib (TLM_CFM-F_OSM) combination has a superior anti-cancer effect in the treatment of non-small-cell lung cancers (NSCLC) by affecting multiple resistant markers that regulate mitochondrial homeostasis, inflammation, oxidative stress, and apoptosis [13]. EGFR-tyrosine kinase inhibitors (TKIs) are the leading therapy for a substantial percentage of NSCLCs. This group studied OSM (which targets EGFR T790M mutation and inhibits activation of AMPK/Lamin-B2/MAPK and PI3K/AKT) in combination with CFM 4.17 NLPFs (CARP-1 signaling and EGFR activity is inhibited by interacting with EGFR's ATP binding site) and TLM (disrupts tumor stromal barriers and leads to enhanced permeation of drugs) and proposed that it will provide superior anti-cancer effects in NSCLC and identify novel targets in tumor regression by using RNA sequence and quantitative proteomics. [13]. The comprehensive review by Plaunt et al. [14] highlighted the recent examples of how the barriers of pulmonary delivery can be overcome using formulation technologies or modifying the chemistry of the compound (drug).

Through decades of effort, scientists, chemists, biologists, toxicologists, engineers, etc., have developed solutions to overcome, and in some cases, even capitalize on, the numerous barriers of the human body as described above. Nonetheless, the relevance of these biological barriers differs by disease, and strategies to overcome barriers are specific to the target-site or treatment. Altogether, this Special Issue incorporates recent advances in overcoming these biological barriers by various research groups. This compilation will bring great opportunities to the scientific community engaged in the research and development of advanced drug delivery systems, and we expect that readers will find this issue an interesting addition to the existing literature.

Funding: This research received no external finding.

Conflicts of Interest: The authors declare no conflict of interest.

References

1. Hugon, G.; Goutal, S.; Dauba, A.; Breuil, L.; Larrat, B.; Winkeler, A.; Novell, A.; Tournier, N. [^{18}F]2-Fluoro-2-deoxy-sorbitol PET Imaging for Quantitative Monitoring of Enhanced Blood-Brain Barrier Permeability Induced by Focused Ultrasound. *Pharmaceutics* **2021**, *13*, 1752. [CrossRef]
2. El Taweel, M.M.; Aboul-Einien, M.H.; Kassem, M.A.; Elkasabgy, N.A. Intranasal Zolmitriptan-Loaded Bilosomes with Extended Nasal Mucociliary Transit Time for Direct Nose to Brain Delivery. *Pharmaceutics* **2021**, *13*, 1828. [CrossRef]
3. Chen, T.C.; da Fonseca, C.O.; Levin, D.; Schönthal, A.H. The Monoterpenoid Perillyl Alcohol: Anticancer Agent and Medium to Overcome Biological Barriers. *Pharmaceutics* **2021**, *13*, 2167. [CrossRef]
4. Jafari, S.; Baum, I.S.; Udalov, O.G.; Lee, Y.; Rodriguez, O.; Fricke, S.T.; Jafari, M.; Amini, M.; Probst, R.; Tang, X.; et al. Opening the Blood Brain Barrier with an Electropermanent Magnet System. *Pharmaceutics* **2022**, *14*, 1503. [CrossRef] [PubMed]
5. Corti, A.; Calimeri, T.; Curnis, F.; Ferreri, A.J.M. Targeting the Blood–Brain Tumor Barrier with Tumor Necrosis Factor-α. *Pharmaceutics* **2022**, *14*, 1414. [CrossRef] [PubMed]
6. Choi, H.; Choi, K.; Kim, D.-H.; Oh, B.-K.; Yim, H.; Jo, S.; Choi, C. Strategies for Targeted Delivery of Exosomes to the Brain: Advantages and Challenges. *Pharmaceutics* **2022**, *14*, 672. [CrossRef]
7. Todorovski, T.; Mendonça, D.A.; Fernandes-Siqueira, L.O.; Cruz-Oliveira, C.; Guida, G.; Valle, J.; Cavaco, M.; Limas, F.I.V.; Neves, V.; Cadima-Couto, I.; et al. Targeting Zika Virus with New Brain- and Placenta-Crossing Peptide–Porphyrin Conjugates. *Pharmaceutics* **2022**, *14*, 738. [CrossRef] [PubMed]

8. Alshammari, R.A.; Aleanizy, F.S.; Aldarwesh, A.; Alqahtani, F.Y.; Mahdi, W.A.; Alquadeib, B.; Alqahtani, Q.H.; Haq, N.; Shakeel, F.; Abdelhady, H.G.; et al. Retinal Delivery of the Protein Kinase C-beta Inhibitor Ruboxistaurin Using Non-Invasive Nanoparticles of Polyamidoamine Dendrimers. *Pharmaceutics* **2022**, *14*, 1444. [CrossRef] [PubMed]
9. Wang, Z.; Xue, Y.; Zhu, Z.; Hu, Y.; Zeng, Q.; Wu, Y.; Wang, Y.; Shen, C.; Jiang, C.; Liu, L.; et al. Quantitative Structure-Activity Relationship of Enhancers of Licochalcone A and Glabridin Release and Permeation Enhancement from Carbomer Hydrogel. *Pharmaceutics* **2022**, *14*, 262. [CrossRef] [PubMed]
10. Zafar, A.; Alruwaili, N.K.; Imam, S.S.; Yasir, M.; Alsaidan, O.A.; Alquraini, A.; Rawaf, A.; Alsuwayt, B.; Anwer, K.; Alshehri, S.; et al. Development and Optimization of Nanolipid-Based Formulation of Diclofenac Sodium: In Vitro Characterization and Preclinical Evaluation. *Pharmaceutics* **2022**, *14*, 507. [CrossRef] [PubMed]
11. Chu, Y.; Sun, T.; Xie, Z.; Sun, K.; Jiang, C. Physicochemical Characterization and Pharmacological Evaluation of Novel Propofol Micelles with Low-Lipid and Low-Free Propofol. *Pharmaceutics* **2022**, *14*, 414. [CrossRef] [PubMed]
12. Tyagi, P.; Koskinen, M.; Mikkola, J.; Sarkhel, S.; Leino, L.; Seth, A.; Madalli, S.; Will, S.; Howard, V.G.; Brant, H.; et al. Injectable Biodegradable Silica Depot: Two Months of Sustained Release of the Blood Glucose Lowering Peptide, Pramlintide. *Pharmaceutics* **2022**, *14*, 553. [CrossRef] [PubMed]
13. Nimma, R.; Kalvala, A.K.; Patel, N.; Surapaneni, S.K.; Sun, L.; Singh, R.; Nottingham, E.; Bagde, A.; Kommineni, N.; Arthur, P.; et al. Combined Transcriptomic and Proteomic Profiling to Unravel Osimertinib, CARP-1 Functional Mimetic (CFM 4.17) Formulation and Telmisartan Combo Treatment in NSCLC Tumor Xenografts. *Pharmaceutics* **2022**, *14*, 1156. [CrossRef] [PubMed]
14. Plaunt, A.J.; Nguyen, T.L.; Corboz, M.R.; Malinin, V.S.; Cipolla, D.C. Strategies to Overcome Biological Barriers Associated with Pulmonary Drug Delivery. *Pharmaceutics* **2022**, *14*, 302. [CrossRef] [PubMed]

pharmaceutics

MDPI

Article

Opening the Blood Brain Barrier with an Electropermanent Magnet System

Sahar Jafari [1], Ittai S. Baum [1], Oleg G. Udalov [1], Yichien Lee [2], Olga Rodriguez [2,3], Stanley T. Fricke [2,3,4], Maryam Jafari [5], Mostafa Amini [6], Roland Probst [7], Xinyao Tang [1], Cheng Chen [1], David J. Ariando [8], Anjana Hevaganinge [1], Lamar O. Mair [1], Christopher Albanese [2,3,4] and Irving N. Weinberg [1,*]

[1] Weinberg Medical Physics, Inc., North Bethesda, MD 20852, USA; sahar.jafari2011@gmail.com (S.J.); ittaisbaum@gmail.com (I.S.B.); udalovog@gmail.com (O.G.U.); xxt81@case.edu (X.T.); cxc717@case.edu (C.C.); anjana.heva@gmail.com (A.H.); lamar.mair@gmail.com (L.O.M.)
[2] Department of Oncology, Georgetown University Medical Center, Washington, DC 20057, USA; yl285@georgetown.edu (Y.L.); rodriguo@georgetown.edu (O.R.); stanley.fricke@gmail.com (S.T.F.); albanese@georgetown.edu (C.A.)
[3] Center for Translational Imaging, Georgetown University Medical Center, Washington, DC 20057, USA
[4] Department of Radiology, Georgetown University Medical Center, Washington, DC 20057, USA
[5] Independent Consultant, Oklahoma City, OK 73134, USA; jafary.maryam@gmail.com
[6] Department of Management Science and Information Systems, Oklahoma State University, Stillwater, OK 74078, USA; moamini@okstate.edu
[7] ACUITYnano LLC, Chevy Chase, MD 20815, USA; probstroland@gmail.com
[8] Department of Electrical and Computer Engineering, University of Florida, Gainesville, FL 32611, USA; dajo.ariando@gmail.com
* Correspondence: inweinberg@gmail.com

Citation: Jafari, S.; Baum, I.S.; Udalov, O.G.; Lee, Y.; Rodriguez, O.; Fricke, S.T.; Jafari, M.; Amini, M.; Probst, R.; Tang, X.; et al. Opening the Blood Brain Barrier with an Electropermanent Magnet System. *Pharmaceutics* **2022**, *14*, 1503. https://doi.org/10.3390/pharmaceutics14071503

Academic Editors: Vibhuti Agrahari and Prashant Kumar

Received: 2 July 2022
Accepted: 18 July 2022
Published: 20 July 2022

Abstract: Opening the blood brain barrier (BBB) under imaging guidance may be useful for the treatment of many brain disorders. Rapidly applied magnetic fields have the potential to generate electric fields in brain tissue that, if properly timed, may enable safe and effective BBB opening. By tuning magnetic pulses generated by a novel electropermanent magnet (EPM) array, we demonstrate the opening of tight junctions in a BBB model culture in vitro, and show that induced monophasic electrical pulses are more effective than biphasic ones. We confirmed, with in vivo contrast-enhanced MRI, that the BBB can be opened with monophasic pulses. As electropermanent magnets have demonstrated efficacy at tuning B0 fields for magnetic resonance imaging studies, our results suggest the possibility of implementing an EPM-based hybrid theragnostic device that could both image the brain and enhance drug transport across the BBB in a single sitting.

Keywords: blood brain barrier; electropermanent magnet; magnetic resonance imaging

1. Introduction

The blood brain barrier (BBB) is composed of brain endothelial cells, pericytes, and astrocytes in tight junctions without fenestrations [1–4]. The BBB prevents 98% of small molecules, and an even greater percentage of large molecules, from reaching their intended brain targets [5,6] and is therefore considered the most significant barrier to the efficient and targeted delivery of therapeutics to the brain [3]. Due to its significance, numerous approaches have focused on safely and temporarily opening the BBB. To date, heat [7–9], light [10–12], sound [13], electric fields [14], and magnetic fields [15] have all shown promise as BBB-opening techniques. Moving towards increased spatial specificity, image-guided BBB opening may be achieved using MRI-guided focused ultrasound (MRgFUS) [16]. Other techniques aim to bypass the BBB altogether by the delivery of therapeutic payloads to the spinal cord or via the nasal delivery of magnetic nanoparticles [5].

In cell culture models of the BBB, pulsed electric fields have been shown to be capable of destabilizing cell membranes and inducing the formation of nanoscale aqueous pores in the membranes, which may reseal (i.e., reversible electroporation) or may lead to cell death (irreversible electroporation) [6,14,16,17]. Drug infusion during reversible electroporation (using electric fields in the $(5-7) \times 10^4$ V/m range) has been used to improve survival and reduce tumor growth in glioma-bearing rats and dogs [18–20]. In a cell culture model, Sharabi et al. demonstrated that electric fields with significantly lower magnitudes (i.e., as low as 1500 V/m) could reversibly open the BBB [14]. These electric fields are similar in magnitude to those induced by clinical transcranial magnetic stimulation (TMS), as demonstrated by Hedarheydari et al. in mouse experiments involving components of a clinical TMS system [15].

Variations in electric field waveforms can have different effects on the brain. For example, Reilly et al. provided a theoretical basis that explained why monophasic pulses might be more effective at neuromodulation than the biphasic pulses typically used in TMS [21]. Peterchev et al. demonstrated a TMS power supply circuit that could apply currents with rapid rise times to TMS coils with slow fall times, effectively generating primarily monophasic electric pulses [22].

Electropermanent magnets (EPMs) confer users with the ability to specify material properties dynamically (i.e., to operate as programmable matter) [23]. EPMs generally consist of one or more permanent magnet material cores with a low magnetic coercivity (e.g., alnico), surrounded by a current-carrying coil [24,25]. By sending specified electrical currents through the coil, the permanent magnet component of the EPMs can be tuned to specific magnetizations [26]. Once tuned to a specific magnetization, the core material retains this magnetization without the need for the further application of current through the coil, and can be reset to a different magnetization with one or more additional current pulses. Appropriate control software allows these magnetizations to be programmed with a high spatial and temporal specificity. Udalov et al. modeled a control method using EPMs to generate electric fields in brain tissue, in which the magnetization status of the core would affect the rise- and fall-times of the magnetic field produced by the EPM (and hence also the waveform of the electric field induced by the magnetic field) [27]. Udalov et al. also presented models showing that the phases of current pulses in EPMs placed in arrays around the head could be adjusted such that superficial portions of the brain would be exposed to electric fields with different waveforms versus other parts of the brain. Such differential waveforms address regulatory limitations on scalp stimulation [28]. In earlier work on EPMs, Ropp et al. showed that EPMs could be used to perform nuclear magnetic resonance imaging [26]. In this work, we demonstrate the temporary opening of the BBB in both an in vitro cell culture model and in live mice using an array of four electropermanent magnets. We demonstrate variations in BBB opening for two different electric waveforms induced by the EPMs. This work represents the first use of EPMs with relevance to neuromodulation, BBB disruption, and drug delivery.

2. Materials and Methods

2.1. In Vitro Opening of a BBB Model System

In vitro experiments were performed on cell cultures containing tight junctions formed by Caco-2 cell monolayers (ReadyCell, Barcelona, Spain). Previous work has validated these Caco-2 cultures as BBB models [29,30]. Caco-2 cells were passaged in Eagle's minimum essential medium (EMEM, ATCC, Manassas, VA, USA), then cultured on permeable transwell (TW) inserts in a 24-well plate at a density of 2×10^5 cells/mL. Transwell dishes make use of inserts with track-etched membranes (Product #353096, Falcon, Corning Inc., Corning, NY, USA) for cell culture. After 21 days of culture in EMEM, Caco-2 cells form tight junction monolayers at the base surface of the insert in the culture well. We cultured and tested 18 TW samples possessing cell-loaded inserts with intact tight junction monolayers.

The cultures were exposed to electric fields induced by an array of four electropermanent magnets (described below). Prior to and after the electric field exposures, tight junction integrity was tested using transepithelial electrical resistance (TEER). TEER measurements were obtained with an EVOM^2 epithelial volt/Ohm meter (World Precision Instruments, Sarasota, FL, USA).

Each EPM was composed of 200 Alnico-5 rods (each rod being 2 mm in diameter and 100 mm in length) bundled together into a rectangular bundle (measuring 3 cm × 3 cm × 20 cm). The EPM bundles were housed as assemblies in custom 3D-printed holders, around which were wound 40 turns of magnet wire (14 HML NEMA MW16-C, MWS Wire Industries, Oxnard, CA, USA) for applying current pulses. An array of four EPM assemblies is shown in Figure 1. The distance between the magnets is of the order of 1 cm. The sample is placed in the center between the magnets. Thus, the distance between the magnets and the samples is also of the order of 1 cm.

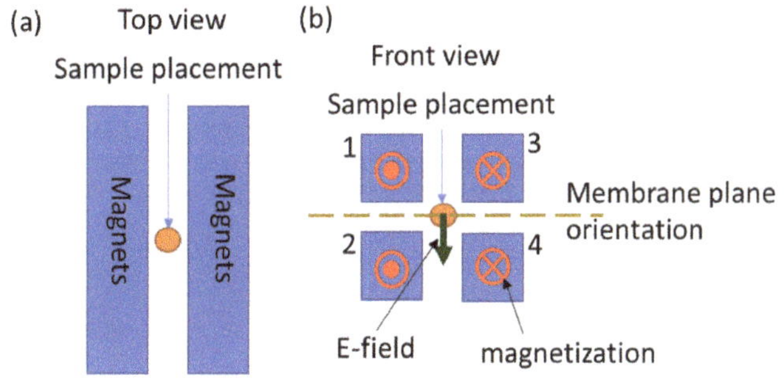

Figure 1. Experimental geometry. (**a**) Top view of the EPM array with a centrally positioned sample (orange circle). (**b**) Front view of the EPM array, showing four EPM assemblies with magnetizations directed along the length of each EPM assembly. The direction of the electric field is shown by an arrow, and a dotted line depicts the orientation of the transwell membrane (on which the Caco-2 cells are grown) for in vitro experiments. The EPM magnet assemblies are numbered 1 through 4.

Pulsing the coils of the EPM assemblies with 1 kiloampere currents was achieved using an H-bridge circuit. The EPM array was able to generate magnetic fields of up to 150 mT at the sample position. The duration of the current pulse was about 50 µs as shown in Figure 2. Experiments with a single EPM assembly were performed to measure the electric field produced by a single EPM assembly (Figure 2a,b). These experiments showed that the single EPM assembly produced an electric field in the range of 1000 V/m at 1 cm distance from the EPM assembly's surface.

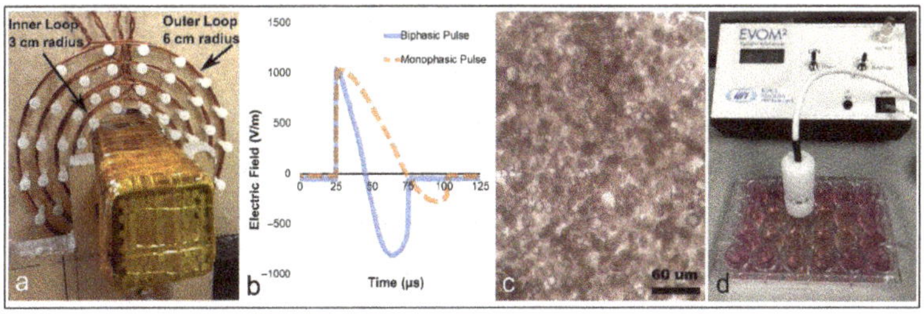

Figure 2. EPM assembly electric field measurements, Caco-2 cultures, and TEER measurement apparatus. (**a**) Electropermanent magnet assembly and coated copper wire windings, centered in an electric-field measurement device composed of concentric coils. The electric field generated by pulsing the EPM assembly is quantified by measuring the voltage induced across the coils. (**b**) The induced electric field for biphasic and monophasic pulses. As can be seen in (**b**), the monophasic pulses (orange dotted line) induce only a one-directional electric field, while the biphasic pulses (solid blue line) induce bi-directional electric fields. (**c**) Caco-2 cells cultured on transwell membranes prior to TEER measurements. (**d**) Apparatus and technique for TEER measurements of the BBB tight junction model.

In the four EPM assembly array (Figure 1), the direction of the electric field produced in the sample during the pulse can vary depending on the magnetization direction of the magnets and on the sign of the electric current pulses. For the experiments reported here, the electric field was oriented perpendicularly to the cell culture membrane plane.

Depending on the initial magnetization states of the EPM assemblies, two different kinds of electric field pulses can be produced. If the magnets are saturated and the current pulses apply a magnetic field in the direction of the magnets' magnetization, then the EPM assembly's magnetization state before and after the current pulse will not change. In this case, the electric field pulse will be a biphasic (BP) pulse, where both positive and negative electric fields are generated during the pulse and the time integral of the electric field in the sample is zero. If the EPM assemblies were initially saturated, but the coil field during the pulse is opposite to this initial magnetization state, then the EPM assemblies will become demagnetized during the pulse. In this case, the electric field pulse is a mono-phasic (MP) pulse, meaning that the time integral of the electric field is non-zero, and the sample is primarily exposed to an electric field with a single polarity.

A single EPM assembly and corresponding electric field measuring setup are shown in Figure 2a. Coils of varying diameter were set up to measure the induced currents, with the smallest diameter being 3 cm and the largest diameter 6 cm. Measurements of the electric field for both MP and BP pulses are shown in Figure 2b. As shown in Figure 2b, the electric field produced by the BP pulse lasted 50 μs, with approximately equal positive and negative electrical lobe magnitudes and durations. The MP pulses were below 75 μs, but primarily produced a unipolar electric field.

We separated the 18 Caco-2 TW cultures into three groups of equal size (n = 6 TW cultures per group): control (no magnetic field exposure), biphasic pulse (BP) electric field exposure, and monophasic pulse (MP) electric field exposure. For all three groups, the tight junctions of the cells were assessed using the EVOM^2 to measure the TEER [31]. We used an STX2-PLUS electrode (World Precision Instruments), calibrated using a 1000 Ω probe. The STX2-PLUS electrodes were treated with chloride (4.5% sodium hypochlorite, CLOROX, California USA) for >10 min prior to TEER measurements. Before and after each experiment, the probe was rinsed with isopropanol and deionized water, then dried in air.

For groups 2 and 3, a series of 40 pulses (BP or MP) was applied over 5 min. Then, the TEER measurements were repeated. The controls, biphasic pulse exposure, and monophasic pulse exposure samples were each tested six times (n = 6).

2.2. *In Vivo Experiments on Mice*

In vivo experiments were performed in the Preclinical Imaging Research Laboratory at Georgetown University Medical Center, with all experiments being performed in accordance with the USA standards for animal well-being set by the Office of Laboratory Animal Welfare, and in accordance with the Georgetown University Medical Center Institutional Animal Care and Use Committee (IACUC, protocol #2019-0048).

A total of 16 healthy C57Bl/6 male mice (~1 year of age, weighing between 28 and 30 g) were divided into two groups (sham and treated). The mice in the treatment group were anesthetized with isoflurane, injected intra-peritoneally with the gadolinium-based contrast agent Gadovist (BayerHealthCare AG, Leverkusen, Germany) at a dose of 0.1 mmol/kg and exposed to 40 MP pulses (as described above in the in vitro studies section) at a comparable distance from the mouse's brain (Figure 3). The mice in the sham group received only the contrast agent injection. Twenty minutes after injection, all animals underwent magnetic resonance imaging (MRI) in the Georgetown-Lombardi Preclinical Imaging Research Laboratory on a 7 tesla Bruker Biospec Avance NEO magnet run by ParaVision 360 software. Briefly, the mice were anesthetized (1.5% isoflurane in a gas mixture of 30% oxygen and 68.5% nitrous oxide) and placed on a custom-manufactured stereotaxic device with built-in temperature and cardio-respiratory monitoring (ASI Instruments, Warren, Michigan). The MRI protocol used was a T1-weighted RARE sequence with TE: 8.75 ms, TR: 850 ms, rare factor: 2, matrix: 256 × 256, and FOV: 20 × 20 mm. BBB permeability was evaluated by measuring T1 signal intensity enhancement in two regions of interest (ROI): one was localized on the right brain cortex, the other on the right neck muscles (which served as a positive control for contrast agent uptake) and background air (which was used to normalize for image intensity). Four of the treated mice were randomly selected for follow-up studies to assess the duration of BBB opening. These mice were re-injected with the contrast agent and re-imaged by MRI again 24 h after their initial testing.

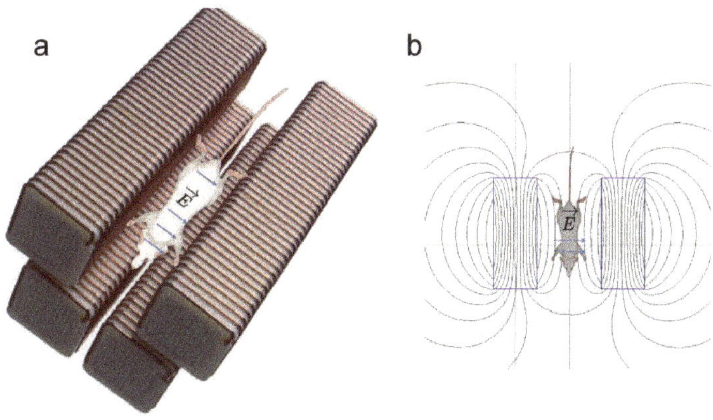

Figure 3. Murine experimental setup. (**a**) For in vivo experiments, a mouse was placed inside the four-magnet EPM array, with the length of the mouse oriented along the length of the EPM assemblies. (**b**) The EPM assemblies, shown as blue rectangles, generate magnetic fields, shown here as black lobe-shaped lines. The magnetic pulses generate electric fields (blue arrows) to which the mouse is exposed.

2.3. Statistical Analysis

The TEER data were evaluated for normality through Shapiro–Wilk and Anderson–Darling tests. One-way analysis of variance (ANOVA) and Fisher's least significant difference (LSD) tests were performed for statistical investigation between the three groups. A statistical analysis of the MRI signal intensity over the two regions of interest (ROIs) was performed using JMP statistical software V16.1 (SAS, Cary, NC, USA). Shapiro–Wilk and Anderson–Darling tests were applied to test the normality of the distribution. JMP provides the Shapiro–Wilk test in the distribution platform for a departure from a normal distribution within each group of experiments. This test has been shown to be more powerful than alternative tests, including the Anderson–Darling test [32]. ANOVAs followed by Fisher's LSD (where we had more than two experimental groups) were used to compare the efficiency of different pulsing regimes. Here, $p < 0.05$ was considered significant in the rejection of the null hypothesis. Fisher's LSD method is more commonly used to compare means from multiple processes, as it compares all pairs of means and controls for error rate for each individual pairwise comparison but does not control the family error rate. Both error rates are given in the output. A t-test analysis was used to compare the ROI measurement of MRI signal intensities between the control and test groups of mice. Here, $p < 0.05$ was considered significant in the rejection of the null hypothesis that there was a difference between the control and test groups. Due to the small sample size (four mice) for the 24-h delayed mouse studies, observational assessment only was performed for this experiment.

3. Results

3.1. Pulse Characterization and In Vitro Model BBB Culture Experiments

Initial measurements of resistance in all 18 cultures confirmed the existence of tight junctions across the transwell membranes, indicating that the cultures were intact and had formed sufficiently conformal layers with accompanying tight junction connections, as in prior work describing this in vitro BBB model [33–36]. All of the initial resistance measurements reported resistances of approximately 2000 $\Omega{\cdot}cm^2$ or greater, confirming the formation of tight junctions. The TEER measurements of the control group (no magnetic field) showed a change of less than 200 $\Omega{\cdot}cm^2$ in resistance over the course of the experimental timeframe. Samples exposed to biphasic pulses exhibited non-significant changes in TEER values versus controls ($p = 0.4$), while samples exposed to MP pulses experienced the highest change in TEER resistance as compared with controls ($p < 0.01$) (Figure 4).

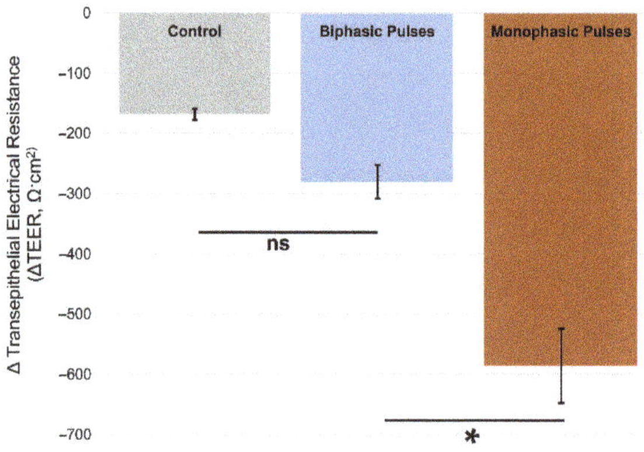

Figure 4. TEER measurement results. Samples exposed to monophasic electric field pulses demonstrate statistically relevant changes in TEER measurements. Here, ns indicates results which are not statistically significant, while * indicates statistical significance.

3.2. *In Vivo BBB Opening Experiments*

As only MP pulses were used in vivo, we simply refer to groups as sham or treated. Figure 5 depicts MRI slices taken from mice, showing locations for comparing Gadovist uptake in the brain cortex versus Gadovist uptake in the muscle. Figure 6 shows data on the averaged Gadovist uptake in the brain cortex and facial muscle, comparing the control group (sham) with the treated group (MP pulses). Data, in the form of the average MR image intensity across a circular region of a single slice for each mouse (Figure 5), at specified locations (muscle, cortex), were first evaluated for normality through Shapiro–Wilk and Anderson–Darling tests. The p-values obtained from the Shapiro–Wilk tests were 0.49 and 0.16 for the brain-cortex-to-muscle ratio for the control and treated groups, respectively. The p-values from the Anderson–Darling normality tests for the cortex-to-muscle ratio were 0.51 and 0.23 for the control and treated groups, respectively. The p-values for the brain cortex of the control and treated groups from the Shapiro–Wilk tests were 0.6 and 0.5, respectively. The p-values from the Anderson–Darling normality tests for the brain cortex were 0.6 and 0.5 for the control and treated groups, respectively. The p-values from the Shapiro–Wilk tests for the muscle of the control and treated groups were 0.6 and 0.08, respectively. The p-values from the Anderson–Darling normality tests for the muscle control and treated groups were 0.6 and 0.1, respectively. Here, p-values > 0.05 indicated that the normal distribution was a good fit for each group. A t-test analysis was performed for statistical investigation between the groups of experiments. A p-value of less than 0.05 (typically < 0.05) was considered statistically significant.

There was a significant difference between the contrast agent uptake of the brain cortex ($p < 0.0002$) in the animals of the treated group and the control group. There was a significant difference ($p < 0.0003$) between the cortex-to-muscle ratio in the animals of the treated group and the control group as well. No significant difference ($p < 0.2$) was observed in the contrast agent uptake by the muscles of the treated group and the control group. The number of animals kept for 24 h was too small to make statistically significant observations. We infer that the BBB stays open for a time greater than the initial scan (20 min), but less than 24 h.

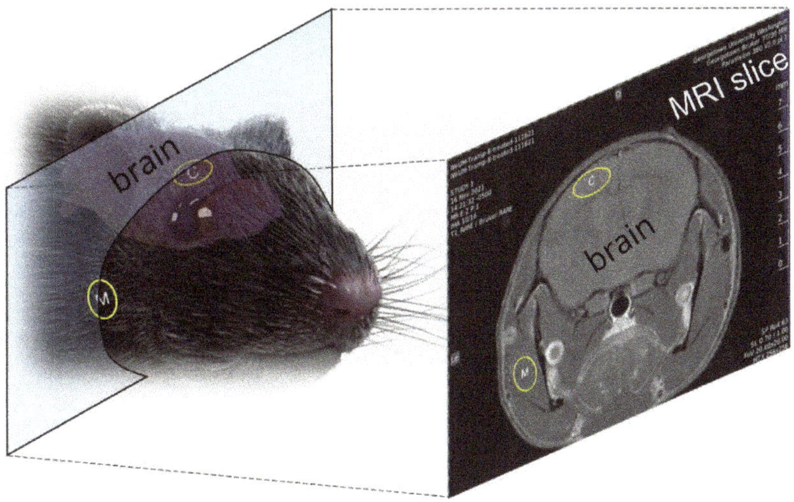

Figure 5. Mouse brain MRI for assessing Gadovist uptake. MRI slices collected of the mouse head were analyzed at two distinct locations, shown above (yellow circles). Gadovist uptake, as characterized by a change in signal intensity before and after EPM pulses, was measured in regions of the cortex (yellow circle with (**C**)) and regions of muscle (yellow circle with (**M**)) for comparison.

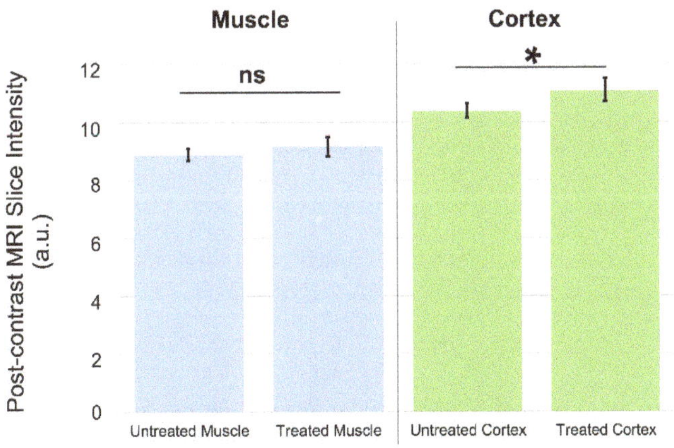

Figure 6. In vivo Gadovist uptake results for muscle and cortex. Comparison of MRI region-of-interest signal in muscle and brain cortex for untreated and treated mice. The muscle shows no statistically significant difference in post-contrast MRI intensity for untreated and treated animals. The cortex shows a statistically significant difference in post-contrast MRI intensity for untreated animals as compared with treated animals. Here, ns indicates results which are not statistically significant, while * indicates statistical significance.

Comparing ratios for the treated and untreated animals, a cortex-to-muscle ratio was calculated for the treated and untreated groups (Figure 7). The ratio simply takes the post-contrast MRI slice intensities for the cortex and divides by the post-contrast slice intensities for the muscle, separately for treated and untreated animals.

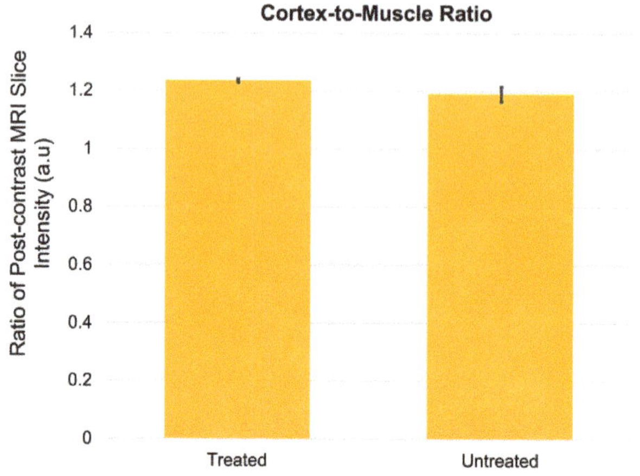

Figure 7. Ratio of cortex-to-muscle post-contrast MRI intensity in mice. Mice treated with MP pulses showed a greater ratio of cortex-to-muscle post-contrast intensity as compared with untreated mice.

4. Discussion

Our in vitro results demonstrate that a monophasic electric field is more than twice as effective at opening tight junctions in a BBB model as compared with a biphasic electric field, consistent with prior theoretical results for TMS efficacy [21]. Consistent with prior work [6,14,15,18], the increased MRI signal in the cortex of treated mice likely derives from the disruption of the BBB (and the release of Gadovist from the local vasculature, see right side of Figure 6) by rapid magnetic pulses generated by our electropermanent magnet system. No significant increase in MRI signal was noted for non-brain tissues (i.e., muscle, see left side of Figure 6). The results of the murine in vivo experiments demonstrate that a monophasic electric field produced by EPMs is effective in temporarily opening the BBB. It should be noted that the MP pulse is not strictly monophasic, but does include a short ~25 µs negative voltage component (Figure 2b). This negative voltage component of the MP may or may not be implicated in the BBB opening results observed. Future experiments will determine if the small negative component of the MP pulse is significant or not. As the phase control of the EPM-generated magnetic fields can create different waveforms (i.e., monophasic versus biphasic) at different locations in the brain, and can also be used to create magnetic resonance images, these results demonstrate that EPMs hold promise as novel devices for enhancing drug delivery via localized BBB opening [27]. Since EPM arrays have previously demonstrated use in novel methods of field-tunable NMR and MRI [26], we envision systems built with such arrays used as tools for combined imaging and therapy. A popular technique for disrupting the BBB is focused ultrasound, which may have the disadvantage of causing permanent neuronal damage and therefore has a relatively low therapeutic ratio [37,38]. Based on literature showing that the electrical field required for permanent neuronal damage is at least 100 times higher than the fields we are realizing with electropermanent magnets [39], we expect a more favorable therapeutic ratio. An additional potential advantage is the use of the same electropermanent magnet array to collect MRI images with the same apparatus, which will be convenient for clinicians [27]. Finally, the data demonstrate that BBB disruption is dependent on the waveform of the electrical pulses generated by the electropermanent magnets. We expect that this principle can be taken advantage of by selectively actuating the electropermanent magnets with appropriate phases, thereby implementing spatially selective BBB opening over preselected tracts and regions of the brain with arbitrary shapes and sizes.

5. Conclusions

Our results demonstrate that the BBB may be opened selectively and temporarily through an array of electropermanent magnets that can be dynamically controlled to yield monophasic or biphasic electric fields. The findings are promising as a proof-of-principle for the construction of a hybrid EPM-based device with multiple functionalities, including MRI, TMS, and drug delivery. The ability to tailor electrical waveforms, and hence selectively affect BBB permeability according to the location in the brain, would be useful in focal drug delivery in the brain (enabling a reduction the off-target effects of such drugs). Additional studies will need to be conducted to establish the limits of such a system in terms of drug size and localization efficiency.

Author Contributions: Conceptualization, S.J., I.S.B., O.G.U., O.R., C.A., X.T., C.C., D.J.A., A.H. and I.N.W.; methodology, S.J., I.S.B., O.G.U., Y.L., O.R., S.T.F., C.A., M.J., M.A., X.T., C.C., D.J.A., A.H. and I.N.W.; software, I.S.B., O.G.U., R.P., X.T., C.C., D.J.A. and A.H.; validation, S.J., I.S.B., O.G.U., Y.L., O.R., C.A., X.T., C.C., D.J.A., A.H. and I.N.W.; formal analysis, S.J., I.S.B., O.G.U., M.J., M.A. and I.N.W.; investigation, S.J., I.S.B., O.G.U., Y.L., O.R., C.A. and I.N.W.; resources, O.R., S.T.F., C.A. and I.N.W.; data curation, S.J., I.S.B., O.G.U., Y.L., O.R., S.T.F., C.A., M.J. and M.A.; writing—original draft preparation, S.J., I.S.B., O.G.U., O.R., C.A., R.P., L.O.M. and I.N.W.; writing—review and editing, S.J., I.S.B., O.G.U., Y.L., O.R., S.T.F., C.A., M.J., M.A., X.T., C.C., D.J.A., A.H., L.O.M., R.P. and I.N.W.; visualization, S.J., I.S.B., O.G.U., Y.L., O.R., R.P., L.O.M. and I.N.W.; supervision, O.R., C.A. and I.N.W.; project administration, I.N.W.; funding acquisition, O.R., C.A. and I.N.W. All authors have read and agreed to the published version of the manuscript.

Funding: This research was supported by the National Institutes of Health's National Institute on Aging, grant #R44AG066386, as well as NIH S10 OD025153 (CA) and NIH-P30 CA051008.

Institutional Review Board Statement: All in vivo imaging was performed in the Georgetown-Lombardi Preclinical Imaging Research Laboratory, and the animal study protocol was approved by the Institutional Review Board of Georgetown University, as well as Georgetown University Medical Center Institutional Animal Care and Use Committee (approval #2019-0048, 7 approved October 2019). Gadovist was kindly provided by Bayer HealthCare AG, D-51368 Leverkusen, Germany.

Data Availability Statement: Data is contained within the article.

Conflicts of Interest: Several authors (S.J., I.S.B., O.G.U., X.T., C.C., A.H., L.O.M., and I.N.W.) were employed by Weinberg Medical Physics, who constructed the electropermanent arrays used in the experiments and funded the study under a subcontract to Georgetown University from the NIH.

References

1. Ballabh, P.; Braun, A.; Nedergaard, M. The blood–brain barrier: An overview. *Neurobiol. Dis.* **2004**, *16*, 1–13. [CrossRef] [PubMed]
2. Abbott, N.J.; Patabendige, A.A.K.; Dolman, D.E.M.; Yusof, S.R.; Begley, D.J. Structure and function of the blood–brain barrier. *Neurobiol. Dis.* **2010**, *37*, 13–25. [CrossRef] [PubMed]
3. Wong, A.D.; Ye, M.; Levy, A.F.; Rothstein, J.D.; Bergles, D.E.; Searson, P.C. The blood-brain barrier: An engineering perspective. *Front. Neuroeng.* **2013**, *6*, 7. [CrossRef] [PubMed]
4. Daneman, R.; Prat, A. The Blood–Brain Barrier. *Cold Spring Harb. Perspect. Biol.* **2015**, *7*, a020412. [CrossRef]
5. Jafari, S.; Mair, L.O.; Weinberg, I.N.; Baker-McKee, J.; Hale, O.; Watson-Daniels, J.; English, B.; Stepanov, P.Y.; Ropp, C.; Atoyebi, O.F.; et al. Magnetic drilling enhances intra-nasal transport of particles into rodent brain. *J. Magn. Magn. Mater.* **2018**, *469*, 302–305. [CrossRef]
6. Sharabi, S.; Last, D.; Daniels, D.; Fabian, I.; Atrakchi, D.; Bresler, Y.; Liraz-Zaltsman, S.; Cooper, I.; Mardor, Y. Non-Invasive Low Pulsed Electrical Fields for Inducing BBB Disruption in Mice—Feasibility Demonstration. *Pharmaceutics* **2021**, *13*, 169. [CrossRef]
7. McDannold, N.; Vykhodtseva, N.; Jolesz, F.A.; Hynynen, K. MRI investigation of the threshold for thermally induced blood-brain barrier disruption and brain tissue damage in the rabbit brain. *Magn. Reson. Med.* **2004**, *51*, 913–923. [CrossRef]
8. Tabatabaei, S.N.; Girouard, H.; Carret, A.-S.; Martel, S. Remote control of the permeability of the blood–brain barrier by magnetic heating of nanoparticles: A proof of concept for brain drug delivery. *J. Control. Release* **2015**, *206*, 49–57. [CrossRef]
9. Patel, B.; Yang, P.H.; Kim, A.H. The effect of thermal therapy on the blood-brain barrier and blood-tumor barrier. *Int. J. Hyperth.* **2020**, *37*, 35–43. [CrossRef]
10. Semyachkina-Glushkovskaya, O.; Kurths, J.; Borisova, E.; Sokolovski, S.; Mantareva, V.; Angelov, I.; Shirokov, A.; Navolokin, N.; Shushunova, N.; Khorovodov, A.; et al. Photodynamic opening of blood-brain barrier. *Biomed. Opt. Express* **2017**, *8*, 5040–5048. [CrossRef]

11. Semyachkina-Glushkovskaya, O.; Chehonin, V.; Borisova, E.; Fedosov, I.; Namykin, A.; Abdurashitov, A.; Shirokov, A.; Khlebtsov, B.; Lyubun, Y.; Navolokin, N.; et al. Photodynamic opening of the blood-brain barrier and pathways of brain clearing. *J. Biophotonics* **2018**, *11*, e201700287. [CrossRef] [PubMed]
12. Madsen, S.J.; Hirschberg, H. Site-specific opening of the blood-brain barrier. *J. Biophotonics* **2010**, *3*, 356–367. [CrossRef] [PubMed]
13. Aryal, M.; Arvanitis, C.D.; Alexander, P.M.; McDannold, N. Ultrasound-mediated blood–brain barrier disruption for targeted drug delivery in the central nervous system. *Adv. Drug Deliv. Rev.* **2014**, *72*, 94–109. [CrossRef] [PubMed]
14. Sharabi, S.; Bresler, Y.; Ravid, O.; Shemesh, C.; Atrakchi, D.; Schnaider-Beeri, M.; Gosselet, F.; Dehouck, L.; Last, D.; Guez, D.; et al. Transient blood–brain barrier disruption is induced by low pulsed electrical fields in vitro: An analysis of permeability and trans-endothelial electric resistivity. *Drug Deliv.* **2019**, *26*, 459–469. [CrossRef] [PubMed]
15. Heydarheydari, S.; Firoozabadi, S.M.; Mirnajafi-Zadeh, J.; Shankayi, Z. Pulsed high magnetic field-induced reversible blood-brain barrier permeability to enhance brain-targeted drug delivery. *Electromagn. Biol. Med.* **2021**, *40*, 361–374. [CrossRef]
16. Rodriguez, A.; Tatter, S.B.; Debinski, W. Neurosurgical Techniques for Disruption of the Blood–Brain Barrier for Glioblastoma Treatment. *Pharmaceutics* **2015**, *7*, 175–187. [CrossRef]
17. Yarmush, M.L.; Golberg, A.; Serša, G.; Kotnik, T.; Miklavčič, D. Electroporation-Based Technologies for Medicine: Principles, Applications, and Challenges. *Annu. Rev. Biomed. Eng.* **2014**, *16*, 295–320. [CrossRef]
18. Garcia, P.A.; Rossmeisl, J.H.; Robertson, J.L.; Olson, J.D.; Johnson, A.J.; Ellis, T.L.; Davalos, R.V. 7.0-T Magnetic Resonance Imaging Characterization of Acute Blood-Brain-Barrier Disruption Achieved with Intracranial Irreversible Electroporation. *PLoS ONE* **2012**, *7*, e50482. [CrossRef]
19. Sharabi, S.; Last, D.; Guez, D.; Daniels, D.; Hjouj, M.I.; Salomon, S.; Maor, E.; Mardor, Y. Dynamic effects of point source electroporation on the rat brain tissue. *Bioelectrochemistry* **2014**, *99*, 30–39. [CrossRef]
20. Sharabi, S.; Last, D.; Daniels, D.; Zaltsman, S.L.; Mardor, Y. The effects of point-source electroporation on the blood-brain barrier and brain vasculature in rats: An MRI and histology study. *Bioelectrochemistry* **2020**, *134*, 107521. [CrossRef]
21. Reilly, J.P.; Freeman, V.T.; Larkin, W.D. Sensory Effects of Transient Electrical Stimulation—Evaluation with a Neuroelectric Model. *IEEE Trans. Biomed. Eng.* **1985**, *BME-32*, 1001–1011. [CrossRef] [PubMed]
22. Peterchev, A.V.; Murphy, D.L.; Lisanby, S.H. Repetitive transcranial magnetic stimulator with controllable pulse parameters. *J. Neural Eng.* **2011**, *8*, 036016. [CrossRef]
23. Knaian, A.N. Electropermanent Magnetic Connectors and Actuators: Devices and Their Application in Programmable Matter. Ph.D. Thesis, Electrical Engineering and Computer Science, Massachusetts Insitute of Technology, Cambridge, MA, USA, 2010.
24. Gilpin, K.; Knaian, A.; Rus, D. Robot pebbles: One centimeter modules for programmable matter through self-disassembly. In Proceedings of the 2010 IEEE International Conference on Robotics and Automation, Anchorage, AK, USA, 3–7 May 2010; pp. 2485–2492. [CrossRef]
25. Knaian, A.N.; Cheung, K.C.; Lobovsky, M.B.; Oines, A.J.; Schmidt-Neilsen, P.; Gershenfeld, N.A. The Milli-Motein: A self-folding chain of programmable matter with a one centimeter module pitch. In Proceedings of the 2012 IEEE/RSJ International Conference on Intelligent Robots and Systems, Vilamoura-Algarve, Portugal, 7–12 October 2012; pp. 1447–1453. [CrossRef]
26. Ropp, C.; Chen, C.; Greer, M.; Glickstein, J.; Mair, L.; Hale, O.; Ariando, D.; Jafari, S.; Hevaganinge, A.; Mandal, S.; et al. Electropermanent magnets for variable-field NMR. *J. Magn. Reson.* **2019**, *303*, 82–90. [CrossRef] [PubMed]
27. Udalov, O.G.; Weinberg, I.N.; Baum, I.; Chen, C.; Tang, X.; Petrillo, M.; Probst, R.; Seward, C.; Jafari, S.; Stepanov, P.Y.; et al. Combined TMS/MRI with deep brain stimulation capability. In *Neurotherapeutics*; Springer: New York, NY, USA, 2021; Volume 18, p. 2150.
28. Deng, Z.-D.; Lisanby, S.H.; Peterchev, A.V. Electric field depth–focality tradeoff in transcranial magnetic stimulation: Simulation comparison of 50 coil designs. *Brain Stimul.* **2013**, *6*, 1–13. [CrossRef] [PubMed]
29. Lohmann, C.; Hüwel, S.; Galla, H.-J. Predicting Blood-Brain Barrier Permeability of Drugs: Evaluation of Different In Vitro Assays. *J. Drug Target.* **2002**, *10*, 263–276. [CrossRef]
30. Garberg, P.; Ball, M.; Borg, N.; Cecchelli, R.; Fenart, L.; Hurst, R.D.; Lindmark, T.; Mabondzo, A.; Nilsson, J.E.; Raub, T.J.; et al. In vitro models for the blood–brain barrier. *Toxicol. In Vitro* **2005**, *19*, 299–334. [CrossRef]
31. Elbrecht, D.H.; Long, C.J.; Hickman, J.J. Transepithelial/endothelial Electrical Resistance (TEER) theory and applications for microfluidic body-on-a-chip devices. *J. Rare Dis. Res. Treat.* **2016**, *1*, 46–52. [CrossRef]
32. Razali, N.M.; Wah, Y.B. Power Comparisons of Shapiro-Wilk, Kolmogorov-Smirnov, Lilliefors and Anderson-Darling Tests. *J. Stat. Modeling Anal.* **2011**, *2*, 21–33.
33. Rubin, L.L.; Hall, D.E.; Porter, S.; Barbu, K.; Cannon, C.; Horner, H.C.; Janatpour, M.; Liaw, C.W.; Manning, K.; Morales, J. A cell culture model of the blood-brain barrier. *J. Cell Biol.* **1991**, *115*, 1725–1735. [CrossRef]
34. Cucullo, L.; Couraud, P.-O.; Weksler, B.; Romero, I.; Hossain, M.; Rapp, E.; Janigro, D. Immortalized Human Brain Endothelial Cells and Flow-Based Vascular Modeling: A Marriage of Convenience for Rational Neurovascular Studies. *J. Cereb. Blood Flow Metab.* **2007**, *28*, 312–328. [CrossRef]
35. Stone, N.L.; England, T.J.; O'Sullivan, S.E. A Novel Transwell Blood Brain Barrier Model Using Primary Human Cells. *Front. Cell. Neurosci.* **2019**, *13*, 230. [CrossRef] [PubMed]
36. Srinivasan, B.; Kolli, A.R.; Esch, M.B.; Abaci, H.E.; Shuler, M.L.; Hickman, J.J. TEER Measurement Techniques for In Vitro Barrier Model Systems. *J. Lab. Autom.* **2015**, *20*, 107–126. [CrossRef] [PubMed]

37. Burgess, A.; Shah, K.; Hough, O.; Hynynen, K. Focused ultrasound-mediated drug delivery through the blood–brain barrier. *Expert Rev. Neurother.* **2015**, *15*, 477–491. [CrossRef]
38. Darrow, D.P.; O'Brien, P.; Richner, T.J.; Netoff, T.I.; Ebbini, E.S. Reversible neuroinhibition by focused ultrasound is mediated by a thermal mechanism. *Brain Stimul.* **2019**, *12*, 1439–1447. [CrossRef] [PubMed]
39. Hjouj, M.; Last, D.; Guez, D.; Daniels, D.; Sharabi, S.; Lavee, J.; Rubinsky, B.; Mardor, Y. MRI Study on Reversible and Irreversible Electroporation Induced Blood Brain Barrier Disruption. *PLoS ONE* **2012**, *7*, e42817. [CrossRef]

pharmaceutics

MDPI

Article

Retinal Delivery of the Protein Kinase C-β Inhibitor Ruboxistaurin Using Non-Invasive Nanoparticles of Polyamidoamine Dendrimers

Rehab A. Alshammari [1,2], Fadilah S. Aleanizy [2,*], Amal Aldarwesh [3], Fulwah Y. Alqahtani [2], Wael A. Mahdi [2], Bushra Alquadeib [2], Qamraa H. Alqahtani [4], Nazrul Haq [2], Faiyaz Shakeel [2], Hosam G. Abdelhady [5] and Ibrahim A. Alsarra [2]

[1] Department of Pharmaceutical Sciences, College of Pharmacy, AlMaarefa University, Ad Diriyah 13713, Saudi Arabia; rshammari@mcst.edu.sa
[2] Department of Pharmaceutics, College of Pharmacy, King Saud University, Riyadh 11451, Saudi Arabia; fyalqahtani@ksu.edu.sa (F.Y.A.); wmahdi@ksu.edu.sa (W.A.M.); bquadeib@ksu.edu.sa (B.A.); nazrulhaq59@gmail.com (N.H.); faiyazs@fastmail.fm (F.S.); ialsarra@ksu.edu.sa (I.A.A.)
[3] Department of Optometry, College of Applied Medical Sciences, King Saud University, Riyadh 11451, Saudi Arabia; aaldarweesh@ksu.edu.sa
[4] Department of Pharmacology and Toxicology, College of Pharmacy, King Saud University, Riyadh 11451, Saudi Arabia; ghamad@ksu.edu.sa
[5] Department of Physiology & Pharmacology, College of Osteopathic Medicine, Sam Houston State University, 925 City Central Avenue, Conroe, TX 77304, USA; hosam.abdelhady@shsu.edu
* Correspondence: faleanizy@ksu.edu.sa

Citation: Alshammari, R.A.; Aleanizy, F.S.; Aldarwesh, A.; Alqahtani, F.Y.; Mahdi, W.A.; Alquadeib, B.; Alqahtani, Q.H.; Haq, N.; Shakeel, F.; Abdelhady, H.G.; et al. Retinal Delivery of the Protein Kinase C-β Inhibitor Ruboxistaurin Using Non-Invasive Nanoparticles of Polyamidoamine Dendrimers. *Pharmaceutics* **2022**, *14*, 1444. https://doi.org/10.3390/pharmaceutics14071444

Academic Editors: Vibhuti Agrahari and Prashant Kumar

Received: 2 June 2022
Accepted: 6 July 2022
Published: 11 July 2022

Abstract: Ruboxistaurin (RBX) is an anti-vascular endothelial growth factor (anti-VEGF) agent that is used in the treatment of diabetic retinopathy and is mainly given intravitreally. To provide a safe and effective method for RBX administration, this study was designed to develop RBX nanoparticles using polyamidoamine (PAMAM) dendrimer generation 5 for the treatment of diabetic retinopathy. Drug loading efficiency, and in vitro release of proposed complexes of RBX: PAMAM dendrimers were determined and the complexation ratio that showed the highest possible loading efficiency was selected. The drug loading efficiency (%) of 1:1, 2.5:1, and 5:1 complexes was 89.2%, 96.4%, and 97.6%, respectively. Loading capacities of 1:1, 2.5:1, and 5:1 complexes were 1.6%, 4.0%, and 7.2% respectively. In comparison, the 5:1 complex showed the best results in the aforementioned measurements. The in vitro release studies showed that in 8 h, the RBX release from 1:1, 2.5:1, and 5:1 complexes was 37.5%, 35.9%, and 77.0%, respectively. In particular, 5:1 complex showed the highest drug release. In addition, particle size measurements showed that the diameter of empty PAMAM dendrimers was 214.9 $\pm$ 8.5 nm, whereas the diameters of loaded PAMAM dendrimers in 1:1, 2.5:1, 5:1 complexes were found to be 461.0 $\pm$ 6.4, 482.4 $\pm$ 12.5, and 420.0 $\pm$ 7.1 nm, respectively. Polydispersity index (PDI) showed that there were no significant changes in the PDI between the free and loaded PAMAM dendrimers. The zeta potential measurements showed that the free and loaded nanoparticles possessed neutral charges due to the presence of anionic and cationic terminal structures. Furthermore, the safety of this formulation was apparent on the viability of the MIO-M1 cell lines. This nanoformulation will improve the therapeutic outcomes of anti-VEGF therapy and the bioavailability of RBX to prevent vision loss in patients with diabetic retinopathy.

Keywords: polyamidoamine dendrimers; diabetic retinopathy; protein kinase C-β inhibitor; nanoparticles; ruboxistaurin

1. Introduction

Diabetic retinopathy (DR) is a well-known consequence of poorly controlled hyperglycemia. It is responsible for significant blindness in diabetes mellitus (DM) patients [1]. When DR progresses to a vision-threatening complication, vitreous surgery and laser photocoagulation are the only effective procedures in restoring or maintaining the vision. Nevertheless, the laser-treated retina usually loses its function and develops scarring tissue [2]. The main drug classes used for the management of DR and other DM related complications are anti-vascular endothelial growth factor (anti-VEGF) drugs, protein kinase C (PKC) inhibitors, corticosteroids, and somatostatin analogues [1]. The development of anti-VEGF therapy as a new approach for treating proliferative DR (PDR) has recently been adopted [3]. Anti-VEGF agents have been identified to reduce or prevent neovascularization and vessel drainage through antagonization of VEGF's effects as they bind to VEGF, and prevent its cellular action [3–6]. Ranibizumab, bevacizumab, and pegaptanib intravitreal (IVT) injections are currently being used in the treatment of DR [1].

A modern anti-VEGF therapy which relies on using PKC ß-inhibitor has been developed for the treatment of DR. Ruboxistaurin (RBX) is an investigational drug that has recently attracted a great deal of attention as a potent drug for treating DR. It acts as a selective PKC ß-inhibitor that is still pending for the United States Food and Drug Administration (FDA) and European Medicines Agency (EMA) approval. In diabetic rats, RBX has been found to inhibit PKCβ activity when given orally or intravitreally [7,8]. The findings reported by Aldeweesh (2016) demonstrated that RBX is very potent at lowering VEGF release from human retinal macroglial Müller cells (MIO-M1) in the first 24 h under simulated conditions of hyperglycemia. Furthermore, prolonged exposure to RBX resulted in a continued reduction which could indicate the breakdown of VEGF over time [9]. This medicine could slow down or prevent DR progression and which will lead to better quality of life for DM patients. Therefore, this potential candidate needs to be formulated in an appropriate dosage form to be available upon approval by the FDA and EMA [10]. The ideal route for RBX administration can be attained through reaching the retina at a constant rate. In recent years, invasive drug delivery systems (DDSs) have been chosen to deliver anti-VEGFs to the retina, to reduce the risk of systemic side effects and provide better drug targeting for oral and systemic drug delivery [11]. Delivering RBX to the retina via invasive methods can successfully slow down the progression of DR by exposing the retina to a high level of RBX, but unfortunately, will lead to the appearance of unwanted side effects. As a consequence, these side effects will not be tolerated which affects the compliance of patients and thus minimizes the efficacy of the therapy. In this case, microvascular complications of DR remain advanced over time, causing vision to be distorted and quality of life to be reduced. Non-invasive dosage forms, however, are self-administered by the patient and therefore well tolerated as they do not involve injections or invasive equipment. Hopefully, they would increase the patient compliance toward the treatment without experiencing the ocular discomfort and complications associated with IVT injections [12]. If the non-invasive delivery of retinal drugs is achievable and efficient, RBX eye drops could be used as prophylactic approach to lessen the formation of new fragile vessels in the retina [13]. In recent years, researchers have been studying topical drug delivery for their potential in the treatment of retinal diseases [13,14]. The distribution of dexamethasone (DEX) in the ocular tissue was studied by Bessonova et al. (2011). In fact, DEX was found in the eyelid, cornea, aqueous humor, iris, lens, vitreous cavity, retina, and choroid at a range of concentrations following topical application. However, the highest levels of DEX were found in the anterior structures of the eye. This study has shown that DEX cannot be transported to the posterior chamber of the eye via topical application, resulting in a lack of therapeutic responses to treat retinal diseases [14].

Likewise, delivery of oral drugs has been investigated as a non-invasive alternative; however, it has largely been ineffective [15]. Hence, the ideal method is to develop a DDS that can passively deliver RBX from the ocular surface, through the layers of the eye and reside in the retinal tissues [11–13]. This can be achieved by the production of nanocarriers that are capable of encasing and delivering therapeutic agents to their site of action [11–13]. In the past years, a number of nanocarriers have been investigated for ocular drug delivery, especially degradable nanoparticles (NPs) made with polymers, such as dendrimers, liposomes, polylactic-co-glycolic acid (PLGA) nanoparticles, and chitosan nanoparticles [11–13]. These studies suggested that the properties of nanocarriers could influence their application in both segments of the eye [11–13]. In fact, dendrimers are exceptional polymers, which offer various advantages over conventional linear or branched polymers [1]. These advantages are better solubility in common solvents, monodisperse distribution, controlled particle size, and higher area/volume ratio [1,12]. These nanocarriers have proved themselves to be very effective to be used as bioavailability, permeability, and solubility enhancers for different routes of administration [1]. For that reason, the goal of this study was to formulate and characterize RBX nanoparticles by encapsulating RBX within the internal cavities of polyamidoamine (PAMAM) dendrimer generation 4.5 and 5, respectively. Out of different generation PAMAM dendrimers, only intermediate generation 3.5–5 dendrimers are suitable for drug delivery carriers. Due to the application of generation 4.5 and 5 as drug delivery carriers, these carriers were developed in this study [12]. Generation 4.5 dendrimers are anionic in nature; however, generation 5 dendrimers are neutral in nature [1,13].

2. Materials and Methods

2.1. Materials

RBX (LY-333531 hydrochloride, 1 mg vial), dimethyl sulfoxide (DMSO), dialysis cellulose membrane (MWCO 14,000 Da), reusable plastic sample cuvette, folded capillary ζ-cells, and human vascular endothelial growth factor (Hu VEGF) ELISA were obtained from Sigma Aldrich (St. Louis, MO, USA). Polyamidoamine dendrimer generation 4.5 (PAMAM dendrimers G4.5, 1 g vial) and polyamidoamine dendrimer generation 5 (PAMAM dendrimers G5, 1 g vial) were purchased from Nanosynthons (Mt. Pleasant, MI, USA). All chemicals and reagents were of analytical grade.

2.2. Formulation of Anionic G4.5 and Neutral G5 Complexes

To achieve loading of RBX into anionic G4.5 and neutral G5 PAMAM dendrimers, RBX (1 mg) was dispersed into 1 mL of dimethyl sulfoxide (DMSO) making a concentration of (0.1% w/v). The obtained PAMAM dendrimers G4.5 or G5 (1 g) were further dispersed into 10 mL of purified water to achieve a concentration of (10% w/v). A number of formulations were prepared for the optimization of the best one. In this study, a molar ratio of 1:1, 2.5:1, 5:1, and 25:1 PAMAM dendrimers G4.5: RBX and PAMAM dendrimers G5: RBX were prepared and coded as G4.5 1:1, G4.5 2.5:1, G4.5 5:1, and G4.5 25:1, respectively for G4.5 complexes and G5 1:1, G5 2.5:1, G5 5:1, and G5 25:1, respectively for G5 counterparts. The amounts of these complexes were calculated and added to the reaction mixture. In each one of these mixtures, the volume was completed with deionized water to 1 mL. Briefly, RBX and amounts for each proposed complex are shown in Table 1. After preparation, the reaction mixtures were stirred for 24 h in the dark at 4 °C [16]. The formulated complexes were extracted by removing the excess amounts of the undissolved drug by cold dialysis using cellulose membrane (MWCO 14,000 Da) against distilled water for 24 h [17,18]. The complexes were then lyophilized for 72 h using Labcono Free Zone 6 Liter Benchtop Freeze Dry System and stored at −30 °C for further use [19].

Table 1. Calculated amounts of G4.5 and G5 complexes.

Formulation	Amount of RBX (0.1% w/v)	Amount of PAMAM Dendrimers G4.5 (10% w/v)	Amount of PAMAM Dendrimers G5 (10% w/v)
		G4.5 complexes	
G4.5 complex 1:1	50 µL	25 µL	-
G4.5 complex 2.5:1	50 µL	10 µL	-
G4.5 complex 5:1	50 µL	5 µL	-
G4.5 complex 25:1	50 µL	1 µL	-
		G5 complexes	
G5 complex 1:1	50 µL	-	28 µL
G5 complex 2.5:1	50 µL	-	11.2 µL
G5 complex 5:1	50 µL	-	5.6 µL
G5 complex 25:1	50 µL	-	1.1 µL

2.3. Measurement of Particle Size (PS), Polydispersity Index (PDI), and ζ-Potential

PS and PDI of G4.5 and G5 complexes and the empty PAMAM dendrimers G4.5 and G5 were measured by Zetasizer (Malvern Instruments Ltd., Malvern, UK) [20], which was based on dynamic light scattering (DLS). DLS analysis was performed in triplicate at 25 °C and scattering angle of 90°. The volume-average PS was determined for each sample. The surface charge of G4.5 and G5 complexes and the empty PAMAM dendrimers G4.5 and G5 was determined using Zetasizer (Malvern Instruments Ltd., Malvern, UK) [20]. The ζ-potential of these nanoparticles was determined in an electric field. The velocity and direction of the nanoparticle movement was measured and was demonstrated to be proportional to their ζ-potential. Analysis was performed in triplicate at 25 °C [21].

2.4. Determination of Drug Loading Efficiency (DE%)

The loading of different amounts of the drug into the dendritic structure of PAMAM dendrimers G4.5 and G5 was studied to estimate the maximum drug loading efficiency of each complex. To achieve this, DE% of G4.5 and G5 complexes was determined by using the dialysis method. G4.5 and G5 complexes were placed into a cellulose membrane (MWCO 14,000 Da), then immersed in deionized water and stirred for 24 h at 4 °C [22]. After that, a sample from the surrounding media (i.e., deionized water) was withdrawn and measured by Nanodrop UV spectrophotometer at 254 nm. This was carried out to indirectly determine the amount of the drug loaded in PAMAM dendrimers. The measured amount of free drug from the surrounding media was referred as amount of free drug, and the original amount of drug added in the mixture was called amount of total drug. The DE% was calculated by the following equation:

$$DE\% = \frac{\text{Amount of total drug} - \text{amount of free drug}}{\text{Amount of total drug}} \times 100 \qquad (1)$$

2.5. Transmission Electron Microscopy

The loading visual pattern as well as the morphology of G4.5 and G5 complexes and the empty PAMAM dendrimers, G4.5 and G5, was determined by transmission electron microscopy (TEM) (JEM1230EX; Tokyo, Japan). The image of the nanoparticles was created by using scattered electrons. These electrons were transmitted through the sample, and then the image was formed by detecting the reflected electrons [21].

2.6. In Vitro Drug Release of G4.5 and G5 Complexes

In vitro drug release study was carried out to determine the amount of drug released from G4.5 and G5 complexes. To conduct this study, a phosphate buffer solution (PBS) media (pH 7.4) was prepared and used as a dissolution media [23,24]. A total of 200 μL of each studied complex containing 10 μg of RBX was placed into a cellulose membrane with a molecular weight cut-off (MWCO) 14,000 Da, then was immersed in 20 mL of PBS media (pH 7.4). In vitro drug release of G4.5 and G5 complexes was tested at 37 ± 0.5 °C with slow magnetic stirring for a period of 8 h. Aliquots of 500 μL were withdrawn from the solution and replaced with the same volume of fresh PBS at predetermined time points (i.e., 1, 2, 3, 4, 5, 6, 7, and 8 h). After that, RBX amounts in the withdrawn samples was determined by Nanodrop UV spectrophotometer at 254 nm. Throughout the experiments, sink conditions were maintained [1,16].

2.7. Stability Studies

According to the manufacturer, PAMAM dendrimers should be stored in the dark at 2–8 °C, while RBX is a light sensitive drug and should be kept at −20 °C. In this work, the effect of light and temperature on the stability of the formulated nanoparticles was investigated. Samples of G4.5 and G5 complexes were stored in the dark and daylight and kept at different temperatures ranging from (4–50) °C as shown in Supplementary Table S1. In addition, the stability of G4.5 and G5 complexes was studied at periods of 1, 3, and 6 months.

2.7.1. Physical Stability

At the end of the 6-month study period, the nanoparticles were observed and signs of color changes, precipitation, or turbidity were recorded [25]. The most physically stable complex was then visualized using scanning electron microscopy (SEM) (JSM 7610F; Tokyo, Japan) to confirm that the complex still preserves its shape and size under certain storage conditions.

2.7.2. Chemical Stability

In addition to the physical stability of G4.5 and G5 complexes, drug content was also assessed under storage conditions mentioned in Table S1. This was carried out by calculating the percent content of RBX remaining in each tested complex. Drug content was quantified by ultra-performance liquid chromatography coupled to the mass spectrometry (UPLC-MS/MS) method as reported in the literature [26].

2.8. Cell Culture

2.8.1. Moorfield's/Institute of Ophthalmology-Müller-1 (MIO-M1) Cells

In this work, cell culture studies were carried out to assess the viability of macroglial Müller cells when exposed to RBX, PAMAM dendrimers, and the proposed complexes as well. The viability of these cells was assessed in controlled and high glucose treatment with and without the tested complexes. The cell line used in this study is MIO-M1; a spontaneously immortalized human cell line. These cell lines were obtained from UCL institute of Ophthalmology, London, UK. These cells were named after the institution where they were isolated, MIO-M1 [27].

2.8.2. Culture of the MIO-M1 Glial Cell Line

MIO-M1 cells were cultured in Dulbecco's Minimal Essential Medium (DMEM) containing GLUTAMAX and physiological glucose levels of 5.55 mM. The medium was supplemented with 10% fetal bovine serum (FBS) and 50 mg/L penicillin/streptomycin. Prior to experimental work, cells were seeded at 5000 cells per well in 96 well plates (100 μL medium). After that, cells were grown for three days to achieve >80% confluence and were starved with serum-free DMEM for at least 24 h before the experiment [9].

2.8.3. Cell Viability Studies

Cell viability was assessed using (Cell Titer 96 Aqueous Proliferation Assay, Promega, Southampton, UK). This assay was carried out according to the manufacturer's protocol. This test is a colorimetric assay used to determine the number of viable cells. It is based on the conversion of a 3-(4,5-dimethylthiazol-2-yl)-5-(3-carboxymethoxyphenyl)-2-(4-sulfophenyl)-2H-tetrazolium (MTS) into a brown formazan product when reduced by active cells [28]. The tetrazolium reduction takes place in the mitochondria and measures mitochondrial metabolic rate as a measure of cell viability [29]. Briefly, after exposing cells to experimental conditions, the medium was removed from the 96 well plate and replaced with 100 μL MTS solution. At the end of each tested period (i.e., 24, 48, and 72 h), the fluorescence of formazan was measured at 490 nm with a micro-plate reader [30].

2.8.4. High Glucose Experiments

In this work, MIO-M1 cells were exposed to simulated conditions of hyperglycemia to test the cells' behavior in the presence of RBX, PAMAM dendrimers, and the proposed complexes. This was achieved by incubating the cells in controlled DMEM (5.55 mM glucose) and high glucose DMEM of (25 mM glucose) for 24, 48, and 72 h with and without the tested compounds. Then, the medium was collected for subsequent cell viability studies [9].

2.8.5. High Glucose Treatment of PAMAM Dendrimers and Complexes

In this study, a drug-dose–response study of RBX, PAMAM dendrimers, and the proposed complexes was carried out in MIO-M1 cells cultured in controlled and high glucose medium. In hyperglycemic conditions, the viability of MIO-M1 cells was assessed using an

MTS assay at the end of each tested period (i.e., 24, 48, and 72 h). Two concentrations (200 and 500 nM) of pure RBX were tested. In addition, two concentrations (200 and 500 nM) of RBX formulated as nanoparticles (G4.5 and G5 complexes 25:1) were tested as well. Moreover, PAMAM dendrimers G4.5 and G5 were tested in both cell mediums in the same amount available in G4.5 and G5 complex respectively. This was carried out to examine whether PAMAM dendrimers in the presented concentrations could cause any cytotoxicity to the cells. Furthermore, this step was performed to investigate the safety of the tested compounds in simulated conditions of hyperglycemia and also, to determine the most tolerable doses by MIO-M1 cells.

2.8.6. In Vitro Permeability Study

The integrity of the monolayer cell membrane of MIO-M1 was evaluated via an in vitro permeability study on Transwell® and transendothelial electrical resistance (TEER). The in vitro studies were performed in a 24-well plate format on a polyester membrane (PET) Transwell® (0.33 cm^2, 0.4 μm pore size). MIO-M1 cells were seeded at a density of 0.5×10^6 cells/insert in the apical (upper) compartment with 300 μL media, and the basolateral (lower) compartment was filled with 900 μL media. The cells were grown in Dulbecco's Modified Eagle's medium (DMEM) containing glutamine supplemented with 10% fetal bovine serum and 1% penicillin-streptomycin. MIO-M1 cells were incubated at 37 °C at 5% CO_2, along with DMEM media of well and insert replenished every two days [31,32].

It is important that MIO-M1 make confluent monolayers so that they require monolayer integrity and will function as a barrier. To evaluate monolayer integrity, the measurement of TEER was performed using an endothelial volt-ohmmeter (EVOM) (World Precision Instruments, Sarasota, FL, USA) according to the manufacturer's instructions. The resistance value (R_{Blank}) in units of (Ω) measured for each insert (no cells) was subtracted from the resistance (R_{Total}) across the cell layer on the membrane to obtain the cell specific resistance ($R_{MIO\text{-}M1}$):

$$R_{MIO\text{-}M1}\ (\Omega) = R_{Total} - R_{Blank} \quad (2)$$

$$\text{TEER resistance}\ (\Omega\cdot cm^2) = R_{MIO\text{-}M1}\ (\Omega) \times SA_{\text{semipermeable membrane surface Area}}\ (cm^2) \quad (3)$$

$R_{MIO\text{-}M1}$ value was then multiplied by the surface area of the insert (0.33 cm^2) to obtain the value of TEER resistance of MIO-M1 ($\Omega\cdot cm^2$). Each filter was measured three times, and each culture condition was carried out at least with triplicate filters [33–36].

At the time of the experiments, MIO-M1 was cultured for at least 14 days to reach the highest and constant TEER value of the membrane. Transwells® were washed twice with sterile PBS without calcium and magnesium and transferred to a serum-free medium for the duration of the experiments. At 37 °C in 5% CO_2 in a humidified incubator, pure drug (RBX), or dendrimers (with or without RBX), at 500 nM of RBX concentration, was incubated for 24 h. The monolayer membrane's integrity was evaluated by quantifying tracer permeability of solution containing fluorescein isothiocyanate conjugate (FITC)-dextran at an initial concentration of 100 μg/mL, which was added to the apical (upper) compartment. At 1, 3, 6, 12, and 24 h, samples were drawn from the basolateral compartment, which was replaced with an equal volume of fresh medium each time. The fluorescence intensities were measured using a Synergy H1 plate reader (BioTek) at emission/excitation wavelengths of 495/520 nm and were converted to the concentrations of FITC-dextran with the calibration curve [31,32,37–39]. The apparent permeability coefficient (Papp) was calculated based on the following equation [38,40]:

$$\text{Papp (cm/s)} = J/(AC_D) \quad (4)$$

where, J is the rate of appearance of the compounds in the receiver compartment, A is the surface area of the filter membrane, and C_D is the initial concentration in the donor compartment.

2.9. Statistical Analysis

Values were expressed as the means and standard error of the mean (SEM). Differences among treated groups and control (MIO-M1 only) were evaluated by one-way analysis of variance (ANOVA) followed by *post-hoc* comparisons using Tukey's multiple comparisons using Graph Pad Prism (version 9.0, GraphPad Inc., La Jolla, San Diego, CA, USA). A p value of 0.05 or less was considered statistically significant.

3. Results

3.1. Characterization of G4.5 Complexes

3.1.1. Measurement of PS and PDI

PS and PDI measurements were carried out for both G4.5 complexes and the empty PAMAM dendrimers G4.5 and results of PS and PDI for the G4.5 complexes and the empty PAMAM dendrimers G4.5 are demonstrated in Table 2, Figure S1A and Figure S2A, respectively. According to the manufacturer, PS of free PAMAM G4.5 is 143.0 ± 19.6 nm. Results obtained from Zetasizer demonstrated that PS of the empty PAMAM dendrimers G4.5 was 186.0 ± 2.3 nm. When loaded with RBX, the measurements revealed that PS of G4.5 complexes 1:1, 2.5:1, 5:1, and 25:1 was increased to 367.0, 416.0, 289.0, and 301.0 nm, respectively. However, G4.5 complex 25:1 possessed less PS among all studied complexes. PAMAM dendrimers possess lower PDI when compared to other nanoparticles. PDI was measured for G4.5 complexes and the empty PAMAM dendrimers G4.5 and revealed that there is no significant change in PDI measurement of the dendrimers after loading it with RBX ($p > 0.05$). However, G4.5 complex 25:1 possessed the least PDI among all studied nanoformulations (PDI ≤ 0.35).

Table 2. PS, PDI and ζ-potential of blank and loaded PAMAM dendrimers G4.5 and G5 (mean ± SD, $n = 3$).

RBX-PAMAM Nanoparticles	PS (nm) ± SD	PDI ± SD	ζ-Potential in (mV) ± SD
Empty PAMAM dendrimers G4.5	186.0 ± 2.3	0.297 ± 0.040	−44.0 ± 2.0
G4.5 complex 1:1	367.0 ± 13.0	0.335 ± 0.010	−16.2 ± 3.1
G4.5 complex 2.5:1	416.0 ± 4.3	0.337 ± 0.030	−5.1 ± 10.4
G4.5 complex 5:1	289.0 ± 14.9	0.361 ± 0.030	−6.4 ± 1.8
G4.5 complex 25:1	301.0 ± 7.1	0.304 ± 0.010	−13.0 ± 1.6
Empty PAMAM dendrimers G5	214.0 ± 8.5	0.356 ± 0.010	−0.2 ± 0.0
G5 complex 1:1	461.0 ± 6.4	0.394 ± 0.010	4.3 ± 1.3
G5 complex 2.5:1	482.0 ± 9.5	0.388 ± 0.020	5.5 ± 0.2
G5 complex 5:1	669.0 ± 2.0	0.587 ± 0.100	9.7 ± 4.9 **
G5 complex 25:1	307.0 ± 6.9	0.380 ± 0.030	−0.0 ± 0.0

** $p \leq 0.01$.

3.1.2. Measurement of ζ-Potential of G4.5 Complexes

ζ-potential measurements were carried out for G4.5 complexes and the empty PAMAM dendrimers G4.5, and results are demonstrated in Table 2. In this study, ζ-potential measurements demonstrated that ζ-potential of empty PAMAM dendrimers G4.5 is −44.0 ± 2.0 mV. After the loading process, ζ-potential measurements of G4.5 complexes 1:1, 2.5:1, 5:1 and 25:1 was −16.2, −5.1, −6.4, and −13.0 mV, respectively. In fact, the surface charge of PAMAM dendrimers plays an important role in permeability of these nanoparticles through the negatively charged ocular barriers. In this work, it was found that the loaded G4.5 complex 25:1 have preserved its negative charge after the loading process. In summary, the previous features demonstrated with G4.5 complex 25:1 are needed for the non-invasive ocular delivery of RBX.

3.1.3. Determination of DE%

The DE% of G4.5 complexes were determined and results are presented in Figure S3A. In this study, DE% of the studied nanoparticles was similar. However, G4.5 complex 25:1 showed the best DE% among all the other proposed complexes though statistically not significant.

3.1.4. In Vitro Drug Release of G4.5 Complexes

Release profiles of G4.5 complexes were studied in order to evaluate the amount of RBX that will be released following the topical instillation of the nanoparticles. As indicated in Figure 1, most of the G4.5 complexes presented a sustained release of RBX. It was shown that at pH 7.4 in a period of 8 h, RBX release of G4.5 complexes 1:1, 2.5:1, and 5:1 was 47.3%, 72.5%, and 79.0%, respectively. In particular, it was observed that the RBX release rate of G4.5 complexes 25:1 was distinctly higher than all the other studied complexes. For a period of 8 h, this complex possessed an initial release of 11.9%. After that, RBX release was gradually increased in a sustained manner up to 86.1%. Moreover, the previous in vitro characterizations of the proposed complexes demonstrated that G4.5 complex 25:1 has revealed the best in vitro release as well as the highest DE% among all other proposed nanoparticles. Because of these remarkable results of G4.5 complex 25:1, this complex was chosen for the next experiments.

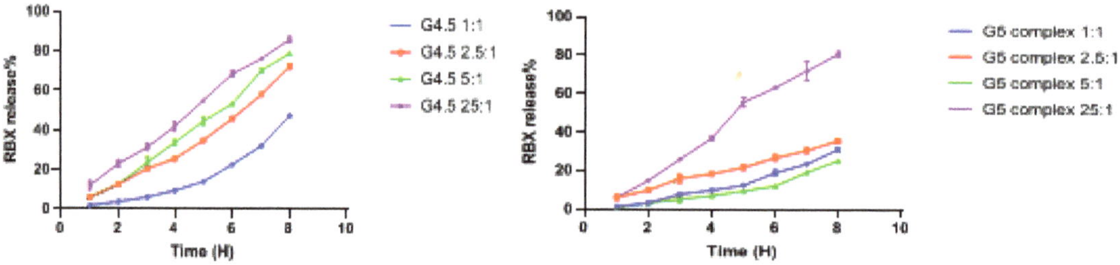

Figure 1. In vitro release profiles of different complexes (mean ± SD, $n = 6$).

3.1.5. Stability Studies of G4.5 Complex

Physical Stability

The stability of the G4.5 25:1 was studied at daylight and in the dark in different temperature conditions ranging from (4–50 °C). For a period of 6 months, the nanoformulations were stored in colorless Eppendorfs and observed for any sign of color change, precipitation, or turbidity. Results are presented in Table S2. After the study period ended, the nanoformulations stored in the dark at 4 °C were examined by the eye inspection and did not show any signs of physical change. In daylight, the sample kept at 25 °C was visualized and showed a color change from pink to colorless while the sample kept in the dark did not show any physical changes. Moreover, a precipitate and a color change were also observed at higher temperatures, 37 °C and 50 °C, respectively. The previous investigation indicated that it is suitable to store the nanoparticles in amber containers at 4 °C. In addition, these nanoparticles were visualized using SEM to assess their shape and size. As seen in Figure 2A, the complex possessed an almost spherical shape and particle size equivalent to those measured by Zetasizer Nano ZS.

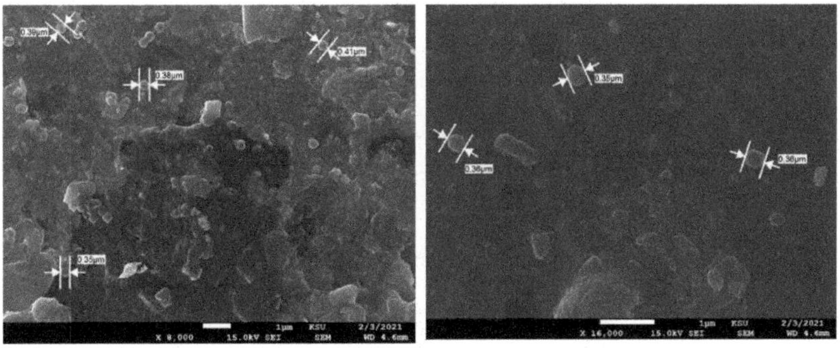

(A) **(B)**

Figure 2. Scanning electron microscope (SEM) overview image of (**A**) G4.5 complex 25:1 and (**B**) G5 complex 25:1.

Chemical Stability

The present work is a quantitative study of the stability of RBX to assess the effect of light source and temperature overtime. This test will help in choosing the best storing conditions for the nanoparticles. Samples of G4.5 complex 25:1 containing 1 µg of RBX was stored at the dark and daylight at different temperatures (4–50 °C). Each one of these samples was kept for 1, 3, and 6 months and analyzed by UPLC MS/MS after the end of each tested period. To determine percent content of RBX for each studied sample, the remaining amount of RBX was quantified from the equation of calibration curve using peak area values and then percent content of RBX was calculated. Results obtained from the stability studies are shown in Figure S4A. Data indicated that RBX is more stable when stored in amber containers. Upon protecting the nanoformulation from light, higher percent content of RBX was demonstrated. In addition, it was observed that the stability of RBX in PAMAM dendrimers G4.5 was slightly decreased with time. In a duration of 6 months, measurements of percent content of RBX in G4.5 complex 25:1 remain above 80.0% in this time period. Moreover, data show that RBX is more stable within PAMAM dendrimers at 4 > 25 > 37 > 50 °C. In fact, the highest percent content of RBX was achieved when storing the nanoparticles in the dark at 4 °C.

TEM

G4.5 complex 25:1 and the empty PAMAM dendrimers G4.5 were visualized by TEM to determine their morphology and to confirm the loading of RBX. Figure 3 displays the morphology of empty PAMAM dendrimers G4.5 as well as G4.5 complex 25:1.

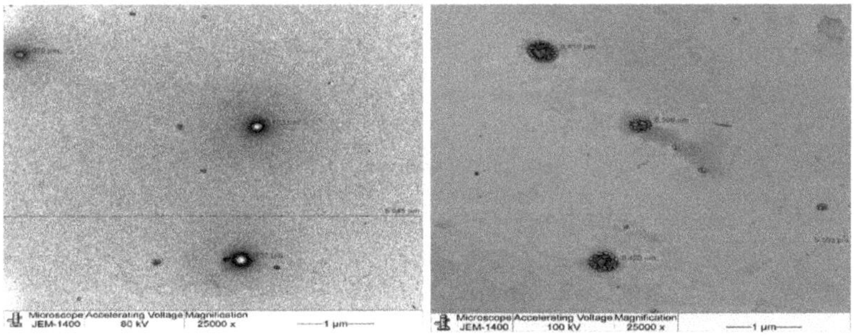

(A) **(B)**

Figure 3. Transmission electron microscope (TEM) overview images of (**A**) empty PAMAM dendrimers G4.5 and (**B**) G4.5 complex 25:1.

3.2. *Characterization of G5 Complexes*

3.2.1. Measurement of PS and PDI

PS and PDI measurements were carried out for both G5 complexes and the empty PAMAM dendrimers, and results are demonstrated in Table 2, Figure S1B, and Figure S2B. According to the manufacturer, the PS of free PAMAM G5 dendrimers is 224.0 ± 13.0 nm. Results obtained from Zetasizer demonstrated that PS of the empty PAMAM dendrimers G5 was 214.9 ± 8.5 nm. When loaded with RBX, the measurements revealed that PS of G5 complexes 1:1, 2.5:1, 5:1, and 25:1 was increased to 461.2, 482.4, 669.8 and 307.1 nm, respectively. Indeed, PS increase of loaded PAMAM dendrimers may be attributed to RBX entrapment within the internal cavities of PAMAM dendrimers. However, G4.5 complex 25:1 possessed the lowest PS among all studied nanoformulations. PDI was measured for the free and loaded PAMAM dendrimers and revealed that there are no significant changes in PDI of the dendrimers after loading it with RBX except for G5 complex 5:1. In fact, G5 complex 25:1 possessed the least PDI among all studied nanoformulations (PDI $\leq$ 0.39). However, a significant increase in PDI was demonstrated with G5 complex 5:1 (Table 2 and Figure S2B).

3.2.2. Measurements of ζ-Potential of G5 Complexes

ζ-potential provided by the manufacturer indicated that the neutral PAMAM G5 dendrimers possesses a neutral charge. In this study, ζ-potential measurements demonstrated that the surface charge of the empty PAMAM dendrimers G5 was −0.1 ± 0.0 mV. Table 2 demonstrates ζ-potential of G5 complexes. After the loading process, ζ-potential of G5 complexes 1:1, 2.5:1, 5:1, and 25:1 was 4.3, 5.5, 9.7, and −0.0 mV, respectively. Indeed, the free and loaded PAMAM G5 dendrimers possessed a neutral charge even after the loading process. Results indicated that ζ-potential of PAMAM dendrimers G5 were not affected by the drug loading process ($p > 0.05$).

3.2.3. Determination of DE%

DE% of the studied nanoparticles showed similar percent content between G5 complexes. Although not statistically significant, G5 complex 25:1 showed the highest DE% among all the other proposed complexes. Results of DE% are presented in Figure S3B.

3.2.4. In Vitro Drug Release of G5 Complexes

As indicated in Figure 1, nearly all G5 complexes possessed a sustained release of RBX. It was shown that at pH 7.4 in a period of 8 h, in vitro release of G5 complexes 1:1, 2.5:1, and 5:1 was 31.3%, 35.8%, and 25.3%, respectively. In particular, RBX release rate of G5 complexes 25:1 was distinctly higher than all the other studied complexes. For a period of 8 h, this complex possessed an initial release of 6.3%. After that, RBX release was gradually increased in a sustained manner up to 81.0%. In fact, among the proposed complexes, G5 25:1 has demonstrated the best in vitro characterizations. Because of these remarkable results of G4.5 complex 25:1, the next studies were manipulated for this complex.

3.2.5. Stability Studies of G5 Complex

Physical Stability

The stability of the G5 25:1 was studied at daylight and in the dark in different temperature conditions ranging from (4–50 °C). For a period of 6 months, the nanoformulations were stored in colorless Eppendorfs and observed for any sign of color change, precipitation, or turbidity. Results are presented in Table S3. This study was performed to investigate which storing condition is suitable for G5 complex 25:1. Based on the result of this investigation, it is clearly indicated that G5 complex 25:1 must be stored in amber containers at 4 °C. In addition, these nanoparticles were visualized using SEM to assess their shape and size. As seen in Figure 2B, the complex possessed an almost spherical shape and particle size equivalent to those measured by Zetasizer Nano ZS (Malvern, UK).

Drug Content

The results for the stability of RBX in G5 25:1 complex were similar to the results obtained from the G4.5 complex 25:1 stability study. It was noticed that there were no significant differences in RBX peak area between G4.5 and G5 samples. Percent content of RBX in G5 complex 25:1 was calculated and demonstrated in Figure S4B.

TEM

G5 complex 25:1 and the empty PAMAM dendrimers G5 were visualized by TEM to determine their morphology and to confirm the loading of RBX. Figure 4 displays the morphology of empty PAMAM dendrimers G5 as well as G5 complex 25:1 complex.

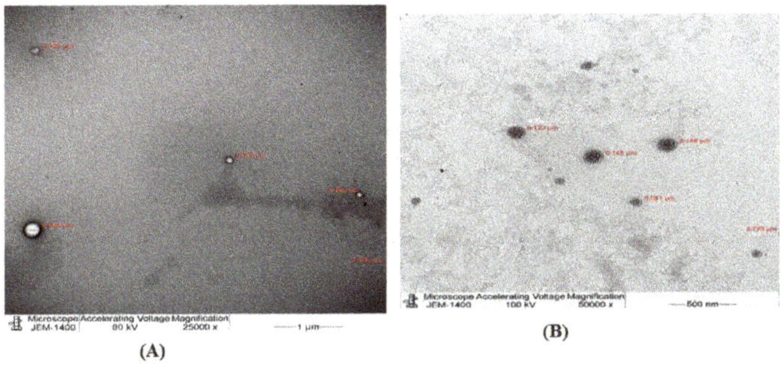

Figure 4. TEM overview images of (**A**) empty PAMAM dendrimers G5 and (**B**) G5 complex 25:1.

3.3. Cell Viability Studies (MTS Assay)

3.3.1. Dose–Response Studies in Controlled Mediums

Dose–Response of RBX

In this work, the safety of RBX was assessed by cell viability studies using MIO-M1 cell line. These investigations were carried out using MTS assay. MIO-M1 cells were cultured in a controlled glucose medium (5.55 mM glucose media) and treated with a range of doses of RBX (100 nM–1 μM). After 24 h, viability (%) of the treated cells was assessed and compared to the viability of untreated cells that were cultured in the same controlled conditions. As seen in Figure 5, viability of the treated cells with RBX did not show any significant reduction when compared to viability of untreated cells ($p > 0.05$). This finding indicates that RBX is safe and the investigated doses are tolerable by MIO-M1 cell line in normal conditions.

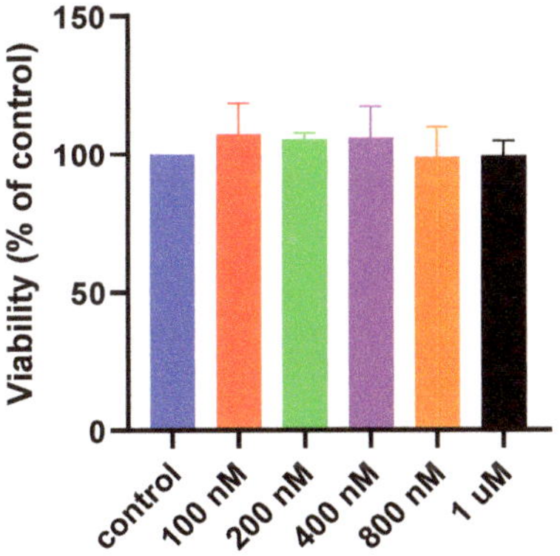

Figure 5. Effect of RBX after 24 h exposure on the cell viability of MIO-M1 cells under controlled conditions (mean ± SD, $n = 3$).

Dose–Response of PAMAM Dendrimers G4.5

Similar to the previous work, the safety of PAMAM dendrimers G4.5 was assessed using different concentrations ranging from (1–50 nM). These investigations were carried out using MTS assay. After 24 h, viability of the treated cells was assessed and compared to the viability of untreated cells that were cultured in the same controlled conditions. As seen in Figure 6A, viability of the treated cells with PAMAM dendrimers G4.5 did not show any significant reduction when compared to viability of untreated cells ($p > 0.05$). These finding indicates that PAMAM dendrimers G4.5 is safe and the investigated doses are tolerable by MIO-M1 cell line in normal conditions.

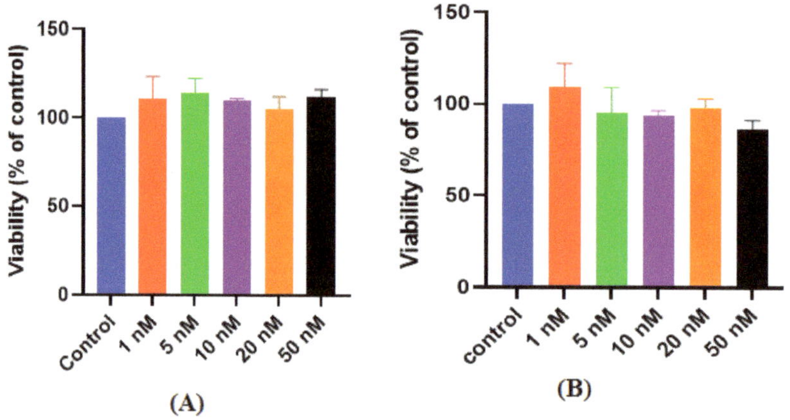

Figure 6. Effect of (**A**) PAMAM dendrimers G4.5 and (**B**) PAMAM dendrimers G5 after 24 h. Exposure on the cell viability of MIO-M1 cells under controlled conditions (mean ± SD, $n = 3$).

Dose–Response of PAMAM dendrimers G5

Similar to the previous work, the safety of PAMAM dendrimers G5 was assessed using different concentrations ranging from (1–50 nM). These investigations were carried out using MTS assay. After 24 h, viability of the treated cells was assessed and compared to the viability% of untreated cells that were cultured in the same controlled conditions. As seen in Figure 6B, viability of the treated cells with PAMAM dendrimers G5 did not show any significant reduction when compared to viability of untreated cells ($p > 0.05$). These findings indicate that the PAMAM dendrimer G5 is safe and the investigated doses are tolerable by MIO-M1 cell line in normal conditions.

Dose–Response of G4.5 Complex 25:1

It was clearly indicated that RBX and PAMAM dendrimers are well tolerated by MIO-M1 cells. More investigations were carried out to assess the safety of the formulated G4.5 complex 25:1. This was carried out using MTS assay. After 24 h, viability of the treated cells was assessed using different concentrations ranging from (100 nM–1 µM) and compared to the viability of untreated cells that were cultured in the same controlled conditions. As seen in Figure 7A, viability of the treated cells with PAMAM dendrimers G4.5 did not show any significant reduction when compared to the viability of untreated cells ($p > 0.05$). These finding indicates that G4.5 complex 25:1 is safe and the investigated doses are tolerable by MIO-M1 cell line in normal conditions.

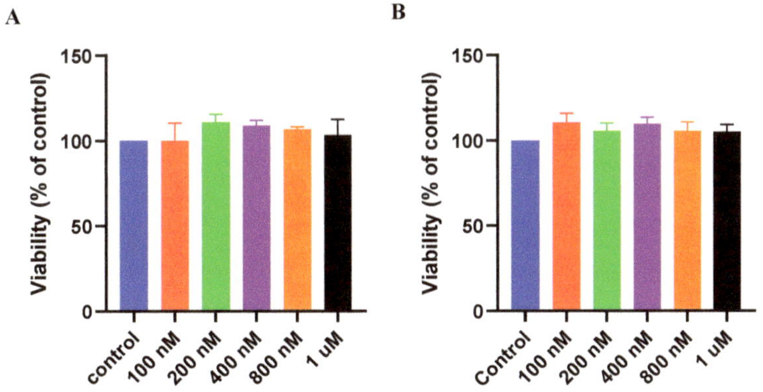

Figure 7. Effect of G4.5 complex 25:1 (**A**) and G5 complex 25:1 (**B**) after 24 h exposure on the cell viability of MIO-M1 cells under controlled conditions (mean ± SD; $n = 3$).

Dose–Response of RBX G5 Complex 25:1

Similarly, the safety of G5 complex 25:1 was assessed using MTS assay. After 24 h, viability of the treated cells was assessed using different concentrations ranging from (100 nM–1 µM) and compared to the viability of untreated cells that were cultured in the same controlled conditions. As seen in Figure 7B, viability of the treated cells with G5 complex 25:1 did not show any significant reduction when compared to viability of untreated cells ($p > 0.05$). This finding indicates that G5 complex 25:1 is safe and the investigated doses are tolerable by MIO-M1 cell line in normal conditions.

3.3.2. Effect of High Glucose Treatment on the Viability of MIO-M1 Cells

A series of experiments were conducted to test the effect of RBX, PAMAM dendrimers, and the proposed complexes on the viability of MIO-M1 cells in two different culture mediums; the controlled medium (5.55 mM) and high glucose medium were approximately five times normal levels of glucose to simulate hyperglycemia for MIO-M1 cells (25 mM). To test the effect of the tested compounds in high glucose treatment, MIO-M1 cells were incubated with the tested compounds for 24, 48, and 72 h. Then, viability was calculated and compared to the relevant controlled medium of that particular time point. As seen in Figure 8, in the presence of the tested compounds, there is no significant loss in cell viability of MIO-M1 cells cultured in high glucose media when compared to relevant controlled media of each studied time point ($p > 0.05$).

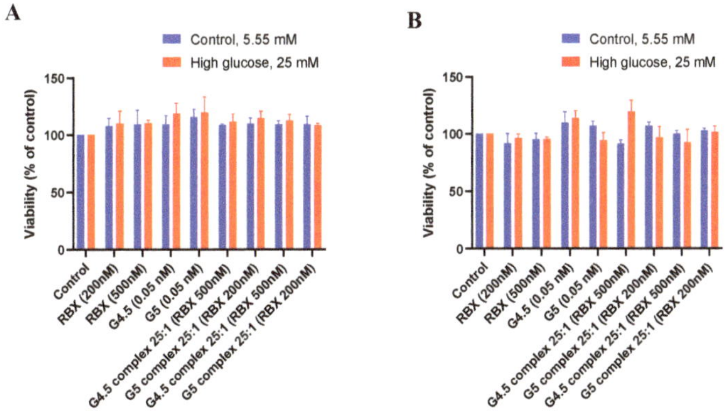

Figure 8. Effect of the tested compounds after (**A**) 24 h and (**B**) 48 h. Exposure on the cell viability of MIO-M1 cells under controlled and high glucose mediums (mean ± SD, $n = 3$).

3.3.3. In Vitro Permeability Study

The effect of RBX and dendrimers (with or without RBX) on the monolayer integrity of MIO-M1 was examined by measuring TEER values across the cell monolayer membrane in the upper Transwell® chamber before and after treatments (Figure 9). At the beginning of this experiment, the MIO-M1 monolayer was developed on a porous membrane of Transwell® inserts before TEER values were measured to evaluate the monolayer integrity. TEER values across the cell monolayer were measured every other day until the cell monolayers exhibited constant TEER values of more than 8 Ω*cm^2. These values were used as controls for each particular insert. A total of 500 nM of RBX and dendrimers (with or without RBX) was incubated for 24 h, and then TEER values were measured again to investigate the influence of complexes on monolayer integrity of MIO-M1 cells as compared to RBX and dendrimers alone. A paired *t*-test was used to determine whether there was a statistically significant difference between TEER values when the MIO-M1 monolayer was treated compared to non-treated cells. As highlighted in Figure 9, TEER values were shown to be approximately 13.0 %, which is the highest reduction ($9.7 \pm 1.7 \rightarrow 8.4 \pm 0.7$) across the cell monolayer membrane following 24 h of treatment with G4.5 (0.05 nM). Even though the TEER values of G4.5 (0.05 nM) showed the highest reduction across the cell monolayer membrane, it was not statistically significant when compared to TEER values before treatment at a *p*-value less than 0.01. Indeed, the reduction in TEER value of MIO-M1 monolayer, following the treatment of G5 complex 25:1, G4.5 complex 25:1, and RBX, was not statistically significant according to paired student *t*-test (p value < 0.01). As detailed in Figure 10, the data exhibited a high Papp ($4.0 \pm 0.1 \times 10^{-6}$ cm/s) of the groups without the MIO-M1 monolayer. However, the Papp ($1.9 \pm 0.0 \times 10^{-6}$ cm/s) of the developed MIO-M1 without treatment was hardly distinguishable from that observed by Papp of G5 complex and G4.5 complex, at the same condition, were $1.8 \pm 0.0 \times 10^{-6}$ cm/s and $1.7 \pm 0.0 \times 10^{-6}$ cm/s, respectively. In the in vitro permeability assessment, the collected data of cell treated with G5 complex and G4.5 complex showed that the permeability of MIO-M1 did not significantly change compared to that of non-treated MIO-M1 cells. One-way ANOVA analysis revealed that no statistically significant differences were detected among the permeability of the MIO-M1 monolayer with or without treatment of G5 complex, G4.5 complex, and RBX alone. Further statistical analysis by a *post-hoc* test showed that the difference between dendrimers with or without RBX on MIO-M1 permeability was not statistically significant at a p value < 0.01.

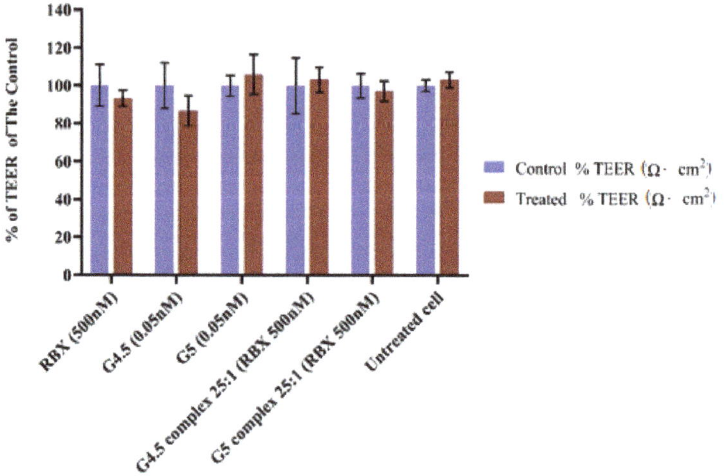

Figure 9. TEER measurements of monolayer cell membrane 24 h after exposure to treatments. Data represent % of TEER mean of the control ± SEM (n = 3–4).

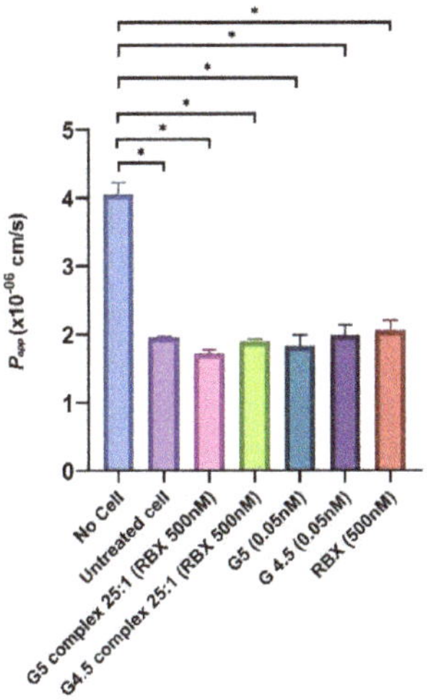

Figure 10. Apparent permeability coefficient (Papp) of the MIO-M1 monolayer cell after 24 treatments * p value < 0.01.

4. Discussion

PAMAM dendrimers have recently been studied to determine their ability to provide an effective and noninvasive drug delivery to the retina. Recent findings of Chang Liu et al. (2016) found that PAMAM dendrimers could rapidly penetrate from the surface of the eye into the vitreous and resided in the retina. This new approach is considered to be important in the development of a safe and noninvasive drug delivery for posterior segment diseases [41]. Herein, we aimed to develop a retinal delivery system by which RBX would be passively delivered from the surface of the eye to the retina. This was achieved through the development of RBX nanoparticles using PAMAM dendrimers. To achieve our aim, several complexes were formulated using 2 different generations and surface functional groups (i.e., anionic PAMAM dendrimers G4.5 and neutral PAMAM dendrimers G5). Then, these complexes were characterized and assessed for their cytotoxicity effects using the MIO-M1 cell line. The ideal nanosystem for ocular therapy formulations must have high loading efficiency, small particle size, and fast drug release [42]. In the current study, the diameter of PAMAM G4.5 and G5 was found to be 186.6 ± 2.3 and 214.9 ± 8.5 nm, respectively, supported by the findings of Yavuz (2015) [1]. Furthermore, nanoparticles with a size range typically < 400.0 nm are suitable for ophthalmic use according to Gorantla et al. (2020) [43]. In addition, the results of this study revealed that the mean particle size values of G4.5 and G5 loaded with RBX varied from 289.4 ± 39.9 nm to 482.4 ± 28.7 nm, indicating the loaded polymer is suitable as an ophthalmic formulation. Results indicated that the proposed complexes have significantly increased particle size when compared to the empty PAMAM dendrimers ($p < 0.05$), which is attributed to entrapment of RBX molecules within the internal cavities of PAMAM dendrimers. Sizes of both complex formulations of each generation were enlarged in a range approximately between 100.0–280.0 nm with the exception of PAMAM G5 5:1 complex which was measured as 669.8 ± 35.3 nm. High particle size of this formulation might be a result of aggregation. Such results were in line with the findings of Yavuz et al. [1].

The PDI is usually measured to determine the heterogeneity of a sample based on the size. PDI is the potential result of size distribution or aggregation of the particles in a sample during isolation or analysis [44,45]. It was demonstrated that PDI values of empty PAMAM dendrimers G4.5 and G5 were 0.297 ± 0.055 and 0.350 ± 0.008, respectively. Surfing the literature revealed that PDI < 0.35 is suitable for ocular drug delivery [46]. G4.5 and G5 complexes possessed a PDI value ranging from (0.335–0.394). Such findings revealed that there are no significant changes in PDI of the dendrimers after loading it with RBX ($p > 0.05$). Findings of this work were indicative of monodispersity of PAMAM dendrimers. Specifically, G4.5 and G5 complex 25:1 possessed the least PDI among all studied nanoformulations (PDI ≤ 0.35) indicating high particle homogeneity. In fact, the lower PDI value is much closer to achieving a monodisperse system; so, the latter complexes were considered the most monodisperse systems that is suitable for ocular drug delivery of RBX. However, an exception to the aforesaid findings was observed with G5 complex 5:1. This complex possessed a significantly high PDI value (0.587 $\pm$ 0.106), which was previously discussed in possessing a high particle size as well. This observation could be related to the aggregation of the nanoparticles. According to Tawfik et al. (2018), PDI measurements of all studied vardenafil/PAMAM complexes were characterized by small PDI values ≤ 0.25 [21]. Another study by Peng et al. demonstrated that the PDI of the PAMAM formulation was found to be in a range of (0.230–0.339), which supports our findings [47].

ζ-potential measurements determine the electrostatic potential at the electrical double layer surrounding a nanoparticle in a solution. In fact, ζ-potential plays an important role in determining the stability of nanoparticles as well as knowing the intensity of electrostatic attraction between biomolecules and the nanoparticles. Nanoparticles with a ζ-potential between −10.0 and +10.0 mV are considered approximately neutral, while nanoparticles with ζ-potentials of greater than +30.0 mV or less than −30.0 mV are considered to be strongly cationic and strongly anionic, respectively. Since most of eye cellular membranes are negatively charged, ζ-potential can affect a nanoparticle's tendency to permeate membranes, with cationic particles generally displaying more toxicity associated with cell wall disruption [48]. A study carried out by Yavuz (2015) found that ζ-potential values of blank dendrimer generations G4.5 was strongly anionic (−45.9 + 8.8) [1]. On the other hand, nanosynthons; manufacturer of PAMAM dendrimers G5, has stated that PAMAM dendrimers G5 possesses a neutral charge as they were synthesized with aminoethanol surface. In the current work, the ζ-potential measurement of G4.5 was −44.0 mV, which is similar to the result demonstrated by Yavuz [1]. Additionally, it was found that the surface charge of G5 was −0.2 mV which is in line with the information provided by nanosynthons. In this work, measurements of ζ-potential for G4.5 and G5 complexes showed that, ζ-potential values, either negative or neutral, were increased in the presence of RBX. Moreover, G4.5 complexes 25:1 and 1:1 remained anionic in contrast to PAMAM dendrimers used in complex 2.5:1 and 5:1, which exhibited a neutral charge after the loading process. Results obtained from this work also showed that zeta potential values for neutral complexes (i.e., G5 complexes) increased yet did not significantly change after the loading process ($p > 0.05$). However, it was clear that the loading of RBX, a weakly basic drug, into PAMAM dendrimers had a positive impact on these ζ-potential findings. Results demonstrated by Tawfik et al. (2018) supported our findings as vardenafil, a weakly basic drug (similar to RBX), was encapsulated within PAMAM dendrimers and ζ-potential measurements were increased after the loading process [21]. Drugs, such as RBX, could be encapsulated or conjugated to dendrimers. The morphology of G4.5 and G5 complexes was observed by TEM. It was shown that complexes as well as blank PAMAM dendrimers showed a discrete spherical morphology. Investigation of drug–polymer binding revealed that RBX was encapsulated within PAMAM dendrimers and no binding to PAMAM surface occurred. Furthermore, the ability of a fixed amount of RBX to be incorporated into various dendrimer generations and concentrations was investigated to estimate DE%. The drug loading efficiency is influenced by certain factors. These include the nature of the polymer, the encapsulated drug molecules, and polymer–drug ratio [25]. DE% of RBX in G4.5 and G5 complexes varied from 88.8% to 98.68%. It was demonstrated that drug loading efficiency of RBX did not show any significant differences among the proposed nanoparticles ($p > 0.05$). However, increasing the amount of RBX did not significantly show any differences compared to lower concentrations in the proposed nanoparticles ($p > 0.05$). Nabavizadeh et al. (2016) prepared different concentrations of 5:1, 5:2, 5:3, 5:4, and 5:5 of capecitabine: PAMAM dendrimers and studied DE% of these formulations. They found that DE% of capecitabine decreased with higher PAMAM dendrimer concentration. Increasing PAMAM dendrimer concentration has led to stronger electrostatic interactions between capecitabine and PAMAM dendrimers as a result [22,23]. In contrast to the findings reported by the later study, no significant differences occurred between DE% of G4.5 complexes as well as G5 complexes. Our findings were not similar to Nabavizadeh et al. (2016) results and were not affected by the factor of conjugation [22]. We supported our findings by visualizing the loading pattern of the complexes under TEM, which showed that RBX was only encapsulated within PAMAM dendrimers and not conjugated to PAMAM surface. Tawfik et al. (2018) studied vardenafil DE% among the proposed nanoparticles and revealed that direct correlation between the dendrimer concentration and vardenafil DE% was not held true for all concentrations. Statistically, no significant differences in vardenafil DE% were observed between the proposed nanoformulations [21]. These finding are in line with our results, which showed no significant differences in DE% were observed between 1:1, 2.5:1, 5:1, and 25:1 RBX: PAMAM.

Based on the results of DE%, the appropriate ratio of RBX-PAMAM dendrimer was selected for stability studies and ex vivo cell line studies, which was found to be 25:1 for each studied PAMAM generation. Moreover, Yavuz et al. (2015) studied the in vitro drug release of dexamethasone nanoparticles using different generations of PAMAM dendrimers. Since the nanoparticles are expected to be cleared from the eye in approximately an hour, it was desired that dexamethasone should be immediately released to penetrate to the posterior segment of the eye. Thus, a 3 h long in vitro drug release study was conducted in PBS at 37 °C. In a period of 3 h, the studied complexes released dexamethasone in a range of 40.0 to 80.0% [1]. In our work, a period of 8 h in vitro release study was carried out since the complex formulations were designed as fast release nanoparticles to be applied topically and their ocular retention time is suggested to be shorter. After the release study period has ended, it was found that G4.5 complexes released RBX in a range from 47.0–86.0%, while G5 complexes released RBX in a range of 25.0–81.0%. Cumulative release (%) of RBX from the studied nanoparticles showed that the drug was released in a sustained manner. In this study, it was clearly noticed that the highest release of RBX was demonstrated with G4.5 complex 25:1 and G5 complex 25:1 up to 86.0% and 81.0% respectively ($p < 0.05$). The release of RBX from the suggested complexes was compared to other in vitro release studies of PAMAM dendrimers. Gothwal et al. (2017) formulated bendamustine nanoparticles of PAMAM dendrimers G4. In this study, PAMAM dendrimers released the drug in a sustained manner up to 72 h [49,50]. Another study presented by Yesil-Celiktas et al. (2017) reported that PAMAM dendrimers provided a sustained release of BCA for six consecutive days [51]. All of these studies are in line with our findings of this study which demonstrated that PAMAM dendrimers are found to provide a sustained release of RBX in all studied formulations. In another study, Kesharwani et al. (2015) observed that the curcumin release decreased as PAMAM generation increased despite having a higher loading capacity [52]. The result of this study supports our findings in which RBX was released in higher percentages from the lower generation (G4.5) when compared to RBX release from the higher generation (G5).

Furthermore, the stability of G4.5 and G5 25:1 complexes was inspected visually to evaluate the appearance of any color change, precipitation, or turbidity. This was carried out to determine the disintegration of the proposed nanoparticles when exposed to light and/or high temperatures. Results obtained from this work showed that after the study period has ended, it was clearly observed that with increasing the storage temperature, physical changes such as color change and precipitation were recorded. Our findings revealed that the nanoformulations were found to be physically stable at 4 °C, whether kept in the dark or the light. Shadrack et al. (2015) has investigated physical stability of tetramethylscutellarein nanoparticles using PAMAM dendrimers at different temperature conditions (i.e., 0, 27 and 40 °C) for two months. Investigations showed a sign of color change, turbidity and precipitate formation were observed for formulations stored in light indicating that light had an influence on their stability [25]. These findings come in agreement with results obtained from our study that suggested that light exposure have can influence the stability of RBX nanoparticles. Findings of the later study found that nanoparticles were relatively stable when kept in the dark at high temperature (i.e., 40 °C). In contrast to these findings, we have observed physical changes of the nanoformulation at higher temperatures even when kept in the dark. This phenomenon was described by Prajapati et al. (2009) who explained that the formation of precipitates observed may be attributed to the opening of dendritic structures at higher temperatures [53]. By that means, we suggest that RBX complexes should be kept in the dark at 4 °C to provide the maximum stability of the proposed formulations. Also, another measurement was carried out to investigate the stability of RBX in the proposed complexes when exposed to different storage conditions. When each study period has ended, drug content was determined in each studied complex by using UPLC MS/MS. After that, percent content of RBX was calculated to estimate the loss of RBX in each tested complex. Results obtained from UPLC-MS/MS showed that RBX in G4.5 complex 25:1 remained above 90% stability at 4 °C for 6 months, the stability was slightly decreased over time from one month to 6 months. Moreover, percent content of RBX was apparently decreased by more than 20% with increasing the temperature. The results of this experiment revealed that the percent content of RBX is higher at 4 > 25 > 37 > 50 °C. Similar finding were observed with G5 complex 25:1. All studied nanoformulations were more stable when stored in the dark despite the influence of temperature over time. As a result of these observations, it is suggested that RBX nanoparticles should be stored in amber containers at 4 °C for maximum stability. RBX is a very sensitive drug that should be kept away from light and higher temperatures. To avoid RBX degradation, this drug must be stored in an amber container at −20 °C. In this work, it was observed that formulating RBX in a nanoparticulate system using PAMAM dendrimers can improve the stability of RBX in addition to its tendency to provide a facile retinal drug delivery.

Furthermore, ex vivo cell line studies were conducted to evaluate the safety of the formulated nanoparticles in MIO-M1 cells. It was found that the drug RBX in a range of concentrations did not affect the cell viability in both controlled and high glucose mediums. Similar results were observed with the work of Aldarwesh (2016) [9]. Also, empty and loaded PAMAM dendrimers G4.5 and G5 were investigated for their cytotoxicity effect in MIO-M1 cell line. The nanoparticles, in different concentrations, did not affect the viability of these cells, despite the type of cell medium (i.e., controlled or high glucose medium). To our knowledge, this is the first cytotoxicity study that was carried out to assess ex vivo behavior of PAMAM dendrimers using the MIO-M1 cell line. To assess the negative effect of complexes on the MIO-M1 monolayer integrity as a simple blood–retinal barrier (BRB) model, an in vitro permeability study on Transwell® and TEER was carried out. The cells were developed on the upper surface of the semi-permeable membrane in the Transwell® culture chambers in order to quantify the disruption level of new complexes on a monolayer of MIO-M1 cells. The difference in the TEER values of dendrimers and complexes was not statistically significant compared to TEER values before treatment at a p-value less than 0.01. Indeed, the reduction in TEER value of MIO-M1 monolayer, following the treatment of G5 complex 25:1, G4.5 complex 25:1, RBX, was not statistically significant according to paired Student t-test ($p < 0.01$). These findings suggest that both G5 complex 25:1 and G4.5 complex 25:1 did not significantly damage the monolayer integrity of MIO-M1 cells. The value of apparent permeability of developed MIO-M1 monolayers was confirmed by comparing it to the literature value for MIO-M1 cells [54]. Furthermore, the permeability values of about 10–6 cm/s have been previously observed in various in vitro BRB studies [32,38]). After confirmation of the monolayer integrity of MIO-M1, the monolayer integrity of MIO-M1 was inspected by calculating Papp of the barriers using FITC-dextran. During in vitro permeability assay, the monolayer cells were exposed to one of the G5 complex 25:1, G4.5 complex 25:1, and RBX for 24 h. The effect of the complexes on the barrier integrity was examined and compared to RBX, non-treated cells, and no cell groups with regards to the impact of treatment on the apparent permeability coefficient of the MIO-M1 monolayer. As shown in Figure 10, the Papp value of non-seeded insert was significantly higher than the

Papp value of untreated cell, indicating the formation of MIO-M1 monolayer membrane on the Transwell®. Furthermore, the results showed no statistically significant differences among the permeability value of the MIO-M1 monolayer with or without treatment of dendrimers and complexes. The difference between dendrimers with or without RBX on MIO-M1 permeability was not statistically significant ($p > 0.05$). These findings suggest that both G5 complex and G4.5 complex did not have a negative effect on the monolayer integrity of MIO-M1 cells. In addition, the above mentioned data support the cell viability studies which indicate the safety of G5 complex and G4.5 complex on MIO-M1 cell line in normal conditions.

5. Conclusions

RBX is a newly potent anti-VEGF drug that has been recently investigated for the treatment of DR. At present, anti-VEGF therapy is usually delivered to the retina via intravitreal injections carrying many ocular complications that cause patient noncompliance. To provide the maximum therapeutic outcomes of treating diabetic retinopathy, a non-invasive therapy of RBX was designed. This was carried out using nanoparticles of PAMAM dendrimers. Several methodologies have been implemented and the non-invasive nanoparticles that show the best in vitro characterization were formulated and characterized. The proposed nanoparticles will overcome ocular complications associated with the invasive therapy of diabetic retinopathy and the result will help in increasing patient adherence. The future direction of this study is to assess the in vivo behavior of RBX nanoparticles and to evaluate their permeability properties and ability to provide non-invasive retinal delivery of the potent anti-VEGF, RBX.

Supplementary Materials: The following supporting information can be downloaded at: https://www.mdpi.com/article/10.3390/pharmaceutics14071444/s1, Figure S1: Particle size (PS) of (A) G4.5 and (B) G5 complexes along with the empty PAMAM dendrimers G4.5 and G5 (mean ± SD, $n = 3$; ANOVA* $p \leq 0.05$); Figure S2: Polydispersity index (PDI) of (A) G4.5 complexes and (B) G5 complexes along with the empty PAMAM dendrimers G4.5 and G5 (mean ± SD, $n = 3$; ANOVA* $p \leq 0.05$); Figure S3: Drug loading efficiency (DE%) of (A) G4.5 complexes and (B) G5 complexes (mean ± SD, $n = 3$; ANOVA* $p \leq 0.05$); Figure S4: Stability studies of RBX in (A) G4.5 complexes and (B) G5 complexes under different storage conditions (mean ± SD, $n = 3$); Table S1: Different storage conditions used to assess the stability of G4.5 and G5 complexes; Table S2: Effect of heat and light on the stability of G4.5 complex 25:1; Table S3: Effect of heat and light on the stability of G5 complex 25:1.

Author Contributions: Conceptualization, R.A.A. and I.A.A.; methodology, F.S.A., A.A., F.Y.A., B.A., R.A.A. and N.H.; software, F.S. and W.A.M.; validation, F.S.A., F.Y.A. and H.G.A.; formal analysis, B.A. and N.H.; investigation, F.S., R.A.A. and Q.H.A.; resources, F.S.A.; data curation, W.A.M.; writing—original draft preparation, F.S.; writing—review and editing, B.A., F.S.A., and F.Y.A.; visualization, F.S.A.; supervision, I.A.A. and F.S.A.; project administration, I.A.A.; funding acquisition, F.S.A. All authors have read and agreed to the published version of the manuscript.

Funding: This research project was supported by Researchers Supporting Project number RSP-2021/340, King Saud University, Riyadh, Saudi Arabia.

Institutional Review Board Statement: Not applicable.

Informed Consent Statement: Not applicable.

Data Availability Statement: Not applicable.

Acknowledgments: Authors are thankful to the Researchers Supporting Project number RSP-2021/340, King Saud University, Riyadh, Saudi Arabia for supporting this work.

Conflicts of Interest: The authors declare no conflict of interest.

References

1. Yavuz, B.; Pehlivan, S.B.; Bolu, B.S.; Sanyal, R.N.; Vural, I.; Unlu, N. Dexamethasone–PAMAM dendrimer conjugates for retinal delivery: Preparation, characterization and in vivo evaluation. *J. Pharm. Pharmacol.* **2016**, *68*, 1010–1020. [CrossRef]
2. Gupta, N.; Mansoor, S.; Sharma, A.; Sapkal, A.; Sheth, J.; Falatoonzadeh, P.; Kuppermann, B.D.; Kenney, M.C. Diabetic retinopathy and VEGF. *Open Ophthalmol. J.* **2013**, *7*, 4–10. [CrossRef] [PubMed]
3. Zhao, Y.; Singh, R.P. The role of anti-vascular endothelial growth factor (anti-VEGF) in the management of proliferative diabetic retinopathy. *Drugs Context* **2018**, *7*, E212532. [CrossRef] [PubMed]
4. Del Amo, E.M.; Rimpelä, A.-K.; Heikkinen, E.; Kari, O.K.; Ramsay, E.; Lajunen, T.; Schmitt, M.; Pelkonen, L.; Bhattacharya, M.; Richradson, D.; et al. Pharmacokinetic aspects of retinal drug delivery. *Prog. Retin. Eye Res.* **2017**, *57*, 134–185. [CrossRef] [PubMed]
5. Yau, J.W.; Rogers, S.L.; Kawasaki, R.; Lamoureux, E.L.; Kowalski, J.W.; Bek, T.; Chen, S.-J.; Dekker, J.M.; Fletcher, A.; Grauslund, J.; et al. Global prevalence and major risk factors of diabetic retinopathy. *Diabetes Care* **2012**, *35*, 556–564. [CrossRef]
6. Xia, P.; Aiello, L.P.; Ishii, H.; Jiang, Z.Y.; Park, D.J.; Robinson, G.S.; Takagi, H.; Newsome, W.P.; Jirousek, M.R.; King, G.L. Characterization of vascular endothelial growth factor's effect on the activation of protein kinase C, its isoforms, and endothelial cell growth. *J. Clin. Investig.* **1996**, *98*, 2018–2026. [CrossRef]
7. Nonaka, A.; Kiryu, J.; Tsujikawa, A.; Yamashiro, K.; Miyamoto, K.; Nishiwaki, H.; Honda, Y.; Ogura, Y. PKC-β inhibitor (LY333531) attenuates leukocyte entrapment in retinal microcirculation of diabetic rats. *Investig. Ophthalmol. Vis. Sci.* **2000**, *41*, 2702–2706.
8. Way, K.; Katai, N.; King, G. Protein kinase C and the development of diabetic vascular complications. *Diab. Med.* **2001**, *18*, 945–959. [CrossRef]
9. Aldarwesh, A. Oxygen and Glucose Deprivation on Human Müller Cells (MIO-M1) and Human Organotypic Retinal Cultures (HORCs) in Relation to Glaucoma. Ph.D. Thesis, University of East Anglia, Norwich, UK, 2015.
10. Liu, Y.; Lei, S.; Gao, X.; Mao, X.; Wang, T.; Wong, G.T.; Vanhoutte, P.; Irwin, M.G.; Xia, Z. PKCβ inhibition with ruboxistaurin reduces oxidative stress and attenuates left ventricular hypertrophy and dysfuntion in rats with streptozotocin-induced diabetes. *Clin. Sci.* **2012**, *122*, 161–173. [CrossRef]
11. Edelhauser, H.F.; Rowe-Rendleman, C.L.; Robinson, M.R.; Dawson, D.G.; Chader, G.J.; Grossniklaus, H.E.; Ritetnhouse, K.D.; Wilson, C.G.; Weber, D.E.; Kuppermann, B.D.; et al. Ophthalmic drug delivery systems for the treatment of retinal diseases: Basic research to clinical applications. *Investig. Ophthalmol. Vis. Sci.* **2010**, *51*, 5403–5420. [CrossRef]
12. Jiang, S.; Franco, Y.L.; Zhou, Y.; Chen, J. Nanotechnology in retinal drug delivery. *Int. J. Ophthalmol.* **2018**, *11*, 1038–1044. [PubMed]
13. Patel, A.; Cholkar, K.; Agrahari, V.; Mitra, A.K. Ocular drug delivery systems: An overview. *World J. Pharmacol.* **2013**, *2*, 47–64. [CrossRef] [PubMed]
14. Bessonova, J.; Meyer-Lindenberg, A.; Bäumer, W.; Kietzmann, M. Tissue distribution of dexamethasone in feline ocular structures following single topical application of dexamethasone as an ointment or suspension. *Vet. Ophthalmol.* **2011**, *14*, 109–113. [CrossRef] [PubMed]
15. Gaudana, R.; Ananthula, H.K.; Parenky, A.; Mitra, A.K. Ocular drug delivery. *AAPS J.* **2010**, *12*, 348–360. [CrossRef]
16. Kolhe, P.; Misra, E.; Kannan, R.M.; Kannan, S.; Lieh-Lai, M. Drug complexation, in vitro release and cellular entry of dendrimers and hyperbranched polymers. *Int. J. Pharm.* **2003**, *259*, 143–160. [CrossRef]
17. Ma, P.; Zhang, X.; Ni, L.; Li, J.; Zhang, F.; Wang, Z.; Lian, S.; Sun, K. Targeted delivery of polyamidoamine-paclitaxel conjugate functionalized with anti-human epidermal growth factor receptor 2 trastuzumab. *Int. J. Nanomed.* **2015**, *10*, 2173–2190. [CrossRef]
18. Wang, Y.; Guo, R.; Cao, X.; Shen, M.; Shi, X. Encapsulation of 2-methoxyestradiol within multifunctional poly (amidoamine) dendrimers for targeted cancer therapy. *Biomaterials* **2011**, *32*, 3322–3329. [CrossRef]
19. Dobrovolskaia, M.A.; Patri, A.K.; Simak, J.; Hall, J.B.; Semberova, J.; Lacerda, S.H.D.P.; McNeil, S.E. Nanoparticle size and surface charge determine effects of PAMAM dendrimers on human platelets in vitro. *Mol. Pharm.* **2012**, *9*, 382–393. [CrossRef]
20. Williams, D.B.; Carter, C.B. The transmission electron microscope. In *Transmission Electron Microscopy*; Springer: Berlin/Heidelberg, Germany, 1996; pp. 3–17.
21. Tawfik, M.A.; Tadros, M.I.; Mohamed, M.I. Polyamidoamine (PAMAM) dendrimers as potential release modulators and oral bioavailability enhancers of vardenafil hydrochloride. *Pharm. Dev. Technol.* **2019**, *24*, 293–302. [CrossRef]
22. Nabavizadeh, F.; Fanaei, H.; Imani, A.; Vahedian, J.; Amoli, F.A.; Ghorbi, J.; Sohanaki, H.; Mohammadi, S.M.; Golchoobian, R. Evaluation of nanocarrier targeted drug delivery of Capecitabine-PAMAM dendrimer complex in a mice colorectal cancer model. *Acta Med. Iran.* **2016**, *54*, 485–493.
23. Klajnert, B.; Bryszewska, M. Dendrimers: Properties and applications. *Acta Biochim. Pol.* **2001**, *48*, 199–208. [CrossRef]
24. Vandamme, T.F.; Brobeck, L. Poly (amidoamine) dendrimers as ophthalmic vehicles for ocular delivery of pilocarpine nitrate and tropicamide. *J. Control. Release* **2005**, *102*, 23–38. [CrossRef] [PubMed]
25. Shadrack, D.M.; Mubofu, E.B.; Nyandoro, S.S. Synthesis of polyamidoamine dendrimer for encapsulating tetramethylscutellarein for potential bioactivity enhancement. *Int. J. Mol. Sci.* **2015**, *16*, 26363–26377. [CrossRef]
26. Yeo, K.P.; Lowe, S.L.; Lim, M.T.; Voelker, J.R.; Burkey, J.L.; Wise, S.D. Pharmacokinetics of ruboxistaurin are significantly altered by rifampicin-mediated CYP3A4 induction. *Br. J. Clin. Pharmacol.* **2006**, *61*, 200–210. [CrossRef] [PubMed]
27. Limb, G.A.; Salt, T.E.; Munro, P.M.G.; Moss, S.E.; Khaw, P.T. In vitro characterization of a spontaneously immortalized human Muller cell line (MIO-M1). *Investig. Ophthalmol. Vis. Sci.* **2002**, *43*, 864–869.

28. Cory, A.H.; Owen, T.C.; Barltrop, J.A.; Cory, J.G. Use of an aqueous soluble tetrazolium/formazan assay for cell growth assays in culture. *Cancer Commun.* **1991**, *3*, 207–212. [CrossRef] [PubMed]
29. Riss, T.L.; Moravec, R.A.; Niles, A.L. Cytotoxicity testing: Measuring viable cells, dead cells, and detecting mechanism of cell death. *Methods Mol. Biol.* **2011**, *740*, 103–114.
30. Jafari, F.; Aghazadeh, M.; Jafari, S.; Khaki, F.; Kabiri, F. In vitro cytotoxicity comparison of MTA fillapex, AH-26 and apatite root canal sealer at different setting times. *Iran. Endod. J.* **2017**, *12*, 162–167.
31. Churm, R.; Dunseath, G.J.; Prior, S.L.; Thomas, R.L.; Banerjee, S.; Owens, D.R. Development and characterization of an in vitro system of the human retina using cultured cell lines. *Clin. Exp. Ophthalmol.* **2019**, *47*, 1055–1062. [CrossRef]
32. Namba, R.; Kaneko, H.; Suzumura, A.; Shimizu, H.; Kataoka, K.; Takayama, K.; Yamada, K.; Funahashi, Y.; Ito, S.; Nonobe, N.; et al. In vitro epiretinal membrane model and antibody permeability: Relationship with anti-VEGF resistance in diabetic macular edema. *Investig. Ophthalmol. Vis. Sci.* **2019**, *60*, 2942–2949. [CrossRef]
33. Garcia-Ramírez, M.; Villarroel, M.; Corraliza, L.; Hernández, C.; Simó, R. Measuring permeability in human retinal epithelial cells (ARPE-19): Implications for the study of diabetic retinopathy. *Methods Mol. Biol.* **2011**, *763*, 179–194. [PubMed]
34. Hubatsch, I.; Ragnarsson, E.G.E.; Artursson, P. Determination of drug permeability and prediction of drug absorption in Caco-2 monolayers. *Nat. Prot.* **2007**, *2*, 2111–2119. [CrossRef] [PubMed]
35. Palumbo, P.; Picchini, U.; Beck, B.; Van Gelder, J.; Delbar, N.; DeGaetano, A. A general approach to the apparent permeability index. *J. Pharmacokin. Pharmacodyn.* **2008**, *35*, 235–248. [CrossRef] [PubMed]
36. Helms, H.C.; Abbott, N.J.; Burek, M.; Cecchelli, R.; Couraud, P.-O.; Deli, M.A.; Forster, C.; Galla, H.J.; Romero, I.A.; Shusta, E.V.; et al. In vitro models of the blood-brain barrier: An overview of commonly used brain endothelial cell culture models and guidelines for their use. *J. Cereb. Blood Flow Metab.* **2016**, *36*, 862–890. [CrossRef] [PubMed]
37. Dunn, K.C.; Aotaki-Keen, A.E.; Putkey, F.R.; Hjelmeland, L.M. ARPE-19, a human retinal pigment epithelial cell line with differentiated properties. *Exp. Eye Res.* **1996**, *62*, 155–170. [CrossRef]
38. Ma, B.; Wang, J.; Sun, J.; Li, M.; Xu, H.; Sun, G.; Sun, X. Permeability of rhynchophylline across human intestinal cell in vitro. *Int. J. Clin. Exp. Pathol.* **2014**, *7*, 1957–1966.
39. Yuan, S.Y.; Rigor, R.R. *Regulation of Endothelial Barrier Function*; Morgan & Claypool Life Sciences: San Rafael, CA, USA, 2010. Available online: https://www.ncbi.nlm.nih.gov/books/NBK54124/ (accessed on 20 December 2021).
40. Eigenmann, D.E.; Dürig, C.; Jähne, E.A.; Smieško, M.; Culot, M.; Gosselet, F.; Cecchelli, R.; Helms, H.C.C.; Brodin, B.; Wimmer, L.; et al. In vitro blood-brain barrier permeability predictions for GABAA receptor modulating piperine analogs. *Eur. J. Pharm. Biopharm.* **2016**, *103*, 118–126. [CrossRef]
41. Liu, C.; Jiang, K.; Tai, L.; Liu, Y.; Wei, G.; Lu, W.; Pan, W. Facile noninvasive retinal gene delivery enabled by penetratin. *ACS Appl. Mater. Interf.* **2016**, *8*, 19256–19267. [CrossRef]
42. Mittal, N.; Kaur, G. Investigations on polymeric nanoparticles for ocular delivery. *Adv. Polym. Technol.* **2019**, *2019*, 1316249. [CrossRef]
43. Gorantla, S.; Rapalli, V.K.; Waghule, T.; Singh, P.P.; Dubey, S.K.; Saha, R.N.; Singhvi, G. Nanocarriers for ocular drug delivery: Current status and translational opportunity. *RSC Adv.* **2020**, *10*, 27835–27855. [CrossRef]
44. Mudalige, T.; Qu, H.; Van Haute, D.; Ansar, S.M.; Paredes, A.; Ingle, T. Characterization of nanomaterials: Tools and challenges. *Nanomater. Food Appl.* **2019**, 313–353. [CrossRef]
45. Clayton, K.N.; Salameh, J.W.; Wereley, S.T.; Kinzer-Ursem, T.L. Physical characterization of nanoparticle size and surface modification using particle scattering diffusometry. *Biomicrofluidics* **2016**, *10*, 054107. [CrossRef] [PubMed]
46. Janagam, D.R.; Wu, L.; Lowe, T.L. Nanoparticles for drug delivery to the anterior segment of the eye. *Adv. Drug Deliv. Rev.* **2017**, *122*, 31–64. [CrossRef] [PubMed]
47. Peng, J.; Qi, X.; Chen, Y.; Ma, N.; Zhang, W.; Xing, J.; Zhu, X.; Li, Z.; Wu, Z. Octreotide-conjugated PAMAM for targeted delivery to somatostatin receptors over-expressed tumor cells. *J. Drug Target.* **2014**, *22*, 428–438. [CrossRef]
48. Clogston, J.D.; Patri, A.K. Zeta potential measurement. In *Characterization of Nanoparticles Intended for Drug Delivery*; Springer: Berlin/Heidelberg, Germany, 2011; pp. 63–70.
49. Liu, Y.; Ng, Y.; Toh, M.R.; Chiu, G.N.C. Lipid-dendrimer hybrid nanosystem as a novel delivery system for paclitaxel to treat ovarian cancer. *J. Control. Release* **2015**, *220*, 438–446. [CrossRef] [PubMed]
50. Gothwal, A.; Khan, I.; Kumar, P.; Raza, K.; Kaul, A.; Mishra, A.K.; Gupta, U. Bendamustine–PAMAM conjugates for improved apoptosis, efficacy, and in vivo pharmacokinetics: A sustainable delivery tactic. *Mol. Pharm.* **2017**, *15*, 2084–2097. [CrossRef]
51. Yesil-Celiktas, O.; Pala, C.; Cetin-Uyanikgil, E.O.; Sevimli-Gur, C. Synthesis of silica-PAMAM dendrimer nanoparticles as promising carriers in Neuro blastoma cells. *Anal. Biochem.* **2017**, *519*, 1–7. [CrossRef]
52. Kesharwani, P.; Xie, L.; Banerjee, S.; Mao, G.; Padhye, S.; Sarkar, F.H.; Iyer, A.K. Hyaluronic acid-conjugated polyamidoamine dendrimers for targeted delivery of 3, 4-difluorobenzylidene curcumin to CD44 overexpressing pancreatic cancer cells. *Colloids Surf. B Biointerfaces* **2015**, *136*, 413–423. [CrossRef]
53. Prajapati, R.N.; Tekade, R.K.; Gupta, U.; Gajbhiye, V.; Jain, N.K. Dendimer-mediated solubilization, formulation development and in vitro−in vivo assessment of piroxicam. *Mol. Pharm.* **2009**, *6*, 940–950. [CrossRef]
54. Tretiach, M.; Madigan, M.C.; Gillies, M.C. Conditioned medium from mixed retinal pigmented epithelium and Müller cell cultures reduces in vitro permeability of retinal vascular endothelial cells. *Br. J. Ophthalmol.* **2004**, *88*, 957–961. [CrossRef]

pharmaceutics MDPI

Review

Targeting the Blood–Brain Tumor Barrier with Tumor Necrosis Factor-α

Angelo Corti [1,2,*], Teresa Calimeri [3], Flavio Curnis [1] and Andres J. M. Ferreri [3,*]

1 Tumor Biology and Vascular Targeting Unit, Division of Experimental Oncology, IRCCS San Raffaele Scientific Institute, 20132 Milan, Italy; curnis.flavio@hsr.it
2 Faculty of Medicine, Università Vita-Salute San Raffaele, 20132 Milan, Italy
3 Lymphoma Unit, Department of Onco-Hematology, IRCCS San Raffaele Scientific Institute, 20132 Milan, Italy; calimeri.teresa@hsr.it
* Correspondence: corti.angelo@hsr.it (A.C.); ferreri.andres@hsr.it (A.J.M.F.); Tel.: +39-02-2643-4802 (A.C.); +39-02-2643-7649 (A.J.M.F.); Fax: +39-02-2643-7534 (A.J.M.F.)

Abstract: The blood–brain tumor barrier represents a major obstacle for anticancer drug delivery to brain tumors. Thus, novel strategies aimed at targeting and breaching this structure are of great experimental and clinical interest. This review is primarily focused on the development and use of a derivative of tumor necrosis factor-α (TNF) that can target and alter the blood–brain-tumor-barrier. This drug, called NGR-TNF, consists of a TNF molecule fused to the Cys-Asn-Gly-Arg-Cys-Gly (CNGRCG) peptide (called NGR), a ligand of aminopeptidase N (CD13)-positive tumor blood vessels. Results of preclinical studies suggest that this peptide-cytokine fusion product represents a valuable strategy for delivering TNF to tumor vessels in an amount sufficient to break the biological barriers that restrict drug penetration in cancer lesions. Moreover, clinical studies performed in patients with primary central nervous system lymphoma, have shown that an extremely low dose of NGR-TNF (0.8 $\mu g/m^2$) is sufficient to promote selective blood–brain-tumor-barrier alteration, increase the efficacy of R-CHOP (a chemo-immunotherapy regimen) and improve patient survival. Besides reviewing these findings, we discuss the potential problems related to the instability and molecular heterogeneity of NGR-TNF and review the various approaches so far developed to obtain more robust and homogeneous TNF derivatives, as well as the pharmacological properties of other peptide/antibody-TNF fusion products, muteins and nanoparticles that are potentially useful for targeting the blood–brain tumor barrier. Compared to other TNF-related drugs, the administration of extremely low-doses of NGR-TNF or its derivatives appear as promising non-immunogenic approaches to overcome TNF counter-regulatory mechanism and systemic toxicity, thereby enabling safe breaking of the BBTB.

Keywords: blood–brain tumor barrier; permeabilization; brain tumors; primary central nervous system lymphoma; tumor necrosis factor-alpha; targeted delivery; vascular targeting; CD13; TNF; TNF receptors; NGR-TNF

Citation: Corti, A.; Calimeri, T.; Curnis, F.; Ferreri, A.J.M. Targeting the Blood–Brain Tumor Barrier with Tumor Necrosis Factor-α. *Pharmaceutics* **2022**, *14*, 1414. https://doi.org/10.3390/pharmaceutics14071414

Academic Editors: Vibhuti Agrahari and Prashant Kumar

Received: 30 May 2022
Accepted: 5 July 2022
Published: 6 July 2022

1. Introduction

The prognosis of patients with tumors of the central nervous system (CNS), such as primary lymphomas, gliomas, or brain metastases from neoplasms that originate in other organs, is still poor. This is mainly due to the presence of the blood–brain barrier (BBB), which represents an important obstacle for anticancer drug delivery to brain tumors. Although tumors in the brain compromise the integrity of the BBB in the affected area, this barrier (referred to as the "blood–brain tumor barrier", BBTB) is heterogeneously permeable and represents, therefore, a major obstacle for a homogeneous penetration of anticancer drugs in tumor tissues. The description of structure and function of the BBTB is beyond the scope of this paper, and we refer the readers to an excellent review on this subject, recently published [1]. Thus, patients with tumors affecting the CNS, primary or secondary, would greatly benefit from the development of new tools capable of altering the BBTB and, consequently, enhancing the penetration of anticancer drugs in tumor tissues. The various approaches so far developed to meet this medical need have been recently reviewed [2]. These strategies include approaches based on (a) direct delivery of drugs into the brain parenchyma (e.g., by intraoperative placement of the drug or by convection-enhanced delivery), (b) exploitation of normal transport mechanisms (e.g., by solute carrier-mediated or receptor-mediated transcytosis), and (c) use of tools that increase the BBTB permeability (e.g., osmotic agents, focused ultrasounds, or pharmacological means) [2]. Another strategy recently developed for delivering nanoparticles to brain tumors exploits, in a counter-intuitive manner, the impermeability of the BBB in a two-step approach based on the selective retainment of ligand molecules on the surface of the brain vasculature, thanks to the lower endocytic rate of brain endothelium compared to peripheral endothelial cells, followed, in a second step, by administration of ligand-selective nanoparticles [3]. However, despite the various strategies so far developed, overcoming the BBTB still represents a major problem for brain tumor therapy. The present review is focused on the development and use of NGR-TNF, a genetically engineered derivative of tumor necrosis factor-α (TNF) that can target the tumor blood vessels and increase the permeability of the BBTB. We review here the structural and functional properties of this drug (which consists of TNF fused to the C-terminal residue of the CNGRCG peptide), its receptors, its biological effects on the barriers that limit drug penetration in solid tumors, and its mechanisms of action. In addition, we review the results of preclinical and clinical studies performed with this drug, alone or in combination with chemo- and immuno-therapy, including those of a recent study performed in patients with primary CNS lymphomas (PCNSL) showing that this drug may represent a valuable tool for breaching the BBTB. Finally, we also discuss the problems related to NGR-TNF instability and review the approaches so far developed to obtain more robust TNF derivatives, as well as the potential advantages/disadvantages of other peptide/antibody-TNF conjugates, muteins and TNF-based nanodrugs that could be potentially used for targeting brain neoplasms and other solid tumors.

2. The CNGRCG-TNF Recombinant Protein (NGR-TNF) and Its Receptors

TNF is an inflammatory cytokine originally discovered for its capability to cause massive hemorrhagic necrosis of cancer lesions in mice [4,5]. Unfortunately, despite the impressive anti-cancer effects observed in mice, studies performed in cancer patients in the late 1980s showed that TNF, upon systemic administration, can induce toxic effects and no, or very modest, anti-tumor responses [6,7]. However, clinical studies performed in the 1990s showed that locoregional administration of a high doses of TNF combined with chemotherapy, by isolated limb perfusion, can induce high response rates in subjects with sarcomas of the extremities or with melanomas [8–11]. These results indicate that TNF can be used in a safe and successful manner to treat cancer patients if high levels of cytokine are attained in tumors, locally and not in circulation. These notions stimulated, in the subsequent years, studies aimed at developing targeting strategies for this cytokine, in the attempt to enable systemic administration of therapeutically efficacious doses of TNF without causing toxicity. Among the various approaches that have been pursued for this purpose, targeted delivery of TNF to the tumor-associated vessels (e.g., by fusing this cytokine with peptide or antibody ligands that recognize receptors or molecules expressed by the tumor vasculature) represents a valid strategy [12]. NGR-TNF, a recombinant homo-trimeric protein consisting of CNGRCG fused to the N-terminal residue of TNF and produced in *E. coli*, represents a prototypical example of these class of compounds [13].

The CNGRCG peptide was originally identified by panning peptide-phage libraries in tumor-bearing mice [14]. This compound contains two cysteines and a disulfide-constrained NGR motif that can recognize a specific form of CD13 (a membrane metalloprotease called aminopeptidase N) barely (or not at all) expressed by blood vessels in normal conditions and up-regulated in the angiogenic vasculature [15–18]. In solid tumors this protease is expressed by pericytes and endothelial cells, and, in certain cases, also by fibroblasts and cancer cells. CD13 is also expressed by cells of healthy tissues, such as epithelial cells of the prostate, small intestine, kidney, liver, as well as by mast cells, myeloid cells, antigen-presenting cells, and keratinocytes [19–22]. CD13 is highly expressed by pericytes in the brain vasculature, i.e., on cells that are behind the endothelial barrier and, therefore, poorly accessible to circulating molecules in normal tissues, but potentially accessible in those areas of brain tumors with an altered BBTB. Notably, a recent study performed in PCNSL patients have revealed CD13 expression on the tumor endothelium, i.e., on cells that are accessible to circulating molecules also in areas with an intact BBTB [23,24]. Experimental evidence suggests that compounds containing the CNGRCG sequence can recognize $CD13^+$ tumor vasculature, but not other normal tissues that express high levels of CD13 [13,16].

The molecular bases of this selective recognition are still unclear. CD13 is a dimeric glycoprotein with an archlike structure and with monomers that can assume closed or open conformations [25]. It is possible that different conformations in different tissues, owing to the presence of tissue-specific cofactors, post-translational modifications or signaling molecules, may result in a differential binding affinity for NGR-containing peptides. According to this view, studies on the interaction of a cyclic CNGRC peptide with various CD13-expressing cells (endothelial cells, pericytes, tumor cells, and myeloid cells), by 2D Transferred Nuclear Overhouser Effect Spectroscopy (2D TR-NOESY) and by immunofluorescence techniques, showed that the expression of CD13 was necessary but not sufficient for the binding, as binding was observed to cells that form the tumor vasculature (endothelial cells and pericytes) and to some tumor cell lines, but not to myeloid cells [26].

Because of their tumor vasculature homing properties, CNGRCG and other NGR-peptides have been exploited for delivering a variety of therapeutic or imaging compounds to neoplastic lesions, including liposomes, chemotherapeutic agents, DNA, viruses, anti-angiogenic compounds, fluorescent molecules, contrast agents and also cytokines [12]. In NGR-TNF, which was the first NGR-cytokine conjugate to be developed, the CNGRCG domain does not impair folding, TNF subunit oligomerization and binding to type-1 and type-2 TNF receptors. Furthermore, the TNF domain does not impair the interaction of NGR with its receptor (CD13) [13]. Thus, NGR-TNF can engage high-avidity interactions with TNF-receptors and CD13 on cells that express both types of receptors, as it occurs in endothelial cells of the tumor vasculature, but not in normal vessels (which lack CD13) [13]. For the same reason NGR-TNF is unlikely to engage high-avidity multivalent interactions with the soluble CD13, alone, present in the blood. The high-avidity interactions with both types of receptors in the tumor vasculature can likely account for the tumor-homing properties of NGR-TNF and its capability to exert anti-cancer effects at extremely low doses in mice [27]. This view is supported by the observation that the anti-cancer activity of low-dose NGR-TNF in murine models is abrogated by co-administration of a neutralizing anti-CD13 antibody or by anti-TNF-Rs antibodies [13,27]. However, it is also worth highlighting the fact that the function of CD13 is not limited to NGR-TNF homing to tumor vessels, as upon NGR-TNF binding this membrane protein can also induce co-signaling mechanisms that impair the activation of pro-survival pathways induced by the TNF moiety (Ras, Erk, Akt, NF-kB) without affecting other pathways related to stress and cell death (p38 and JNK), a mechanism that may contribute to the overall biological activity of the fusion protein [26]. In other words, both NGR and TNF domains have a direct role in both cell binding and signaling. Whether or not TNF receptors are internalized, recycled or destroyed after NGR-TNF binding and whether the NGR domain of TNF is cleaved upon binding to CD13 are unknown.

Finally, considering the notion that CD13 is expressed in angiogenic vessels, it is important to highlight the fact that besides targeting the angiogenic vasculature of tumors, off-target delivery of NGR-TNF to non-tumoral angiogenic vessels might occur in the case of concomitant diseases with an angiogenic component.

3. Preclinical Studies of NGR-TNF

3.1. NGR-TNF as a Single Agent in Murine Models of Solid Tumors

Considering that human TNF can efficiently bind murine type-1, but not type-2, TNF receptor [28], most preclinical studies in mice have been performed with murine NGR-TNF. Studies in murine models of lymphoma, fibrosarcoma, and melanoma have shown that the dose–response curve of systemically administered NGR-TNF is markedly different from that of TNF: while both TNF and NGR-TNF have therapeutic anti-cancer activity at doses in the microgram range, only NGR-TNF can induce anti-tumor responses when administered at doses in the picogram range (e.g., 100 pg/mouse). Nanogram doses of NGR-TNF (e.g., 3–10 ng) were paradoxically less active than picograms, pointing to a triphasic-dose–response curve [13,27]. Mechanistic studies have shown that this behavior depends on the shedding of soluble TNF-receptors in circulation (i.e., of TNF inhibitors), which can be triggered by TNF and NGR-TNF at doses >1 ng/mouse. This counter-regulatory mechanism efficiently inhibits the potential anti-cancer and toxic effects of both TNF and NGR-TNF [27]. When doses in the range of micrograms are used, however, both drugs can overcome these counter-regulatory mechanisms and induce strong anti-cancer effects, but, for the same reason, they can also cause systemic toxic reactions. In contrast, doses of NGR-TNF in the range of picograms do not induce the shedding of soluble TNF receptors and can exert pharmacological effects without causing systemic toxicity [27]. Thus, the use of extremely low doses of NGR-TNF may represent a strategy to avoid toxicity as well as systemic counter-regulatory mechanisms.

Studies on the mechanisms of NGR-TNF anti-tumor activity have shown that targeted delivery of low amounts of this drug to tumor blood vessels (e.g., 100 pg/mouse, >100,000-fold lower than the median lethal dose, LD50) can affect the tumor vasculature and microenvironment, causing the up-regulation of intercellular adhesion molecule (ICAM)-2 and vascular cell adhesion molecule (VCAM)-1 in the endothelial lining of tumor vasculature and the release of various chemokines and cytokines involved in the activation and migration T-cells in the tumor tissue, such as MCP-1/CCL-2, MIP-2, oncostatin-M, MCP-3/CCL-7, and stem cell factor [29]. Low-dose NGR-TNF, but not TNF, can affect VE-cadherin dependent adherence junctions and enhance vascular permeability in tumors [30]. Accordingly, magnetic resonance imaging in lymphoma-bearing mice, 2 hours after drug administration, have shown an enhanced leakage of the blood pool contrast agent from tumor blood vessels [12]. Low-dose NGR-TNF can also cause apoptosis of endothelial cells and, at later time points, also apoptosis of tumor cells, likely because of vascular damage and nutrients/oxygen deprivation [12]. It appears, therefore, that a combination of endothelial barrier alteration, vascular damage and inflammatory/immune responses contribute to the overall anti-cancer effects of low-dose NGR-TNF.

3.2. Effect of Low-Dose NGR-TNF on the Barriers That Limit the Penetration of Chemotherapeutic Drugs in Tumors

Low-dose NGR-TNF (100 pg/mouse, systemically administered) can increase the response of tumors to chemotherapeutic drugs, as observed with cisplatin, melphalan, doxorubicin, gemcitabine and paclitaxel in various models of transplantable tumors and in an orthotopic model of prostate cancer (TRAMP) [27,31,32].

Maximal synergism can be obtained with a 2-hour delay between NGR-TNF and chemotherapeutic drug administrations, irrespective of tumor model and drug used. Mechanistic studies performed in mice bearing melanomas or lymphomas have shown that low-dose NGR-TNF can increase the tumor uptake of the anthracycline doxorubicin [27]. This phenomenon can be related to the capability of TNF to reduce the barriers that limit drug penetration in tumor tissues, such as those related to the endothelial barrier function and to the high interstitial pressure, thereby leading to an increase of the convective transport of drugs through the tumor vasculature wall, at least in those areas that are poorly perfused and characterized by low permeability [9,33–40]. Notably, chromogranin A, a neurosecretory glycoprotein capable of inhibiting the vascular leakage induced by TNF, can also inhibit the synergism between NGR-TNF and chemotherapeutic drugs in tumor-bearing mice [30]. This observation is in line with the hypothesis that an increased vascular permeability is a crucial mechanism of the increased chemotherapeutic-drug penetration in tumors, after NGR-TNF administration, and synergism (Figure 1A). NGR-TNF and doxorubicin synergism occurs in immunocompetent mice, but not in interferon-γ (IFNγ)–knock-out or nude mice, suggesting that a fully functional immune system and IFNγ are necessary for the overall anti-tumor effects of this combination [41].

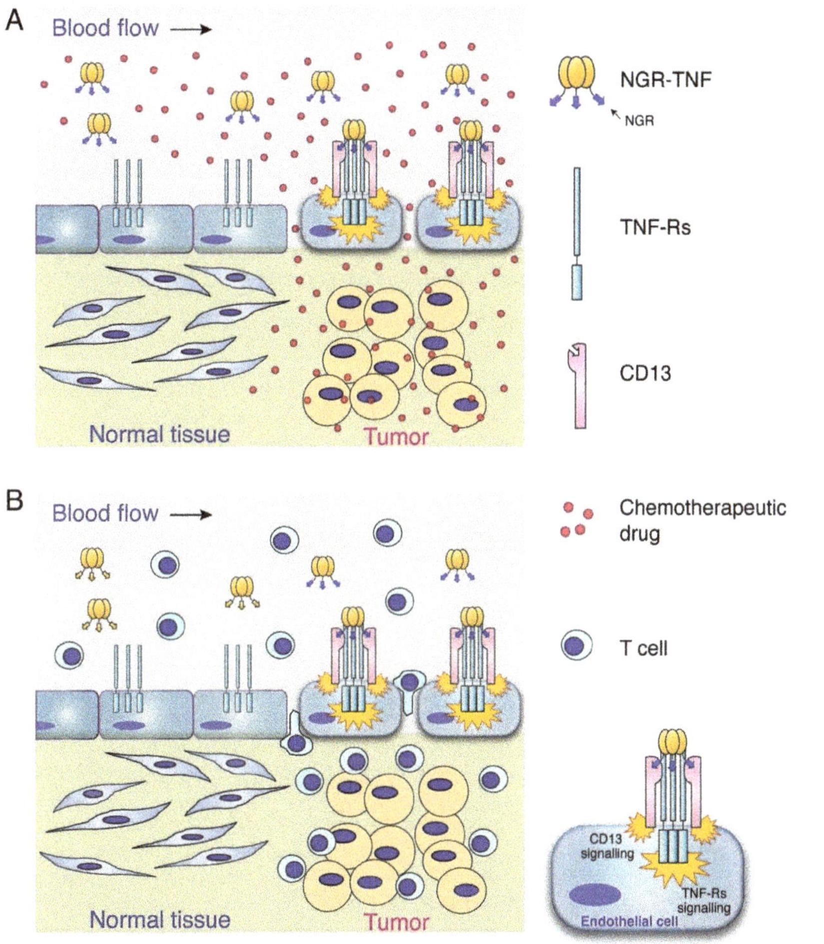

Figure 1. Schematic representation of the primary mechanisms of the synergistic effects of low-dose NGR-TNF with chemo/immunotherapy. Low-dose NGR-TNF recognizes with high avidity CD13 and TNF receptors (TNF-Rs) expressed in the vasculature of solid tumors. This interaction activates TNF-Rs- and CD13-dependent signaling mechanisms that lead to selective activation of endothelial cells and, consequently, to alteration of the endothelial-barrier function and cytokine-chemokine secretion. These mechanisms favor chemotherapeutic drug penetration (**A**) and CD8 T-cells infiltration (**B**) in tumor tissues. These effects are also followed, at later time points, by vascular damage (see text). The selectivity of these effects depends on the fact that CD13 (the NGR receptor) is overexpressed in tumor vessels and little, or not at all, by endothelial cells in normal tissues.

3.3. Effect of Low-Dose NGR-TNF on the Infiltration of Lymphocyte in Tumors

Low-dose NGR-TNF can promote lymphocyte extravasation in tumors [29] (Figure 1B). This phenomenon is likely related to the capability of NGR-TNF to loosen vascular endothelial cadherin-dependent adherence junctions, to up-regulate leukocyte-adhesion molecules on the tumor vasculature, and to promote the secretion of various chemokines in neoplastic tissues (see above paragraphs). Studies performed in murine models of melanoma and in a spontaneous-orthotopic model of prostate cancer (TRAMP) have shown that NGR-TNF can increase tumor-tissue infiltration of either endogenous or adoptively transferred cytotoxic T-cells, without modification of T-cell distribution in blood, spleen or kidney in tumor-bearing mice [29]. Notably, NGR-TNF can increase the efficacy of adoptive or active immunotherapy of tumor-bearing mice, either when administered alone or in combination with chemotherapy [29]. Comparable doses of TNF were marginally or not at all active in the same models, suggesting that the NGR-directed targeted delivery of TNF to the tumor vasculature was necessary for the efficacy of the combined therapies. Low-dose NGR-TNF can also increase the efficacy of TCR-engineered tumor-redirected lymphocytes, leading to tumor eradication in the orthotopic model of prostate cancer [42]. Finally, studies performed in mice bearing prostate cancers or melanomas, have shown that low doses of NGR-TNF can enhance the infiltration of effector T cells in tumors, as well as the therapeutic effects of immune checkpoint blockers combined with adoptive cell therapy [43].

4. Clinical Studies with NGR-TNF

4.1. Clinical Studies with NGR-TNF in Patients with Solid Tumors

Human NGR-TNF (NGR-hTNF) has been evaluated alone or in combination with chemotherapy in several phase-I and -II studies enrolling patients with various types of solid tumors, and in also in a phase-III study in patients with malignant pleural mesothelioma.

The first phase I study, conducted on 69 patients with histologic or cytologic confirmation of advanced cancer, showed for the first time in humans that treatment with NGR-hTNF could cause anti-vascular effects in tumors [44]. NGR-hTNF was administered once every 3 weeks by a 20 to 60 min intravenous infusion using escalating doses (0.2–60 $\mu g/m^2$) with a maximum tolerated dose (MTD) of 45 $\mu g/m^2$ administered in 1 hour. The most frequent observed toxicities were rigors and fever. The terminal half-life of NGR-hTNF was 1 to 2 hours. No objective responses were observed, but 39% of patients had stable disease (SD), with a median duration of response of 12 weeks. Based on the results of another phase-I study, designed to define safety and optimal dose in patients with advanced solid tumors, the dose of 0.8 $\mu g/m^2$ was chosen for subsequent studies, either as single-agent or in combination with chemotherapeutic drugs, considering the favorable toxicity profile observed with this dose, the disease control obtained (44% of SD for a median time of 5.9 months), the lack of stimulation of TNF-receptors shedding and the significant anti-vascular effects observed [45]. Another important Phase I clinical study, performed on 31 patients with advanced solid tumors, showed that the anti-vascular activity of NGR-hTNF was inversely correlated to the tumor dimension, probably because of the presence of a less-mature neovasculature in small lesions [46]. This study also confirmed that the levels of circulating soluble TNF-receptors were not increased by low doses of NGR-hTNF (<1.3 $\mu g/m^2$) and showed that patients did not develop anti-NGR-hTNF antibodies.

Thus, phase II clinical studies with low-dose NGR-TNF (0.8 $\mu g/m^2$, 1 h infusion, weekly or every 3 weeks) as a single agent were then conducted in pre-treated patients with hepatocellular carcinoma (HCC), malignant pleural mesothelioma (MPM), and colorectal cancer (CRC). The results showed again anti-vascular effects and significant disease control [47–49]. The treatment was well-tolerated, as no drug-related grade 3 to 4 toxicities were registered except for 1 grade 3 syncope in the 3-weekly cohort of the MPM study.

Phase I studies on the combination of low-dose NGR-hTNF with doxorubicin (60–75 mg/m^2) [50] or cisplatin (80 mg/m^2) [51] showed that these therapeutic regimens were feasible and well-tolerated. Notably, a promising anti-tumor activity was registered in patients pretreated and refractory to the chemotherapeutic drug used in the combination.

Low-dose NGR-hTNF, combined with doxorubicin, was also evaluated in a phase II study enrolling 37 relapsed ovarian cancer patients with a platinum-free interval lower than 12 months. The overall response rate was 66% (23% PR and 43% SD), median PFS and OS were 5 months and 17 months, respectively [52]. No unexpected toxicities and strong association between baseline-lymphocyte counts and outcomes were reported. Notably, this association was observed also in unselected patients with relapsed small cell lung cancer injected with NGR-hTNF and doxorubicin [53]. In these patients, similar anti-tumor activity was observed in both platinum-sensitive and platinum-resistant patient cohorts. In another phase-II study, two sequential groups of CRC patients who had failed standard treatment received NGR-hTNF, 0.8 or 45 μg/m^2, combined with a fixed dose of capecitabine-oxaliplatin (XELOX). Both these treatments were safe, but apparently a sign of efficacy was evident only with the lower NGR-hTNF dose [54]. This is a remarkable observation, as it supports the concept that "the-more-is-better" principle is not valid for NGR-hTNF (and likely also for other TNF derivatives). As observed in preclinical studies, the lower anti-tumor activity of high-dose NGR-hTNF (45 μg/m^2) seemed to be related to the induction of soluble TNF-receptors shedding in the circulation, i.e., the release of TNF inhibitors. However, the results of a phase I study conducted with doses (60–325 μg/m^2) higher than the MTD previously established in 48 patients with refractory solid tumors (45 μg/m^2) suggest that these doses are tolerated and can induce anti-tumor effects if a more protracted length of infusion (2 h) and mild premedication with paracetamol are used [55]. This behavior observed in patients recapitulates the complex dose–response curve observed in murine models (discussed above).

NGR-hTNF was also combined with a peptide-based vaccination in a pilot phase-I study enrolling patients with metastatic melanoma [56]. Accrual was slow and the trial was closed earlier due to new therapies that became available for metastatic melanoma. However, the combination was associated with an ex-vivo T-cell response and a long-term overall survival (>4 months in six out of eight evaluable patients).

The results of a randomized, double blind, placebo-controlled phase-III clinical trial on 400 previously treated patients with MPM and treated with or without low-dose NGR-hTNF (0.8 μg/m^2, weekly) in combination with the best investigator choice have been published in 2018 [57]. Although the primary end point on the overall survival (OS) was not reached for the entire population of patients treated with NGR-hTNF (n = 200) a significant improvement in progression-free survival (PFS) and OS was observed in patients who progressed more rapidly after first-line treatment (short treatment-free-interval, representing 50% of the entire patient population), suggesting that there could be a benefit from treating patients with more aggressive MPM with NGR-hTNF.

4.2. *Targeting the Blood–Brain Tumor Barrier with NGR-TNF in Patients with PCNSL*

Primary diffuse large B-cell lymphoma (DLBCL) of the CNS (PCNSL), a rare extranodal non-Hodgkin lymphoma confined to brain, eyes, meninges, and other structures of the CNS, is a paradigmatic example of one of the major challenge in the treatment of CNS tumors: the delivery of drugs across the BBB [58]. PCNSL are usually treated with high-dose methotrexate-based combinations, which require hospitalization and large expertise [59]. The use of R-CHOP (rituximab, cyclophosphamide, doxorubicin, vincristine, and prednisone, the standard treatment of systemic DLBCL) might overcome these difficulties, but CNS penetration of these drugs is poor [58]. Thus, strategies aimed at improving drug penetration in this setting are of great interest and many invasive and noninvasive approaches have already been tested [58]. Studies performed in mice bearing brain metastases of breast cancer have shown that systemic administration of relatively high doses of TNF can induce BBTB permeabilization [23] and enhance tumor penetration of therapeutic compounds [60], but, as discussed above, this approach cannot be used in patients because of its inherent systemic toxicity [12]. Based on the idea that these limitations could be overcome by BBTB permeabilization with low-dose NGR-hTNF followed by R-CHOP, a phase-II trial on NGR-hTNF plus R-CHOP in patients with relapsed/refractory PCNSL has been designed and conducted ("INGRID" trial). The trial was designed to include two distinct parts: (a) an exploratory phase on the first 10 enrolled patients, aimed at assessing the feasibility of the NGR-hTNF/R-CHOP combination and obtaining the "proof of principle" of BBTB alteration by NGR-hTNF [24]; and (b) an expansion phase on 28 patients, aimed at assessing the efficacy and safety of this therapy in the whole patients cohort [23]. Treatment schedule consisted of six courses of R-CHOP21 preceded by NGR-hTNF (0.8 μg/m^2 delivered 2 hours before R-CHOP by a 1 h infusion). Per protocol, the first course of R-CHOP was not preceded by NGR-hTNF in the first 10 patients. All subjects who achieved a partial response (PR) or a complete response (CR) at the end of the program, were evaluated for consolidative therapy which, per protocol and accordingly to prior treatments, could be represented by whole-brain radiation therapy (30–36 Gy), carmustine-thiotepa-conditioned autologous stem cell transplantation or oral lenalidomide maintenance. A total of 28 patients were enrolled (median age: 58 years, range 26–78; 14 males); most patients had unfavorable features at trial registration (IELSG risk score intermediate or high in 82%). Tumor response was observed in 21 patients (75%; 95%CI = 59–91), complete in 11 patients, and the predetermined efficacy threshold ($\geq$12 responses) was achieved, indicating that the combination of NGR-hTNF and RCHOP was efficacious in these patients (Figure 2A). At a median follow-up of 34 months (27–44 months), six patients were still alive, and five patients remained relapse free. Of note, the responses observed after R-CHOP alone in the first 10 enrolled patients were not significant, with most patients showing stable disease or progressive disease, excluding, *bona fide*, that responses achieved later were exclusively due to immune-chemotherapy activity. Treatment was well-tolerated. Toxicities were quickly solved with no need of dose reductions or interruptions, and, overall, no treatment related death was observed. A total of 15 systemic adverse events were recorded in 11 patients, with 9 grade 1–2 reactions to NGR-hTNF infusion. Dynamic-contrast enhanced magnetic resonance imaging and single-photon emission computed tomography studies showed an increase of vascular permeability after NGR-hTNF infusion in tumor and perilesional areas (Figure 2B). Notably, immunohistochemical analysis of tumor tissue sections have revealed the presence of CD13 on the luminal side of tumor vasculature in all diagnostic brain biopsies evaluated, suggesting that the NGR receptor target was accessible to NGR-hTNF intravenously delivered [23,24]. The localized action of TNF on tumoral and peritumoral areas, likely mediated by CD13 targeting, is also suggested by the observation that no changes in the cerebrospinal fluid/plasma drug levels occurred after NGR-hTNF infusion. The effect of NGR-hTNF on the blood–retina barrier and the blood–cerebrospinal fluid barrier remains to be established because none of the patients had meningeal disease at trial registration, and only three patients had ocular involvement. Overall, the results obtained in PCNSL patients are in line with the good tolerability of NGR-hTNF observed in previous studies on patients with other solid tumors, thus suggesting that this innovative therapeutic approach deserves to be investigated as first-line treatment in PCNSL patients.

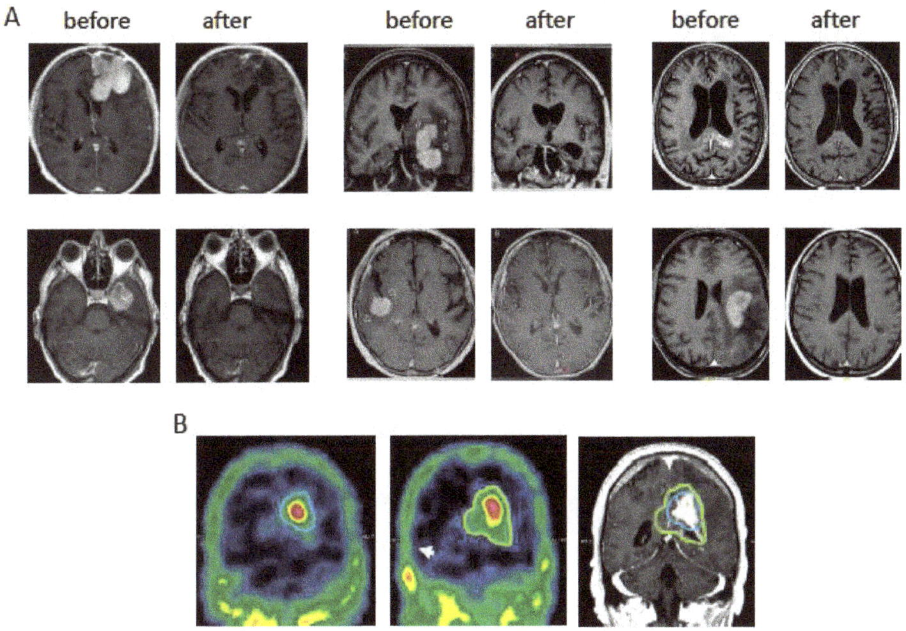

Figure 2. Examples of responses to NGR-hTNF/R-CHOP combination in patients with PCNSL. (**A**) DCE-MRI (gadolinium-enhanced T1-weighted scan) before and after treatment with 2–4 cycles of R-CHOP preceded by NGR-hTNF in 6 PCNSL patients. (**B**) SPECT analysis of a patient before and after the third treatment with NGR-hTNF and R-CHOP, showing an increase of uptake of 99mTc-DTPA. The volume of ≥30% uptake of 99mTc-DTPA is contoured in the two studies performed before (left image, blue line) and after (central image, green line) administration of NGR-hTNF/R-CHOP. The contoured volumes are also reported on the image obtained by gadolinium-enhanced T1-weighted MRI (right image) showing the tumor location. The volume of increased uptake before and after NGR-hTNF/R-CHOP administration was 22 and 40 cm^3, respectively. Part of this research was originally published in *Blood* [24] and *Blood Advances* [23].

4.3. NGR-TNF Immunogenicity

Studies on the immunogenicity of the CNGRCG domain of NGR-TNF, carried out in rabbits and mice injected with NGR-TNF or with various compounds consisting of CNGRCG coupled with immunogenic carrier proteins, have shown that the CNGRCG peptide ligand is poorly, or not at all, immunogenic [61]. Experiments based on molecular dynamics simulation predicted that the most populated structures of CNGRC are superimposable to a GNGRG hairpin structure present in human fibronectin 5th type I repeat (FN-I5) [61]. This can explain the low immunogenicity of the CNGRCG peptide sequence, as it likely mimics a "self" structure. Accordingly, as discussed above, no anti-NGR-TNF antibodies were raised in patients treated with human NGR-TNF, even after repeated injections.

4.4. NGR-TNF Derivatives with Improved Stability and Homogeneity

TNF is a homotrimeric protein. Structural studies of human and murine NGR-TNF, produced by genetic engineering technology in *Escherichia coli* (*E. coli*) cells, have shown that these products consist of trimers made by subunits with different molecular weights, including subunits with the expected molecular weight (17939.39 Da and 17844.25 Da, respectively) and subunits with −17, +1, +42 and +58 Da than expected [62]. The molecular heterogeneity of human and murine NGR-TNF is related to post-translational modifications of their N-terminal domains, including N-terminal acetylation and oxidation (+42 and

+58 Da), asparagine deamidation (+1 Da), and formation of 6–7 membered rings between cysteine α-amino group and asparagine side-chain (−17 kDa). These post-translational modification and degradation reactions need a cysteine (C) in the first position (with a free α-amino group) and an asparagine (N) in second position, as in the CNGRCG domain of NGR-TNF [62].

While the acetylated-CNGRCG domain can recognize CD13 with a binding strength similar to that of the non-acetylated domain, the −17 Da subunits are likely non-functional, as this modification (which involves the reaction of the cysteine α-amino group with the asparagine side-chain of the CNGRCG domain) destroys the NGR motif [62]. Thus, incorporation of these altered subunits in NGR-TNF may have important pharmacological implications.

The asparagine deamidation reaction leads to the formation of aspartate and isoaspartate. The consequent NGR-to-isoDGR transition causes receptor switch from CD13 to αvβ3 integrin, isoDGR being an integrin-binding motif [63]. Notably, αvβ3 is an integrin overexpressed in the tumor neovasculature and for this reason isoDGR-TNF (a degradation product of NGR-TNF) is endowed of potent anti-cancer activity [63]. It is possible, therefore, that the asparagine deamidation reaction (which may occur in low but significant amounts in vitro, during NGR-TNF production and storage, and in vivo, after drug injection in patients) may lead to a dual mechanism of tumor vessel targeting based on CD13 and αvβ3 recognition. The effect of isoDGR-TNF on other αvβ3-expressing cells, such as platelets and myeloid cells (dendritic cells, macrophages, microglia) is unknown.

Considering the molecular heterogeneity of NGR-TNF subunits and assuming a random association of different subunits in trimer formation, different trimers are expected to be present in NGR-TNF preparations. This may represent a major problem in drug development, particularly in terms of lot-to-lot consistency and quality assurance. Thus, various attempts have been made to generate NGR-TNF derivatives more homogeneous and stable. At this regard, an NGR-TNF product lacking the +58 Da and +42 modifications can be obtained by expressing the cDNA encoding this protein in *P. pastoris*, instead of *E. coli* [62]. Furthermore, blockade of the cysteine α-amino group with a serine in first position leads to the expression in *E. coli* of a SCNGRCG-TNF product (called S-NGR-TNF) more homogeneous and stable than NGR-TNF [62]. Finally, a stable nano-formulations of NGR-TNF can be produced using TNF-bearing gold nanoparticles functionalized with a cyclic NGR-peptide having a N-methylated glycine in place of glycine, which completely prevents asparagine deamidation without impairing CD13 recognition [64]. All these products, tested only in animal models so far, may represent more homogeneous, stable, and active second-generation NGR-TNF that deserve further investigation.

4.5. Other TNF-Based Tumor Targeting Agents

The results of preclinical and clinical studies obtained with NGR-TNF indicate that extremely low doses of this drug (e.g., 100 pg/mouse or 0.8 μg/m^2 in patients) are sufficient to affect the tumor vasculature and to induce anti-tumor effects. This also suggests that the CNGRCG peptide (NGR) and the CD13 receptor represent an efficient ligand–receptor system for delivering TNF to the tumor vasculature. However, besides CNGRCG, other ligands and delivery systems can be exploited for increasing the therapeutic index of TNF [12]. For example, a conjugate consisting of TNF coupled to the tumor vasculature-homing peptide CRGRRST was shown to increase tumor vessel stability, vascular perfusion, and T-cell infiltration in a mouse model of pancreatic endocrine tumors, when administered biweekly at doses of 2 μg [65]. The selective advantage of this drug over TNF was lost with a dose of 0.2 μg and no beneficial effects at all were observed with a dose of 0.2 ng [65].

Antibodies can also be exploited as targeting ligands. For example, the single-chain Fv fragment of L19, an antibody against the alternatively spliced EDB domain of fibronectin, has been fused to TNF by genetic engineering technology and used for delivering TNF to various types of solid tumors in animal models and in patients [66,67]. Of note, this product (called L19-TNF) has shown anti-tumor activity in a murine glioblastoma model [68] and is currently investigated in phase I/II trials in glioma patients at relatively high doses (10–13 μg/kg), as a single agent or combined with lomustine (clinicaltrials.gov; NCT03779230 and NCT04573192). Early findings in glioblastoma patients showed that L19-TNF monotherapy could decrease blood perfusion within the tumor, which was associated with increased tumor necrosis and T-cell infiltration [67,69]. Anti-CD13 antibodies have also been used as TNF vehicles [70,71]. An interesting strategy developed to reduce the systemic toxicity of antibody-TNF conjugates is based on the use of conjugates bearing mutations in the TNF moiety that decrease its affinity for TNF receptors, thereby reducing off-target effects on normal cells [70,71]. These de-potentiated TNF versions, thanks to their specific accumulation on the target molecules, such as alternatively spliced EDB domain of fibronectin or CD13, can regain their activity on targeted cells, e.g., by local avidity-driven receptor binding. For example, administration of high doses (375 μg/kg) of a depotentiated version of L19-TNF (I97A) to mice bearing subcutaneous WEHI-164 fibrosarcomas showed a more potent anti-tumor activity, without apparent toxicity, than the wild-type product [71]. Similarly, daily injection of a CD13-specific VHH single-domain antibody fused to a mutated (Y86F) single-chain murine TNF (50 μg/mouse) could selectively activate the tumor neovasculature in a murine melanoma model without detectable toxicity [70,71]. Although these approaches might reduce the systemic toxicity of conjugates, the antibody ligands, the linkers, the mutations, and the markedly high doses necessary to induce anti-tumor effects might negatively impact the immunogenicity of this class of compounds, a point that should be carefully considered.

Other approaches used by different investigators for delivering TNF to tumors are based on the use of nanomaterials capable of exploiting the "passive" targeting mechanism consequent to the "enhanced permeability and retention effects (EPR)" of neoplastic tissues [72,73], such as gold nanoparticles [74–80], superparamagnetic iron oxide nanoparticles decorated exosome [81], magnetite (Fe_3O_4) nanoparticles [82], dendritic mesoporous silica nanoparticles [83], lactoferrin-bearing polypropylenimine dendriplexes [83], carbon dot festooned and surface-passivated graphene-reinforced chitosan nanoparticles [84], and poly-lactic acid microspheres [85]. Notably, recent studies have shown that the functionalization of TNF-bearing gold nanoparticles with NGR- or isoDGR-containing ligands can enable also the "active" targeted delivery of extremely low, but pharmacologically active, doses of nanodrug (e.g., equivalent to 5 pg of biologically active TNF/mouse) to the tumor vasculature in murine models [64,86]. Finally, genetically modified viruses, bacteria, and bacteriophages, engineered to express TNF alone or in combination with other cytokines, have also been developed [87–93]. For example, a recent study performed in a murine model of human glioblastoma have shown that an RGD4C-directed hybrid virus of adeno-associated virus and phage (AAVP) can deliver the TNF gene to the tumors, and induce damage of tumor-associated neovessels and cell death [94].

All these strategies are promising, but their clinical utility in safely breaching the BBB in cancer patients is yet to be demonstrated.

5. Conclusions

The results of studies performed with NGR-TNF in animal models of solid tumors and in PCNSL patients suggest that coupling TNF with the CNGRCG peptide (NGR) is a valuable strategy for delivering an amount of cytokine to tumor blood vasculature sufficient to alter the biological barriers that limit drug penetration in cancer lesions, including the BBTB. Remarkably, the dose of NGR-TNF necessary for BBTB alteration in patients (0.8 μg/m^2) is well-tolerated. The results of these studies have also shown that the use of an extremely low dose of NGR-TNF can overcome, on the one hand, the problem of TNF systemic toxicity, and, on the other hand, systemic counter-regulatory mechanisms that limit the therapeutic efficacy of this cytokine. This is made possible by the excellent accessibility of the CD13 target (the luminal side of the endothelial lining of tumor vasculature, thus not beyond the BBTB) and the high avidity of the interactions among NGR-TNF, CD13 and TNF-receptors, co-expressed on the endothelium of the tumor vasculature. The NGR targeting domain, besides delivering TNF effector molecules to CD13-positive tumor vessels, can also induce co-signaling mechanisms that impair the activation of pro-survival pathways by the TNF moiety, a mechanism that may contribute to the biological effects observed with extremely low doses of the fusion protein.

The low dose of drug necessary for BBTB breaching, the target accessibility, the small size and the poor (or null) immunogenicity of the NGR peptide, may represent important advantages compared to other ligands and vehicles so far developed for delivering TNF (protein or gene) to tumors, e.g., those based on antibodies, nanoparticles, viral agents, or genetically engineered cells, particularly in the case of therapies that need repeated treatments.

In conclusion, the results achieved so far in animal models and in PCNSL patients suggest that targeted delivery of low amounts of NGR-TNF (or its more homogeneous derivatives) to CD13-positive tumor neovasculature represents a valuable strategy for breaching the BBTB and for enhancing anticancer drug delivery to neoplastic cells in patients with PCNSL. Further studies are warranted to assess the potential use of NGR-TNF (or its more stable and homogeneous derivative S-NGR-TNF), in combination with chemo/immunotherapy, for the treatment of other primary and secondary brain tumors, such as glioblastoma multiforme and brain metastases of breast and lung cancer.

Author Contributions: A.C., T.C., F.C. and A.J.M.F. performed the literature research, data interpretation, clinical trials analysis, figures, and wrote and approved the submitted manuscript. All authors have read and agreed to the published version of the manuscript.

Funding: This research was funded by Associazione Italiana per la Ricerca sul Cancro (AIRC) under IG 2019–ID. 23470 project–P.I. Angelo Corti and by Fondazione AIRC 5 per Mille 2019 (ID 22737) program, P.I. MC Bonini, Group Leader A Corti).

Institutional Review Board Statement: Not applicable.

Informed Consent Statement: Not applicable.

Conflicts of Interest: A.C., F.C. and A.J.M.F. are the inventors of patents on NGR-TNF and its use in PCNSL.

References

1. Steeg, P.S. The blood-tumour barrier in cancer biology and therapy. *Nat. Rev. Clin. Oncol.* **2021**, *18*, 696–714. [CrossRef]
2. Marcucci, F.; Corti, A.; Ferreri, A.J.M. Breaching the Blood-Brain Tumor Barrier for Tumor Therapy. *Cancers* **2021**, *13*, 2391. [CrossRef] [PubMed]
3. Gonzalez-Carter, D.; Liu, X.; Tockary, T.A.; Dirisala, A.; Toh, K.; Anraku, Y.; Kataoka, K. Targeting nanoparticles to the brain by exploiting the blood-brain barrier impermeability to selectively label the brain endothelium. *Proc. Natl. Acad. Sci. USA* **2020**, *117*, 19141–19150. [CrossRef] [PubMed]
4. Carswell, E.A.; Old, L.J.; Kassel, R.L.; Green, S.; Fiore, N.; Williamson, B. An endotoxin-induced serum factor that causes necrosis of tumors. *Proc. Natl. Acad. Sci. USA* **1975**, *72*, 3666–3670. [CrossRef] [PubMed]
5. Helson, L.; Green, S.; Carswell, E.; Old, L.J. Effect of tumor necrosis factor on cultured human melanoma cells. *Nature* **1975**, *258*, 731–732. [CrossRef] [PubMed]
6. Lejeune, F.J.; Lienard, D.; Matter, M.; Ruegg, C. Efficiency of recombinant human TNF in human cancer therapy. *Cancer. Immun.* **2006**, *6*, 6. [PubMed]
7. Fraker, D.L.; Alexander, H.R.; Pass, H.I. Biologic therapy with TNF: Systemic administration and isolation-perfusion. In *Biologic Therapy of Cancer: Principles and Practice*; De Vita, V., Hellman, S., Rosenberg, S., Eds.; J.B. Lippincott Company: Philadelphia, PA, USA, 1995; pp. 329–345.
8. Lienard, D.; Ewalenko, P.; Delmotte, J.J.; Renard, N.; Lejeune, F.J. High-dose recombinant tumor necrosis factor alpha in combination with interferon gamma and melphalan in isolation perfusion of the limbs for melanoma and sarcoma. *J. Clin. Oncol.* **1992**, *10*, 52–60. [CrossRef] [PubMed]
9. Eggermont, A.M.; Schraffordt Koops, H.; Lienard, D.; Kroon, B.B.; van Geel, A.N.; Hoekstra, H.J.; Lejeune, F.J. Isolated limb perfusion with high-dose tumor necrosis factor-alpha in combination with interferon-gamma and melphalan for nonresectable extremity soft tissue sarcomas: A multicenter trial. *J. Clin. Oncol.* **1996**, *14*, 2653–2665. [CrossRef] [PubMed]
10. Fraker, D.L.; Alexander, H.R.; Andrich, M.; Rosenberg, S.A. Treatment of patients with melanoma of the extremity using hyperthermic isolated limb perfusion with melphalan, tumor necrosis factor, and interferon gamma: Results of a tumor necrosis factor dose-escalation study. *J. Clin. Oncol.* **1996**, *14*, 479–489. [CrossRef] [PubMed]

11. Eggermont, A.M.; de Wilt, J.H.; ten Hagen, T.L. Current uses of isolated limb perfusion in the clinic and a model system for new strategies. *Lancet Oncol.* **2003**, *4*, 429–437. [CrossRef]
12. Corti, A.; Curnis, F.; Rossoni, G.; Marcucci, F.; Gregorc, V. Peptide-mediated targeting of cytokines to tumor vasculature: The NGR-hTNF example. *BioDrugs* **2013**, *27*, 591–603. [CrossRef] [PubMed]
13. Curnis, F.; Sacchi, A.; Borgna, L.; Magni, F.; Gasparri, A.; Corti, A. Enhancement of tumor necrosis factor alpha antitumor immunotherapeutic properties by targeted delivery to aminopeptidase N (CD13). *Nat. Biotechnol.* **2000**, *18*, 1185–1190. [CrossRef] [PubMed]
14. Arap, W.; Pasqualini, R.; Ruoslahti, E. Cancer treatment by targeted drug delivery to tumor vasculature in a mouse model. *Science* **1998**, *279*, 377–380. [CrossRef]
15. Pasqualini, R.; Koivunen, E.; Kain, R.; Lahdenranta, J.; Sakamoto, M.; Stryhn, A.; Ashmun, R.A.; Shapiro, L.H.; Arap, W.; Ruoslahti, E. Aminopeptidase N is a receptor for tumor-homing peptides and a target for inhibiting angiogenesis. *Cancer Res.* **2000**, *60*, 722–727. [PubMed]
16. Curnis, F.; Arrigoni, G.; Sacchi, A.; Fischetti, L.; Arap, W.; Pasqualini, R.; Corti, A. Differential binding of drugs containing the NGR motif to CD13 isoforms in tumor vessels, epithelia, and myeloid cells. *Cancer Res.* **2002**, *62*, 867–874.
17. Lahdenranta, J.; Sidman, R.L.; Pasqualini, R.; Arap, W. Treatment of hypoxia-induced retinopathy with targeted proapoptotic peptidomimetic in a mouse model of disease. *FASEB J.* **2007**, *21*, 3272–3278. [CrossRef]
18. Buehler, A.; van Zandvoort, M.A.; Stelt, B.J.; Hackeng, T.M.; Schrans-Stassen, B.H.; Bennaghmouch, A.; Hofstra, L.; Cleutjens, J.P.; Duijvestijn, A.; Smeets, M.B.; et al. cNGR: A novel homing sequence for CD13/APN targeted molecular imaging of murine cardiac angiogenesis in vivo. *Arter. Thromb. Vasc. Biol.* **2006**, *26*, 2681–2687. [CrossRef]
19. Taylor, A. Aminopeptidases: Structure and function. *FASEB J.* **1993**, *7*, 290–298. [CrossRef]
20. Shipp, M.A.; Look, A.T. Hematopoietic differentiation antigens that are membrane-associated enzymes: Cutting is the key. *Blood* **1993**, *82*, 1052–1070. [CrossRef]
21. Dixon, J.; Kaklamanis, L.; Turley, H.; Hickson, I.D.; Leek, R.D.; Harris, A.L.; Gatter, K.C. Expression of aminopeptidase-n (CD 13) in normal tissues and malignant neoplasms of epithelial and lymphoid origin. *J. Clin. Pathol.* **1994**, *47*, 43–47. [CrossRef]
22. Di Matteo, P.; Arrigoni, G.L.; Alberici, L.; Corti, A.; Gallo-Stampino, C.; Traversari, C.; Doglioni, C.; Rizzardi, G.P. Enhanced Expression of CD13 in Vessels of Inflammatory and Neoplastic Tissues. *J Histochem. Cytochem.* **2010**, *59*, 47–59. [CrossRef] [PubMed]
23. Ferreri, A.J.M.; Calimeri, T.; Ponzoni, M.; Curnis, F.; Conte, G.M.; Scarano, E.; Rrapaj, E.; De Lorenzo, D.; Cattaneo, D.; Fallanca, F.; et al. Improving the antitumor activity of R-CHOP with NGR-hTNF in primary CNS lymphoma: Final results of a phase 2 trial. *Blood Adv.* **2020**, *4*, 3648–3658. [CrossRef] [PubMed]
24. Ferreri, A.J.M.; Calimeri, T.; Conte, G.M.; Cattaneo, D.; Fallanca, F.; Ponzoni, M.; Scarano, E.; Curnis, F.; Nonis, A.; Lopedote, P.; et al. R-CHOP preceded by blood-brain barrier permeabilization with engineered tumor necrosis factor-alpha in primary CNS lymphoma. *Blood* **2019**, *134*, 252–262. [CrossRef] [PubMed]
25. Wong, A.H.; Zhou, D.; Rini, J.M. The X-ray crystal structure of human aminopeptidase N reveals a novel dimer and the basis for peptide processing. *J. Biol. Chem.* **2012**, *287*, 36804–36813. [CrossRef] [PubMed]
26. Valentinis, B.; Porcellini, S.; Asperti, C.; Cota, M.; Zhou, D.; Di Matteo, P.; Garau, G.; Zucchelli, C.; Avanzi, N.R.; Rizzardi, G.P.; et al. Mechanism of Action of the Tumor Vessel Targeting Agent NGR-hTNF: Role of Both NGR Peptide and hTNF in Cell Binding and Signaling. *Int. J. Mol. Sci.* **2019**, *20*, 4511. [CrossRef]
27. Curnis, F.; Sacchi, A.; Corti, A. Improving chemotherapeutic drug penetration in tumors by vascular targeting and barrier alteration. *J. Clin. Investig.* **2002**, *110*, 475–482. [CrossRef]
28. Lewis, M.; Tartaglia, L.A.; Lee, A.; Bennet, L.G.; Rice, G.R.; Wong, G.H.W.; Chen, E.Y.; Goeddel, D.V. Cloning and expression of cDNA for two distinct murine tumor necrosis factor receptors demonstrate one receptor is species specific. *Proc. Natl. Acad. Sci. USA* **1991**, *88*, 2830–2834. [CrossRef]
29. Calcinotto, A.; Grioni, M.; Jachetti, E.; Curnis, F.; Mondino, A.; Parmiani, G.; Corti, A.; Bellone, M. Targeting TNF-alpha to Neoangiogenic Vessels Enhances Lymphocyte Infiltration in Tumors and Increases the Therapeutic Potential of Immunotherapy. *J. Immunol.* **2012**, *188*, 2687–2694. [CrossRef]
30. Dondossola, E.; Gasparri, A.M.; Colombo, B.; Sacchi, A.; Curnis, F.; Corti, A. Chromogranin A Restricts Drug Penetration and Limits the Ability of NGR-TNF to Enhance Chemotherapeutic Efficacy. *Cancer Res.* **2011**, *71*, 5881–5890. [CrossRef]
31. Sacchi, A.; Gasparri, A.; Gallo-Stampino, C.; Toma, S.; Curnis, F.; Corti, A. Synergistic antitumor activity of cisplatin, paclitaxel, and gemcitabine with tumor vasculature-targeted tumor necrosis factor-alpha. *Clin. Cancer Res.* **2006**, *12*, 175–182. [CrossRef]
32. Bertilaccio, M.T.; Grioni, M.; Sutherland, B.W.; Degl'Innocenti, E.; Freschi, M.; Jachetti, E.; Greenberg, N.M.; Corti, A.; Bellone, M. Vasculature-targeted tumor necrosis factor-alpha increases the therapeutic index of doxorubicin against prostate cancer. *Prostate* **2008**, *68*, 1105–1115. [CrossRef]
33. Brett, J.; Gerlach, H.; Nawroth, P.; Steinberg, S.; Godman, G.; Stern, D. Tumor necrosis factor/cachectin increases permeability of endothelial cell monolayers by a mechanism involving regulatory G proteins. *J. Exp. Med.* **1989**, *169*, 1977–1991. [CrossRef] [PubMed]
34. Goldblum, S.E.; Sun, W.L. Tumor necrosis factor-alpha augments pulmonary arterial transendothelial albumin flux in vitro. *Am. J. Physiol.* **1990**, *258*, L57–L67. [CrossRef] [PubMed]
35. van der Veen, A.H.; de Wilt, J.H.; Eggermont, A.M.; van Tiel, S.T.; Seynhaeve, A.L.; ten Hagen, T.L. TNF-alpha augments intratumoural concentrations of doxorubicin in TNF-alpha-based isolated limb perfusion in rat sarcoma models and enhances anti-tumour effects. *Br. J. Cancer* **2000**, *82*, 973–980. [CrossRef] [PubMed]

36. Lejeune, F.J. High dose recombinant tumour necrosis factor (rTNF alpha) administered by isolation perfusion for advanced tumours of the limbs: A model for biochemotherapy of cancer. *Eur. J. Cancer* **1995**, *31A*, 1009–1016. [CrossRef]
37. Kristensen, C.A.; Nozue, M.; Boucher, Y.; Jain, R.K. Reduction of interstitial fluid pressure after TNF-alpha treatment of three human melanoma xenografts. *Br. J. Cancer* **1996**, *74*, 533–536. [CrossRef]
38. Suzuki, S.; Ohta, S.; Takashio, K.; Nitanai, H.; Hashimoto, Y. Augmentation for intratumoral accumulation and anti-tumor activity of liposome-encapsulated adriamycin by tumor necrosis factor-alpha in mice. *Int. J. Cancer* **1990**, *46*, 1095–1100. [CrossRef] [PubMed]
39. de Wilt, J.H.; ten Hagen, T.L.; de Boeck, G.; van Tiel, S.T.; de Bruijn, E.A.; Eggermont, A.M. Tumour necrosis factor alpha increases melphalan concentration in tumour tissue after isolated limb perfusion. *Br. J. Cancer* **2000**, *82*, 1000–1003. [CrossRef]
40. Jain, R.K. Barriers to drug delivery in solid tumors. *Sci. Am.* **1994**, *271*, 58–65. [CrossRef]
41. Sacchi, A.; Gasparri, A.; Curnis, F.; Bellone, M.; Corti, A. Crucial role for interferon-gamma in the synergism between tumor vasculature-targeted tumor necrosis factor alpha (NGR-TNF) and doxorubicin. *Cancer Res.* **2004**, *64*, 7150–7155. [CrossRef]
42. Manzo, T.; Sturmheit, T.; Basso, V.; Petrozziello, E.; Hess Michelini, R.; Riba, M.; Freschi, M.; Elia, A.R.; Grioni, M.; Curnis, F.; et al. T Cells Redirected to a Minor Histocompatibility Antigen Instruct Intratumoral TNFalpha Expression and Empower Adoptive Cell Therapy for Solid Tumors. *Cancer Res.* **2017**, *77*, 658–671. [CrossRef] [PubMed]
43. Elia, A.R.; Grioni, M.; Basso, V.; Curnis, F.; Freschi, M.; Corti, A.; Mondino, A.; Bellone, M. Targeting Tumor Vasculature with TNF Leads Effector T Cells to the Tumor and Enhances Therapeutic Efficacy of Immune Checkpoint Blockers in Combination with Adoptive Cell Therapy. *Clin. Cancer Res.* **2018**, *24*, 2171–2181. [CrossRef] [PubMed]
44. van Laarhoven, H.W.; Fiedler, W.; Desar, I.M.; van Asten, J.J.; Marreaud, S.; Lacombe, D.; Govaerts, A.S.; Bogaerts, J.; Lasch, P.; Timmer-Bonte, J.N.; et al. Phase I clinical and magnetic resonance imaging study of the vascular agent NGR-hTNF in patients with advanced cancers (European Organization for Research and Treatment of Cancer Study 16041). *Clin. Cancer Res.* **2010**, *16*, 1315–1323. [CrossRef] [PubMed]
45. Gregorc, V.; Citterio, G.; Vitali, G.; Spreafico, A.; Scifo, P.; Borri, A.; Donadoni, G.; Rossoni, G.; Corti, A.; Caligaris-Cappio, F.; et al. Defining the optimal biological dose of NGR-hTNF, a selective vascular targeting agent, in advanced solid tumours. *Eur. J. Cancer* **2010**, *46*, 198–206. [CrossRef] [PubMed]
46. Desar, I.M.; van Herpen, C.M.; van Asten, J.J.; Fiedler, W.; Marreaud, S.; Timmer-Bonte, J.N.; ter Voert, E.G.; Lambiase, A.; Bordignon, C.; Heerschap, A.; et al. Factors affecting the unexpected failure of DCE-MRI to determine the optimal biological dose of the vascular targeting agent NGR-hTNF in solid cancer patients. *Eur. J. Radiol.* **2011**, *80*, 655–661. [CrossRef]
47. Gregorc, V.; Zucali, P.A.; Santoro, A.; Ceresoli, G.L.; Citterio, G.; De Pas, T.M.; Zilembo, N.; De Vincenzo, F.; Simonelli, M.; Rossoni, G.; et al. Phase II study of asparagine-glycine-arginine-human tumor necrosis factor alpha, a selective vascular targeting agent, in previously treated patients with malignant pleural mesothelioma. *J. Clin. Oncol.* **2010**, *28*, 2604–2611. [CrossRef] [PubMed]
48. Santoro, A.; Pressiani, T.; Citterio, G.; Rossoni, G.; Donadoni, G.; Pozzi, F.; Rimassa, L.; Personeni, N.; Bozzarelli, S.; Colombi, S.; et al. Activity and safety of NGR-hTNF, a selective vascular-targeting agent, in previously treated patients with advanced hepatocellular carcinoma. *Br. J. Cancer* **2010**, *103*, 837–844. [CrossRef] [PubMed]
49. Santoro, A.; Rimassa, L.; Sobrero, A.F.; Citterio, G.; Sclafani, F.; Carnaghi, C.; Pessino, A.; Caprioni, F.; Andretta, V.; Tronconi, M.C.; et al. Phase II study of NGR-hTNF, a selective vascular targeting agent, in patients with metastatic colorectal cancer after failure of standard therapy. *Eur. J. Cancer* **2010**, *46*, 2746–2752. [CrossRef] [PubMed]
50. Gregorc, V.; Santoro, A.; Bennicelli, E.; Punt, C.; Citterio, G.; Timmer-Bonte, J.; Caligaris Cappio, F.; Lambiase, A.; Bordignon, C.; van Herpen, C. Phase Ib study of NGR-hTNF, a selective vascular targeting agent, administered at low doses in combination with doxorubicin to patients with advanced solid tumours. *Br. J. Cancer* **2009**, *101*, 219–224. [CrossRef] [PubMed]
51. Gregorc, V.; De Braud, F.G.; De Pas, T.M.; Scalamogna, R.; Citterio, G.; Milani, A.; Boselli, S.; Catania, C.; Donadoni, G.; Rossoni, G.; et al. Phase I study of NGR-hTNF, a selective vascular targeting agent, in combination with cisplatin in refractory solid tumors. *Clin. Cancer Res.* **2011**, *17*, 1964–1972. [CrossRef] [PubMed]
52. Lorusso, D.; Scambia, G.; Amadio, G.; di Legge, A.; Pietragalla, A.; De Vincenzo, R.; Masciullo, V.; Di Stefano, M.; Mangili, G.; Citterio, G.; et al. Phase II study of NGR-hTNF in combination with doxorubicin in relapsed ovarian cancer patients. *Br. J. Cancer* **2012**, *107*, 37–42. [CrossRef] [PubMed]
53. Gregorc, V.; Cavina, R.; Novello, S.; Grossi, F.; Lazzari, C.; Capelletto, E.; Genova, C.; Salini, G.; Lambiase, A.; Santoro, A. NGR-hTNF and Doxorubicin as Second-Line Treatment of Patients with Small Cell Lung Cancer. *Oncologist* **2018**, *23*, 1133.e106–1133.e112. [CrossRef] [PubMed]
54. Mammoliti, S.; Andretta, V.; Bennicelli, E.; Caprioni, F.; Comandini, D.; Fornarini, G.; Guglielmi, A.; Pessino, A.; Sciallero, S.; Sobrero, A.F.; et al. Two doses of NGR-hTNF in combination with capecitabine plus oxaliplatin in colorectal cancer patients failing standard therapies. *Ann. Oncol.* **2011**, *22*, 973–978. [CrossRef] [PubMed]
55. Zucali, P.A.; Simonelli, M.; De Vincenzo, F.; Lorenzi, E.; Perrino, M.; Bertossi, M.; Finotto, R.; Naimo, S.; Balzarini, L.; Bonifacio, C.; et al. Phase I and pharmacodynamic study of high-dose NGR-hTNF in patients with refractory solid tumours. *Br. J. Cancer* **2013**, *108*, 58–63. [CrossRef] [PubMed]
56. Parmiani, G.; Pilla, L.; Corti, A.; Doglioni, C.; Cimminiello, C.; Bellone, M.; Parolini, D.; Russo, V.; Capocefalo, F.; Maccalli, C. A pilot Phase I study combining peptide-based vaccination and NGR-hTNF vessel targeting therapy in metastatic melanoma. *Oncoimmunology* **2014**, *3*, e963406. [CrossRef]

57. Gregorc, V.; Gaafar, R.M.; Favaretto, A.; Grossi, F.; Jassem, J.; Polychronis, A.; Bidoli, P.; Tiseo, M.; Shah, R.; Taylor, P.; et al. NGR-hTNF in combination with best investigator choice in previously treated malignant pleural mesothelioma (NGR015): A randomised, double-blind, placebo-controlled phase 3 trial. *Lancet Oncol.* **2018**, *19*, 799–811. [CrossRef]
58. Calimeri, T.; Marcucci, F.; Corti, A. Overcoming the blood-brain barrier in primary central nervous system lymphoma: A review on new strategies to solve an old problem. *Ann. Lymphoma* **2021**, *5*, 20–30. [CrossRef]
59. Batchelor, T.T. Primary central nervous system lymphoma. *Hematol. Am. Soc. Hematol. Educ. Program* **2016**, *2016*, 379–385. [CrossRef] [PubMed]
60. Connell, J.J.; Chatain, G.; Cornelissen, B.; Vallis, K.A.; Hamilton, A.; Seymour, L.; Anthony, D.C.; Sibson, N.R. Selective permeabilization of the blood-brain barrier at sites of metastasis. *J. Natl. Cancer Inst.* **2013**, *105*, 1634–1643. [CrossRef] [PubMed]
61. Di Matteo, P.; Curnis, F.; Longhi, R.; Colombo, G.; Sacchi, A.; Crippa, L.; Protti, M.P.; Ponzoni, M.; Toma, S.; Corti, A. Immunogenic and structural properties of the Asn-Gly-Arg (NGR) tumor neovasculature-homing motif. *Mol. Immunol.* **2006**, *43*, 1509–1518. [CrossRef] [PubMed]
62. Corti, A.; Gasparri, A.M.; Sacchi, A.; Colombo, B.; Monieri, M.; Rrapaj, E.; Ferreri, A.J.M.; Curnis, F. NGR-TNF Engineering with an N-Terminal Serine Reduces Degradation and Post-Translational Modifications and Improves Its Tumor-Targeting Activity. *Mol. Pharm.* **2020**, *17*, 3813–3824. [CrossRef] [PubMed]
63. Curnis, F.; Sacchi, A.; Gasparri, A.; Longhi, R.; Bachi, A.; Doglioni, C.; Bordignon, C.; Traversari, C.; Rizzardi, G.P.; Corti, A. Isoaspartate-glycine-arginine: A new tumor vasculature-targeting motif. *Cancer Res.* **2008**, *68*, 7073–7082. [CrossRef]
64. Corti, A.; Gasparri, A.M.; Ghitti, M.; Sacchi, A.; Sudati, F.; Fiocchi, M.; Buttiglione, V.; Perani, L.; Gori, A.; Valtorta, S.; et al. Glycine N-methylation in NGR-Tagged Nanocarriers Prevents Isoaspartate formation and Integrin Binding without Impairing CD13 Recognition and Tumor Homing. *Adv. Funct. Mater.* **2017**, *27*, 1701245. [CrossRef] [PubMed]
65. Johansson, A.; Hamzah, J.; Payne, C.J.; Ganss, R. Tumor-targeted TNFalpha stabilizes tumor vessels and enhances active immunotherapy. *Proc. Natl. Acad. Sci. USA* **2012**, *109*, 7841–7846. [CrossRef] [PubMed]
66. Hutmacher, C.; Neri, D. Antibody-cytokine fusion proteins: Biopharmaceuticals with immunomodulatory properties for cancer therapy. *Adv. Drug. Deliv. Rev.* **2019**, *141*, 67–91. [CrossRef] [PubMed]
67. Murer, P.; Neri, D. Antibody-cytokine fusion proteins: A novel class of biopharmaceuticals for the therapy of cancer and of chronic inflammation. *New Biotechnol.* **2019**, *52*, 42–53. [CrossRef] [PubMed]
68. Weiss, T.; Puca, E.; Silginer, M.; Hemmerle, T.; Pazahr, S.; Bink, A.; Weller, M.; Neri, D.; Roth, P. Immunocytokines are a promising immunotherapeutic approach against glioblastoma. *Sci. Transl. Med.* **2020**, *12*, eabb2311. [CrossRef] [PubMed]
69. Papadia, F.; Basso, V.; Patuzzo, R.; Maurichi, A.; Di Florio, A.; Zardi, L.; Ventura, E.; Gonzalez-Iglesias, R.; Lovato, V.; Giovannoni, L.; et al. Isolated limb perfusion with the tumor-targeting human monoclonal antibody-cytokine fusion protein L19-TNF plus melphalan and mild hyperthermia in patients with locally advanced extremity melanoma. *J. Surg. Oncol.* **2013**, *107*, 173–179. [CrossRef] [PubMed]
70. Huyghe, L.; Van Parys, A.; Cauwels, A.; Van Lint, S.; De Munter, S.; Bultinck, J.; Zabeau, L.; Hostens, J.; Goethals, A.; Vanderroost, N.; et al. Safe eradication of large established tumors using neovasculature-targeted tumor necrosis factor-based therapies. *EMBO Mol. Med.* **2020**, *12*, e11223. [CrossRef] [PubMed]
71. Dakhel, S.; Lizak, C.; Matasci, M.; Mock, J.; Villa, A.; Neri, D.; Cazzamalli, S. An Attenuated Targeted-TNF Localizes to Tumors In Vivo and Regains Activity at the Site of Disease. *Int. J. Mol. Sci.* **2021**, *22*, 10020. [CrossRef] [PubMed]
72. Matsumura, Y.; Maeda, H. A new concept for macromolecular therapeutics in cancer chemotherapy: Mechanism of tumoritropic accumulation of proteins and the antitumor agent smancs. *Cancer Res.* **1986**, *46*, 6387–6392. [PubMed]
73. Chithrani, B.D.; Ghazani, A.A.; Chan, W.C. Determining the size and shape dependence of gold nanoparticle uptake into mammalian cells. *Nano Lett.* **2006**, *6*, 662–668. [CrossRef] [PubMed]
74. Powell, A.C.; Paciotti, G.F.; Libutti, S.K. Colloidal gold: A novel nanoparticle for targeted cancer therapeutics. *Methods Mol. Biol.* **2010**, *624*, 375–384. [CrossRef] [PubMed]
75. Shenoi, M.M.; Iltis, I.; Choi, J.; Koonce, N.A.; Metzger, G.J.; Griffin, R.J.; Bischof, J.C. Nanoparticle delivered vascular disrupting agents (VDAs): Use of TNF-alpha conjugated gold nanoparticles for multimodal cancer therapy. *Mol. Pharm.* **2013**, *10*, 1683–1694. [CrossRef]
76. Libutti, S.K.; Paciotti, G.F.; Byrnes, A.A.; Alexander, H.R., Jr.; Gannon, W.E.; Walker, M.; Seidel, G.D.; Yuldasheva, N.; Tamarkin, L. Phase I and pharmacokinetic studies of CYT-6091, a novel PEGylated colloidal gold-rhTNF nanomedicine. *Clin. Cancer Res.* **2010**, *16*, 6139–6149. [CrossRef]
77. Paciotti, G.F.; Zhao, J.; Cao, S.; Brodie, P.J.; Tamarkin, L.; Huhta, M.; Myer, L.D.; Friedman, J.; Kingston, D.G. Synthesis and Evaluation of Paclitaxel-Loaded Gold Nanoparticles for Tumor-Targeted Drug Delivery. *Bioconjug. Chem.* **2016**, *27*, 2646–2657. [CrossRef]
78. Koonce, N.A.; Quick, C.M.; Hardee, M.E.; Jamshidi-Parsian, A.; Dent, J.A.; Paciotti, G.F.; Nedosekin, D.; Dings, R.P.; Griffin, R.J. Combination of Gold Nanoparticle-Conjugated Tumor Necrosis Factor-alpha and Radiation Therapy Results in a Synergistic Antitumor Response in Murine Carcinoma Models. *Int. J. Radiat. Oncol. Biol. Phys.* **2015**, *93*, 588–596. [CrossRef]
79. Paciotti, G.F.; Myer, L.; Weinreich, D.; Goia, D.; Pavel, N.; McLaughlin, R.E.; Tamarkin, L. Colloidal gold: A novel nanoparticle vector for tumor directed drug delivery. *Drug Deliv.* **2004**, *11*, 169–183. [CrossRef]
80. Farma, J.M.; Puhlmann, M.; Soriano, P.A.; Cox, D.; Paciotti, G.F.; Tamarkin, L.; Alexander, H.R. Direct evidence for rapid and selective induction of tumor neovascular permeability by tumor necrosis factor and a novel derivative, colloidal gold bound tumor necrosis factor. *Int. J. Cancer* **2007**, *120*, 2474–2480. [CrossRef]

81. Zhuang, M.; Chen, X.; Du, D.; Shi, J.; Deng, M.; Long, Q.; Yin, X.; Wang, Y.; Rao, L. SPION decorated exosome delivery of TNF-alpha to cancer cell membranes through magnetism. *Nanoscale* **2020**, *12*, 173–188. [CrossRef]
82. Teo, P.; Wang, X.; Chen, B.; Zhang, H.; Yang, X.; Huang, Y.; Tang, J. Complex of TNF-alpha and Modified Fe3O4 Nanoparticles Suppresses Tumor Growth by Magnetic Induction Hyperthermia. *Cancer Biother. Radiopharm.* **2017**, *32*, 379–386. [CrossRef] [PubMed]
83. Altwaijry, N.; Somani, S.; Parkinson, J.A.; Tate, R.J.; Keating, P.; Warzecha, M.; Mackenzie, G.R.; Leung, H.Y.; Dufes, C. Regression of prostate tumors after intravenous administration of lactoferrin-bearing polypropylenimine dendriplexes encoding TNF-alpha, TRAIL, and interleukin-12. *Drug Deliv.* **2018**, *25*, 679–689. [CrossRef] [PubMed]
84. Jaleel, J.A.; Ashraf, S.M.; Rathinasamy, K.; Pramod, K. Carbon dot festooned and surface passivated graphene-reinforced chitosan construct for tumor-targeted delivery of TNF-alpha gene. *Int. J. Biol. Macromol.* **2019**, *127*, 628–636. [CrossRef] [PubMed]
85. Sabel, M.S.; Su, G.; Griffith, K.A.; Chang, A.E. Intratumoral delivery of encapsulated IL-12, IL-18 and TNF-alpha in a model of metastatic breast cancer. *Breast Cancer Res. Treat.* **2010**, *122*, 325–336. [CrossRef] [PubMed]
86. Curnis, F.; Fiocchi, M.; Sacchi, A.; Gori, A.; Gasparri, A.; Corti, A. NGR-tagged nano-gold: A new CD13-selective carrier for cytokine delivery to tumors. *Nano Res.* **2016**, *9*, 1393–1408. [CrossRef] [PubMed]
87. Jiang, Y.Q.; Zhang, Z.; Cai, H.R.; Zhou, H. Killing effect of TNF-mediated by conditionally replicating adenovirus on esophageal cancer and lung cancer cell lines. *Int. J. Clin. Exp. Pathol.* **2015**, *8*, 13785–13794. [PubMed]
88. Havunen, R.; Siurala, M.; Sorsa, S.; Gronberg-Vaha-Koskela, S.; Behr, M.; Tahtinen, S.; Santos, J.M.; Karell, P.; Rusanen, J.; Nettelbeck, D.M.; et al. Oncolytic Adenoviruses Armed with Tumor Necrosis Factor Alpha and Interleukin-2 Enable Successful Adoptive Cell Therapy. *Mol. Ther. Oncolytics* **2017**, *4*, 77–86. [CrossRef]
89. Kurena, B.; Muller, E.; Christopoulos, P.F.; Johnsen, I.B.; Stankovic, B.; Oynebraten, I.; Corthay, A.; Zajakina, A. Generation and Functional In Vitro Analysis of Semliki Forest Virus Vectors Encoding TNF-alpha and IFN-gamma. *Front. Immunol.* **2017**, *8*, 1667. [CrossRef]
90. Christie, J.D.; Appel, N.; Canter, H.; Achi, J.G.; Elliott, N.M.; de Matos, A.L.; Franco, L.; Kilbourne, J.; Lowe, K.; Rahman, M.M.; et al. Systemic delivery of TNF-armed myxoma virus plus immune checkpoint inhibitor eliminates lung metastatic mouse osteosarcoma. *Mol. Ther. Oncolytics* **2021**, *22*, 539–554. [CrossRef]
91. Mukai, H.; Takahashi, M.; Watanabe, Y. Potential usefulness of Brevibacillus for bacterial cancer therapy: Intratumoral provision of tumor necrosis factor-alpha and anticancer effects. *Cancer Gene Ther.* **2018**, *25*, 47–57. [CrossRef]
92. Fan, J.X.; Li, Z.H.; Liu, X.H.; Zheng, D.W.; Chen, Y.; Zhang, X.Z. Bacteria-Mediated Tumor Therapy Utilizing Photothermally-Controlled TNF-alpha Expression via Oral Administration. *Nano Lett.* **2018**, *18*, 2373–2380. [CrossRef] [PubMed]
93. Chongchai, A.; Waramit, S.; Suwan, K.; Al-Bahrani, M.; Udomruk, S.; Phitak, T.; Kongtawelert, P.; Pothacharoen, P.; Hajitou, A. Bacteriophage-mediated therapy of chondrosarcoma by selective delivery of the tumor necrosis factor alpha (TNFalpha) gene. *FASEB J.* **2021**, *35*, e21487. [CrossRef] [PubMed]
94. Staquicini, F.I.; Smith, T.L.; Tang, F.H.F.; Gelovani, J.G.; Giordano, R.J.; Libutti, S.K.; Sidman, R.L.; Cavenee, W.K.; Arap, W.; Pasqualini, R. Targeted AAVP-based therapy in a mouse model of human glioblastoma: A comparison of cytotoxic versus suicide gene delivery strategies. *Cancer Gene Ther.* **2020**, *27*, 301–310. [CrossRef] [PubMed]

pharmaceutics

MDPI

Article

Combined Transcriptomic and Proteomic Profiling to Unravel Osimertinib, CARP-1 Functional Mimetic (CFM 4.17) Formulation and Telmisartan Combo Treatment in NSCLC Tumor Xenografts

Ramesh Nimma [1,†], Anil Kumar Kalvala [1,†], Nilkumar Patel [1], Sunil Kumar Surapaneni [1], Li Sun [2], Rakesh Singh [3], Ebony Nottingham [1], Arvind Bagde [1], Nagavendra Kommineni [1], Peggy Arthur [1], Aakash Nathani [1], David G. Meckes, Jr. [2] and Mandip Singh [1,*]

[1] College of Pharmacy and Pharmaceutical Sciences, Florida A&M University, Tallahassee, FL 32307, USA; ramesh.nimma@famu.edu (R.N.); anil.kalvala@famu.edu (A.K.K.); nealpatel442@gmail.com (N.P.); sunil30.niper@gmail.com (S.K.S.); ebony1.nottingham@famu.edu (E.N.); bagde.arvind02@gmail.com (A.B.); nagavendra.kommineni@famu.edu (N.K.); peggyart33@gmail.com (P.A.); aakash1.nathani@famu.edu (A.N.)

[2] Department of Biomedical Sciences, College of Medicine, Florida State University, 1115 West Call Street, Tallahassee, FL 32306, USA; li.sun@med.fsu.edu (L.S.); david.meckes@med.fsu.edu (D.G.M.J.)

[3] Department of Translational Science Laboratory, College of Medicine, Florida State University, 1115 West Call St., Tallahassee, FL 32306, USA; rsingh3@fsu.edu

* Correspondence: mandip.sachdeva@famu.edu or mandip.sachdeva@gmail.com; Tel.: +1-850-561-2790; Fax: +1-850-599-3813

† These authors contributed equally to this work.

Citation: Nimma, R.; Kalvala, A.K.; Patel, N.; Surapaneni, S.K.; Sun, L.; Singh, R.; Nottingham, E.; Bagde, A.; Kommineni, N.; Arthur, P.; et al. Combined Transcriptomic and Proteomic Profiling to Unravel Osimertinib, CARP-1 Functional Mimetic (CFM 4.17) Formulation and Telmisartan Combo Treatment in NSCLC Tumor Xenografts. *Pharmaceutics* **2022**, *14*, 1156. https://doi.org/10.3390/pharmaceutics14061156

Academic Editors: Vibhuti Agrahari and Prashant Kumar

Received: 15 March 2022
Accepted: 11 May 2022
Published: 28 May 2022

Abstract: The epidermal growth factor receptor (EGFR) is highly expressed in many non-small cell lung cancers (NSCLC), necessitating the use of EGFR-tyrosine kinase inhibitors (TKIs) as first-line treatments. Osimertinib (OSM), a third-generation TKI, is routinely used in clinics, but T790M mutations in exon 20 of the EGFR receptor lead to resistance against OSM, necessitating the development of more effective therapeutics. Telmisartan (TLM), OSM, and cell cycle and apoptosis regulatory protein 1 (CARP-1) functional mimetic treatments (CFM4.17) were evaluated in this study against experimental H1975 tumor xenografts to ascertain their anti-cancer effects. Briefly, tumor growth was studied in H1975 xenografts in athymic nude mice, gene and protein expressions were analyzed using next-generation RNA sequencing, proteomics, RT-PCR, and Western blotting. TLM pre-treatment significantly reduced the tumor burden when combined with CFM-4.17 nanoformulation and OSM combination (TLM_CFM-F_OSM) than their respective single treatments or combination of OSM and TLM with CFM 4.17. Data from RNA sequencing and proteomics revealed that TLM_CFM-F_OSM decreased the expression of Lamin B2, STAT3, SOD, NFKB, MMP-1, TGF beta, Sox-2, and PD-L1 proteins while increasing the expression of AMPK proteins, which was also confirmed by RT-PCR, proteomics, and Western blotting. According to our findings, the TLM_CFM-F_OSM combination has a superior anti-cancer effect in the treatment of NSCLC by affecting multiple resistant markers that regulate mitochondrial homeostasis, inflammation, oxidative stress, and apoptosis.

Keywords: epidermal growth factor receptor; non-small cell lung cancer; Lamin B2; AMPK; Osimertinib; RNA seq; proteomics; RT-PCR

1. Introduction

Lung cancer is still the deadliest cancer globally, and the World Health Organization estimates that 2.09 million new cases are reported each year, with 1.76 million deaths (18.4 percent of all cancer deaths) [1]. Non-small cell lung cancer (NSCLC) accounts for over 85% of lung cancer cases, and its incidence is increasing every year, seriously threatening human health [2].

Tyrosine kinase inhibitors (TKIs) are the majorly front-line agents for treating NSCLC over platinum doublet chemotherapy [3]. Resistance to chemotherapy develops in many patients, and more than 20 percent of NSCLC patients show epidermal growth factor receptor (EFGR) mutations [4,5]. Erlotinib and Gefitinib, which are the first-generation EGFR targeted TKIs, bind to EGFR reversibly, leading cells to acquire resistance by inducing mutations that enhance the affinity to Adenosine triphosphate (ATP) (T790M-mutation), resulting in decreased interaction with its receptors following therapy [6]. Afatinib and Dacomitinib are second-line EGFR TKIs that bind to EGFR permanently and show beneficial effects in cancer therapy, but there have been toxicity concerns due to elevated wild-type EGFR off-target binding [7]. Osimertinib (OSM) is a third-generation EGFR-TKI, irreversibly binds EGFR protein activating mutations (such as L858R and Exon19 del) and also targets EGFR TKIs resistant mutations that reduce interaction with wild-type EGFR [8]. The EGFR C797S mutation has been linked to OSM resistance by enhancing receptor affinity to ATP. Additionally, the combination therapy with various TKIs has been suggested as an excellent way to combat resistance, though there are some drawbacks, such as enhanced toxicity [9]. Even though radiotherapy and chemotherapy can help advanced patients to improve their survival rate [10–16], these approaches are toxic to normal cells resulting in impaired immunity, bone marrow suppression and neurotoxicity [17]. Molecular targeted therapy has gradually become a new choice because of its low dosage, remarkable effect, strong specificity, and low side effects [18].

Several reports suggested that OSM inhibits the activation of several downstream pathways, such as RAS/RAF/MAPK and PI3K/AKT, and regulates different cellular processes, including DNA synthesis and proliferation [19]. Cell cycle and apoptosis regulator protein 1 (CARP-1/CCAR1) is a perinuclear phosphoprotein that co-activates the anaphase-promoting complex/cyclosome (APC/C), an E3-ubiquitin ligase, which affects cell cycle and tumor growth [20,21]. Through p53 co-activation, it also regulates chemotherapy-induced apoptosis [21]. CARP-1 functional mimetics (CFMs) inhibit cell growth in various cancer cells and cause apoptosis via lowering CARP-1 binding to the APC/C component APC2 [22]. Previous research on CARP-1 functional mimetics has primarily investigated their role in CARP-1 signaling, ignoring their ability to suppress EGFR activation. According to molecular docking studies, both CFM4.16 and CFM4.17 have been shown to bind with EGFR's ATP binding site [6]. This is consistent with the work of other investigators who have demonstrated that compounds with the ability to target numerous components in the EGFR signaling cascade are more inhibited than those with only one target [23].

Many anti-cancer drugs are ineffective due to high interstitial pressure or tumor stromal barriers. In addition to its role in decreasing tumor interstitial barriers, telmisartan (TLM) has also been shown to aid in the delivery of nanoparticles and liposomes to tumor cells [24–31]. TLM promotes the peroxisome proliferator-activated receptor (PPAR) pathways by inhibiting PI3K signaling [32,33]. In our laboratory, we have demonstrated that TLM could enhance the anti-cancer effects of sorafenib and CFM 4.16 in the rociletinib-resistant H1975 NSCLC xenograft model, lowering the protein expression of p-EGFR/EGFR, Nanog, Sox2, Oct4, pMET/MET, TGF-beta, and MMP9 while raising the expression of E-cadherin protein [34].

Gene mutations are a substantial barrier to lung cancer treatment, and the ability to directly measure the expression levels of molecular drug targets and profile the activation of key molecular pathways allows the personalized prioritization of all molecular-targeted therapies [35]. For high-throughput quantitative transcriptomics, it has been observed that RNA sequencing is the most reliable tool [36]. Our studies used RNA seq analysis to investigate the downstream targets contributing to cancer cell growth in NSCLC.

A thorough understanding of molecular communication will provide new insights into the molecular process behind the disease's medication action. Proteomics, a powerful method for a detailed analysis of protein changes in response to medication therapy, has been widely used to investigate molecular pathways and identify anti-cancer therapeutic targets [37]. A recent study using proteomic analysis observed potential tyrosine kinase inhibitor (OSM) sensitivity indicators in EGFR-mutated lung cancer and identified novel targets for future therapy options [38]. In our studies, proteomics was used to explore the expression of all the proteins in H1975 tumor xenografts treated with various drugs and formulations.

EGFR TKIs are still the leading therapy for a substantial percentage of NSCLCs, and the need for resistance to TKIs remains a critical breakthrough. Herein, we hypothesize that OSM (i.e., which targets EGFR T790M mutation and inhibits activation of AMPK/Lamin-B2/MAPK and PI3K/AKT) in combination with CFM 4.17 NLPFs (i.e., CARP-1 signaling and EGFR activity is inhibited by interacting with EGFR's ATP binding site) and TLM (i.e., disrupts tumor stromal barriers and leads to enhanced permeation of drugs) will provide superior anti-cancer effects in NSCLC, and by using RNA sequence and the quantitative proteomics, we can identify novel targets that have a role to play in tumor regression.

2. Materials and Methods

2.1. Materials

CFM 4.17 was synthesized by Otava chemicals (Concord, ON, Canada), DMSO, Tween 80, Ethanol, PBS was obtained from VWR International, LLC, (Radnor, PA, USA). All additional components and reagents were bought from Sigma-Aldrich (St. Louis, MI, USA). Cell Signaling Technology provided all primary and secondary antibodies utilized in our research.

2.2. Formulation of CFM 4.17 Lipid Formulation (CFM-F)

CFM-F was formulated in our laboratory, thereby using an already published procedure that consists of a melt dispersion process (optimized with Design Expert and MATLAB utilizing the Box–Behnken developed surface response methodology). CFM-F showed enhanced efficacy and increased oral bioavailability [6].

2.3. Cell Culture

The NSCLC cell lines H1975 (E746-A750 deletion) and HCC827 were purchased from ATCC. The cells were cultured in RPMI-1640 media with 10% heat-inactivated fetal bovine serum (FBS) and (5000 units/mL penicillin, 5 mg/mL streptomycin, and 10 mg/mL neomycin; GIBCO) at 37 °C in 5% CO_2.

2.4. H1975 Xenograft Model of Non-Small Cell Lung Cancer

The Institutional Animal Use and Care Committee of Florida Agricultural and Mechanical University evaluated and approved all animal experiment procedures as per the NIH standards and all applicable national legislation. Mice were randomly divided into 5 groups, 5 in each group. The H1975 xenograft NSCLC model was developed by injecting 2.5 million H1975 cells (in a 1:1 ratio, suspended in matrigel) into the right flank of athymic female nude mice (Foxn1nu; 20–25 grams' body weight, 5–6 weeks old). When the tumor volume reached 1500 mm^3, the animals were treated for 2 weeks with CFM-F (40 mg/kg body weight) and OSM (25 mg/kg body weight) alone. For the CFM 4.17 solution, TLM, and OSM combination, animals were pre-treated with TLM (10 mg/kg body weight) three times per week, followed by two weeks of CFM4.17-solution (40 mg/kg body weight) and OSM (25 mg/kg body weight). For the TLM, CFM-F, and OSM combination, animals were given TLM (10 mg/kg body weight) three times a week for two weeks before receiving CFM-F (40 mg/kg body weight) and OSM (25 mg/kg body weight) for two weeks. During the course of the drug treatments, tumor volumes were measured twice a week. The digital vernier calliper was used to measure the width and length of the tumor. The formula used to calculate the tumor volume (TV) was: $TV = \frac{1}{2} ab^2$, where 'a' and 'b' denotes the tumor's length and width, respectively. The animals were then monitored regularly for their health and mobility, and when the tumor burden increased beyond 6000 mm^3, the animals were sacrificed, and tumor and blood sample was collected from all animals for proteomic, RNA-seq, and Western blot experiments. Throughout the treatment, the tumor volume was measured twice weekly. The blood samples were further processed to collect the serum, then processed for TotalSeq analysis.

2.5. RNA Sequencing and Data Analysis

The manufacturer's instructions were followed to isolate total RNAs from tumor samples using the Trizol reagent (ThermoFisher, Waltham, MA, USA; 15596018). The DNase I treatment aids in the removal of traces of genomic DNA contamination in the samples. The mRNA library was created using the NEBNext Ultra RNA Library Prep Kit (NEB, E7530) and the NEBNext Poly (A) mRNA Magnetic Isolation Module (NEB, E7490). For quality control, the library was processed on an Agilent Bioanalyzer with HS DNA chip (5067-4626), and the quantification was conducted with the KAPA Library Quantification Kit (KR0405). The library was then pooled at the requisite equal molar concentrations and transferred to the Florida State University (FSU), College of Medicine Translational Laboratory for Illumina NovaSeq 6000 sequencing.

Network Analyst 3.0 software (Guangyan Zhou, Quebec, QC, Canada)was used to analyze the RNA sequencing data; genes with a count of 10%, a variance of 10%, and unannotated were separated and standardized using Log2 counts per million [39]. DEseq2 was used to find the differentially expressed genes [40]. The heatmap aids in the visualization of differentially expressed genes and gene enriched pathways, which may be seen using the same web application. The volcano graphing was conducted using a DESeq2 data set and the log10 (FDR corrected *p*-value) to the log2 (fold change).

2.6. Proteomics

As per the manufacturer's protocol, in-solution digestion was carried out on an S-trap microcolumn (Prod # CO2-micro-80, Protifi). Briefly, 100 µg of lyophilized protein was resuspended in sodium dodecyl sulphate (5%), TEAB (50 mM) pH 8.5 and reduced by adding 1 µL of TCEP (5 mM final concentration) and incubating for 15 min at 55 °C. This was followed by alkylating the mixture by adding 1 µL of alkylating agent (Iodoacetamide, final concentration 20 mM) and incubating at RT in the dark for over 10 min. The mixture was acidified by adding 2.5 µL of phosphoric acid (final concentration ~2.5%) and vortexed thoroughly. Wash/Binding buffer (TEAB-100 mM (final) in 90% methanol, 165 µL) was added to the sample and mixed well. This mixture was transferred onto the S-Trap and placed in a 1.7 mL Eppendorf tube for flow-through (waste). Proteins were trapped onto the column by centrifuging at 4000× *g* for 30 s. Trapped protein was washed thrice with 150 µL of wash buffer (TEAB-100 mM (final) in 90% methanol). To fully remove wash/binding buffer, S-Trap columns were spun at 4000 g for 1 min and transferred to a new 1.7 mL Eppendorf tube for digestion. The protein was digested by adding 5 µg of trypsin in 20 µL of digestion buffer (100 mM TEAB) and incubating the tube at 37 °C overnight. Peptides were eluted sequentially by adding 40 µL of 50 mM TEAB in water, followed by formic acid (0.2%) in purified water and finally 50% acetonitrile in purified water and spinning the column at 4000 g for 1 min. Peptides from elution solution dried in a speed vac and dissolved at 1 µg/µL in formic acid (0.1%) and transferred into auto sampler glass vials.

The peptides were analyzed on an Exploris 480 Orbitrap mass spectrometer (Thermo Fischer Scientific, Bremen, Germany) connected to an Easy-nLC-1200 nanoflow liquid chromatography system (Thermo Scientific). One microgram of the peptide was loaded onto a 2 cm trap column (nanoViper, 3 µm C18 Aq) (Thermo Fisher Scientific). The samples were then analyzed on the 100 C18 HPLC Analytical Column (Acclaim™ PepMap™, 0.075 mm internal diameter, 2 mM C18 particle size, and 150 mm long Cat# 164534) using a 180 min linear gradient of buffer B (90% acetonitrile and 0.1% formic acid) at the flow rate of 300 nL/min. Full MS scans were obtained in the range of 350–1700 m/z at a resolution of 60,000 with a threshold intensity of 5000 and dynamic exclusion of 20 s using the topN method, taking the MS2 of the top 40 ions at 15,000 resolution.

Proteomic raw data were acquired from mass spectrometry by data-dependent acquisition (DDA) method and analyzed by Proteome Discoverer software (Version 2.5,

(Thermo Fisher Scientific, Waltham, MA, USA)) using the Mascot software search engine to search against the uniport homo sapiens database [41,42]. The following criteria were applied to obtain differentially expressed proteins: (a) peptides with peptide score ≥ 10; (b) high protein false discovery rate (FDR) confidence < 0.01; and (c) unique peptides after digestion, and a *p*-value at ≤ 0.05 was used for protein grouping and significantly differentially expressed proteins were identified by setting the threshold fold change value ≥ 1.5. Differentially expressed proteins were organized into different groups with the approach: biological process and molecular functions using Gene Ontology (GO) assignments and Kyoto Encyclopedia of Genes and Genomes (KEGG) pathways by DAVID software [43].

2.7. RNA Isolation

Total RNA was extracted from tissues using TRIzol reagent (Invitrogen, California, USA) and purified using an RNeasy Mini kit (Qiagen, Germantown, MD, USA). Each sample's A260/280 absorbance ratio was measured using a Nanodrop spectrophotometer to evaluate its RNA quality and integrity (ND-1000).

2.8. Reverse Transcription and RT-qPCR

To examine the mRNA levels of specific genes, cDNA synthesis from total RNA was performed according to the manufacturer's instructions using the Maxima H Minus First-strand cDNA Synthesis Kit (Thermo Fisher Scientific, Waltham, MA, USA). Various gene primers (Lamin B2, SOX2, STAT3, NFKB, SOD, MRC-1, and Histone 1 were purchased from Integrated DNA Technologies, Inc. (Redwood City, CA, USA) (Table 1). Quantitative PCR was used to detect gene expression using SsoAdvanced^{TM} Universal SYBR Green Supermix (Bio-Rad) and the CFX96 TouchTM Real-Time PCR Detection System (Bio-Rad Laboratories). Post amplification, a melt curve analysis was used to determine the reaction's specificity. The whole mean expression level of both 18S rRNA and GAPDH genes was used as a reference for comparison when assessing relative mRNA expression using the comparative Ct (ΔCt) technique.

Table 1. Primer list.

Gene	Primer
Lamin B2	F: CGGAGAGTCCTGGATGAGAC
	R: TCTTCTTGGCGCTCTTGTTG
EGFR	F: AACACCCTGGTCTGGAAGTACG
	R: TCGTTGGACAGCCTTCAAGACC
GAPDH	GTCTCCTCTGACTTCAACAGCG
	ACCACCCTGTTGCTGTAGCCAA

2.9. TotalSeq Assay for Serum EVs

A thawed mouse serum sample was then mixed with sterile-filtered PBS (1:1) and centrifuged at 10,000× *g* for 15 min to remove debris. For ultracentrifugation, the collected serum was further diluted with 1 mL PBS (particle-free) and centrifuged for one hour at 100,000× *g*. The serum was further diluted and combined with an 8% polyethylene glycol (PEG) solution for 30 min for the Extra PEG procedure. The pellet was resuspended in PBS after a 3000× *g* centrifugation and purified further with ultracentrifugation at 100,000× *g* for 1 h. They were all resuspended to their original volume to make the ultracentrifuged pellets comparable. The isolated EVs were used for TotalSeq assays.

Protein from the EVs sample was lysed with 0.1 percent SDS for the TotalSeq antibody assay. One microgram of EV protein was blotted onto a nitrocellulose membrane strip. On the same strip, 1 microliter of 2.5% casein blocking buffer (sheared salmon sperm ssDNA (100 g/mL and 0.05 percent tween-20 in PBS) was blotted and air-dried. Then, the strip was placed in a 1.7 mL Eppendorf tube, and a casein-blocking buffer was used for blocking for 1 h at RT. TotalSeq-A antibodies were used in this assay including TotalSeq-A0404 anti-human CD63 Antibody (353035), TotalSeq-A0132 anti-human EGFR Antibody (352923), TotalSeq-A0190 anti-mouse CD274 (PD-L1) Antibody, TotalSeq-A0373 anti-human CD81 (TAPA-1) Antibody (349521) in 100 µL casein blocking solution, a dilution of 1:2000, a TotalSeq-A antibody pool was added and incubated overnight at 4 °C. The strips were washed 5 times with PBST (0.05% tween 20 in PBS) and one time with sterile water. Using absorbent paper, excess liquid was collected from the strip and then transferred to a fresh PCR tube. The extension mix consisted of 1X buffer 2, 1 U Klenow enzyme, dNTP, and 3′-Adaptor (500 nM working concentration). Fifteen microliters extension mix was added to the fresh PCR tube to immerse the strip thoroughly. The PCR tube was then incubated for 5 min at RT before being heat-inactivated for 5 min at 95 °C on an Eppendorf PCR machine. In a 15 µL qPCR experiment, TotalSeq DNA full-length products were measured using TotalSeq forward primer and universal R primer. For all of the TotalSeq antibodies that had been tested, the supernatant was utilized as a qPCR template. In a 15 µL qPCR run, the TotalSeq DNA full-length products were measured using TotalSeq forward primer and universal-R primer [44].

2.10. Western Blot Analysis

The whole-cell lysates were prepared from tissues in radioimmunoassay buffer (RIPA) (Cell Signaling, Danvers, MA, USA), which consists of 1:100 protease and phosphatase inhibitors. The supernatant was recovered after centrifuging the tissue homogenates at 10,000× *g* for 20 min at 4° C. The bicinchoninic acid (BCA) assay was used to estimate protein levels. The samples (40 µg) were loaded on a precast gel with 10% SDS-PAGE (Mini-PROTEAN® TGX™ Precast Gels) at 80 V, 100 mA for 2 h. The proteins were then transferred into the PVDF membrane (Bio-Rad Laboratories, Hercules, CA, USA) and further blocked with 3% BSA PBS-T for 1 h at RT. The blot was then incubated with primary antibody (Table 2, 1:1000) overnight and washed thrice with 10 mL of PBS-T for 10 min. The blot was then incubated for 1 h at room temperature with the secondary antibody (1:8000). The blots were washed three times with PBS-T for ten minutes each time and then incubated with SuperSignal West Pico Chemiluminescent substrate, and pictures were recorded with a Chemidoc. The blots were also quantified using the NIH ImageJ software's densitometry.

Table 2. Antibody list.

S.No	Antibody Name	Company	Catalog No.
1	Lamin B2	Cell Signaling Technology	12255
2	SOD	Cell Signaling Technology	13141
3	SOX2	Cell Signaling Technology	3579
4	EGFR	Cell Signaling Technology	54359
5	AMPK	Cell Signaling Technology	2532
6	TGF-beta	Cell Signaling Technology	3709
7	Bcl2	Cell Signaling Technology	4223
8	Bax	Cell Signaling Technology	5023
9	p38	Cell Signaling Technology	8690
10	P53	Cell Signaling Technology	2527
11	HSC 70	Santa Cruz Biotechnology	sc-7298
12	TSG 101	Cell Signaling Technology	28405
13	CD 63	Cell Signaling Technology	28405
14	Calnexin	Cell Signaling Technology	2679
15	Flotillin-2	Cell Signaling Technology	3436
16	Caveolin-1	Cell Signaling Technology	3267

2.11. Statistical Analysis

The mean ± standard error is used to describe all of the data presented. GraphPad Prism version 5.0 (Dr. Harvey Motulsky, San Diego, CA, USA) was used to evaluate a significant difference between the treatment groups using either a Student *t*-test or a one-way ANOVA. When the one-way ANOVA demonstrated statistical significance, Bonferroni's multiple comparisons test was used for post hoc analysis. Statistical significance was defined as a p-value < 0.05.

3. Results

3.1. Effect of TLM_CFM-F_OSM on Tumor Volume in the In Vivo Mouse Model

After the 14th day post-treatment, TLM_CFM-F_OSM ($p < 0.001$) and TLM_CFM-S_OSM ($p < 0.001$) combination treatment group substantially reduced the tumor volume when compared to the control, as shown in Figure 1. Further, we observed that TLM_CFM-F_OSM demonstrated a superior anti-cancer effect in reducing the tumor burden compared to TLM_CFM-S_OSM ($p < 0.05$). However, when compared to normal control, OSM and CFM-F did reduce the tumor volume ($p < 0.05$) on the 14th day (Figure 1).

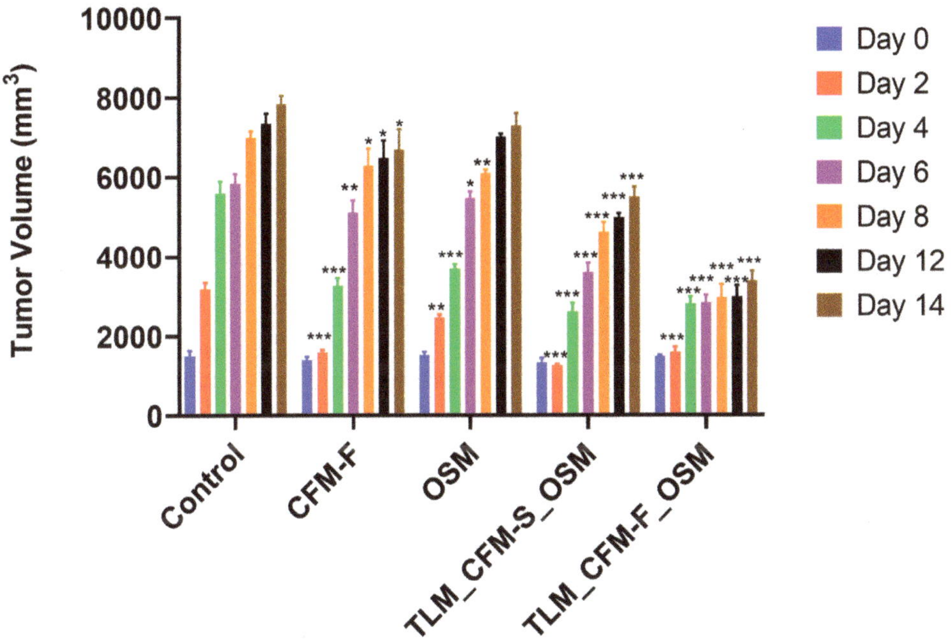

Figure 1. The effect of Telmisartan, CFM-F, and Osimertinib on tumor volume in experimental NSCLC. Histogram demonstrating the H1975 tumor volumes in athymic nude mice after treatment with Osimertinib (OSM), CFM4.17 lipid formulation (CFM-F), CFM4.17 solution (CFM-S), Telmisartan (TLM) and their combinations. Data were represented as the mean ± SD of three separate experiments ($n = 3$). *** $p < 0.001$, ** $p < 0.01$ and * $p < 0.05$ vs. control.

3.2. RNA Sequencing and Differential Gene Expression Analysis in Lung Cancer

When compared to normal control tissue, RNA sequencing suggested differential regulation of numerous genes after various treatments. The determination of differentially expressed genes (p-value < 0.05 and FC > 1.0) between normal control and treated tissues was conducted using a heatmap (Figure 2A), which demonstrated that 950 genes were upregulated, and 1240 were downregulated after treatment. The linkage of biological pathways was determined using the KEGG pathway analysis, demonstrating differentially elevated genes. According to KEGG pathway analysis, differentially expressed genes after therapy were found to be engaged in many pathways, including spliceosome, metabolic, immunological, inflammation, mitochondrial function, apoptosis, RNA transport, and signaling. Among these, metabolic pathways (AMPK), immunological pathways (PD-L1), mitochondrial function (SOD), inflammation pathway (NFKB, STAT3, TGF beta), and apoptotic pathways (Lamin-B2, Macrophage mannose receptor 1) drew our attention because of their significance in cancer mediation shown in Figure 2. RNA seq data revealed that TLM_CFM-F_OSM induces downregulation of Lamin B2, MMP1, EGFR, NFKB, PD-L1, and TGF-beta genes. TLM_CFM-F_OSM treatment induced downregulation of Lamin B2 (i.e., 1.4-fold lower), MMP1 (i.e., 3.6-fold), EGFR (i.e., 1.8-fold), NFKB (i.e., 1.4-fold), PD-L1 (i.e., 3.46-fold), and TGF beta (i.e., 2.33-fold), in comparison to control (Figure 2H–M).

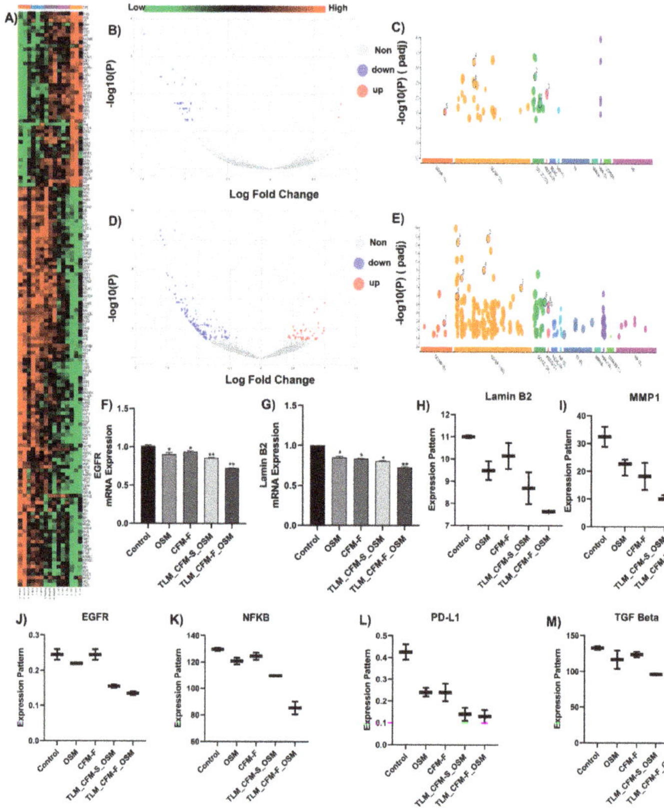

Figure 2. RNA-Seq identified differential mRNA expressions and their RTPCR validation in NSCLC tumor tissues isolated from athymic nude mice (**A**) Heat map illustrations of hierarchical clustering analysis of differentially expressed mRNA in tissues of control and treated H1975 Xenograft mice. Representative volcano plots of differentially expressed genes (DEGs) in between (**B**) control and TLM_CFM-F_OSM groups, (**C**) control and TLM_CFM-S_OSM groups. Representative Gene ontology (GO) and Kyoto Encyclopedia of Genes and Genomes (KEGG) annotation analysis in between (**D**) control and TLM_CFM-F_OSM groups and (**E**) control and TLM_CFM-S_OSM groups. Representative bar graphs show RT-PCR analysis of (**F**) Lamin B2 and (**G**) EGFR. Representative box plots show transcriptomic expressions of (**H**) Lamin B2, (**I**) MMP1, (**J**) EGFR, (**K**) NFKB, (**L**) PD-L1, and (**M**) TGF beta. Data were represented as the mean ± SD of three separate experiments ($n = 3$). ** $p < 0.01$, * $p < 0.05$ vs. control.

3.3. Validation of Differentially Expressed Transcripts via qRT-PCR

We performed qRT-PCR to validate RNA-Seq data and proteomics data. Here, we selected genes that showed a highly differential expression in the treatment group compared to the control group. The qRT-PCR showed that Lamin B2 (i.e., 1.33-fold) and EGFR (1.38-fold) were significantly down-regulated (p < 0.05) in the TLM_CFM-F_OSM group compared with control, not only at the proteome level (Figure 3) but also at the transcriptome level (Figure 2). As compared to the control group, every treatment group (OSM, CFM-F, and TLM_CFM-F_OSM) significantly downregulated the EGFR and Lamin B2 mRNA expression level (p < 0.05) but did not show significant difference across different treatment groups (Figure 2F,G). At the transcriptional level, genes showed variable expression, which would lead to changes in their protein expression.

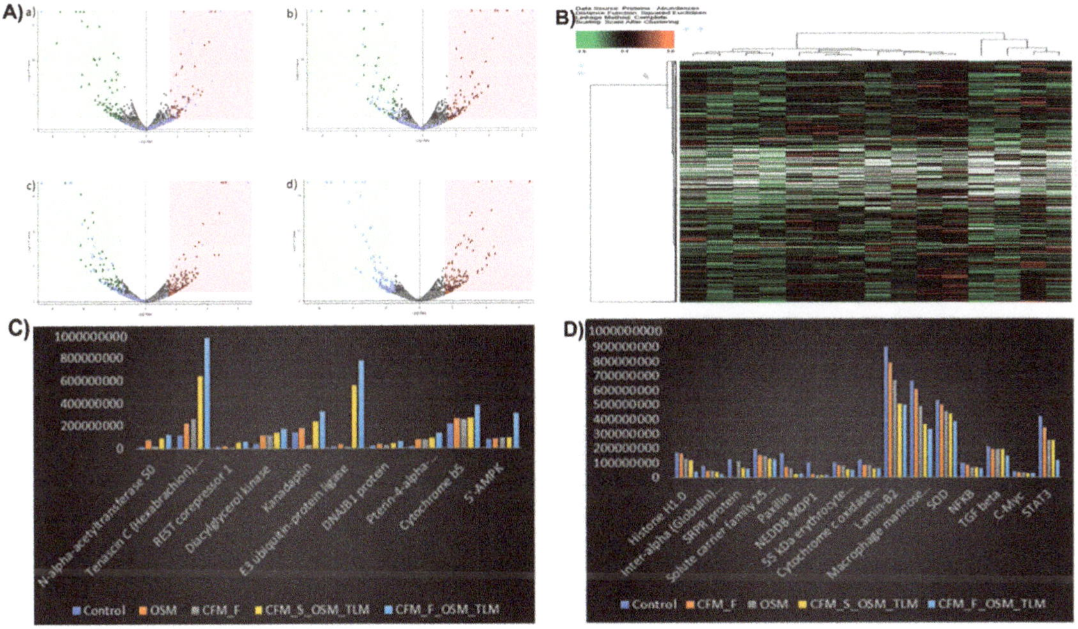

Figure 3. Proteomic identified differentially expressed proteins (DEPs) in lung cancer after treatment. (**A**) Representative Volcano plots of DEPs in between (a) Control and Osimertinib (OSM) groups, (b) Control and CFM4.17 nanolipid formulation (CFM-F), (c) Control and CFM-F_OSM_ telmisartan (TLM) combination, and (d) Control and CFM4.17 solution (CFM-S) OSM_TLM combination (**B**) Representing illustrations of hierarchical clustering analysis of differentially expressed proteins in control and treatment groups and proteins with the highest abundance alterations. (**C**) Schematic representation showing proteins with the largest overall increase in expression and (**D**) the proteins with the greatest reduction in expression upon treatment are represented.

3.4. Proteomics and Differential Gene Expression Analysis in Drug-Treated H1975 Tumors

Briefly, 4299 proteins were identified, and among those, 3948 proteins were quantified under both the control and treatment groups. The statistical significance level was set at p < 0.05 with the treatment/control group (considerably equal or greater than 1.5-fold, adjusted with the p-value). This parameter gave us 212 (down) and 184 (up) proteins in OSM, 175 (down) and 221 (Up) proteins in CFM-F, 214 (down) and 261 (up) proteins in TLM_CFM-F_OSM, 188 (down) and 224 (up) proteins in TLM_CFM_F_OSM when compared with the control (Figure 3A). The quantitative proteome data were used for hierarchical clustering, and the biological functions of H1975 samples are shown in Figure 3B.

The functional alterations in the treatment group were determined using the Kyoto Encyclopedia of Genes and Genomes (KEGG) enrichment analysis. Differentially expressed proteins were organized into different groups using DAVID software. KEGG enrichment analysis software was used to identify differentially expressed proteins (DEPs) and those significantly enriched KEGG pathways (based on p-value). The upregulated and downregulated proteins in the treatment group led to various pathways: spliceosome, metabolic, inflammation, immunological, and RNA transport. Based on all the pathways given, SOD, NFKB, TGF beta, C-Myc, STAT3, Lamin-B2, Macrophage mannose receptor 1, and Histone H1.0 proteins attracted attention, which was also observed in RNA-seq, and they have also been implicated in mediating lung cancer (Table 3).

Table 3. Proteins with high abundance values and role in cancer.

Protein Name	Role in Cancer	Expression in Treatment Group
Histone H1.0	Histone H1.0 overexpression in all cancer cells promotes differentiation during tumor development [45].	Downregulated
Lamin-B2	By upregulating demethylation of histone 3 lysine 9, Lamin B2 increases the malignant phenotype of non-small cell lung cancer cells [46].	Downregulated
Macrophage mannose receptor 1	Tumor-associated macrophages (TAMs) that express the multi-ligand endocytic receptor mannose receptor (CD206/MRC1) have a role in angiogenesis, metastasi, tumor immunosuppression, and recurrence [47].	Downregulated
SOD2	High superoxide dismutase 2 (SOD2) expression is associated with a poor prognosis at many cancer sites, the presence of metastases, and more advanced cancer [48].	Downregulated
NFKB	The oncogenesis process is influenced by the pleiotropic transcription factor NFKB, which upregulates genes involved in cell proliferation, metastasis, apoptosis suppression and angiogenesis [49]	Downregulated
TGF beta	TGF- is the most potent inducer of epithelial-mesenchymal transition in non-small cell lung cancer cells, and it is essential for the establishment of a tumor-promoting microenvironment in lung cancer tissue [50].	Downregulated
STAT3	Many malignancies have constitutively active STAT3, which plays a key role in tumor development and metastasis [51].	Downregulated
AMPK	In cancer, AMPK plays a tumor suppressor role. Activation of AMPK reduces tumor growth by targeting several tumorigenesis-related signaling pathways at various phases of tumor formation [52].	Upregulated

The treatment groups were analyzed individually for differentially expressed proteins with a threshold limit of 1.5-fold change. The conclusive results of the upregulated and downregulated proteins from the treatment groups and the control group are listed in Table 2. Among these, only 4–7% were identified, and differentially expressed proteins were commonly regulated in all the treatment groups and had a high abundance ratio. The high abundance of upregulated proteins is shown in Figure 3C and also the downregulated proteins in Figure 3D. The TLM_CFM-F_OSM group showed significantly downregulated proteins; Lamin B2, Macrophage mannose receptor 1, Histone H1.0, SOD2, TGF-beta, NFKB, C-Myc, STAT3, NEDD8-MDP1, Solute carrier family 25, Paxillin, and Inter-alpha inhibitor H4 as compared to TLM_CFM-S_OSM, CFM-F, OSM, and control group. Among high-abundance upregulated proteins, overexpression of AMPK, REST corepressor 1, DNAJB1 protein, and Cytochrome b5 were more significantly upregulated in the TLM_CFM-F_OSM group as compared to the TLM_CFM-S_OSM, CFM-F, OSM, and control group.

3.5. Combination of TLM_CFM-F_OSM Induces Anti-Cancer Effect via the LAMIN B2/STAT3/NF-κB Signaling Pathways in Lung Cancer

Western blot analysis was performed to evaluate the protein expression of Lamin B2, SOD, STAT3, and NFKB. TLM_CFM-F_OSM treatment group significantly reduced the expression of Lamin B2 when compared to the control ($p < 0.0001$). TLM_CFM-F_OSM significantly downregulated the expression of Lamin B2 as compared to TLM_CFM-S_OSM ($p < 0.01$) and single treatment groups OSM ($p < 0.05$), CFM-F ($p < 0.01$). Further, the TLM_CFM-F_OSM combination significantly decreased the expression of SOD2 ($p < 0.01$), NFκB ($p < 0.0001$), STAT3 ($p < 0.0001$) protein as compared to control and single treatments (CFM-F). Collectively TLM_CFM-F_OSM demonstrated a superior anti-cancer effect, thereby decreasing the protein expression of lamin B2, SOD, STAT3, and NFKB (Figure 4).

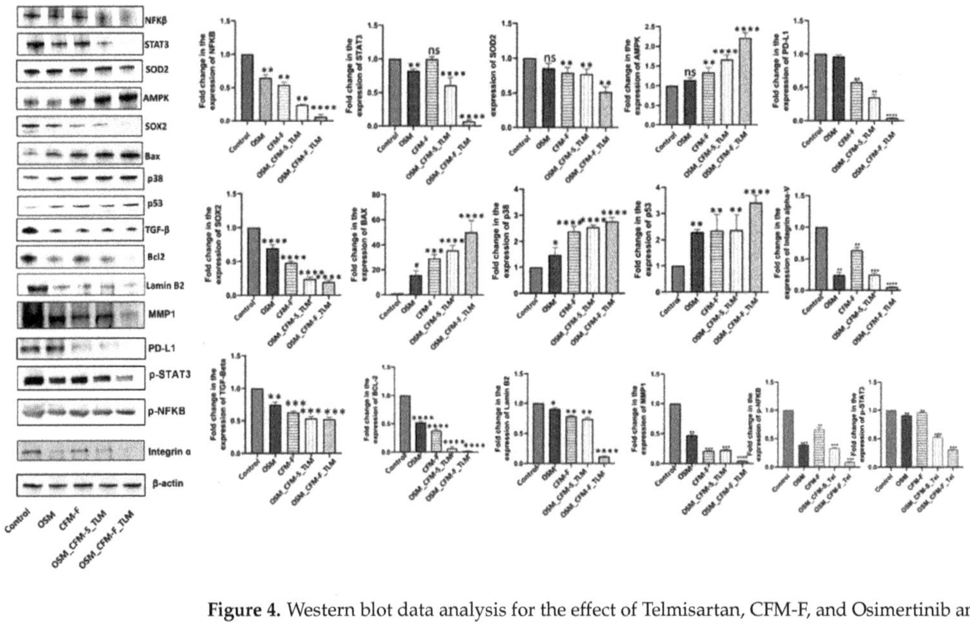

Figure 4. Western blot data analysis for the effect of Telmisartan, CFM-F, and Osimertinib and their combinations against H1975 lung cancer. Western blots and densitometric analysis of various proteins in the H1975 xenograft model of lung cancer. Data are representative of three different experiments and presented as mean, and error bars refer to SEM. ns $p > 0.05$ * $p < 0.05$, ** $p < 0.01$, *** $p < 0.001$, **** $p < 0.0001$ was considered significant when compared to the control.

3.6. Combination of TLM_CFM-F_OSM Reduced the Protein Expression of Lung Cancer Stem Cells, Fibrosis, and Migration

We examined the effects of CFM-F, TLM, and OSM on lung cancer stem cell (SOX2), migration (MMP1), and fibrosis (TGF-β) markers, since cancer stem cells, fibrosis and migration play a certain role in drug resistance development and cancer cell proliferation. It was observed that CFM-F, OSM, and TLM alone groups did not reduce the expression of TGF-β, MMP1, Oct 4, and Sox2 in H1975 lung tumors. The combination of TLM_CFM-F_OSM significantly reduced the protein expression of TGF-β ($p < 0.0001$), Sox2 ($p < 0.0001$), and MMP1 ($p < 0.01$) levels in H1975 xenografts as compared to control and TLM_CFM-S_OSM. Pre-treatment with CFM-F, followed by therapy with OSM, resulted in a significant reduction in the expression of lung cancer stem cell markers, migration, and fibrosis. Pre-treatment with TLM and CFM-F enhanced OSM sensitivity (Figure 4).

3.7. Combination of TLM_CFM-F_OSM Effects on the Protein Expression of Tumor Suppressor Proteins and Apoptotic Proteins

The tumor suppressor proteins (p38 and p53), AMPK, and the Bax protein all appear to affect cell apoptosis susceptibility. The combination of TLM CFM-F OSM significantly enhanced protein expression of p38 ($p < 0.0001$), p53 ($p < 0.0001$), AMPK ($p < 0.0001$) and Bax ($p < 0.0001$) in the H1975 tumors as compared to control. Here, the combination of TLM_CFM-F_OSM leads to the induction of apoptosis by increasing the protein expression of p38, p53, AMPK, and Bax in H1975 lung tumors (Figure 4).

3.8. The Effects of TLM_CFM-F_OSM Combination on Exosomal Markers Expression in H1975 Lung Cancer

Exosomes (EVs) are intercellular messengers that play a key role in cancer formation. CD63, TSG 101, Flotilin-2, calnexin, Syntenin-1, and Caveolin-1 are commonly used exosomal markers. TotalSeq assay from mouse serum EVs revealed that TLM_CFM-F_OSM induced the downregulation of exosomal marker CD63, CD81, and oncogenic proteins (EGFR and PD-L1) in lung cancer, and we further validated these results by checking the protein expression through Western blotting in lung cancer tissues after their respective treatments. Exosomal markers CD63 ($p < 0.0001$), TSG 101 ($p < 0.001$), Flotillin-2 ($p < 0.0001$), Calnexin ($p < 0.0001$), Syntenin-1 ($p < 0.0001$) were significantly downregulated and Caveolin-1 ($p < 0.0001$), HSC 70 ($p < 0.001$) protein expression were significantly upregulated as compared to control group as shown in Figure 5.

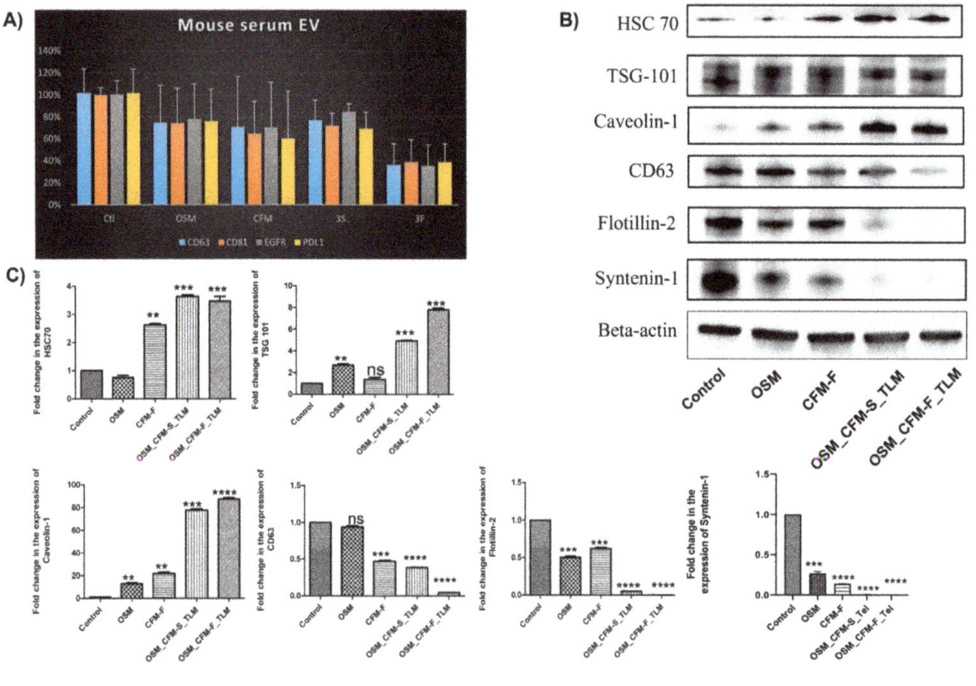

Figure 5. Analysis of exosomal markers in H1975 xenografts and serum samples: (**A**) Bar graph represents the TotalSeq assay in serum samples of H1975 tumor bearing athymic nude mice after treatment with different drugs and their combinations; (**B**) Representative Western blots showing expressions of exosomal protein markers after treatment in H1975 tumor tissue homogenates; (**C**) bar graphs represent the densitometric analysis of respective Western blots. Data represented as three different experiments and presented as mean ± SEM. ns $p > 0.05$ ** $p < 0.01$, and *** $p < 0.001$, **** $p < 0.0001$ was considered significant when compared to control.

4. Discussion

Lung cancer with EGFR gene mutations has been observed in over 15% of NSCLC adenocarcinomas, with a frequency of around 62 percent in Asian populations [4,5,53]. TKIs are the first-line treatment for NSCLC, though resistance can develop due to hyperactivation or mutations in a variety of oncogenic proteins (in various cancers), including EGFR, fibroblast growth factor receptor, BRAF, MET, Anaplastic lymphoma kinase, vascular endothelial growth factor receptor (VEGFR), and tyrosine-protein kinase Src [54–56]. Different EGFR-dependent and EGFR-independent mechanisms are responsible for developing the third-generation OSM (TKI) resistance in EGFR mutant NSCLC, and the molecular mechanisms underlying TKI resistance are still being investigated [57–59]. There is a need to combat OSM resistance in NSCLC, and presently, there are very limited options. Hence, finding new therapeutic targets and treatment options that enhance TKI anti-cancer effects while also overcoming TKI resistance is a critical clinical need for NSCLC. To our knowledge, this is the first study to demonstrate that a combination of TLM, CFM 4.17F, and OSM has anti-cancer potential in H1975 xenografts of athymic nude mice and to understand their mechanisms using proteomics and RNA-seq studies.

The formulation of CFM 4.17 in a lipid formulation has already been established in our laboratory, and we have already demonstrated that a combination of OSM and CFM4.17 formulation inhibited the growth of H1975 cells in vitro more effectively than OSM alone, with an IC_{50} value that was 2-fold lower [6]. We did not conduct any in vitro studies for these studies since we have already published extensively with them in an earlier communication [6].

Our in vivo studies revealed that the TLM_CFM-F_OSM formulation outperformed CFM-F and CFM-S, as well as their combinations with TLM, in terms of reducing tumor burden. Based on our earlier reports, these observations are not surprising but were expected [6]. For example, in our laboratory, we demonstrated that TLM, when used in combination with CFM 4.16 and Sorafenib, significantly enhanced the anti-cancer effects of sorafenib in rociletinib resistant NSCLC xenografts ($p < 0.01$), which was attributed to disrupting tumor-stromal barriers, allowing sorafenib to penetrate deeper into tumors when administered in vivo [35]. However, in the present study, we used RNA-seq and proteomic analysis to uncover molecular changes in genes and proteins in H1975 cells to investigate the possible anti-cancer mode of action of the triple combination (TLM_CFM-F_OSM). RNA-seq (KEGG Pathway) revealed differential regulation of several genes, including metabolic (AMPK), immunological (PD-L1), mitochondrial function (SOD), inflammatory pathways (NFKB, STAT3, TGF beta), and apoptotic pathways (Lamin-B2, Macrophage mannose receptor 1). In the treatment of lung cancers, these pathways are linked to adhesion, invasion, evasion, proliferation, migration, differentiation, angiogenesis, apoptosis, and resistance to growth suppressors. In addition, we performed proteomics in the same samples to confirm the RNA-seq results and identified the upregulated (AMPK, P53, P38 and BAX) and downregulated (Lamin B2, STAT3, BCL2, SOX2, MMP-1, PDL-1, SOD, NFKB, TGF beta, and C-Myc) proteins in a sequence that matched the gene expression pattern shown in RNA sequencing data.

Adenosine monophosphate kinase (AMPK) is a bioenergetic sensor that activates in response to an elevation in the AMP/ATP ratio and is phosphorylated at Thr172 of the catalytic subunit by upstream kinases, such as liver kinase B1 (LKB1) or calmodulin kinase 1 (CAMK1), regulating metabolic homeostasis in the cell [60–63]. AMPK activation has been shown to induce tumor regression in neuroblastoma, B-cell chronic lymphocytic leukemia and breast and prostate cancer cells. This is attributed to the multiple signaling pathways, including mTOR inhibition to block protein synthesis, stabilizing p53, and cyclin-dependent kinase inhibitors to induce cell cycle arrest [64]. Similarly, we observed increased AMPK gene and protein expression levels in H1975 lung cancers in vivo after TLM, OSM, and CFM-F, and their combination showed the most superior efficacy in upregulating AMPK expression. OSM stimulates apoptosis, activating the AMPK pathway in colorectal cancer cells [65]. TLM has been demonstrated to inhibit cell growth by inducing apoptosis in a variety of cancer cell lines, including hepatocellular carcinoma (HLF cells) and gastric cancer (MKN45 cells) [66,67]. Our earlier studies have demonstrated that CFM-1, -4, and -5, CARP-1 functional mimetics, suppressed malignant pleural mesothelioma cell growth by triggering apoptosis in vitro. Further, CFM4.16 has been demonstrated to cause apoptosis via activating pro-apoptotic stress-activated protein kinases (SAPKs) such as p38 and JNK and enhanced CARP-1 production loss of the oncogene c-myc, PARP1 cleavage, and mitotic cyclin B1 [68,69]. However, while CFM 4.17-F treatment increased AMPK expression, the specific mechanism behind its activation of AMPK has to be further investigated through knockdown or knock-in studies. Based on these findings, we hypothesize that TLM_CFM-F_OSM induces apoptosis in H1975 tumors by activating AMPK.

MAPK pathways have been shown to regulate cancer growth and progression by modulating gene expression, mitosis, proliferation, metabolism, and apoptosis [70]. AMPK activity has recently been linked to p38 MAPK in several studies. AICAR, an AMPK activator that activates the p38 MAPK pathway, increases glucose uptake in skeletal muscle, but the p38 MAPK inhibitor did not affect AICAR activation [71]. Furthermore, AMPK phosphorylation of P38 MAPK induces P53 protein in various cancer cells [72]. Many cancer studies have shown that the AMPK/P38/P53 pathway increases apoptosis by regulating the expressions of BAX and caspases [73,74]. In the current study, H1975 xenografts treated with the TLM_CFM-F_OSM combination had higher levels of AMPK, p38, p53, and Bax proteins (Figure 4). Further, TLM_CFM-F_OSM significantly reduced cell proliferation and induced apoptotic cell death in H1975 lung tumors via the AMPK/p38 pathway in a p53-dependent manner compared to other treatments.

The intermediate filaments, known as Lamins, line the inner nuclear membrane, provide structural support for the nucleus and regulate gene expression [75]. Lamin B2 promotes the malignant phenotype of non-small cell lung cancer cells by interacting with micro chromosome maintenance protein 7 and Cyclin D1, both of which increase tumor motility and tumor cell epithelial-mesenchymal transition [76]. In a Drosophila laminopathy model, Chandran et al. demonstrated activating AMPK suppresses Lamin mutations and thus regulates laminopathies [77]. However, the precise relationship found between Lamin B2 and AMPK is unknown in cancer studies, and only very few studies have been conducted to investigate the role of Lamin B2 in cancer progression. The most interesting finding in our study is that Lamin B2 is the most differentially expressed protein and is highly under-expressed in the TLM_CFM-F_OSM combination treatment. Based on these findings, we hypothesize that AMPK activation by TLM_CFM-F_OSM combination controls Lamin B2 expression and thus cell proliferation, migration, and invasion in H1975 tumors.

The pleiotropic transcription factor nuclear factor-κB (NF-κB) influences lung carcinogenesis, thereby upregulating genes involved in cell proliferation, metastasis, cell migration, invasion, and apoptosis suppression [78]. Although tissue heterogeneity exists in lung cancers, the samples collected from the patients always showed an increased level of NF-κB in NSCLC [79]. In line with these findings, we discovered increased NF-κB gene and protein expression levels in H1975 tumors in the current study. Interestingly, the combination of TLM, CFM 4.17, and OSM outperformed their individual treatments in decreasing NF-κB expression in H1975 tumors. In a recent study, Jiang et al. revealed that NCI-H1975/OSM-resistant cells were highly dependent on the NF-κB pathway for survival; the treatment with the NF-κB pathway inhibitor BAY 11-7082 or genetic silencing of p65 resulted in a significantly greater number of cell deaths when compared to parental NCI-H1975/OSM resistant cells [80]. The same study demonstrated that OSM resistance was achieved through TGFβ2-mediated epithelial-mesenchymal transition and NF-κB pathway activation. In our laboratory, we have already demonstrated that CFM-4.16 formulation in combination with sorafenib inhibited the growth of tumor xenografts formed from rociletinib-resistant H1975 NSCLC cells by inhibiting the NF-κB pathway [35] and TLM treatment significantly reduced the inflammatory and hyperproliferative changes in lung tissue after ovalbumin challenge in rats [81]. Based on these findings, we hypothesize that

TLM and the CFM 4.17F increase OSM antitumor effects in H1975 cancers by decreasing NF-κB activity.

TGF-β regulates the proliferation, differentiation, apoptosis, migration, adhesion, immune surveillance, and survival of many cancer cells. According to Mingze ma et al., TGF-β promotes epithelial-mesenchymal transition in A549 human lung cancer cells via the NF-κB/nox4/ROS signaling pathway [82]. In line with these findings, the current study demonstrated considerable TGF-β expression in H1975 tumors and treatment with the TLM_CFM-F_OSM combination significantly reduced its expression in H1975 tumors, as evidenced by Western blotting, RNA sequencing, and proteomics analysis. TLM reduced TGF-β levels in NSCLC lung tumors, which was linked to PPAR-γ activation, VEGF, and MMP-9 inhibition, resulting in more nanoparticle penetration into the tumor [28,31,32]. As a result, TLM, in combination with any other anti-cancer drug, would be more effective in treating metastatic lung cancers. In addition, MMP-9 is involved in lung cancer invasion, metastasis, angiogenesis, and progression [83]. It negatively affects cancer immune modulation via TGF-β activation and intercellular adhesion molecule-1 shedding (ICAM-1) [84]. Indeed, we believe that the TLM_CFM-F_OSM combination's superior anti-cancer properties against NSCLC lung tumors are due to increased TGF-β and MMP-9 expression as well as increased CFM-F penetration into the tumors in this study.

STAT3 is one of the potential therapeutic targets for NSCLC. The level of constitutive STAT3 activation has been linked to lung cancer metastasis, angiogenesis, and resistance to a variety of anti-cancer drugs [85]. The chemotherapeutic sensitivity of OSM against non-small cell lung cancer cells was increased when STAT3 was suppressed by chemically modified siRNAs. STAT3 and NF-κB activation and interaction are crucial in controlling cancer cell-inflammatory cell communication. NF-κB and STAT3 are critical regulators of tumor angiogenesis and invasiveness in pre-neoplastic and malignant lung cancer cells [86]. We noted a significant reduction in STAT3 expression in H1975 tumors post-treatment with the TLM_CFM-F_OSM combination, which is consistent with these reports. Based on these findings, we hypothesize that NF-κB inhibition by the TLM_CFM-F_OSM combination regulates STAT3 expression and thus tumor growth and metastasis in H1975 tumors. Collectively TLM_CFM-F_OSM affects multiple pathways, including the AMPK, NF-κB, Lamin B2, and JAK-STAT pathways, as shown in Figure 6.

EVs from cancer cells contain microRNA, long non-coding RNA, small interfering RNA, DNA, protein, and lipids, which are all being studied for use in cancer diagnosis and treatment [87]. Shimada Y et al. investigated serum exosomal PD-L1 as a quantitative marker for predicting anti-PD-1 response and evaluating clinical outcomes in NSCLC patients [88]. In line with this study, EV markers from NSCLC tumors and serum showed significantly lower levels of exosomal markers (CD63, CD81, EGFR, and PD-L1) after treatment with the TLM_CFM-F_OSM combination in the present study. According to a growing body of evidence, EVs derived from NSCLC tumors also increased PD-L1 expression and, thus, tumor development, decreased CD8+ T-cell function, and induced CD8+ T cell death [89]. Furthermore, exosomal wild-type EGFR has been shown to cause OSM resistance in NSCLC (H1975) cancers [90], and exosomal EGFR was downregulated in this study by TLM_CFM-F_OSM treatment, suggesting that combination treatment affecting exosomal PD-L1 and EGFR expression could be helpful in reversing NSCLC tumor growth and OSM resistance.

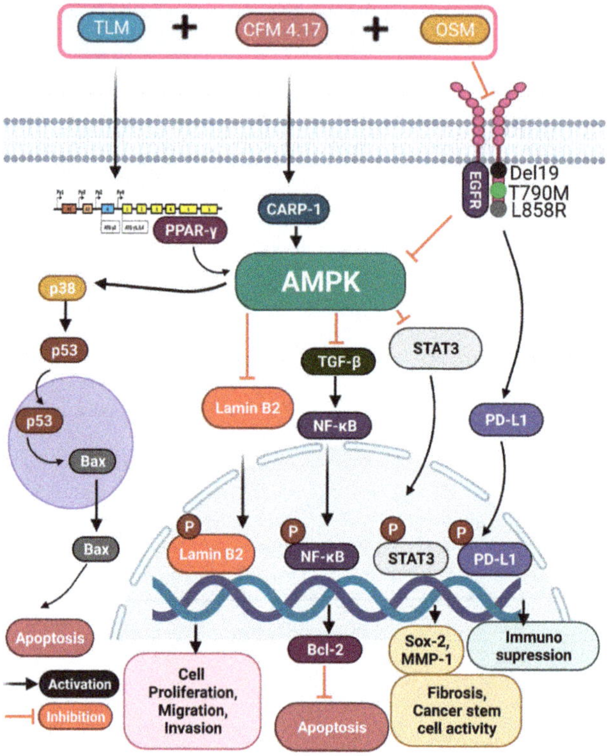

Figure 6. Plausible mechanism of action of CFM4.17, Telmisartan and Osimertinib combination against non-small cell lung cancers in athymic nude mice. Telmisartan activates the PPAR-γ nuclear receptor, CFM4.17 acts on CARP-1, and Osimertinib inhibits the EGFR mutated gene, increasing AMPK activity and thus regulating the p38 MAPkinase pathway, Lamin B2 protein, JAK-STAT pathway, PDL-1, and NF-κB pathway to maintain apoptosis, cancer metastasis, and immune suppression. Bcl-2: B-cell lymphoma 2, Bax: BCL2-associated X protein, CARP-1: Cell cycle and apoptosis regulatory protein 1, EGFR: epidermal growth factor receptor, CFM-F: lipid formulation of CFM4.17, MMP-1: Matrix metalloproteinase-1, OSM: Osimertinib, PD-L1: Programmed cell death 1 ligand 1, STAT3: Signal transducer and activator of transcription 3, SOX2: SRY-Box Transcription Factor 2, TLM: Telmisartan.

5. Conclusions

TLM_CFM-F_OSM showed a significant anti-cancer effect against H1975 tumor xenografts in athymic nude mice. Further, our in vivo studies with H1975 lung cancer cells demonstrated that this combination is effective through multiple pathways, including AMPK, NF-κB, Lamin B2, and JAK-STAT, which regulates mitochondrial homeostasis, inflammation, oxidative stress, and apoptosis. One novel mechanism of this triple combination in reducing the tumor burden of H1975 xenografts was the effect on serum exosome production and PDL1 and EGFR expressions. In addition, extensive molecular research is required to identify the specific molecular targets of these anti-cancer drugs for lung cancer treatment.

Author Contributions: R.N. and A.K.K. designed, performed, and analyzed the results and wrote the manuscript. N.P., S.K.S., L.S., A.B., N.K., E.N., R.S., P.A. and A.N. performed part of the experimental work and/or analyzed the results. D.G.M.J. performed TotalSeq assay from mouse serum EVs. M.S. conceptualized the study, wrote, and revised the manuscript. All authors have read and agreed to the published version of the manuscript.

Funding: National Institute on Minority Health and Health disparities (National Institutes of Health), Grant/Award Number: U54 MD007582 and NSF-CREST Center for Complex Materials Design for Multidimensional Additive Processing (CoManD), Grant/Award Number: 1735968 for providing the funding for this research work.

Institutional Review Board Statement: The animal study was conducted according to the guidelines of the NIH, and approved by the Institutional Animal Use and Care Committee of Florida Agricultural and Mechanical University (**020-07** and 10 December 2021).

Informed Consent Statement: Not applicable.

Data Availability Statement: The data that support the findings of this study are available on request from the corresponding author.

Acknowledgments: We thank the Florida A&M University and Florida State University for providing all kind of support, resources and excellent infrastructure to carry out this research work.

Conflicts of Interest: The authors declare that there are no conflict of interest.

References

1. Siegel, R.L.; Miller, K.D.; Goding Sauer, A.; Fedewa, S.A.; Butterly, L.F.; Anderson, J.C.; Cercek, A.; Smith, R.A.; Jemal, A. Colorectal cancer statistics, 2020. *CA Cancer J. Clin.* **2020**, *70*, 145–164. [CrossRef] [PubMed]
2. Cruz, C.S.D.; Tanoue, L.T.; Matthay, R.A. Lung cancer: Epidemiology, etiology, and prevention. *Clin. Chest Med.* **2011**, *32*, 605–644. [CrossRef] [PubMed]
3. Mitsudomi, T.; Morita, S.; Yatabe, Y.; Negoro, S.; Okamoto, I.; Tsurutani, J.; Seto, T.; Satouchi, M.; Tada, H.; Hirashima, T.; et al. Gefitinib versus cisplatin plus docetaxel in patients with non-small-cell lung cancer harbouring mutations of the epidermal growth factor receptor (WJTOG3405): An open label, randomised phase 3 trial. *Lancet Oncol.* **2009**, *11*, 121–128. [CrossRef]
4. Rosell, R.; Moran, T.; Queralt, C.; Porta, R.; Cardenal, F.; Camps, C.; Majem, M.; Lopez-Vivanco, G.; Isla, D.; Provencio, M.; et al. Screening for Epidermal Growth Factor Receptor Mutations in Lung Cancer. *N. Engl. J. Med.* **2009**, *361*, 958–967. [CrossRef] [PubMed]
5. D'Angelo, S.P.; Pietanza, M.C.; Johnson, M.L.; Riely, G.J.; Miller, V.A.; Sima, C.S.; Zakowski, M.F.; Rusch, V.W.; Ladanyi, M.; Kris, M.G. Incidence of *EGFR* Exon 19 Deletions and L858R in Tumor Specimens From Men and Cigarette Smokers with Lung Adenocarcinomas. *J. Clin. Oncol.* **2011**, *29*, 2066–2070. [CrossRef]
6. Kommineni, N.; Nottingham, E.; Bagde, A.; Patel, N.; Rishi, A.K.; Dev, S.R.; Singh, M. Role of nano-lipid formulation of CARP-1 mimetic, CFM-4.17 to improve systemic exposure and response in OSM resistant non-small cell lung cancer. *Eur. J. Pharm. Biopharm.* **2021**, *158*, 172–184. [CrossRef]
7. Tan, C.-S.; Gilligan, D.; Pacey, S.C. Treatment approaches for EGFR-inhibitor-resistant patients with non-small-cell lung cancer. *Lancet Oncol.* **2015**, *16*, e447–e459. [CrossRef]
8. Thress, K.S.; Paweletz, C.P.; Felip, E.; Cho, B.C.; Stetson, D.; Dougherty, B.; Lai, Z.; Markovets, A.; Vivancos, A.; Kuang, Y.; et al. Acquired EGFR C797S mutation mediates resistance to AZD9291 in non–small cell lung cancer harboring EGFR T790M. *Nat. Med.* **2015**, *21*, 560–562. [CrossRef]
9. Cross, D.; D'Cruz, C.; Eberlein, C.; Spitzler, P.; Ichihara, E.; Meador, C.; Ashton, S.; Mellor, M.; Stewart, R.; Smith, P.; et al. Targeting Resistance in Egfr-Mutant Non-Small Cell Lung Cancer (Nsclc): Preclinical Evidence Supporting the Combination of Egfr Tyrosine Kinase Inhibitors (Tkis) Azd9291 and Gefitinib with Molecularly Targeted Agents and Immunotherapeutics. *Ann. Oncol.* **2014**, *25*, iv155. [CrossRef]
10. Patel, A.R.; Chougule, M.; Singh, M. EphA2 targeting pegylated nanocarrier drug delivery system for treatment of lung cancer. *Pharm. Res.* **2014**, *31*, 2796–2809. [CrossRef]
11. Ichite, N.; Chougule, M.; Patel, A.R.; Jackson, T.; Safe, S.; Singh, M. Inhalation delivery of a novel diindolylmethane derivative for the treatment of lung cancer. *Mol. Cancer Ther.* **2010**, *9*, 3003–3014. [CrossRef] [PubMed]
12. Chougule, M.B.; Patel, A.; Sachdeva, P.; Jackson, T.; Singh, M. Enhanced anticancer activity of gemcitabine in combination with noscapine via antiangiogenic and apoptotic pathway against non-small cell lung cancer. *PLoS ONE* **2011**, *6*, e27394. [CrossRef] [PubMed]
13. Singh, M.; Ferdous, A.J.; Jackson, T.L. Stealth monensin liposomes as a potentiator of adriamycin in cancer treatment. *J. Control. Release* **1999**, *59*, 43–53. [CrossRef]
14. Fulzele, S.V.; Shaik, M.S.; Chatterjee, A.; Singh, M. Anti-cancer effect of celecoxib and aerosolized docetaxel against human non-small cell lung cancer cell line, A549. *J. Pharm. Pharmacol.* **2006**, *58*, 327–336. [CrossRef] [PubMed]

15. Patel, A.R.; Chougule, M.B.; Townley, I.; Patlolla, R.; Wang, G.; Singh, M. Efficacy of aerosolized celecoxib encapsulated nanostructured lipid carrier in non-small cell lung cancer in combination with docetaxel. *Pharm. Res.* **2013**, *30*, 1435–1446. [CrossRef] [PubMed]
16. Haynes, A.; Shaik, M.S.; Chatterjee, A.; Singh, M. Evaluation of an aerosolized selective COX-2 inhibitor as a potentiator of doxorubicin in a non-small-cell lung cancer cell line. *Pharm. Res.* **2003**, *20*, 1485–1495. [CrossRef]
17. Verma, V.; Simone, C.B.; Werner-Wasik, M. Acute and late toxicities of concurrent chemoradiotherapy for locally-advanced non-small cell lung cancer. *Cancers* **2017**, *9*, 120. [CrossRef]
18. Sun, G.; Rong, D.; Li, Z.; Sun, G.; Wu, F.; Li, X.; Cao, H.; Cheng, Y.; Tang, W.; Sun, Y. Role of Small Molecule Targeted Compounds in Cancer: Progress, Opportunities, and Challenges. *Front. Cell Dev. Biol.* **2021**, *9*, 2043. [CrossRef]
19. Zhang, H. OSM making a breakthrough in lung cancer targeted therapy. *OncoTargets Ther.* **2016**, *9*, 5489. [CrossRef]
20. Puliyappadamba, V.T.; Wu, W.; Bevis, D.; Zhang, L.; Polin, L.; Kilkuskie, R.; Finley, R., Jr.; Larsen, S.D.; Levi, E.; Miller, F.R.; et al. Antagonists of Anaphase-promoting Complex (APC)-2-Cell Cycle and Apoptosis Regulatory Protein (CARP)-1 Interaction Are Novel Regulators of Cell Growth and Apoptosis. *J. Biol. Chem.* **2011**, *286*, 38000–38017. [CrossRef]
21. Lehman, N.L.; Tibshirani, R.; Hsu, J.Y.; Natkunam, Y.; Harris, B.T.; West, R.B.; Masek, A.; Montgomery, K.; van de Rijn, M.; Jackson, P.K. Oncogenic Regulators and Substrates of the Anaphase Promoting Complex/Cyclosome Are Frequently Overexpressed in Malignant Tumors. *Am. J. Pathol.* **2007**, *170*, 1793–1805. [CrossRef] [PubMed]
22. Muthu, M.; Cheriyan, V.T.; Rishi, A.K. CARP-1/CCAR1: A biphasic regulator of cancer cell growth and apoptosis. *Oncotarget* **2015**, *6*, 6499. [CrossRef] [PubMed]
23. Ding, H.-W.; Deng, C.-L.; Li, D.-D.; Liu, D.-D.; Chai, S.-M.; Wang, W.; Zhang, Y.; Chen, K.; Li, X.; Wang, J.; et al. Design, synthesis and biological evaluation of novel 4-aminoquinazolines as dual target inhibitors of EGFR-PI3Kα. *Eur. J. Med. Chem.* **2018**, *146*, 460–470. [CrossRef] [PubMed]
24. Swick, A.D.; Prabakaran, P.J.; Miller, M.C.; Javaid, A.M.; Fisher, M.M.; Sampene, E.; Ong, I.M.; Hu, R.; Iida, M.; Nickel, K.P.; et al. Cotargeting mTORC and EGFR Signaling as a Therapeutic Strategy in HNSCC. *Mol. Cancer Ther.* **2017**, *16*, 1257–1268. [CrossRef]
25. Marcucci, F.; Corti, A. How to improve exposure of tumor cells to drugs—Promoter drugs increase tumor uptake and penetration of effector drugs. *Adv. Drug Deliv. Rev.* **2012**, *64*, 53–68. [CrossRef]
26. Chauhan, V.P.; Martin, J.D.; Liu, H.; Lacorre, D.A.; Jain, S.R.; Kozin, S.V.; Stylianopoulos, T.; Mousa, A.S.; Han, X.; Adstamongkonkul, P.; et al. Angiotensin inhibition enhances drug delivery and potentiates chemotherapy by decompressing tumour blood vessels. *Nat. Commun.* **2013**, *4*, 2516. [CrossRef] [PubMed]
27. Curnis, F.; Sacchi, A.; Corti, A. Improving chemotherapeutic drug penetration in tumors by vascular targeting and barrier alteration. *J. Clin. Investig.* **2002**, *110*, 475–482. [CrossRef] [PubMed]
28. Godugu, C.; Patel, A.R.; Doddapaneni, R.; Marepally, S.; Jackson, T.; Singh, M. Inhalation delivery of Telmisartan enhances intratumoral distribution of nanoparticles in lung cancer models. *J. Control. Release* **2013**, *172*, 86–95. [CrossRef]
29. Patel, K.; Doddapaneni, R.; Chowdhury, N.; Boakye, C.H.; Behl, G.; Singh, M. Tumor stromal disrupting agent enhances the anticancer efficacy of docetaxel loaded PEGylated liposomes in lung cancer. *Nanomedicine* **2016**, *11*, 1377–1392. [CrossRef]
30. Chen, Q.; Liu, G.; Liu, S.; Su, H.; Wang, Y.; Li, J.; Luo, C. Remodeling the Tumor Microenvironment with Emerging Nanotherapeutics. *Trends Pharmacol. Sci.* **2018**, *39*, 59–74. [CrossRef]
31. Green, R.; Howell, M.; Khalil, R.; Nair, R.; Yan, J.; Foran, E.; Katiri, S.; Banerjee, J.; Singh, M.; Bharadwaj, S.; et al. Actinomycin D and Telmisartan Combination Targets Lung Cancer Stem Cells Through the Wnt/Beta Catenin Pathway. *Sci. Rep.* **2019**, *9*, 18177. [CrossRef] [PubMed]
32. Patel, K.; Doddapaneni, R.; Sekar, V.; Chowdhury, N.; Singh, M. Combination approach of YSA peptide anchored docetaxel stealth liposomes with oral antifibrotic agent for the treatment of lung cancer. *Mol. Pharm.* **2016**, *13*, 2049–2058. [CrossRef] [PubMed]
33. Li, J.; Chen, L.; Yu, P.; Liu, B.; Zhu, J.; Yang, Y. Telmisartan exerts anti-tumor effects by activating peroxisome proliferator-activated receptor-γ in human lung adenocarcinoma A549 cells. *Molecules* **2014**, *19*, 2862–2876. [CrossRef] [PubMed]
34. Zhang, S.; Wang, Y. Telmisartan inhibits NSCLC A549 cell proliferation and migration by regulating the PI3K/AKT signaling pathway. *Oncol. Lett.* **2018**, *15*, 5859–5864. [CrossRef]
35. Surapaneni, S.K.; Nottingham, E.; Mondal, A.; Patel, N.; Arthur, P.; Gebeyehu, A.; Kalvala, A.K.; Rishi, A.K.; Singh, M. Telmisartan Facilitates the Anticancer Effects of CARP-1 Functional Mimetic and Sorafenib in Rociletinib Resistant Non-small Cell Lung Cancer. *Anticancer Res.* **2021**, *41*, 4215–4228. [CrossRef]
36. Collins, I.; Workman, P. New approaches to molecular cancer therapeutics. *Nat. Chem. Biol.* **2006**, *2*, 689–700. [CrossRef]
37. Leonetti, A.; Sharma, S.; Minari, R.; Perego, P.; Giovannetti, E.; Tiseo, M. Resistance mechanisms to OSM in EGFR-mutated non-small cell lung cancer. *Br. J. Cancer* **2019**, *121*, 725–737. [CrossRef]
38. Cho, W.C. Proteomics technologies and challenges. *Genom. Proteom. Bioinform.* **2007**, *5*, 77–85. [CrossRef]
39. Zhou, G.; Soufan, O.; Ewald, J.; Hancock, R.E.; Basu, N.; Xia, J. NetworkAnalyst 3.0: A visual analytics platform for comprehensive gene expression profiling and meta-analysis. *Nucleic Acids Res.* **2019**, *47*, W234–W241. [CrossRef]
40. Love, M.I.; Huber, W.; Anders, S. Moderated estimation of fold change and dispersion for RNA-seq data with DESeq2. *Genome Biol.* **2014**, *15*, 550. [CrossRef]
41. Orsburn, B.C. Proteome Discoverer—A Community Enhanced Data Processing Suite for Protein Informatics. *Proteomes* **2021**, *9*, 15. [CrossRef] [PubMed]
42. Simpson, H. The MASCOT method. *Softw. Eng. J.* **1986**, *1*, 103–120. [CrossRef]

43. Huang, D.W.; Sherman, B.T.; Tan, Q.; Collins, J.R.; Alvord, W.G.; Roayaei, J.; Stephens, R.; Baseler, M.W.; Lane, H.C.; Lempicki, R.A. The DAVID Gene Functional Classification Tool: A novel biological module-centric algorithm to functionally analyze large gene lists. *Genome Biol.* **2007**, *8*, R183. [CrossRef] [PubMed]
44. Sun, L.; Meckes, D.G. Multiplex protein profiling method for extracellular vesicle protein detection. *Sci. Rep.* **2021**, *11*, 12477. [CrossRef]
45. Di Liegro, C.M.; Schiera, G.; Di Liegro, I. H1. 0 linker histone as an epigenetic regulator of cell proliferation and differentiation. *Genes* **2018**, *9*, 310. [CrossRef]
46. Zhang, M.-Y.; Han, Y.-C.; Han, Q.; Liang, Y.; Luo, Y.; Wei, L.; Yan, T.; Yang, Y.; Liu, S.-L.; Wang, E.-H. Lamin B2 promotes the malignant phenotype of non-small cell lung cancer cells by upregulating dimethylation of histone 3 lysine 9. *Exp. Cell Res.* **2020**, *393*, 112090. [CrossRef]
47. Kielbassa, K.; Vegna, S.; Ramirez, C.; Akkari, L. Understanding the origin and diversity of macrophages to tailor their targeting in solid cancers. *Front. Immunol.* **2019**, *10*, 2215. [CrossRef]
48. Talarico, M.; Nunes, R.; Silva, G.; Costa, L.; Cardoso, M.; Esteves, S.; Sarian, L.Z.; Zeferino, L.; Termini, L. High Expression of SOD2 Protein Is a Strong Prognostic Factor for Stage IIIB Squamous Cell Cervical Carcinoma. *Antioxidants* **2021**, *10*, 724. [CrossRef]
49. Xia, Y.; Shen, S.; Verma, I.M. NF-κB, an active player in human cancers. *Cancer Immunol. Res.* **2014**, *2*, 823–830. [CrossRef]
50. Syed, V. TGF-β Signaling in Cancer. *J. Cell. Biochem.* **2016**, *117*, 1279–1287. [CrossRef]
51. Zou, S.; Tong, Q.; Liu, B.; Huang, W.; Tian, Y.; Fu, X. Targeting STAT3 in cancer immunotherapy. *Mol. Cancer* **2020**, *19*, 145. [CrossRef] [PubMed]
52. Wang, Z.; Wang, N.; Liu, P.; Xie, X. AMPK and Cancer. *AMP-Act. Protein Kinase* **2016**, 203–226. [CrossRef]
53. Collisson, E.; Campbell, J.; Brooks, A.; Berger, A.; Lee, W.; Chmielecki, J.; Beer, D.; Cope, L.; Creighton, C.; Ding, L. Comprehensive molecular profiling of lung adenocarcinoma: The cancer genome atlas research network. *Nature* **2014**, *511*, 543–550.
54. Rosenzweig, S.A. Acquired resistance to drugs targeting tyrosine kinases. *Adv. Cancer Res.* **2018**, *138*, 71–98. [PubMed]
55. Wang, S.; Song, Y.; Yan, F.; Liu, D. Mechanisms of resistance to third-generation EGFR tyrosine kinase inhibitors. *Front. Med.* **2016**, *10*, 383–388. [CrossRef]
56. Botting, G.M.; Rastogi, I.; Chhabra, G.; Nlend, M.; Puri, N. Mechanism of resistance and novel targets mediating resistance to EGFR and c-Met tyrosine kinase inhibitors in non-small cell lung cancer. *PLoS ONE* **2015**, *10*, e0136155. [CrossRef] [PubMed]
57. Walter, A.O.; Sjin, R.T.T.; Haringsma, H.J.; Ohashi, K.; Sun, J.; Lee, K.; Dubrovskiy, A.; Labenski, M.; Zhu, Z.; Wang, Z.; et al. Discovery of a Mutant-Selective Covalent Inhibitor of EGFR that Overcomes T790M-Mediated Resistance in NSCLC. *Cancer Discov.* **2013**, *3*, 1404–1415. [CrossRef] [PubMed]
58. Tung, Y.-C.; Hsiao, A.Y.; Allen, S.G.; Torisawa Y-s Ho, M.; Takayama, S. High-throughput 3D spheroid culture and drug testing using a 384 hanging drop array. *Analyst* **2011**, *136*, 473–478. [CrossRef]
59. Cheriyan, V.T.; Alsaab, H.; Sekhar, S.; Venkatesh, J.; Mondal, A.; Vhora, I.; Sau, S.; Muthu, M.; Polin, L.A.; Levi, E.; et al. A CARP-1 functional mimetic compound is synergistic with BRAF-targeting in non-small cell lung cancers. *Oncotarget* **2018**, *9*, 29680–29697. [CrossRef]
60. Sanders, M.J.; Grondin, P.O.; Hegarty, B.D.; Snowden, M.A.; Carling, D. Investigating the mechanism for AMP activation of the AMP-activated protein kinase cascade. *Biochem. J.* **2007**, *403*, 139–148. [CrossRef]
61. Suter, M.; Riek, U.; Tuerk, R.; Schlattner, U.; Wallimann, T.; Neumann, D. Dissecting the role of 5′-AMP for allosteric stimulation, activation, and deactivation of AMP-activated protein kinase. *J. Biol. Chem.* **2006**, *281*, 32207–32216. [CrossRef] [PubMed]
62. Woods, A.; Johnstone, S.R.; Dickerson, K.; Leiper, F.C.; Fryer, L.G.; Neumann, D.; Schlattner, U.; Wallimann, T.; Carlson, M.; Carling, D. LKB1 is the upstream kinase in the AMP-activated protein kinase cascade. *Curr. Biol.* **2003**, *13*, 2004–2008. [CrossRef] [PubMed]
63. Shaw, R.J.; Kosmatka, M.; Bardeesy, N.; Hurley, R.L.; Witters, L.A.; DePinho, R.A.; Cantley, L.C. The tumor suppressor LKB1 kinase directly activates AMP-activated kinase and regulates apoptosis in response to energy stress. *Proc. Natl. Acad. Sci. USA* **2004**, *101*, 3329–3335. [CrossRef] [PubMed]
64. Hawley, S.A.; Boudeau, J.; Reid, J.L.; Mustard, K.J.; Udd, L.; Mäkelä, T.P.; Alessi, D.R.; Hardie, D.G. Complexes between the LKB1 tumor suppressor, STRADα/β and MO25α/β are upstream kinases in the AMP-activated protein kinase cascade. *J. Biol.* **2003**, *2*, 28. [CrossRef]
65. Motoshima, H.; Goldstein, B.J.; Igata, M.; Araki, E. AMPK and cell proliferation–AMPK as a therapeutic target for atherosclerosis and cancer. *J. Physiol.* **2006**, *574*, 63–71. [CrossRef] [PubMed]
66. Jin, P.; Jiang, J.; Xie, N.; Zhou, L.; Huang, Z.; Zhang, L.; Qin, S.; Fu, S.; Peng, L.; Gao, W.; et al. MCT1 relieves OSM-induced CRC suppression by promoting autophagy through the LKB1/AMPK signaling. *Cell Death Dis.* **2019**, *10*, 615. [CrossRef] [PubMed]
67. Hwang, Y.-J.; Park, J.-H.; Cho, D.-H. Activation of AMPK by Telmisartan Decreases Basal and PDGF-stimulated VSMC Proliferation via Inhibiting the mTOR/p70S6K Signaling Axis. *J. Korean Med. Sci.* **2020**, *35*, e289. [CrossRef]
68. Oura, K.; Tadokoro, T.; Fujihara, S.; Morishita, A.; Chiyo, T.; Samukawa, E.; Yamana, Y.; Fujita, K.; Sakamoto, T.; Nomura, T.; et al. Telmisartan inhibits hepatocellular carcinoma cell proliferation in vitro by inducing cell cycle arrest. *Oncol. Rep.* **2017**, *38*, 2825–2835. [CrossRef]

69. Jamal, S.; Cheriyan, V.T.; Muthu, M.; Munie, S.; Levi, E.; Ashour, A.; Pass, H.I.; Wali, A.; Singh, M.; Rishi, A.K. CARP-1 Functional Mimetics Are a Novel Class of Small Molecule Inhibitors of Malignant Pleural Mesothelioma Cells. *PLoS ONE* **2014**, *9*, e89146. [CrossRef]
70. Dhillon, A.S.; Hagan, S.; Rath, O.; Kolch, W. MAP kinase signalling pathways in cancer. *Oncogene* **2007**, *26*, 3279–3290. [CrossRef]
71. Nader, N.; Ng, S.S.M.; Lambrou, G.I.; Pervanidou, P.; Wang, Y.; Chrousos, G.P.; Kino, T. AMPK regulates metabolic actions of glucocorticoids by phosphorylating the glucocorticoid receptor through p38 MAPK. *Mol. Endocrinol.* **2010**, *24*, 1748–1764. [CrossRef] [PubMed]
72. Lee, C.-W.; Wong, L.L.-Y.; Tse, E.Y.-T.; Liu, H.-F.; Leong, V.Y.-L.; Lee, J.M.-F.; Hardie, D.G.; Ng, I.O.-L.; Ching, Y.-P. AMPK Promotes p53 Acetylation via Phosphorylation and Inactivation of SIRT1 in Liver Cancer Cells. *Cancer Res.* **2012**, *72*, 4394–4404. [CrossRef] [PubMed]
73. Porras, A.; Zuluaga, S.; Black, E.; Valladares, A.; Álvarez, A.M.; Ambrosino, C.; Benito, M.; Nebreda, A.R. p38α Mitogen-activated Protein Kinase Sensitizes Cells to Apoptosis Induced by Different Stimuli. *Mol. Biol. Cell* **2004**, *15*, 922–933. [CrossRef] [PubMed]
74. Taylor, C.A.; Zheng, Q.; Liu, Z.; Thompson, J.E. Role of p38 and JNK MAPK signaling pathways and tumor suppressor p53 on induction of apoptosis in response to Ad-eIF5A1 in A549 lung cancer cells. *Mol. Cancer* **2013**, *12*, 35. [CrossRef] [PubMed]
75. Naetar, N.; Ferraioli, S.; Foisner, R. Lamins in the nuclear interior— life outside the lamina. *J. Cell Sci.* **2017**, *130*, 2087–2096. [CrossRef] [PubMed]
76. Ma, Y.; Fei, L.; Zhang, M.; Zhang, W.; Liu, X.; Wang, C.; Luo, Y.; Zhang, H.; Han, Y. Lamin B2 binding to minichromosome maintenance complex component 7 promotes non-small cell lung carcinogenesis. *Oncotarget* **2017**, *8*, 104813–104830. [CrossRef] [PubMed]
77. Chandran, S.; Suggs, J.A.; Wang, B.J.; Han, A.; Bhide, S.; Cryderman, D.E.; Moore, S.A.; Bernstein, S.I.; Wallrath, L.L.; Melkani, G.C. Suppression of myopathic lamin mutations by muscle-specific activation of AMPK and modulation of downstream signaling. *Hum. Mol. Genet.* **2019**, *28*, 351–371. [CrossRef]
78. Baud, V.; Karin, M. Is NF-κB a good target for cancer therapy? Hopes and pitfalls. *Nat. Rev. Drug Discov.* **2009**, *8*, 33–40. [CrossRef]
79. Basseres, D.; Baldwin, A. Nuclear factor-κ B and inhibitor of κ B kinase pathways in oncogenic initiation and progression. *Oncogene* **2006**, *25*, 6817–6830. [CrossRef]
80. Jiang, X.-M.; Xu, Y.-L.; Yuan, L.-W.; Huang, M.-Y.; Ye, Z.-H.; Su, M.-X.; Chen, X.P.; Zhu, H.; Ye, R.D.; Lu, J.J. TGFβ2-mediated epithelial–mesenchymal transition and NF-κB pathway activation contribute to OSM resistance. *Acta Pharmacol. Sin.* **2021**, *42*, 451–459. [CrossRef]
81. Abdel-Fattah, M.M.; Salama, A.A.; Shehata, B.A.; Ismaiel, I.E. The potential effect of the angiotensin II receptor blocker telmisartan in regulating OVA-induced airway remodeling in experimental rats. *Pharmacol. Rep.* **2015**, *67*, 943–951. [CrossRef] [PubMed]
82. Ma, M.; Shi, F.; Zhai, R.; Wang, H.; Li, K.; Xu, C.; Yao, W.; Zhou, F. TGF-β promote epithelial-mesenchymal transition via NF-κB/NOX4/ROS signal pathway in lung cancer cells. *Mol. Biol. Rep.* **2021**, *48*, 2365–2375. [CrossRef] [PubMed]
83. Merchant, N.; Nagaraju, G.P.; Rajitha, B.; Lammata, S.; Jella, K.K.; Buchwald, Z.S.; Lakka, S.S.; Ali, A.N. Matrix metalloproteinases: Their functional role in lung cancer. *Carcinogenesis* **2017**, *38*, 766–780. [CrossRef] [PubMed]
84. Suzuki, Y.; Tanigaki, T.; Heimer, D.; Wang, W.; Ross, W.G.; Murphy, G.A.; Sakai, A.; Sussman, H.H.; Vu, T.H.; Raffin, T.A. TGF-beta 1 causes increased endothelial ICAM-1 expression and lung injury. *J. Appl. Physiol.* **1994**, *77*, 1281–1287. [CrossRef]
85. Harada, D.; Takigawa, N.; Kiura, K. The role of STAT3 in non-small cell lung cancer. *Cancers* **2014**, *6*, 708–722. [CrossRef]
86. Fan, Y.; Mao, R.; Yang, J. NF-κB and STAT3 signaling pathways collaboratively link inflammation to cancer. *Protein Cell* **2013**, *4*, 176–185. [CrossRef]
87. Silva, M.; AMelo, S. Non-coding RNAs in exosomes: New players in cancer biology. *Curr. Genom.* **2015**, *16*, 295–303. [CrossRef]
88. Shimada, Y.; Matsubayashi, J.; Kudo, Y.; Maehara, S.; Takeuchi, S.; Hagiwara, M.; Kakihana, M.; Ohira, T.; Nagao, T.; Ikeda, N. Serum-derived exosomal PD-L1 expression to predict anti-PD-1 response and in patients with non-small cell lung cancer. *Sci. Rep.* **2021**, *11*, 7830. [CrossRef]
89. Ye, L.; Zhu, Z.; Chen, X.; Zhang, H.; Huang, J.; Gu, S.; Zhao, X. The Importance of Exosomal PD-L1 in Cancer Progression and Its Potential as a Therapeutic Target. *Cells* **2021**, *10*, 3247. [CrossRef]
90. Wu, S.; Luo, M.; To, K.K.; Zhang, J.; Su, C.; Zhang, H.; An, S.; Wang, F.; Chen, D.; Fu, L. Intercellular transfer of exosomal wild type EGFR triggers OSM resistance in non-small cell lung cancer. *Mol. Cancer* **2021**, *20*, 17. [CrossRef]

pharmaceutics

Article

Targeting Zika Virus with New Brain- and Placenta-Crossing Peptide–Porphyrin Conjugates

Toni Todorovski [1,†], Diogo A. Mendonça [2,†], Lorena O. Fernandes-Siqueira [3], Christine Cruz-Oliveira [2], Giuseppina Guida [1], Javier Valle [1], Marco Cavaco [2], Fernanda I. V. Limas [3], Vera Neves [2], Íris Cadima-Couto [2], Sira Defaus [1], Ana Salomé Veiga [2], Andrea T. Da Poian [3,*], Miguel A. R. B. Castanho [2,*] and David Andreu [1,*]

[1] Department of Medicine and Life Sciences, Universitat Pompeu Fabra, 08003 Barcelona, Spain; toni.todorovski@upf.edu (T.T.); giuseppina.guida@upf.edu (G.G.); javier.valle@upf.edu (J.V.); sira.defaus@upf.edu (S.D.)

[2] Instituto de Medicina Molecular, Faculdade de Medicina, Universidade de Lisboa, 1649-028 Lisbon, Portugal; diogo.mendonca@medicina.ulisboa.pt (D.A.M.); christine.oliveira@medicina.ulisboa.pt (C.C.-O.); mcavaco@medicina.ulisboa.pt (M.C.); veraneves@medicina.ulisboa.pt (V.N.); cicouto@medicina.ulisboa.pt (Í.C.-C.); aveiga@medicina.ulisboa.pt (A.S.V.)

[3] Instituto de Bioquímica Médica Leopoldo de Meis, Universidade Federal do Rio de Janeiro, Rio de Janeiro 21941-902, Brazil; losiqueira@bioqmed.ufrj.br (L.O.F.-S.); fernanda.ignaciovl@gmail.com (F.I.V.L.)

* Correspondence: dapoian@bioqmed.ufrj.br (A.T.D.P.); macastanho@medicina.ulisboa.pt (M.A.R.B.C.); david.andreu@upf.edu (D.A.)

† These authors contributed equally to this work.

Citation: Todorovski, T.; Mendonça, D.A.; Fernandes-Siqueira, L.O.; Cruz-Oliveira, C.; Guida, G.; Valle, J.; Cavaco, M.; Limas, F.I.V.; Neves, V.; Cadima-Couto, Í.; et al. Targeting Zika Virus with New Brain- and Placenta-Crossing Peptide–Porphyrin Conjugates. *Pharmaceutics* **2022**, *14*, 738. https://doi.org/10.3390/pharmaceutics14040738

Academic Editors: Vibhuti Agrahari and Prashant Kumar

Received: 5 January 2022
Accepted: 25 March 2022
Published: 29 March 2022

Abstract: Viral disease outbreaks affect hundreds of millions of people worldwide and remain a serious threat to global health. The current SARS-CoV-2 pandemic and other recent geographically-confined viral outbreaks (severe acute respiratory syndrome (SARS), Ebola, dengue, zika and ever-recurring seasonal influenza), also with devastating tolls at sanitary and socio-economic levels, are sobering reminders in this respect. Among the respective pathogenic agents, Zika virus (ZIKV), transmitted by *Aedes* mosquito vectors and causing the eponymous fever, is particularly insidious in that infection during pregnancy results in complications such as foetal loss, preterm birth or irreversible brain abnormalities, including microcephaly. So far, there is no effective remedy for ZIKV infection, mainly due to the limited ability of antiviral drugs to cross blood–placental and/or blood–brain barriers (BPB and BBB, respectively). Despite its restricted permeability, the BBB is penetrable by a variety of molecules, mainly peptide-based, and named BBB peptide shuttles (BBBpS), able to ferry various payloads (e.g., drugs, antibodies, etc.) into the brain. Recently, we have described peptide–porphyrin conjugates (PPCs) as successful BBBpS-associated drug leads for HIV, an enveloped virus in which group ZIKV also belongs. Herein, we report on several brain-directed, low-toxicity PPCs capable of targeting ZIKV. One of the conjugates, PP-P1, crossing both BPB and BBB, has shown to be effective against ZIKV (IC_{50} 1.08 μM) and has high serum stability ($t_{1/2}$ ca. 22 h) without altering cell viability at all tested concentrations. Peptide–porphyrin conjugation stands out as a promising strategy to fill the ZIKV treatment gap.

Keywords: peptide-drug conjugates; blood–brain barrier; blood–placental barrier; Zika virus; BBB shuttles; porphyrins; antivirals

1. Introduction

Among human-targeting viruses, brain-penetrating ones such as Zika virus (ZIKV), Dengue virus, or HIV pose formidable hurdles to pathogen targeting, ZIKV being a particularly illustrative case in this regard.

ZIKV, a member of the *Flaviviridae* family, [1] causes the namesake zika fever, a zoonosis transmitted by *Aedes* mosquito bites [2,3]. The direst consequences of ZIKV infection concern pregnant women, as virus transmission to the foetus causes irreversible congenital brain abnormalities, including microcephaly [4]—a predicament involving over 1400 cases during the 2016 outbreak in Brazil [5]. ZIKV infection can also result in further complications such as foetal loss, preterm birth or other birth defects, and can also trigger Guillain–Barré syndrome [4], encephalomyelitis [6], and similar conditions in adults. ZIKV was detected in a microcephalic foetus ca. 32 weeks after maternal exposure, suggesting long persistence in the foetal brain [3].

The World Health Organization (WHO) has classified ZIKV amongst the viruses posing the greatest public health risk due to its epidemic potential. WHO recommendations have focused on the development of inactive and/or other "non-live" vaccines [7], with a number of vaccine candidates showing some promise in human clinical trials [8]. An alternative approach, involving genetic modification of the *Aedes* mosquito transmission vector, has also raised attention, though conclusive data on its effectiveness is lacking [9]. In more conventional therapeutic approaches, any anti-ZIKV drug development effort must face the challenge of moving the drug across the blood–placental (BPB) and blood–brain (BBB) barriers to reach ZIKV at its most sensitive sites of action: the brain or the foetus [10,11]. The BBB is a natural protective barrier made up by endothelial cells (ECs), astrocytes and pericytes, whose unique composition allows tight regulation of central nervous system (CNS) homeostasis, which is critical for proper neuronal function, as well as for protection from toxins, pathogens, inflammation, injury, and disease. BBB fulfils this role by having very selective transporters for a limited number of specific molecular entities circulating in the blood. For its part, the BPB, consisting of trophoblastic epithelium, is a "leakier" barrier, blocking mainly the diffusion of large molecules.

In the last two decades, a variety of molecules, broadly described as BBB shuttles, have been shown to successfully overcome BBB permeability [12–15]. The "BBB shuttle" term was first introduced by Pardridge [16] to denote the ability of such agents, chemically modified or not, to ferry brain-targeting drug payloads into and out of the brain through the BBB. As many such shuttles are peptide-based, the term "BBB peptide shuttle" [BBBpS] has been more recently coined [17].

Strategies for conjugating BBBpS to drug payloads have been actively explored over recent decades, with the number of new shuttles steadily increasing [12–15,18–20]. Some recent entries, moreover, have shown to be capable not only of carrying drugs into but also removing toxins from the brain, preventing their accumulation [21,22]. For our part, we have reported that peptide–porphyrin conjugates (PPCs), where a BBBpS and an antiviral porphyrin are covalently linked by an amide bond (amino and carboxyl groups in BBBpS and porphyrin, respectively) can successfully pass the BBB and act against brain-targeting viruses such as HIV [23]. As for the BPB, the literature is scarce, with only a few described examples of peptides able to pass it [24].

Herein, we report our results in developing new PPCs able to penetrate both BPB and BBB and act against ZIKV. The PPC production strategy, involving porphyrin (P), *C*- or *N*-terminal conjugation to a BBBpS, has been detailed in a recent publication and is illustrated in Scheme 1 and Scheme S1 [23]. In this paper we describe eight PPCs (Table 1) resulting from the combination of four BBBpS (Table S1) and two porphyrins, and their evaluation in terms of barrier crossing and anti-ZIKV activity. One of the conjugates, PP-P1, emerges as particularly effective against ZIKV, having also the ability to translocate across BPB and BBB.

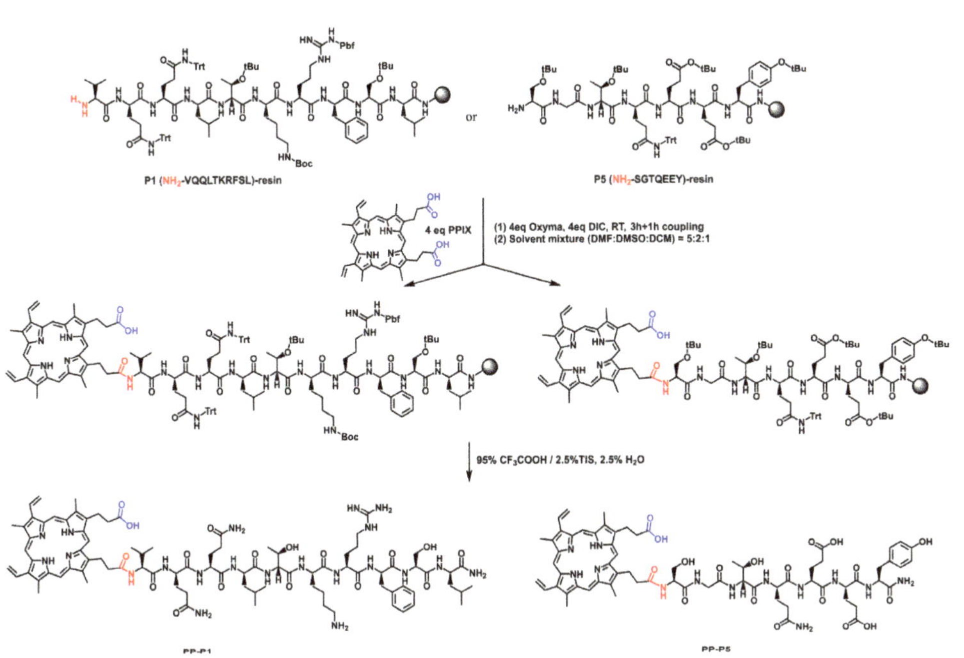

Scheme 1. On-resin conjugation strategy at the N-terminus of a BBBpS.

Table 1. PPCs used in the study.

Abbreviation	Structure	$[M + H^+]^+$
MP-P1	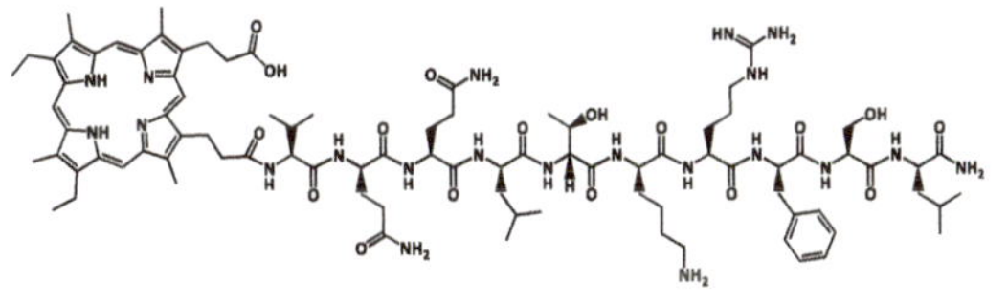	1767.0
PP-P1	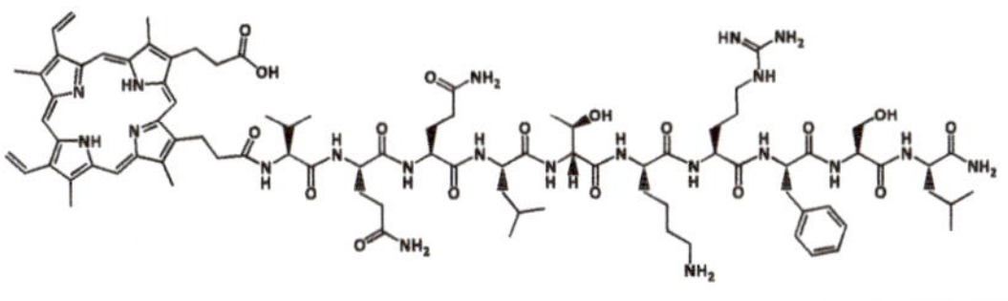	1762.9
P2-MP	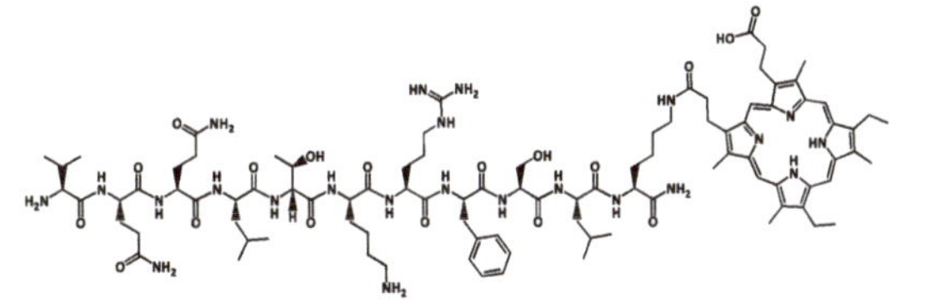	1895.1

Table 1. *Cont.*

Abbreviation	Structure	[M + H+]+
P2-PP	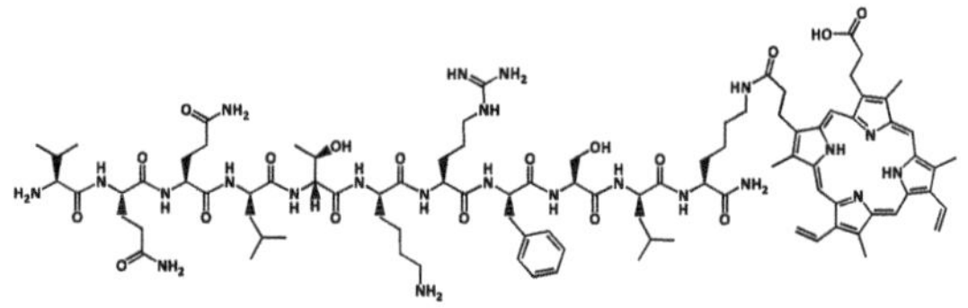	1891.1
MP-P5	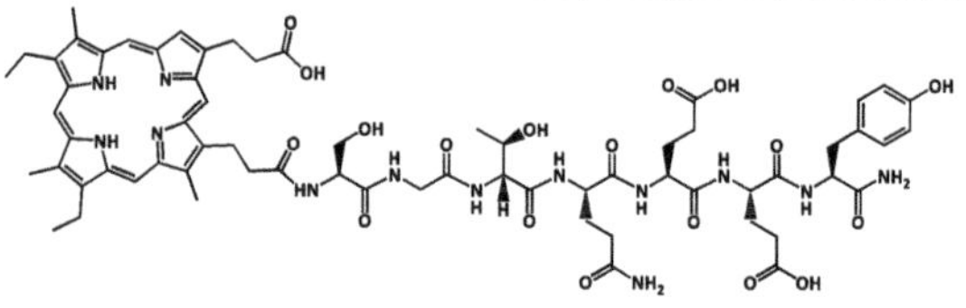	1360.6
PP-P5	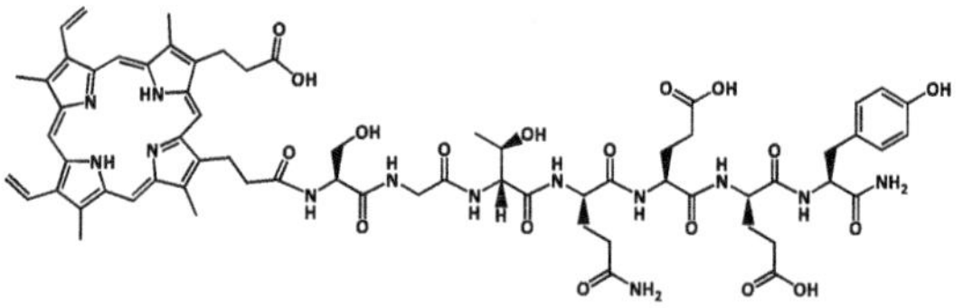	1356.6
P6-MP	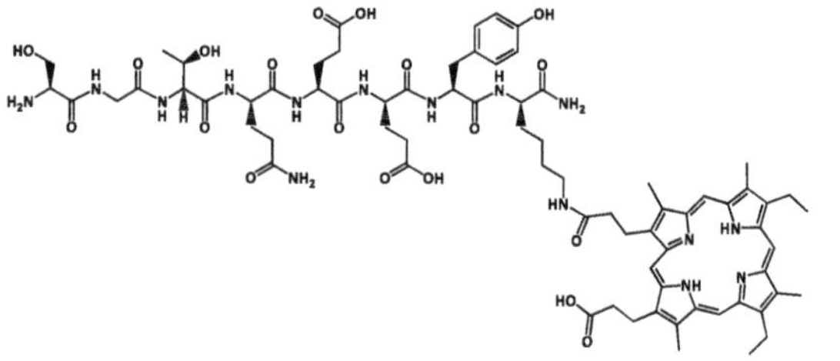	1488.7
P6-PP	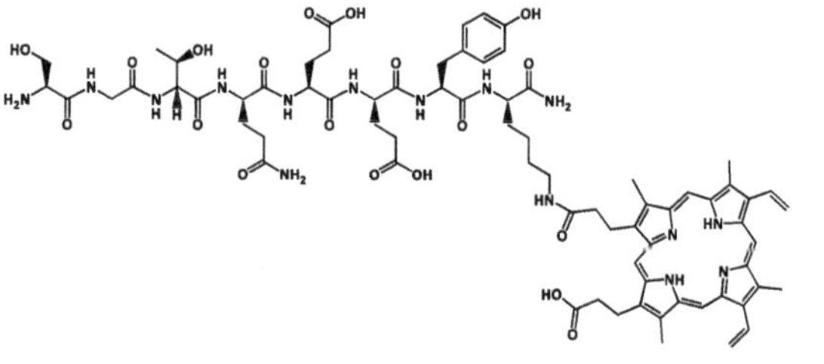	1484.7

2. Materials and Methods

2.1. Chemicals and Reagents

Mesoporphyrin IX dihydrochloride and protoporphyrin IX were from Frontier Scientific, Inc (Logan, UT, USA). HPLC-grade DMF, DCM and MeCN were from Fisher (Madrid, Spain), and NMP was from Sigma-Aldrich (Madrid, Spain). Fmoc-amino acids, DIC and Oxyma were from Iris Biotech (Marktredwitz, Germany).

2.2. Cells and Cell Culture Reagents

HBEC-5i human brain endothelia (ATCC-CRL-3245) and JEG-3 placental trophoblast (ATCC-HTB-36) cell lines, and Eagle's Minimal Essential Medium (EMEM) were from ATCC (Manassas, VA, USA). Dulbecco's Modified Eagle Medium: Nutrient Mixture F-12

(DMEM:F12), foetal bovine serum (FBS), penicillin-streptomycin (Pen-Strep), attachment factor protein and trypsin-EDTA were from Gibco (Thermo-Fisher, Waltham, MA, USA). AlamarBlue® reagent was from Invitrogen (Thermo-Fisher). Endothelial cell growth supplement from bovine neural tissue (ECGS) was from Sigma-Aldrich (Merck, Darmstadt, Germany). Penicillin and streptomycin were from LGC Biotecnologia (Cotia, SP, Brazil).

2.3. Peptide Synthesis

P1, P2, P5 and P6 were made by Fmoc solid phase synthesis on a Liberty Blue (CEM Matthews, NC, USA) instrument using Protide resin (0.54 mmol/g) at 0.1 mmol scale. The P2 and P6 sequences are variants of P1 and P5 (Table S1), respectively, elongated at their *C*-termini with an extra Lys residue, orthogonally protected with the monomethoxytrityl (Mmt) group. Other side chain protecting groups were *tert*-butyl (Ser, Thr, Glu), trityl (Gln), Boc (Lys) and 2,2,4,6,7-pentamethyldihydrobenzofuran-5-sulfonyl (Arg). The identity of the resin-bound peptides prior to porphyrin conjugation was assessed by resin test cleavage (RTC) combined with LC-MS analysis. Briefly, ca. 2 mg of peptide resin were reacted with 170 μL of TFA-TIS-H_2O (95:2.5:2.5, *v*/*v*/*v*) for 90 min at r.t. Then, 1 mL of cold diethyl ether was added, and the suspension was centrifuged at 12,400 rpm for 8 min. The supernatant was removed and the pellet, after drying, was dissolved in 15% MeCN/0.1% TFA (P1 and P2) or 0.1 % TEA (P5 and P6) and analysed by LC-MS (see below).

2.4. Conjugation Chemistry

Reactions were performed at 50 μM scale (1 eq in all further calculations) as reported [23]. Briefly, 4 eq of porphyrin (MPIX or PPIX), mixed with 4 eq oxyma, were dissolved, respectively, in NMP:DCM:DMF (3:2:1, *v*/*v*/*v*) or DMF:DMSO:DCM (5:2:1, *v*/*v*/*v*), at a final 0.05 M concentration. The solution was mixed with 4 eq DIC (plus 8 eq DIPEA in the case of MPIX) and added to the peptide resin. In C-terminal conjugations (P2 and P6), prior to porphyrin coupling, the Mmt group at the C-terminal Lys side chain was selectively removed by 1% TFA in DCM (5 × 1 min) followed by DCM washes: the cycle was repeated until no more yellow colour (presence of Mmt) was observed. After 3 h at r.t., conjugation with fresh reagents was repeated for an additional 1 h. A slightly modified RTC on a small aliquot of the PPC-resin (cleavage as above), with N_2 flush evaporation instead of ether precipitation and the residue dissolved in 20% MeCN for LC-MS analysis, was used to confirm conjugate identity. Next, the bulk PPC-resin was likewise cleaved, the resulting solution was N_2 flush-evaporated, dissolved in H_2O/MeCN (80:20 *v*/*v*) and lyophilized.

2.5. PPC Purification

Conjugates were purified by semi-preparative HPLC on an LC20-AP instrument (Shimadzu, Kyoto, Japan) using a Gemini C_{18} column (10 μm, 110 Å, 10 × 250 mm, Phenomenex, Torrance, CA, USA). Each conjugate was dissolved in 22% MeCN/25% DMF/H_2O and a linear 15-95% MeCN gradient in H_2O (0.1 % TFA) over 40 min at 6 mL/min flow rate was applied. The fractions were analysed by LC-MS and those with >90% homogeneity were collected, combined, lyophilized and stored at −20 °C.

2.6. LC-MS Analysis

Crude peptides or conjugates after RTC were dissolved in 15% or 20% MeCN, respectively, and analysed on a LCMS-2010 EV instrument (Shimadzu). For the analysis, 15 μL of a ~1 mg/mL solution were injected on an Aeris XB-C_{18} column (3.6 μm, 150 × 4.6 mm, Phenomenex) eluted with a linear 5–95% MeCN gradient into 0.1 % FA in H_2O over 15 min at 1 mL/min flow rate. MS detection was set to 200–2000 *m/z*. Purified conjugates were dissolved at 1 mg/mL in 20% MeCN and analysed by LC-MS using a linear 10–60% MeCN gradient into 0.1% FA in H_2O over 15 min, other parameters as above.

2.7. In Vitro BBB Translocation Assay

HBEC-5i cells were cultured as a monolayer on T-flasks in DMEM:F12 supplemented with 10% (*v*/*v*) FBS, 1% (*v*/*v*) Pen-Strep and 1% (*v*/*v*) ECGS. Cells were grown in a humidified atmosphere of 5% CO_2 at 37 °C (MCO-18AIC (UV), Sanyo, Japan) with the medium changed every other day. Cells were allowed to grow until confluence in a culture T-flask, then carefully harvested with trypsin-EDTA and seeded (8000 cells/well) into tissue culture 24-well inserts (transparent polyester membrane with 1.0 µm pores) (BD Falcon-Corning, Corning, NY, USA) pre-coated with attachment factor protein solution. The medium was changed every other day for 5–8 days, afterwards cells were washed with 1 × PBS, followed by DMEM:F12 medium without phenol red. Next, PPCs diluted in DMEM:F12 without phenol red, at a final 10 µM concentration, were added to the apical side of the in vitro BBB model. Experiments were performed on different days using independently grown cell cultures.

PPC translocation was determined by fluorescence intensity (λ_{ex} = 410 nm, λ_{em} = 625 nm for MP conjugates: λ_{ex} = 410 nm, λ_{em} = 635 nm for PP conjugates). P1-carboxyfluorescein (CF-P1) and P5-carboxyfluorescein (CF-P5) were used as positive translocation controls (λ_{ex} = 492 nm and λ_{em} = 517 nm). After 24 h incubation, samples from the basolateral side were collected and analysed. Fluorescence was measured in a Varioskan Lux plate reader (Thermo Scientific). PPC translocation (%) was calculated as follows:

$$\text{PPC translocation } (\%) = \frac{F_i - Fcells}{F_{PPC} - F_{Medium}} \times 100 \tag{1}$$

where F_i is the fluorescence intensity of the sample collected at the basolateral side, F_{cells} is the intrinsic fluorescence intensity of cells without *PPC* incubation, F_{PPC} is the intensity of total *PPC* initially added to the transwell apical side, and F_{Medium} is the intensity of DMEM:F12 medium without phenol red. Three independent replicates were performed.

2.8. In Vitro BBB Integrity Assay

After 24 h incubation with PPCs, cells were washed with PBS and DMEM:F12 medium without phenol red. Then, 4 kDa fluorescein isothiocyanate-dextran (FD4) (Sigma-Aldrich, Madrid, Spain) in DMEM:F12 without phenol red, previously diluted to an absorbance of 0.1, was added to the apical side and incubated for 2 h. Samples were collected at the basolateral side, and fluorescence intensity was measured at λ_{ex} = 493 nm and λ_{em} = 520 nm. Barrier integrity was evaluated from FD4 permeability as follows:

$$FD4 \text{ Permeability } (\%) = \frac{F_i - F_{cells}}{F_{FD4} - F_{Medium}} \times 100 \tag{2}$$

where F_i is the fluorescence intensity of the sample at the basolateral side, F_{cells} is the intrinsic fluorescence intensity of cells without FD4 incubation, F_{FD4} is the intensity of FD4 stock initially added to the apical side, and F_{Medium} is the intensity of DMEM:F12 medium without phenol red. Three independent replicates were performed.

2.9. In Vitro BPB Translocation and Integrity Assay

JEG-3 cells were cultured as a monolayer on T-flasks in EMEM supplemented with 10% (*v*/*v*) FBS and 1% (*v*/*v*) Pen-Strep. Cells were grown in a humidified atmosphere of 5% CO_2 at 37 °C with the medium changed every other day. Cells were allowed to grow until confluence in a culture T-flask, then carefully harvested with trypsin-EDTA and seeded (3000 cells/well) onto rat-tail collagen-coated tissue culture 24-well inserts. A cellular monolayer with low permeability was formed 5 days after the incubation on the tissue culture insert. BPB translocation and integrity measurement methods are identical to those for the BBB in vitro model. Three independent replicates were performed.

2.10. Virus Samples

ZIKV^{BR} was isolated from a febrile case in the state of Pernambuco, Brazil (gene bank ref. number KX197192) and was kindly provided by Dr. Ernesto T. A Marques Jr (Centro de Pesquisas Aggeu Magalhães, Fiocruz, Pernambuco, Brazil). ZIKV^{BR} was propagated in C6/36 cells using a multiplicity of infection (MOI) of 0.01. After infection, cells were cultured for 7 days. The culture medium collected from the infected cultures was centrifuged at 700× *g* to remove cellular debris, stored in aliquots at −80 °C and titrated by plaque assay as described elsewhere [25].

2.11. ZIKV Inactivation Assay

To determine the effect of PPCs on ZIKV^{BR}, 10^5 plaque forming units (PFU) were pre-treated with different PPC concentrations in the 0.01–50 μM range for 1 h at 37 °C, in the dark. After treatment, viral samples were serially diluted (10-fold) for titration [25]. Samples were incubated for 1 h at 37 °C and 5% CO_2 with Vero cells. After infection, the medium was removed and 1 mL DMEM containing 1% (*v*/*v*) FBS, 100 U/mL penicillin, 100 μg/mL streptomycin and 1.5% carboxymethylcellulose was added to each well. The plates were incubated at 37 °C and 5% CO_2. After 5 days, cells were fixed by 1 mL of 4% (*v*/*v*) formaldehyde in H_2O for 30 min. Each plate was washed and stained with a 1% (*v*/*v*) crystal violet, 20% (*v*/*v*) ethanol solution. The number of plaques on each well was counted and corrected for well dilution to determine the pfu/mL number. The half-maximum inhibitory concentration (IC_{50}) was determined by nonlinear regression with sigmoidal profile and variable slope using the software Graphpad Prism (version 6.0, Graphpad Software, San Diego, CA, USA), only on treatments that achieved total inhibition. Three independent replicates were performed.

2.12. Cell Viability Assay

HBEC-5i cells and JEG-3 cells were plated in attachment factor protein and rat-tail collagen, respectively, pre-coated 96-well flat bottom clear, black polystyrene plate (Corning, New York, NY, USA) as previously described [23]. Afterwards cells were cultured in complete medium at 37 °C in a 5% CO_2 atmosphere, with medium replaced every 2 days. When the cellular monolayer was formed, cells were treated with various PPC concentrations in the 6.25–50 μM range, for 24 h at 37 °C in a 5% CO_2 atmosphere. Viability was evaluated by the CellTiter-Blue® assay (Promega, Madison, WI, USA), based on resazurin reduction into highly fluorescent resorufin by metabolically active cells. By distinguishing metabolic from non-metabolic cells, cytotoxicity can be indirectly determined. After incubation, cells were washed with PBS, pH 7.4, and 15 μL of CellTiterBlue® reagent in 100 μL of complete medium was added to the cells and incubated for 1.5 h at 37 °C in 5% CO_2. Fluorescence (λ_{ex} = 560 nm, λ_{em} = 590 nm), was measured in a Varioskan Lux plate reader. Complete medium and medium containing 0.25% Triton X-100 were used as positive and negative controls (100 and 0% viability), respectively. Cell viability (%) was determined as:

$$\text{Cell viability }(\%) = \frac{F_{treated} - F_{blank}}{F_{non\ treated} - F_{blank}} \times 100 \quad (3)$$

where $F_{treated}$ is the fluorescence intensity of PPC-treated cells, $F_{non\ treated}$ is the fluorescence of untreated cells and F_{blank} is the fluorescence of CellTiterBlue® reagent in complete medium without cells. Three independent replicates were performed.

2.13. Serum Stability

Conjugates, peptides P1, P2 and P5 were dissolved at 0.1 mM in HEPES buffer (10 mM, NaCl 150 mM, pH 7.8), with 1.4 % DMSO added for MP-P1 and P2-MP to improve solubility. Next, 600 μL of conjugate/peptide solution were mixed (1:1 *v*/*v*) with 600 μL of human serum, to a 0.05 mM final concentration. The mixture was incubated at 37 °C and, at various time points, 50 μL (in triplicate) were taken and precipitated with 200 μL cold methanol. The samples were centrifuged at 13,000 rpm, 10 min, +4 °C. Afterwards, 50 μL of each supernatant were injected on an LC-20AD instrument (Shimadzu) equipped with a Luna C18 column (4.6 mm × 50 mm, 3 μm, Phenomenex, Torrance, CA, USA) and analysed using a 0–95% linear gradient of MeCN into 0.1% TFA in H_2O over 15 min with 1 mL/min flow rate. PDA detection at 220 nm and 401 nm was used and the half-life times were calculated by peak area integration at 401 nm, the λ_{max} of MP and PP. Controls included blank serum (25 μL each of 1:1 *v*/*v* serum + HEPES buffer, then precipitation with 200 μL cold methanol), untreated conjugate/peptide (25 μL of 0.1 mM stock in HEPES buffer + 25 μL HEPES buffer, then precipitation with 200 μL cold methanol), and a zero-time sample (200 μL cold methanol + 25 μL serum + 25 μL 0.1 mM conjugate/peptide stock); the conjugate/peptide was added last to avoid any contact with protease. Controls were analysed by LC and LC-MS as above. Three independent replicates were performed.

3. Results and Discussion

3.1. BBBpS—Porphyrin Conjugate Design

Peptide–porphyrin conjugates (PPCs) are regarded as promising leads against viral and bacterial infections [26–30]. The antiviral properties of porphyrins make them attractive for treating viral diseases, including those caused by enveloped viruses such as HIV, ZIKV, and DENV [25,31,32], while BBBpS conjugation allows to overcome obstacles such as porphyrin poor water solubility and low cellular uptake. We have recently shown that PPCs involving a covalent (amide) link between amino (*N*-terminal or Lys side chain) groups of a BBBpS and porphyrin carboxyl groups can successfully pass the BBB and act against HIV without significant cytotoxic activity [23]. For HIV, the most plausible inactivation mechanism seems to be envelope targeting with severe perturbation of lipid bilayer integrity. Since ZIKV is also enveloped, we decided to exploit the same approach by means of a PPC library with potential BPB and BBB-crossing abilities. Specifically, the chemistry in Scheme 1 and Scheme S1 [23] has been applied to two different BBBpS conjugation sites (*N*- or *C*-terminal) and two different porphyrins (MP and PP). All the eight conjugates in Table 1 were obtained at >90% purity and in 10–30% final yields after HPLC purification (Table S3).

3.2. In Vitro BBB and BPB Translocation Assays

At variance with the previous studies [23], where a mouse BBB in vitro model was used, here we used a human model, a cellular barrier formed by human endothelial brain cells (HBEC-5i) [33] grown in a cell culture insert, allowing formation of a cell monolayer with restrictive paracellular permeability and expression of essential BBB transporters. Placed into a transwell system, the cellular monolayer divides two chambers mimicking the blood and brain sides (Figure 1A) and allowing quantification of drug translocation. In this device, all PPCs efficiently translocate the monolayer, five of them—MP-P5, PP-P1, PP-P5, P6-MP and P6-PP—reaching values above 43% (Figure 1B). Although lower than those of non-conjugated peptides P1 and P5, the trans-BBB scores for these PPCs are in the range of best-performing leads reported in peptide-drug antiretroviral and anti-Alzheimer therapeutic approaches [34–36]. Conjugation improves translocation for MP bound to BBBpS P5 or P6 relative to free MP (Figure 1B). Moreover, free PP significantly compromises the integrity of the barrier, as shown by the 2.5-fold increase in FD4 permeability over control values (24.7 and 10.3%, respectively), approaching EGTA disruption values, a behaviour not observed with the conjugates.

To evaluate in vitro BPB translocation, the above-described transwell system was modified to mimic a human placental barrier, using trophoblast cultures (JEG-3 cell line) [37] and optimized to ensure cell monolayers with low permeability (Figure S1). In this setup, the same five PPCs shown to better translocate the BBB in vitro were also those with higher trans-BPB capabilities (Figure 1C), although scores were significantly lower than for BBB translocation. It seems, thus, reasonable to assume that translocation mechanisms for PPCs differ between the two barriers. It is worth mentioning at this point that, while adsorptive-mediated transcytosis (AMT) is deemed the preferential BBB translocation mechanism by our BBBpS [21,22], and the most likely mechanism for the PPCs in this study, it has not yet been reported as a BPB transmigration mechanism [38]. Passive diffusion, the preferential transmigration mechanism used by trans-BPB compounds [39], seems to be non-favoured by PPCs, given the disparity in translocation values between the PPCs and the antipyrine positive control (Figure S1C). At any rate, five PPCs with significant BBB and BPB translocation abilities suitable for ZIKV inactivation were identified. It is also worth noting that none of the PPCs altered cell viability (HBEC-5i, JEG-3) at concentrations up to 50 µM (data not shown).

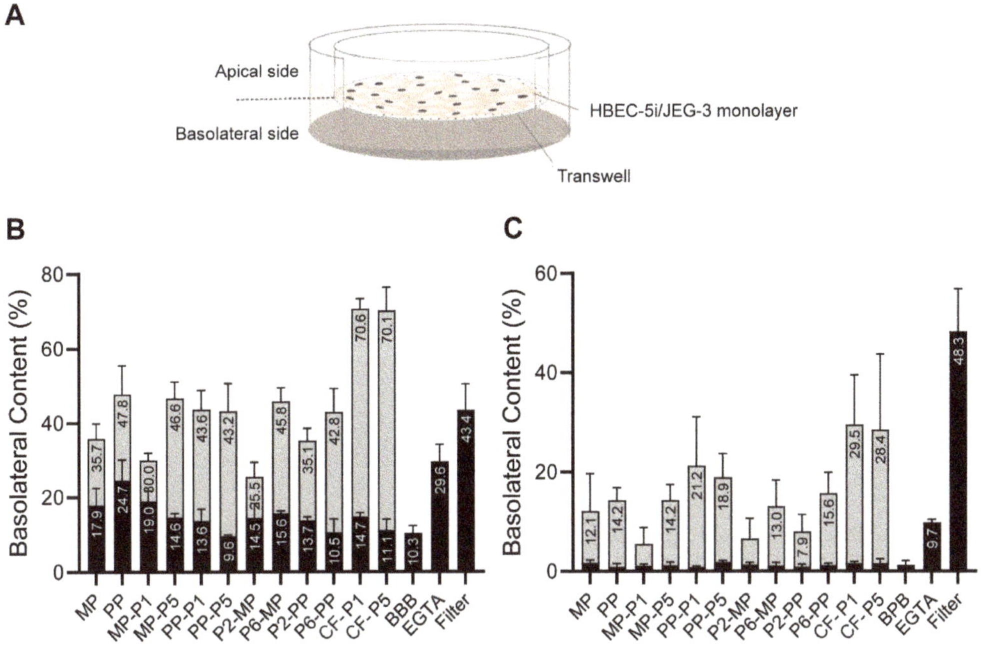

Figure 1. In vitro PPC translocation. (**A**) Schematic representation of the BBB and BPB model transwell system. (**B**,**C**) in vitro BBB and BPB translocation measurements. PPC translocation values are depicted in grey, while FD4 permeability values post-translocation are in black (BBB and BPB—only cells, EGTA—tight junctions disruption control, Filter—no cells).

3.3. ZIKV Inactivation

The five PPCs that successfully translocated BBB and BPB were evaluated for ZIKV inactivation in vitro, using a plaque assay. Of them, two showed significant activity (Table 2 and Table S2), namely MP-P5 (IC_{50} = 25.07 ± 0.05 µM, similar to activity against HIV [23]) and PP-P1 (IC_{50} = 1.08 ± 0.14 µM). Additionally, a treatment assay performed with MP-P5 and PP-P1 revealed that both PPCs efficiently inhibit ZIKV replication when added 1 h and 7 h post-infection (Figure S2). As observed for HIV [23], non-conjugated porphyrins did not show activity against ZIKV, reinforcing the claim that BBBpS conjugation is not only critical for BBB/BPB translocation but also for antiviral activity. On the other hand, and somewhat unexpectedly, PP-P1, shown to be inactive in vitro against HIV [23], emerged as the most active anti-ZIKV conjugate. As described in the literature, the light-independent mechanism of action of porphyrins is based on a direct perturbation of the viral envelope [25,31,32]. Porphyrins interact and accumulate on the envelope lipid membrane, causing a decrease in order and a consequent phase alteration that impairs viral entry processes. Since we ensured no-light conditions and no metal cations are coordinated to the porphyrin rings of the PPCs—avoiding generation of reactive oxygen species—the antiviral light-independent mechanism is the only plausible one. Thus, one may confidently suggest that the PP-P1 specific anti-ZIKV activity is guided by preferential interaction with the ZIKV viral envelope and/or components.

Table 2. PPCs antiviral activity in vitro.

Virus	MP	IC50 (μM) PP	MP-P5	PP-P1
ZIKV	>50	>50	25.07 ± 0.05	1.08 ± 0.14
HIV [a]	>50	>50	33.1 ± 1.38	>50

[a] Values described at [24].

3.4. Serum Stability

The in vitro stability in human serum of all conjugates and their constitutive non-conjugated BBBpS was evaluated by LC and LC-MS as described [40,41]. PP-P1, the conjugate with highest ZIKV inhibitory activity, was remarkably resistant towards serum proteases (Figure 2A, black circles) with $t_{1/2}$ > 22 h. This $t_{1/2}$ is much higher than that of non-conjugated P1 ($t_{1/2}$ = 44.0 min, Figure 2A, white circles), suggesting that the porphyrin payload in PP-P1 causes a steric shielding that occludes protease-sensitive sites in the P1 sequence. Comparably high $t_{1/2}$ values were observed for P5-based conjugates (Figures 2B and S3) which, given the clear differences in amino acid composition and/or charge (P1, cationic; P5, anionic), seem to exclude privileged features in the underlying BBBpS as the basis for preferential stability. Altogether, these data reinforce the view of the porphyrin ring somehow protecting cleavable peptide bonds from protease access. Interestingly, by comparing $t_{1/2}$s, a general trend regarding the attachment site of the porphyrin ring can be discerned, with *N*-terminal conjugates showing higher stability (Figure S3A–D) than *C*-terminal ones (Figure S3E–H). In this last group, conjugation takes place through the side chain of an extra *C*-terminal Lys residue that the *N*-terminal series lacks. This Lys unit, however, cannot be viewed as contributing an additional cleavage point, since the ε-amino group on its side chain is involved in an amide bond with a porphyrin carboxyl and, hence, lacks the requisite positive charge for (trypsin-like) protease susceptibility.

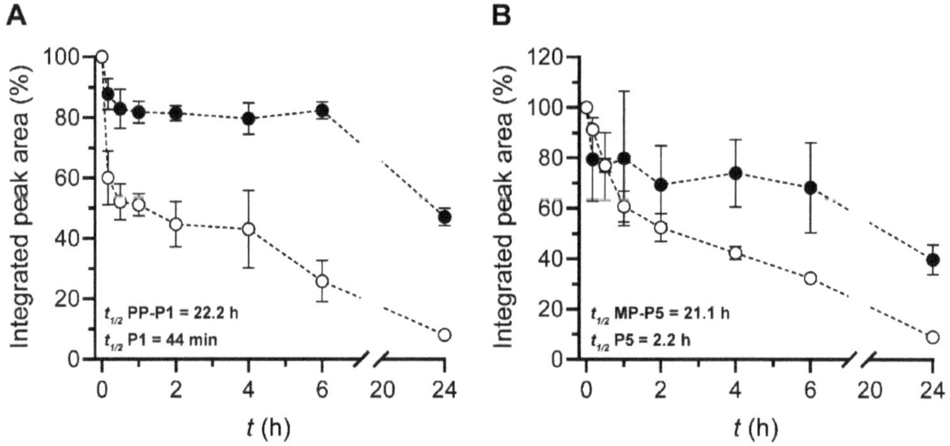

Figure 2. PPCs and peptides serum stability over 24 h. (**A**) PP-P1 (black) and P1 (white). (**B**) MP-P5 (black) and P5 (white).

An alternate explanation for the high $t_{1/2}$s of some conjugates could invoke porphyrin moieties binding and/or blocking the machinery of a crucial set of serum proteases. While this view cannot be excluded outright, it seems less plausible because such an interaction would most likely affect indiscriminately most, if not all, conjugates, in contrast with the protease resistance observed exclusively in the P1 and P5 series (Figure S3). Finally, one may not exclude the aggregation behaviour of the different conjugates also playing a role in stability. In any event, further efforts (e.g., 3D NMR-derived structural models, zeta potential measurements, etc.) are clearly needed to establish either of the above hypotheses, but this exceeds the scope of the present work.

4. Conclusions

The potential of ZIKV to invade adult and foetus brains makes it one of the viruses of global concern. There are no effective drugs against ZIKV yet, mainly because developing molecules capable of overcoming the highly restrictive BPB and BBB to reach and inactivate the virus has proven extremely challenging. PPCs previously described by us [23] exhibited BBB translocation capacity in a mouse BBB in vitro model and promising activity against HIV and can, thus, be viewed as potential leads to fill the ZIKV treatment gap. Herein, we have addressed this issue by evaluating the in vitro BBB and BPB crossing ability and anti-ZIKV activity of eight new PPCs. We have identified PP-P1 as the most promising candidate, with elevated trans-BBB and -BPB scores and the highest antiviral potency. Moreover, PP-P1 has high serum stability, with a $t_{1/2} > 22$ h that bodes well for in vivo application. We do not have an explanation for the unique, manifold activity of PP-P1 among all PPCs examined, although one can conjecture various chemical, membrane and secondary cumulative interactions as a most likely scenario that deserves further in-depth studies. In any event, one may propose peptide–porphyrin conjugation as a promising strategy to tackle brain-resident viruses.

Supplementary Materials: The following supporting information can be downloaded at: https://www.mdpi.com/article/10.3390/pharmaceutics14040738/s1, Table S1: Physicochemical properties of peptide shuttles used in the study; Figure S1: BPB in vitro model optimization. (A) Permeability of the model was evaluated based on the FD4-crossing throughout layers formed by the incubation of JEG-3 cells at densities ranging 1–4 × 10^4 cells/cm^2 in cell culture inserts. (B) Confocal microscopy imaging of BPB in vitro model [JEG-3 density of 1 × 10^4 cells/cm^2, ZO-1 (green) and Hoechst 33342 (blue)]. (C) Translocation capacity of antipyrine across the optimized BPB model (Translocation—grey, FD-4 permeability—black), Figure S2: Treatment of ZIKV-infected cells with PP-P1 and MP-P5. Vero cells were treated at 1 or 7 h post infection (h.p.i.) with 25 µM PP-P1 and MP-P5. After 24 h, the culture medium was collected and the released infectious virus particles were quantified by plaque assay as described in the Material and Methods of the main manuscript. Three independent replicates were performed, Figure S3: Serum stability of *N*-terminal conjugates (A, B, C, D) versus corresponding *C*-terminal conjugates (E, F, G, H). The conjugates labeling are as follows: A (MP-P1), B (PP-P1), C (MP-P5), D (PP-P5), E (P2-MP), F (P2-PP), G (P6-MP) and H (P6-PP), Table S1: Physicochemical properties of peptide shuttles used in the study, Table S2: PPCs global antiviral activity. HIV inhibition assays were performed as described at [2], Table S3: Final yield, HPLC purity and the mass of the synthesized PPCs, Scheme S1: Schematic representation of on-resin conjugation strategy at the *C*-terminus of the corresponding BBBpS.

Author Contributions: Conceptualization, T.T., D.A.M., A.T.D.P., M.A.R.B.C. and D.A.; Methodology, T.T., D.A.M., C.C.-O., M.C., V.N., Í.C.-C., A.T.D.P., M.A.R.B.C. and D.A.; Validation, T.T., D.A.M., L.O.F.-S., C.C.-O., G.G., J.V., Í.C.-C., S.D., A.T.D.P., M.A.R.B.C. and D.A.; Formal Analysis, T.T., D.A.M., L.O.F.-S., C.C.-O., Í.C.-C., A.T.D.P., M.A.R.B.C. and D.A.; Investigation, T.T., D.A.M., L.O.F.-S., C.C.-O. and G.G.; Resources, A.T.D.P., M.A.R.B.C. and D.A.; Writing—Original Draft Preparation, T.T., D.A.M.; Writing—Review and Editing, all authors; Supervision, A.T.D.P., M.A.R.B.C. and D.A.; Project Administration, A.T.D.P., M.A.R.B.C. and D.A.; Funding Acquisition, A.T.D.P., M.A.R.B.C. and D.A. All authors have read and agreed to the published version of the manuscript.

Funding: Work supported by the La Caixa Health Foundation (project HR17_00409, ID 100010434, agreement LCF/PR/HR17/52150011) and by the European Union (H2020-FETOPEN-2018-2019-2020-01 grant no 828774). The Department of Medicine and Life Sciences, Pompeu Fabra University, belongs to the María de Maeztu network of Units of Excellence, funded by the Spanish MICINN and AEI (CEX2018-000792-M). Additional funding from Fundação para a Ciência e Tecnologia (FCT-

MCTES) is also acknowledged for D.A.M. (PD/BD/136752/2018), M.C. (PD/BD/128281/2017), and for C.C.-O. and Í.C.-C. (PTDC/BIAVIR/29495/2017). The grants from Fundação Carlos Chagas Filho de Amparo à Pesquisa do Estado do Rio de Janeiro (FAPERJ), Brazil (grant numbers 201.316/2016, 202.945/2017); and Conselho Nacional de Desenvolvimento Científico e Tecnológico (CNPq), Brazil (grant number 309028/2017-5) are also acknowledged.

Institutional Review Board Statement: Not applicable.

Informed Consent Statement: Not applicable.

Data Availability Statement: Not applicable.

Acknowledgments: Patricia Guerreiro (Instituto de Medicina Molecular, Faculdade de Medicina, Universidade de Lisboa, Lisbon, Portugal) is acknowledged by her contribution on the BPB in vitro model confocal microscopy imaging.

Conflicts of Interest: The authors declare no conflict of interest.

References

1. Malone, R.W.; Homan, J.; Callahan, M.V.; Glasspool-Malone, J.; Damodaran, L.; Schneider, A.D.B.; Zimler, R.; Talton, J.; Cobb, R.R.; Ruzic, I.; et al. Zika Virus: Medical Countermeasure Development Challenges. *PLoS Negl. Trop. Dis.* **2016**, *10*, e0004530. [CrossRef] [PubMed]
2. Chimelli, L.; Melo, A.S.O.; Avvad-Portari, E.; Wiley, C.A.; Camacho, A.H.S.; Lopes, V.S.; Machado, H.N.; Andrade, C.V.; Dock, D.C.A.; Moreira, M.E.; et al. The spectrum of neuropathological changes associated with congenital Zika virus infection. *Acta Neuropathol.* **2017**, *133*, 983–999. [CrossRef] [PubMed]
3. Mlakar, J.; Korva, M.; Tul, N.; Popović, M.; Poljšak-Prijatelj, M.; Mraz, J.; Kolenc, M.; Resman Rus, K.; Vesnaver Vipotnik, T.; Fabjan Vodušek, V.; et al. Zika Virus Associated with Microcephaly. *N. Engl. J. Med.* **2016**, *374*, 951–958. [CrossRef] [PubMed]
4. Parra, B.; Lizarazo, J.; Jiménez-Arango, J.A.; Zea-Vera, A.F.; González-Manrique, G.; Vargas, J.; Angarita, J.A.; Zuñiga, G.; Lopez-Gonzalez, R.; Beltran, C.L.; et al. Guillain–Barré Syndrome Associated with Zika Virus Infection in Colombia. *N. Engl. J. Med.* **2016**, *375*, 1513–1523. [CrossRef] [PubMed]
5. Peiter, P.C.; Pereira, R.D.S.; Nunes Moreira, M.C.; Nascimento, M.; Tavares, M.d.F.L.; Franco, V.d.C.; Carvajal Cortês, J.J.; Campos, D.d.S.; Barcellos, C. Zika epidemic and microcephaly in Brazil: Challenges for access to health care and promotion in three epidemic areas. *PLoS ONE* **2020**, *15*, e0235010. [CrossRef]
6. Niemeyer, B.; Niemeyer, R.; Borges, R.; Marchiori, E. Acute Disseminated Encephalomyelitis Following Zika Virus Infection. *Eur. Neurol.* **2017**, *77*, 45–46. [CrossRef]
7. WHO and Experts Prioritize Vaccines, Diagnostics and Innovative Vector Control Tools for Zika R&D. Available online: https://www.who.int/news/item/09-03-2016-who-and-experts-prioritize-vaccines-diagnostics-and-innovative-vector-control-tools-for-zika-r-d (accessed on 19 December 2021).
8. Pattnaik, A.; Sahoo, B.R.; Pattnaik, A.K. Current Status of Zika Virus Vaccines: Successes and Challenges. *Vaccines* **2020**, *8*, 266. [CrossRef] [PubMed]
9. Waltz, E. First genetically modified mosquitoes released in the United States. *Nature* **2021**, *593*, 175–176. [CrossRef] [PubMed]
10. Albulescu, I.C.; Kovacikova, K.; Tas, A.; Snijder, E.J.; van Hemert, M.J. Suramin inhibits Zika virus replication by interfering with virus attachment and release of infectious particles. *Antivir. Res.* **2017**, *143*, 230–236. [CrossRef]
11. Sacramento, C.Q.; De Melo, G.R.; De Freitas, C.S.; Rocha, N.; Hoelz, L.V.B.; Miranda, M.; Fintelman-Rodrigues, N.; Marttorelli, A.; Ferreira, A.C.; Barbosa-Lima, G.; et al. The clinically approved antiviral drug sofosbuvir inhibits Zika virus replication. *Sci. Rep.* **2017**, *7*, 1–12. [CrossRef]
12. Demeule, M.; Regina, A.; Ché, C.; Poirier, J.; Nguyen, T.; Gabathuler, R.; Castaigne, J.P.; Béliveau, R. Identification and design of peptides as a new drug delivery system for the brain. *J. Pharmacol. Exp. Ther.* **2008**, *324*, 1064–1072. [CrossRef] [PubMed]
13. Malakoutikhah, M.; Teixidó, M.; Giralt, E. Toward an optimal blood-brain barrier shuttle by synthesis and evaluation of peptide libraries. *J. Med. Chem.* **2008**, *51*, 4881–4889. [CrossRef] [PubMed]
14. Malakoutikhah, M.; Guixer, B.; Arranz-Gibert, P.; Teixidó, M.; Giralt, E. 'À la Carte' Peptide Shuttles: Tools to Increase Their Passage across the Blood-Brain Barrier. *ChemMedChem* **2014**, *9*, 1594–1601. [CrossRef] [PubMed]
15. Oller-Salvia, B.; Sánchez-Navarro, M.; Giralt, E.; Teixidó, M. Blood-brain barrier shuttle peptides: An emerging paradigm for brain delivery. *Chem. Soc. Rev.* **2016**, *45*, 4690–4707. [CrossRef]
16. Pardridge, W.M. Receptor-mediated peptide transport through the blood-brain barrier. *Endocr. Rev.* **1986**, *7*, 314–330. [CrossRef]
17. Cavaco, M.; Frutos, S.; Oliete, P.; Valle, J.; Andreu, D.; Castanho, M.A.R.B.; Vila-Perelló, M.; Neves, V. Conjugation of a Blood Brain Barrier Peptide Shuttle to an Fc Domain for Brain Delivery of Therapeutic Biomolecules. *ACS Med. Chem. Lett.* **2021**, *12*, 1663–1668. [CrossRef]
18. Zhang, B.; Sun, X.; Mei, H.; Wang, Y.; Liao, Z.; Chen, J.; Zhang, Q.; Hu, Y.; Pang, Z.; Jiang, X. LDLR-mediated peptide-22-conjugated nanoparticles for dual-targeting therapy of brain glioma. *Biomaterials* **2013**, *34*, 9171–9182. [CrossRef]

19. Banks, W.A.; Kastin, A.J. Peptides and the blood-brain barrier: Lipophilicity as a predictor of permeability. *Brain Res. Bull.* **1985**, *15*, 287–292. [CrossRef]
20. Kumar, P.; Wu, H.; McBride, J.L.; Jung, K.E.; Hee Kim, M.; Davidson, B.L.; Kyung Lee, S.; Shankar, P.; Manjunath, N. Transvascular delivery of small interfering RNA to the central nervous system. *Nature* **2007**, *448*, 39–43. [CrossRef]
21. Neves, V.; Aires-Da-Silva, F.; Morais, M.; Gano, L.; Ribeiro, E.; Pinto, A.; Aguiar, S.; Gaspar, D.; Fernandes, C.; Correia, J.D.G.; et al. Novel Peptides Derived from Dengue Virus Capsid Protein Translocate Reversibly the Blood-Brain Barrier through a Receptor-Free Mechanism. *ACS Chem. Biol.* **2017**, *12*, 1257–1268. [CrossRef] [PubMed]
22. Neves-Coelho, S.; Eleutério, R.P.; Enguita, F.J.; Neves, V.; Castanho, M.A.R.B. A new noncanonical anionic peptide that translocates a cellular blood-brain barrier model. *Molecules* **2017**, *22*, 1753. [CrossRef] [PubMed]
23. Mendonça, D.A.; Bakker, M.; Cruz-Oliveira, C.; Neves, V.; Jiménez, M.A.; Defaus, S.; Cavaco, M.; Veiga, A.S.; Cadima-Couto, I.; Castanho, M.A.R.B.; et al. Penetrating the Blood-Brain Barrier with New Peptide–Porphyrin Conjugates Having anti-HIV Activity. *Bioconjug. Chem.* **2021**, *32*, 1067–1077. [CrossRef]
24. Sakuma, Y.; Baba, R.; Arita, K.; Morimoto, H.; Fujita, M. Food allergens are transferred intact across the rat blood-placental barrier in vivo. *Med. Mol. Morphol.* **2014**, *47*, 14–20. [CrossRef]
25. Neris, R.L.S.; Figueiredo, C.M.; Higa, L.M.; Araujo, D.F.; Carvalho, C.A.M.; Verçoza, B.R.F.; Silva, M.O.L.; Carneiro, F.A.; Tanuri, A.; Gomes, A.M.O.; et al. Co-protoporphyrin IX and Sn-protoporphyrin IX inactivate Zika, Chikungunya and other arboviruses by targeting the viral envelope. *Sci. Rep.* **2018**, *8*, 1–13. [CrossRef]
26. Delcroix, M.; Riley, L.W. Cell-penetrating peptides for antiviral drug development. *Pharmaceuticals* **2010**, *3*, 448–470. [CrossRef]
27. Li, S.Y.; Cheng, H.; Qiu, W.X.; Liu, L.H.; Chen, S.; Hu, Y.; Xie, B.R.; Li, B.; Zhang, X.Z. Protease-Activable Cell-Penetrating Peptide-Protoporphyrin Conjugate for Targeted Photodynamic Therapy in Vivo. *ACS Appl. Mater. Interfaces* **2015**, *7*, 28319–28329. [CrossRef]
28. Dondi, R.; Yaghini, E.; Tewari, K.M.; Wang, L.; Giuntini, F.; Loizidou, M.; MacRobert, A.J.; Eggleston, I.M. Flexible synthesis of cationic peptide-porphyrin derivatives for light-triggered drug delivery and photodynamic therapy. *Org. Biomol. Chem.* **2016**, *14*, 11488–11501. [CrossRef] [PubMed]
29. Lebedeva, N.S.; Gubarev, Y.A.; Koifman, M.O.; Koifman, O.I. The Application of Porphyrins and Their Analogues for Inactivation of Viruses. *Molecules* **2020**, *25*, 4368. [CrossRef] [PubMed]
30. Biscaglia, F.; Gobbo, M. Porphyrin–peptide conjugates in biomedical applications. *Pept. Sci.* **2018**, *110*, e24038. [CrossRef]
31. Assunção-Miranda, I.; Cruz-Oliveira, C.; Neris, R.L.S.; Figueiredo, C.M.; Pereira, L.P.S.; Rodrigues, D.; Araujo, D.F.F.; Da Poian, A.T.; Bozza, M.T. Inactivation of Dengue and Yellow Fever viruses by heme, cobalt-protoporphyrin IX and tin-protoporphyrin IX. *J. Appl. Microbiol.* **2016**, *120*, 790–804. [CrossRef] [PubMed]
32. Cruz-Oliveira, C.; Almeida, A.F.; Freire, J.M.; Caruso, M.B.; Morando, M.A.; Ferreira, V.N.S.; Assunção-Miranda, I.; Gomes, A.M.O.; Castanho, M.A.R.B.; Da Poian, A.T. Mechanisms of Vesicular Stomatitis Virus Inactivation by Protoporphyrin IX, Zinc-Protoporphyrin IX, and Mesoporphyrin IX. *Antimicrob. Agents Chemother.* **2017**, *61*, e00053-17. [CrossRef] [PubMed]
33. Eigenmann, D.E.; Jähne, E.A.; Smieško, M.; Hamburger, M.; Oufir, M. Validation of an immortalized human (hBMEC) in vitro blood-brain barrier model. *Anal. Bioanal. Chem.* **2016**, *408*, 2095–2107. [CrossRef]
34. Jayant, R.; Atluri, V.; Agudelo, M.; Sagar, V.; Kaushik, A.; Nair, M. Sustained-release nanoART formulation for the treatment of neuroAIDS. *Int. J. Nanomed.* **2015**, *10*, 1077. [CrossRef]
35. Yin, T.; Yang, L.; Liu, Y.; Zhou, X.; Sun, J.; Liu, J. Sialic acid (SA)-modified selenium nanoparticles coated with a high blood-brain barrier permeability peptide-B6 peptide for potential use in Alzheimer's disease. *Acta Biomater.* **2015**, *25*, 172–183. [CrossRef]
36. Niewoehner, J.; Bohrmann, B.; Collin, L.; Urich, E.; Sade, H.; Maier, P.; Rueger, P.; Stracke, J.O.; Lau, W.; Tissot, A.C.; et al. Increased Brain Penetration and Potency of a Therapeutic Antibody Using a Monovalent Molecular Shuttle. *Neuron* **2014**, *81*, 49–60. [CrossRef] [PubMed]
37. Rothbauer, M.; Patel, N.; Gondola, H.; Siwetz, M.; Huppertz, B.; Ertl, P. A comparative study of five physiological key parameters between four different human trophoblast-derived cell lines. *Sci. Rep.* **2017**, *7*, 1–11. [CrossRef]
38. Syme, M.R.; Paxton, J.W.; Keelan, J.A. Drug transfer and metabolism by the human placenta. *Clin. Pharmacokinet.* **2004**, *43*, 487–514. [CrossRef] [PubMed]
39. Schneider, H.; Panigel, M.; Dancis, J. Transfer across the perfused human placenta of antipyrine, sodium, and leucine. *Am. J. Obstet. Gynecol.* **1972**, *114*, 822–828. [CrossRef]
40. Cavaco, M.; Valle, J.; da Silva, R.; Correia, J.D.G.; Castanho, M.A.R.B.; Andreu, D.; Neves, V. $_D$ PepH3, an Improved Peptide Shuttle for Receptor-independent Transport Across the Blood-Brain Barrier. *Curr. Pharm. Des.* **2020**, *26*, 1495–1506. [CrossRef]
41. Gallo, M.; Moreno, E.; Defaus, S.; Ortega-Alvaro, A.; Gonzalez, A.; Robledo, P.; Cavaco, M.; Neves, V.; Castanho, M.A.R.B.; Casadó, V.; et al. Orally Active Peptide Vector Allows Using Cannabis to Fight Pain while Avoiding Side Effects. *J. Med. Chem.* **2021**, *64*, 6937–6948. [CrossRef] [PubMed]

pharmaceutics

MDPI

Review

Strategies for Targeted Delivery of Exosomes to the Brain: Advantages and Challenges

Hojun Choi [1], Kyungsun Choi [1], Dae-Hwan Kim [1], Byung-Koo Oh [1], Hwayoung Yim [1], Soojin Jo [1] and Chulhee Choi [1,2,*]

1 ILIAS Biologics Inc., Daejeon 34014, Korea; hchoi@iliasbio.com (H.C.); kchoi@iliasbio.com (K.C.); dkim@iliasbio.com (D.-H.K.); bkoh@iliasbio.com (B.-K.O.); hyim@iliasbio.com (H.Y.); sjo@iliasbio.com (S.J.)

2 Department of Bio and Brain Engineering, Korea Advanced Institute of Science and Technology (KAIST), Daejeon 34141, Korea

* Correspondence: cchoi@iliasbio.com; Tel.: +82-42-863-4450

Abstract: Delivering therapeutics to the central nervous system (CNS) is difficult because of the blood–brain barrier (BBB). Therapeutic delivery across the tight junctions of the BBB can be achieved through various endogenous transportation mechanisms. Receptor-mediated transcytosis (RMT) is one of the most widely investigated and used methods. Drugs can hijack RMT by expressing specific ligands that bind to receptors mediating transcytosis, such as the transferrin receptor (TfR), low-density lipoprotein receptor (LDLR), and insulin receptor (INSR). Cell-penetrating peptides and viral components originating from neurotropic viruses can also be utilized for the efficient BBB crossing of therapeutics. Exosomes, or small extracellular vesicles, have gained attention as natural nanoparticles for treating CNS diseases, owing to their potential for natural BBB crossing and broad surface engineering capability. RMT-mediated transport of exosomes expressing ligands such as LDLR-targeting apolipoprotein B has shown promising results. Although surface-modified exosomes possessing brain targetability have shown enhanced CNS delivery in preclinical studies, the successful development of clinically approved exosome therapeutics for CNS diseases requires the establishment of quantitative and qualitative methods for monitoring exosomal delivery to the brain parenchyma in vivo as well as elucidation of the mechanisms underlying the BBB crossing of surface-modified exosomes.

Keywords: exosome; brain delivery; BBB crossing; transcytosis

Citation: Choi, H.; Choi, K.; Kim, D.-H.; Oh, B.-K.; Yim, H.; Jo, S.; Choi, C. Strategies for Targeted Delivery of Exosomes to the Brain: Advantages and Challenges. *Pharmaceutics* **2022**, *14*, 672. https://doi.org/10.3390/pharmaceutics14030672

Academic Editors: Vibhuti Agrahari, Prashant Kumar and Maria Carafa

Received: 25 December 2021
Accepted: 16 March 2022
Published: 18 March 2022

1. Introduction

The central nervous system (CNS) is one of the most in-demand areas for the development of new therapeutics owing to the increasing occurrence rate of neurodegenerative disorders. However, it remains the most difficult area for drug development because of the blood–brain barrier (BBB), which prevents most of the currently developed drugs from entering the brain parenchyma. The BBB functions as a tight barrier to protect the CNS from potential neurotoxic substances, and regulates the selective transport of specific molecules and nutrients to maintain CNS homeostasis. Water molecules and small ions cross brain capillaries through channels, and small molecules under 500 Da can cross the BBB via passive diffusion [1]. However, macromolecules require specific receptors or transport proteins to facilitate receptor- or adsorptive-mediated transport for entry into the brain parenchyma. The increasing need for new therapeutics for CNS diseases has prompted the investigation of various endogenous transportation mechanisms that can deliver macromolecules across the BBB. The development of novel therapeutics utilizing these transportation pathways has been actively validated in numerous preclinical and clinical studies.

Among the novel therapeutics, exosomes have recently gained attention because of their role as therapeutic vehicles for delivering various active pharmaceutical ingredients to the brain. Exosomes, or small extracellular vesicles (EVs), are a subtype of EVs defined as single-membrane lipid bilayer vesicles generated by vesicle budding into endosomes that mature into multivesicular bodies or by direct vesicle budding from the plasma membrane [2]. Different subtypes of EVs have been identified based on their size and density, which allows separation by methods such as tangential flow filtration, size exclusion chromatography, and differential centrifugation [3]. Nevertheless, careful interpretation is necessary when analyzing different groups of EVs because most EV purification methods cannot determine EVs based on their biogenesis pathways, but rather isolate subtypes of EVs based on their physical properties. Among EVs, exosomes are natural nanoparticles with low immunogenicity that can deliver diverse biological molecules, such as nucleic acids, proteins, lipids, and carbohydrates to target cells [4]. Compared with cell therapy, exosomes possess similar therapeutic efficacy with improved safety profiles in various diseases, such as cancer and ischemia [5–10]. To induce targeted delivery to the brain, therapeutic exosomes can be engineered to express various targeting moieties via direct modification methods, such as chemical modification of exosomal surfaces, or indirect modification methods via genetic engineering of exosome-producing cells. The aim of this review is to briefly discuss current engineering strategies for delivering therapeutics across the BBB and highlight recent advances in the targeted delivery of exosomes to the brain.

2. Current Strategies for Delivering Therapeutics across the BBB

Noninvasive delivery of therapeutics to the CNS can be achieved by hijacking endogenous transport pathways, such as receptor-mediated transcytosis (RMT) and adsorptive-mediated transcytosis (Figure 1, Table 1) [11,12]. Among these, RMT has been the most investigated and applied route for the transportation of drugs through endothelial cells of the BBB [13]. Various therapeutics, including chemicals, antibodies, polymeric nanoparticles, and exosomes, can incorporate these strategies. Their efficacy in brain delivery has been actively tested in numerous preclinical studies and clinical trials [11].

Table 1. Current strategies for delivering therapeutics across the BBB.

BBB Crossing Strategies	Summary
Receptor-mediated transcytosis	- Transcytosis is the vesicular crossing of macromolecules from one side of the cell membrane to the other [14]. - Therapeutics can achieve RMT-mediated brain delivery by expressing specific ligands that bind to receptors inducing transcytosis, such as TfR, LDLR, and INSR [11]. - TfR is responsible for intracellular transport of transferrin and is the most used and validated receptor for RMT-mediated BBB crossing of therapeutics. - LDLR is a ubiquitously expressing receptor and widely expressed in the brain. It is also responsible for the endocytosis of LDLs, such as apolipoprotein B and apolipoprotein E. - INSR is also a widely expressed receptor in various tissues and in the brain microvessels.
Cell-penetrating peptides	- CPPs are a family of various short peptides (fewer than 30 amino acids) that can induce the translocation of macromolecules across cell membranes without interactions with specific receptors [15,16]. - Several issues need to be addressed when using CPPs for brain delivery of therapeutics, such as low tissue specificity and cellular toxicity.
Neurotropic virus	- Neurotropic viruses can cross the BBB and invade the brain parenchyma using specific viral components, such as rabies virus glycoprotein. - Biological safety and clinical efficacy of viral components in the brain delivery of therapeutics should be investigated in more preclinical studies.

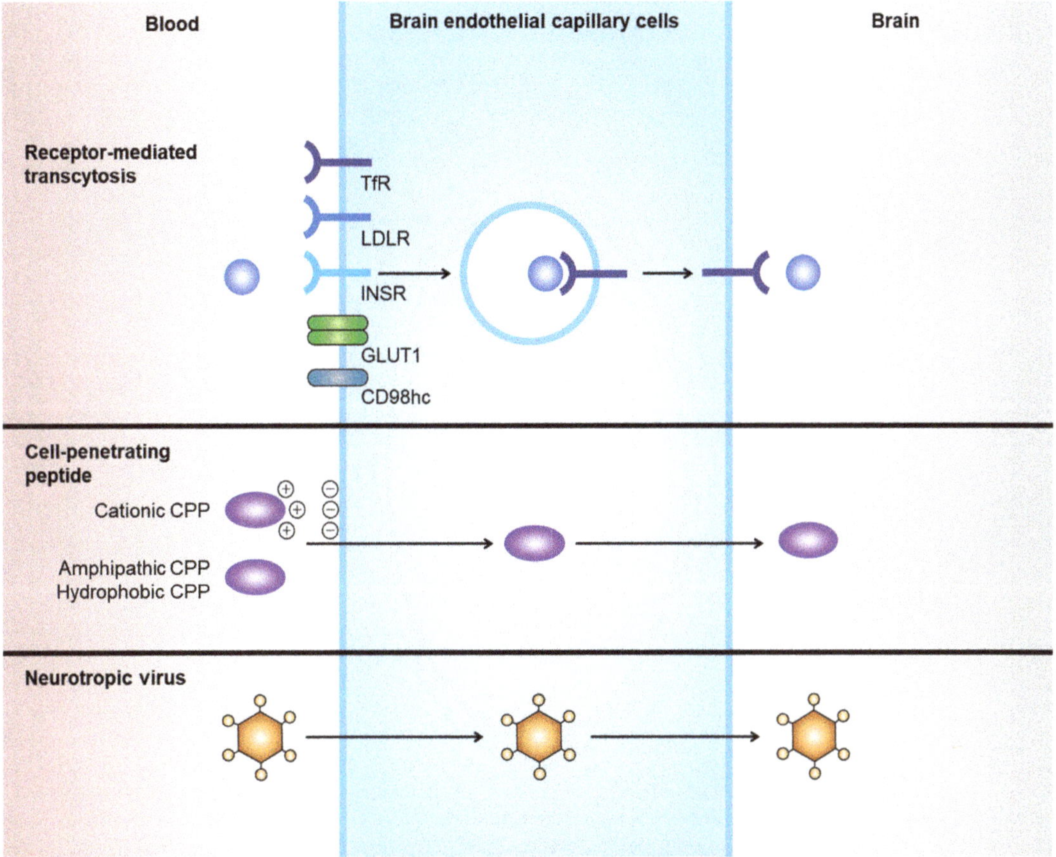

Figure 1. Strategies for delivering therapeutics across the BBB. Noninvasive delivery of therapeutics across the BBB can be achieved by hijacking endogenous transport pathways. RMT-mediated brain delivery of therapeutics can be achieved by expressing specific ligands that bind to receptors and induce transcytosis, such as TfR, LDLR, INSR, GLUT1, and CD98hc. CPPs are a family of various short peptides (fewer than 30 amino acids) that can induce the translocation of macromolecules across cell membranes without interactions with specific receptors. Neurotropic viruses can cross the BBB and invade the brain parenchyma using specific viral components, such as rabies virus glycoprotein.

2.1. Receptor-Mediated Transcytosis

Transcytosis is the vesicular crossing of macromolecules from one side of the cell membrane to another [14]. RMT is mediated by the binding of a ligand to a specific receptor, which subsequently induces receptor-mediated endocytosis and further transports invaginated endosomal compartments to the other side of the membrane. Drugs can hijack RMT by expressing specific ligands that bind to receptors that mediate transcytosis. The optimal receptors to be utilized for RMT-mediated BBB crossing are highly and locally expressed on the membrane of brain capillary endothelial cells (BCECs), with low expression on peripheral endothelial cells. However, to date, no ideal receptor has been identified. Nevertheless, highly and ubiquitously expressed receptors on BCECs have shown promising results in RMT-mediated brain delivery in preclinical studies and several clinical trials.

2.1.1. Transferrin Receptor

The transferrin receptor (TfR) is a widely used and validated receptor for the RMT-mediated BBB crossing of therapeutics. Transferrin is an iron-binding glycoprotein that delivers iron to cells by binding TfR. Although TfR is a ubiquitously expressed receptor, proteomics analysis confirmed that TfR is one of the highest expressed receptors that induces transcytosis in mice [17] and human BCECs [18]. The valency and binding sites of TfR-binding moieties should be carefully considered when developing a TfR-mediated brain delivery system. Recent studies have reported that TfR-targeting antibodies with high valency paradoxically have lower BBB crossing efficacy than low-valency antibodies owing to the lysosomal degradation of antibody-bound TfR [19,20]. Degradation of antibody-bound membrane proteins can also occur in other receptors for RMT-mediated CNS delivery, which warrants further investigation. In addition, it is ideal for TfR-targeting moieties to bind to regions that do not interrupt the endogenous binding of TfR to the receptor. TfR-mediated brain delivery has been applied to various therapeutics, such as liposomes [21–23] and chitosan nanospheres [24]. In addition, several clinical trials of TfR-mediated brain delivery of therapeutics have shown promising results. For example, clinical trials of the lysosomal enzyme iduronate 2-sulfatase conjugated with anti-human TfR antibody have shown positive results in Hunter syndrome (NCT0312893, NCT03568175, and NCT04251026).

2.1.2. Low-Density Lipoprotein Receptor

The low-density lipoprotein receptor (LDLR) family is mainly responsible for the endocytosis of low-density lipoproteins (LDLs), such as apolipoprotein B (ApoB) and apolipoprotein E (ApoE). Each LDL particle contains a single apolipoprotein surrounded by fat molecules, such as cholesterol, phospholipids, and triglycerides, which mediate the delivery of these fatty acids into cells in need. LDLR is not only a ubiquitously expressed receptor, but is also widely expressed in the brain, rendering it an efficient transporter of therapeutics. The conjugation of ApoB- and ApoE-derived peptides to proteins, such as lysosomal enzymes, has been demonstrated to successfully transport proteins across the BBB [25–28]. Nanoparticles, such as liposomes, high-density lipoprotein nanocarriers, and polymersomes, functionalized with ApoE-derived peptides, have also shown enhanced BBB crossing through LDLR- and LDLR-related protein 1 (LRP1)-mediated transcytosis in BCECs [29–35]. ApoB-derived peptides have also exhibited targeted delivery of siRNA and nanoparticles to the brain parenchyma [36,37]. Angiopep-2 is a 19-amino acid peptide originating from the Kunitz domain of bovine protein aprotinin, which binds to LRP1. LRP1 is widely expressed in human and mouse BCECs [18] and gliomas [38], making angiopep-2 an attractive targeting moiety for various nanoparticles for brain delivery and glioma targeting [39–47].

2.1.3. Insulin Receptor

Insulin receptor (INSR) is widely expressed in various tissues. A recent study comparing the expression levels of various receptors mediating transcytosis showed that only INSR was overexpressed in human brain microvessels compared to brain parenchymal and peripheral tissues [48]. A similar pattern was observed in mice, in which INSR, insulin-like growth factor-1 receptor, and LRP8 were highly expressed in brain microvessels compared to those in peripheral tissues [48]. The development of a humanized INSR antibody (HIRMAb), which showed effective delivery in the primate brain after intravenous injection, has accelerated the use of INSR for the brain delivery of drugs [49]. The lysosomal enzyme α-L-iduronidase (IDUA), which is dysfunctional in patients with mucopolysaccharidosis type I, was conjugated to HIRMAb; HIRMAb-conjugated IDUA delivered 1.2% of the injected dose to the brains of rhesus monkeys, whereas IDUA alone resulted in no delivery into the brains [50]. HIRMAb-conjugated IDUA also showed plasma pharmacokinetic profiles comparable to those of human IDUA (laronidase) [51], and an open-label phase 1–2 trial demonstrated a clinical evidence of cognitive and somatic stabilization in patients with mucopolysaccharidosis type I after 52 weeks of intravenous treatment, although few adverse effects, such as infusion-related reactions and transient hypoglycemia, occurred [52].

2.1.4. Other Membrane Proteins

CD98 heavy chain (CD98hc), also known as 4F2 antigen, is a heterodimer membrane protein consisting of a type 2-glycosylated 80-kDa heavy chain linked to a 37-kDa light chain by disulfide bonds [53,54]. CD98hc is highly expressed in human BCECs compared to TfR1, INSR, and LRP1 [18]. CD98hc is expressed on both the apical and basolateral membranes, and can bind and transport amino acids containing CD98 light chains across the BBB [55,56]. A recent study revealed via proteomic analysis that CD98hc is highly expressed in mouse BCECs and that systemic administration of bispecific antibodies targeting CD98hc and β-secretase 1 leads to efficient brain delivery and brain amyloid-beta reduction [17]. This study also showed that targeting CD98hc is more efficient in brain delivery than targeting TfR [17]. CD98hc binding did not alter the endogenous expression and function of CD98hc [17], whereas previous reports have shown that TfR antibodies induce the lysosomal degradation of TfR in an affinity-dependent manner [20].

Glucose transporter 1 (GLUT1), also known as SLC2A1, is a glucose transporter highly expressed on both the apical and basolateral membranes of BCECs [57]. The human brain depends almost entirely on glucose as an energy source, consuming approximately 20% of the total glucose in the body [58], which requires high expression of GLUT1 on the BCECs for efficient glucose transport. Glucose derivatives have been utilized for the BBB crossing of various nanoparticles, such as liposomes [59–63] and micelles [64–66], which implies that GLUT1 could be an attractive target receptor for the CNS delivery of therapeutics.

2.2. Cell-Penetrating Peptides

Cell-penetrating peptides (CPPs), or protein transduction domains, are a family of short peptides (<30 amino acids) that can induce the translocation of biologically active macromolecules across cell membranes without interacting with specific receptors [15,16]. Although no consensus has been reached regarding the taxonomy of CPPs, they can generally be categorized into three classes based on their physicochemical properties: cationic, amphipathic, and hydrophobic [15]. The cationic class is mainly composed of peptides with positive charges, such as arginine and lysine, that can interact with negatively charged plasma membranes. The transactivator of transcription (TAT) protein of HIV-1 was the first CPP observed to be internalized into cells in vitro in 1988 [67,68], and it has since been widely investigated as an inducer of intracellular delivery of therapeutics. Amphipathic CPPs are the most commonly found CPPs in nature, and they contain polar and nonpolar amino acid regions [16]. Hydrophobic CPPs contain nonpolar hydrophobic residues that induce cell penetration by interacting with the hydrophobic domains of plasma membranes. The apical surface of cerebral capillaries is densely covered with a negatively charged glycocalyx, which renders positively charged CPPs an efficient transporter of drugs through the BBB [69]. However, several issues must be addressed when using CPPs for brain delivery, such as their low tissue specificity and cellular toxicity. CPP-conjugated drugs show widespread biodistribution owing to their lack of tissue specificity. In addition, the cytotoxicity of CPPs is a major concern [70], as shown in the case of amphipathic CPP model amphipathic peptide, which induces damage to the cellular membrane, resulting in the leakage of cellular components and subsequent cell death [71].

2.3. Neurotropic Virus

Neurotropic viruses can cross the BBB and invade the brain parenchyma, which prompted the investigation of viruses or viral components as transporters for the brain delivery of therapeutics. For instance, peptides derived from rabies virus glycoprotein (RVG) exhibit efficient penetration through the BBB and target neurons [72]. Although the exact BBB crossing mechanism is unknown, it is expected to occur via neuronal acetylcholine receptor-mediated RMT [72]. RVG has been utilized for the delivery of various nanoparticles through the BBB, including liposomes [73], layered double hydroxide [74], porous silicon nanoparticles [75], and exosomes [76]. However, its biological safety and efficacy should be investigated in preclinical studies for clinical translation.

3. Targeted Delivery of Exosomes to the Brain

3.1. Natural Brain Delivery of Exosomes to the Brain

Unmodified exosomes from various cell types show <1% delivery to the brain after systemic injection [77,78], implying that exosomes have a natural tendency to bypass the BBB. This finding was also observed by our group, although the exact mechanism by which naïve exosomes cross the BBB is unknown. Recent studies have shown that exosomes originating from different parental cells have different organ and tissue tropisms [77,79–81]. Moreover, the specific membrane proteins or molecules of exosomes responsible for the inclination towards specific organs are not fully known. Nevertheless, altering the cell source of exosomes may be a useful strategy to induce brain delivery. Neural stem cell-derived EVs demonstrated enhanced CNS delivery compared with mesenchymal stem cell-derived EVs in a murine stroke model [82]. Based on these observations, exosomes originating from BCECs or brain tumor cells loaded with doxorubicin were tested for the targeted delivery of doxorubicin to brain tumor in a zebrafish model [83].

Transport across the BBB is enhanced under specific pathological conditions. In mice exhibiting brain inflammation, macrophage-derived exosomes showed over three-fold increased delivery to the brain compared to those in normal mice [84]. Enhanced brain delivery is achieved through the interaction of lymphocyte function-associated antigen 1, intercellular adhesion molecule 1, and C-type lectin receptors expressed on macrophage exosomes with BCECs [84]. In an in vitro transwell assay, unmodified naïve exosomes demonstrated enhanced endocytosis and subsequent crossing through BCECs in a tumor necrosis factor-α-induced stroke-like inflammation model [85]. As unmodified exosomes exhibit potential for brain delivery without additional modifications, their efficacy for BBB crossing should be further validated in preclinical studies.

3.2. Brain Delivery of Engineered Exosomes by Receptor-Mediated Transcytosis

Targeted delivery of exosomes to the brain can be achieved through various exosome surface modifications (Figure 2). As hijacking RMT is a widely used strategy for delivering therapeutics across the BBB, it can also be used for transporting exosomes to the brain via labeling of targeting peptides on the surface of exosomes. For example, Kim et al. used a T7 peptide for the delivery of exosomes (T7-exo) [86]. T7 peptide is a TfR-binding peptide with the sequence HAIYPRH, which does not disturb the binding of transferrin to TfR [87,88]. By conjugating T7 peptide to Lamp2b, T7-exo demonstrated superior targeting of intracranial glioblastoma in rat models after intravenous injection compared to unmodified exosomes or RVG-labeled exosomes [86]. Recently, our group utilized the LDLR-mediated transcytosis pathway for the delivery of exosomes by generating ApoB-labeled exosomes via conjugation of ApoB with tetraspanin CD9 (unpublished data). Tetraspanins, such as CD9, CD63, CD81, and CD82, are abundant transmembrane proteins expressed on exosomes, and they consist of four membrane-spanning domains and two extracellular loops termed the short extracellular loop (SEL) and large extracellular loop (LEL) [89]. Tetraspanins can be modified to contain targeting peptides by incorporating the peptides into the extracellular loops of tetraspanin [90]. We transfected Expi293F cells with plasmids encoding *CD9* as a control or *CD9/LEL170-ApoB*, in which ApoB was inserted between the 170–171 amino acid of CD9, to generate ApoB-expressing exosomes. Control exosomes (CD9 exosomes) or ApoB-expressing exosomes (CD9-ApoB exosomes) were isolated and purified from the supernatants of transfected Expi293F cells. To characterize the tissue distribution of the injected exosomes, we labeled CD9 exosomes with DiO and CD9-ApoB exosomes with DiD lipophilic fluorescent dyes, which were injected intravenously into mice. A laser scanning intravital confocal microscope was used to visualize the labeled exosomes in the cerebral cortex of mice by implanting a cranial window. We observed the accumulation of CD9-ApoB exosomes in the cortical blood vessels compared to CD9 exosomes, which were not detected in the vessels (Figure 3a). Next, we examined the biodistribution of surface-engineered exosomes in the mouse brain. DiD-labeled CD9 or CD9-ApoB exosomes were intravenously injected into mice, and the fluorescence intensity was analyzed using a preclinical optical imaging system. As shown in Figure 3b, the fluorescence intensity CD9-ApoB exosomes in the brain was significantly higher than that of the control CD9 exosomes, indicating prolonged retention in the brain for 24 h. These findings revealed the improved CNS-targeting capability of the surface-modified exosomes that hijacked the RMT pathway. Further studies are needed to determine the delivery efficacy of various other receptors for RMT-mediated brain delivery of exosomes.

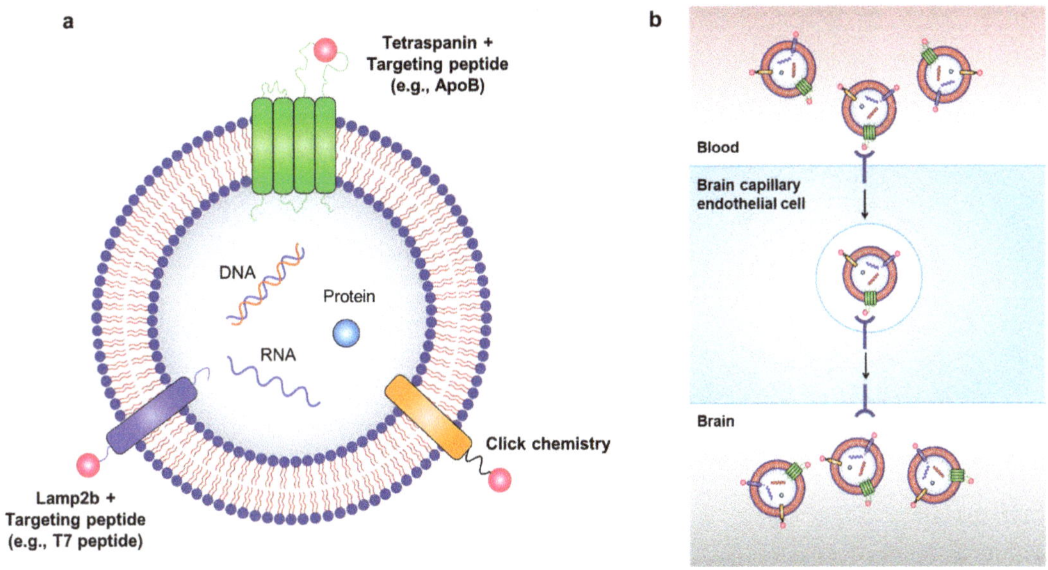

Figure 2. Strategies for targeted delivery of therapeutic exosomes to the brain. (**a**) Targeted delivery of exosomes to the brain can be achieved by labeling various targeting moieties on the surface of exosomes. Therapeutic exosomes can be engineered to express various targeting moieties via chemical modifications, such as click chemistry, or via genetic modification of exosome-producing cells to express targeting peptides fused with exosomal membrane-associated components, such as Lamp2b and tetraspanins. (**b**) RMT can be used to transport exosomes to the brain via labeling of targeting peptides on the surface of exosomes.

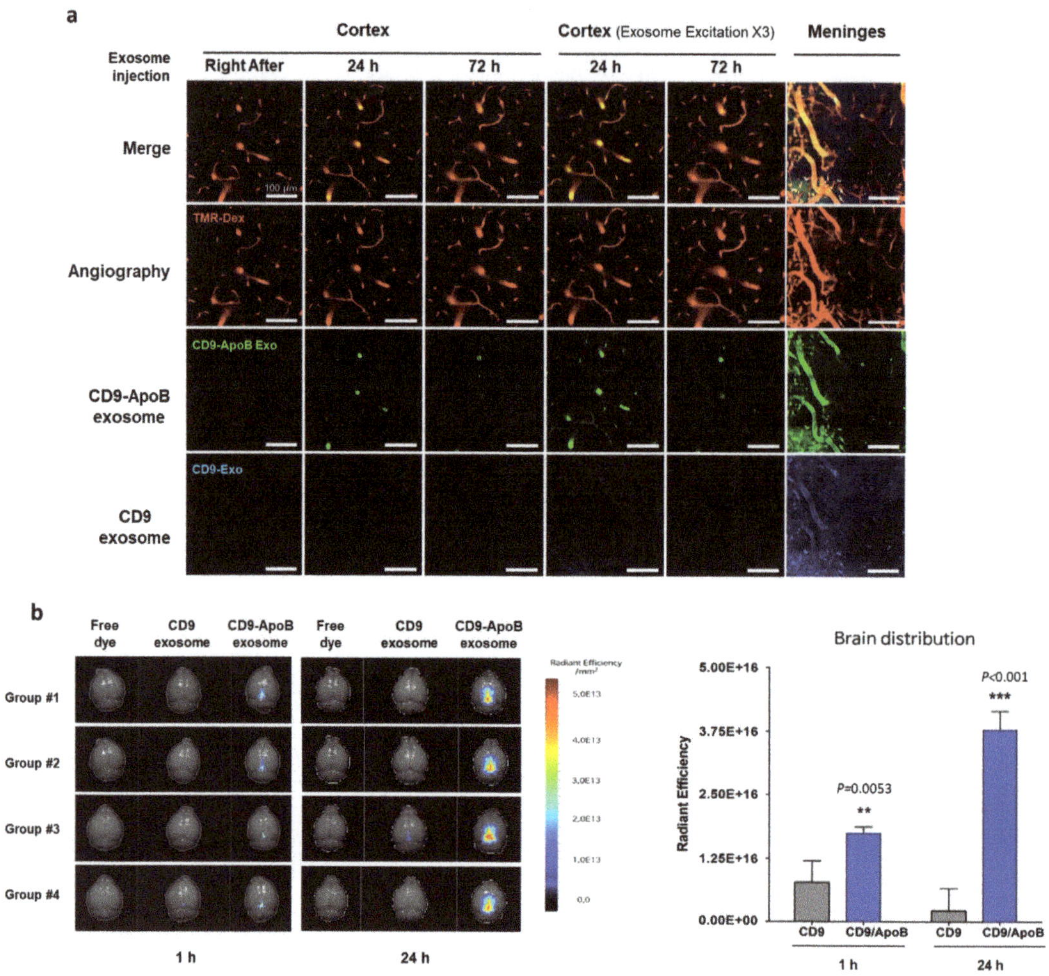

Figure 3. Brain-targeted delivery of exosomes modified with ApoB peptide. (**a**) Exosomes (CD9 or CD9-ApoB) were isolated from transiently transfected Expi293F cells with *CD9* or *CD9/LEL170-ApoB* expression vectors, respectively, and purified using an Amicon Ultra-4 Centrifugal Filter. DiO-labeled CD9 exosomes (blue) and DiD-labeled CD9-ApoB exosomes (green) were intravenously injected (at 1×10^{10} particles each) to C57BL/6 mice. The cortical vascular images of mouse brain in vivo through the cranial window were obtained using intravital confocal microscopy (IVIM Technology, Daejeon, Korea). Cerebral angiography was obtained using TMR-dextran (Red). (**b**) Exosomes (CD9 or CD9-ApoB) were stained with DiD, and labeled exosomes (1×10^{10} particle number/head) were intravenously injected to C57BL/6 mice. The brain distribution of exosomes was determined via fluorescence imaging by VISQUE® InVivo Smart-LF, an in vivo optical imaging system [91]. Differences between groups were compared using two-way analysis of variance with Bonferroni's multiple comparison test. Data are expressed as mean ± SEM. ** $p < 0.01$, *** $p < 0.001$.

3.3. Other Strategies for Brain Delivery

Neurotropic virus-derived peptides, such as RVG, have been used to induce brain-targeting of exosomes in several preclinical studies. In one study, brain delivery of siRNA-loaded exosomes was achieved by expressing RVG at the exosomal membrane and fusing it with Lamp2b, an exosomal membrane protein [76]. The exact BBB crossing pathway has not been shown; however, modified exosomes demonstrated efficient delivery of siRNA to neurons, microglia, and oligodendrocytes in mouse brain [76]. In another study, the same group used a similar approach to deliver siRNA for α-synuclein (α-Syn) to the brain of α-syn transgenic mice [92]. Further studies are needed to identify safety issues associated with the use of virus-derived peptides as therapeutic agents.

Peptides that bind to specific membrane proteins can also be used for exosome modification. For example, c(RGDyK) peptide, which binds to integrin $\alpha_v\beta_3$ that is highly expressed in BCECs under ischemic conditions, was labeled on the surface of mesenchymal stem cell-derived exosomes through click chemistry [93]. Click chemistry, also known as copper-catalyzed azide-alkyne cycloaddition, is an efficient covalent reaction of an alkyne and an azide residue to form a stable triazole linkage, and can be applied to attach various targeting moieties to the surface of exosomes [94–98]. c(RGDyK) peptide-labeled exosomes exhibited 11-fold enhanced delivery to the ischemic region of the brain compared with scrambled peptide-labeled exosomes in a mouse stroke model [93].

4. Conclusions

Exosomes are gaining attention because of their potential as next-generation nanoparticles for treating CNS diseases owing to their potential for natural BBB crossing and broad surface-engineering capability. Various technologies to efficiently incorporate drugs and active pharmaceutical ingredients into exosomes are being actively developed [4,99,100]. In addition, various preclinical studies have investigated engineering strategies for targeted delivery of exosomes to specific organs and tissues [101]. Exosomes carry various membrane proteins (e.g., CD9 [102], CD63 [103], PTGFRN [104], and Lamp2b [76]) and lipids (e.g., phosphatidylserine [105]) that can be utilized for the surface engineering of various targeting moieties. Engineered exosomes possessing targetability to the brain have shown promising results for CNS delivery in preclinical studies; however, they also require intense evaluation through well-designed clinical trials. For the successful development of clinically approved exosome therapeutics for CNS diseases, the establishment of imaging methods for quantitative/qualitative monitoring of exosomal delivery to the brain parenchyma in vivo and uncovering the detailed BBB crossing mechanisms of exosomes is needed.

Author Contributions: Conceptualization, H.C., K.C. and H.Y.; Methodology, H.Y., D.-H.K. and B.-K.O.; Formal analysis, H.Y., D.-H.K., B.-K.O. and S.J.; Data curation, H.C., K.C., H.Y., D.-H.K. and B.-K.O.; Writing—original draft preparation, H.C. and K.C.; Writing—review and editing, C.C.; Supervision, C.C.; Project administration, C.C.; Funding acquisition, C.C. All authors have read and agreed to the published version of the manuscript.

Funding: This work was supported by the Basic Science Research Program through the National Research Foundation (NRF-2016M3A9B6945831) funded by the Ministry of Science and ICT, Republic of Korea.

Institutional Review Board Statement: Animals were purchased from the specific pathogen-free animal facility of Samtako Bio, Inc. (Osan, Korea). All animal experiments were carried out in accordance with an approved protocol (#ILIAS-IACUC-2021-02) by ILIAS Biologics, Inc. and the Institutional Animal Care and Use Committee (IACUC).

Informed Consent Statement: Not applicable.

Data Availability Statement: The datasets generated and/or analyzed during the current study are available from the corresponding author upon reasonable request.

Acknowledgments: We thank Deok-Jin Jang and Cheol Hyoung Park for their constructive suggestions. We also thank Eunjin Kim for performing Nanoparticle Tracking Analysis and DiD labeling of CD9 exosomes and CD9-ApoB exosomes.

Conflicts of Interest: C.C. is the founder and shareholder, and H.C., K.C. and H.Y.Y. are minor shareholders of ILIAS Biologics, Inc. The authors declare no additional financial interest.

References

1. Lipinski, C.A.; Lombardo, F.; Dominy, B.W.; Feeney, P.J. Experimental and computational approaches to estimate solubility and permeability in drug discovery and development settings. *Adv. Drug Deliv. Rev.* **2001**, *46*, 3–26. [CrossRef]
2. Pegtel, D.M.; Gould, S.J. Exosomes. *Annu. Rev. Biochem.* **2019**, *88*, 487–514. [CrossRef]
3. Yang, D.; Zhang, W.; Zhang, H.; Zhang, F.; Chen, L.; Ma, L.; Larcher, L.M.; Chen, S.; Liu, N.; Zhao, Q.; et al. Progress, opportunity, and perspective on exosome isolation—efforts for efficient exosome-based theranostics. *Theranostics* **2020**, *10*, 3684–3707. [CrossRef] [PubMed]
4. Kalluri, R.; LeBleu, V.S. The biology, function, and biomedical applications of exosomes. *Science* **2020**, *367*, eaau6977. [CrossRef] [PubMed]
5. Escudier, B.; Dorval, T.; Chaput, N.; Andre, F.; Caby, M.P.; Novault, S.; Flament, C.; Leboulaire, C.; Borg, C.; Amigorena, S.; et al. Vaccination of metastatic melanoma patients with autologous dendritic cell (DC) derived-exosomes: Results of thefirst phase I clinical trial. *J. Transl. Med.* **2005**, *3*, 10. [CrossRef] [PubMed]
6. Lai, R.C.; Arslan, F.; Lee, M.M.; Sze, N.S.; Choo, A.; Chen, T.S.; Salto-Tellez, M.; Timmers, L.; Lee, C.N.; El Oakley, R.M.; et al. Exosome secreted by MSC reduces myocardial ischemia/reperfusion injury. *Stem Cell Res.* **2010**, *4*, 214–222. [CrossRef] [PubMed]
7. Nikfarjam, S.; Rezaie, J.; Kashanchi, F.; Jafari, R. Dexosomes as a cell-free vaccine for cancer immunotherapy. *J. Exp. Clin. Cancer Res.* **2020**, *39*, 258. [CrossRef]
8. Babaei, M.; Rezaie, J. Application of stem cell-derived exosomes in ischemic diseases: Opportunity and limitations. *J. Transl. Med.* **2021**, *19*, 196. [CrossRef]
9. Ahmadi, M.; Rezaie, J. Ageing and mesenchymal stem cells derived exosomes: Molecular insight and challenges. *Cell Biochem. Funct.* **2021**, *39*, 60–66. [CrossRef]
10. Nam, G.H.; Choi, Y.; Kim, G.B.; Kim, S.; Kim, S.A.; Kim, I.S. Emerging Prospects of Exosomes for Cancer Treatment: From Conventional Therapy to Immunotherapy. *Adv. Mater.* **2020**, *32*, e2002440. [CrossRef]
11. Terstappen, G.C.; Meyer, A.H.; Bell, R.D.; Zhang, W. Strategies for delivering therapeutics across the blood-brain barrier. *Nat. Rev. Drug Discov.* **2021**, *20*, 362–383. [CrossRef] [PubMed]
12. Azarmi, M.; Maleki, H.; Nikkam, N.; Malekinejad, H. Transcellular brain drug delivery: A review on recent advancements. *Int. J. Pharm.* **2020**, *586*, 119582. [CrossRef] [PubMed]
13. Pulgar, V.M. Transcytosis to Cross the Blood Brain Barrier, New Advancements and Challenges. *Front. Neurosci.* **2018**, *12*, 1019. [CrossRef]
14. Tuma, P.; Hubbard, A.L. Transcytosis: Crossing cellular barriers. *Physiol. Rev.* **2003**, *83*, 871–932. [CrossRef] [PubMed]
15. Guidotti, G.; Brambilla, L.; Rossi, D. Cell-Penetrating Peptides: From Basic Research to Clinics. *Trends Pharmcol. Sci.* **2017**, *38*, 406–424. [CrossRef]
16. Xie, J.; Bi, Y.; Zhang, H.; Dong, S.; Teng, L.; Lee, R.J.; Yang, Z. Cell-Penetrating Peptides in Diagnosis and Treatment of Human Diseases: From Preclinical Research to Clinical Application. *Front. Pharmcol.* **2020**, *11*, 697. [CrossRef]
17. Zuchero, Y.J.; Chen, X.; Bien-Ly, N.; Bumbaca, D.; Tong, R.K.; Gao, X.; Zhang, S.; Hoyte, K.; Luk, W.; Huntley, M.A.; et al. Discovery of Novel Blood-Brain Barrier Targets to Enhance Brain Uptake of Therapeutic Antibodies. *Neuron* **2016**, *89*, 70–82. [CrossRef]
18. Uchida, Y.; Ohtsuki, S.; Katsukura, Y.; Ikeda, C.; Suzuki, T.; Kamiie, J.; Terasaki, T. Quantitative targeted absolute proteomics of human blood-brain barrier transporters and receptors. *J. Neurochem.* **2011**, *117*, 333–345. [CrossRef]
19. Niewoehner, J.; Bohrmann, B.; Collin, L.; Urich, E.; Sade, H.; Maier, P.; Rueger, P.; Stracke, J.O.; Lau, W.; Tissot, A.C.; et al. Increased brain penetration and potency of a therapeutic antibody using a monovalent molecular shuttle. *Neuron* **2014**, *81*, 49–60. [CrossRef]
20. Bien-Ly, N.; Yu, Y.J.; Bumbaca, D.; Elstrott, J.; Boswell, C.A.; Zhang, Y.; Luk, W.; Lu, Y.; Dennis, M.S.; Weimer, R.M.; et al. Transferrin receptor (TfR) trafficking determines brain uptake of TfR antibody affinity variants. *J. Exp. Med.* **2014**, *211*, 233–244. [CrossRef]
21. Sharma, G.; Modgil, A.; Layek, B.; Arora, K.; Sun, C.; Law, B.; Singh, J. Cell penetrating peptide tethered bi-ligand liposomes for delivery to brain in vivo: Biodistribution and transfection. *J. Control. Release.* **2013**, *167*, 1–10. [CrossRef] [PubMed]
22. Zhang, Y.; Wang, Y.; Boado, R.J.; Pardridge, W.M. Lysosomal enzyme replacement of the brain with intravenous non-viral gene transfer. *Pharm. Res.* **2008**, *25*, 400–406. [CrossRef] [PubMed]
23. Zhang, Y.; Pardridge, W.M. Near complete rescue of experimental Parkinson's disease with intravenous, non-viral GDNF gene therapy. *Pharm. Res.* **2009**, *26*, 1059–1063. [CrossRef] [PubMed]
24. Karatas, H.; Aktas, Y.; Gursoy-Ozdemir, Y.; Bodur, E.; Yemisci, M.; Caban, S.; Vural, A.; Pinarbasli, O.; Capan, Y.; Fernandez-Megia, E.; et al. A nanomedicine transports a peptide caspase-3 inhibitor across the blood-brain barrier and provides neuroprotection. *J. Neurosci.* **2009**, *29*, 13761–13769. [CrossRef]
25. Spencer, B.J.; Verma, I.M. Targeted delivery of proteins across the blood-brain barrier. *Proc. Natl. Acad. Sci. USA* **2007**, *104*, 7594–7599. [CrossRef]
26. Sorrentino, N.C.; D'Orsi, L.; Sambri, I.; Nusco, E.; Monaco, C.; Spampanato, C.; Polishchuk, E.; Saccone, P.; De Leonibus, E.; Ballabio, A.; et al. A highly secreted sulphamidase engineered to cross the blood-brain barrier corrects brain lesions of mice with mucopolysaccharidoses type IIIA. *EMBO Mol. Med.* **2013**, *5*, 675–690. [CrossRef]

27. Bockenhoff, A.; Cramer, S.; Wolte, P.; Knieling, S.; Wohlenberg, C.; Gieselmann, V.; Galla, H.J.; Matzner, U. Comparison of five peptide vectors for improved brain delivery of the lysosomal enzyme arylsulfatase A. *J. Neurosci.* **2014**, *34*, 3122–3129. [CrossRef]
28. Spencer, B.; Valera, E.; Rockenstein, E.; Trejo-Morales, M.; Adame, A.; Masliah, E. A brain-targeted, modified neurosin (kallikrein-6) reduces alpha-synuclein accumulation in a mouse model of multiple system atrophy. *Mol. Neurodegener.* **2015**, *10*, 48. [CrossRef]
29. Re, F.; Cambianica, I.; Sesana, S.; Salvati, E.; Cagnotto, A.; Salmona, M.; Couraud, P.O.; Moghimi, S.M.; Masserini, M.; Sancini, G. Functionalization with ApoE-derived peptides enhances the interaction with brain capillary endothelial cells of nanoliposomes binding amyloid-beta peptide. *J. Biotechnol.* **2011**, *156*, 341–346. [CrossRef]
30. Re, F.; Cambianica, I.; Zona, C.; Sesana, S.; Gregori, M.; Rigolio, R.; La Ferla, B.; Nicotra, F.; Forloni, G.; Cagnotto, A.; et al. Functionalization of liposomes with ApoE-derived peptides at different density affects cellular uptake and drug transport across a blood-brain barrier model. *Nanomedicine* **2011**, *7*, 551–559. [CrossRef]
31. Wagner, S.; Zensi, A.; Wien, S.L.; Tschickardt, S.E.; Maier, W.; Vogel, T.; Worek, F.; Pietrzik, C.U.; Kreuter, J.; von Briesen, H. Uptake mechanism of ApoE-modified nanoparticles on brain capillary endothelial cells as a blood-brain barrier model. *PLoS ONE* **2012**, *7*, e32568. [CrossRef] [PubMed]
32. Tamaru, M.; Akita, H.; Kajimoto, K.; Sato, Y.; Hatakeyama, H.; Harashima, H. An apolipoprotein E modified liposomal nanoparticle: Ligand dependent efficiency as a siRNA delivery carrier for mouse-derived brain endothelial cells. *Int. J. Pharm.* **2014**, *465*, 77–82. [CrossRef] [PubMed]
33. Song, Q.; Song, H.; Xu, J.; Huang, J.; Hu, M.; Gu, X.; Chen, J.; Zheng, G.; Chen, H.; Gao, X. Biomimetic ApoE-Reconstituted High Density Lipoprotein Nanocarrier for Blood-Brain Barrier Penetration and Amyloid Beta-Targeting Drug Delivery. *Mol. Pharm.* **2016**, *13*, 3976–3987. [CrossRef] [PubMed]
34. Wang, Q.; Kumar, V.; Lin, F.; Sethi, B.; Coulter, D.W.; McGuire, T.R.; Mahato, R.I. ApoE mimetic peptide targeted nanoparticles carrying a BRD4 inhibitor for treating Medulloblastoma in mice. *J. Control. Release* **2020**, *323*, 463–474. [CrossRef]
35. Ouyang, J.; Jiang, Y.; Deng, C.; Zhong, Z.; Lan, Q. Doxorubicin Delivered via ApoE-Directed Reduction-Sensitive Polymersomes Potently Inhibit Orthotopic Human Glioblastoma Xenografts in Nude Mice. *Int. J. Nanomed.* **2021**, *16*, 4105–4115. [CrossRef]
36. Kim, H.R.; Andrieux, K.; Gil, S.; Taverna, M.; Chacun, H.; Desmaele, D.; Taran, F.; Georgin, D.; Couvreur, P. Translocation of poly(ethylene glycol-co-hexadecyl)cyanoacrylate nanoparticles into rat brain endothelial cells: Role of apolipoproteins in receptor-mediated endocytosis. *Biomacromolecules* **2007**, *8*, 793–799. [CrossRef]
37. Spencer, B.; Trinh, I.; Rockenstein, E.; Mante, M.; Florio, J.; Adame, A.; El-Agnaf, O.M.A.; Kim, C.; Masliah, E.; Rissman, R.A. Systemic peptide mediated delivery of an siRNA targeting alpha-syn in the CNS ameliorates the neurodegenerative process in a transgenic model of Lewy body disease. *Neurobiol. Dis.* **2019**, *127*, 163–177. [CrossRef]
38. Baum, L.; Dong, Z.Y.; Choy, K.W.; Pang, C.P.; Ng, H.K. Low density lipoprotein receptor related protein gene amplification and 766T polymorphism in astrocytomas. *Neurosci. Lett.* **1998**, *256*, 5–8. [CrossRef]
39. Demeule, M.; Currie, J.C.; Bertrand, Y.; Che, C.; Nguyen, T.; Regina, A.; Gabathuler, R.; Castaigne, J.P.; Beliveau, R. Involvement of the low-density lipoprotein receptor-related protein in the transcytosis of the brain delivery vector angiopep-2. *J. Neurochem.* **2008**, *106*, 1534–1544. [CrossRef]
40. Regina, A.; Demeule, M.; Che, C.; Lavallee, I.; Poirier, J.; Gabathuler, R.; Beliveau, R.; Castaigne, J.P. Antitumour activity of ANG1005, a conjugate between paclitaxel and the new brain delivery vector Angiopep-2. *Br. J. Pharmcol.* **2008**, *155*, 185–197. [CrossRef]
41. Ren, J.; Shen, S.; Wang, D.; Xi, Z.; Guo, L.; Pang, Z.; Qian, Y.; Sun, X.; Jiang, X. The targeted delivery of anticancer drugs to brain glioma by PEGylated oxidized multi-walled carbon nanotubes modified with angiopep-2. *Biomaterials* **2012**, *33*, 3324–3333. [CrossRef] [PubMed]
42. Xin, H.; Sha, X.; Jiang, X.; Zhang, W.; Chen, L.; Fang, X. Anti-glioblastoma efficacy and safety of paclitaxel-loading Angiopep-conjugated dual targeting PEG-PCL nanoparticles. *Biomaterials* **2012**, *33*, 8167–8176. [CrossRef] [PubMed]
43. Shao, K.; Huang, R.; Li, J.; Han, L.; Ye, L.; Lou, J.; Jiang, C. Angiopep-2 modified PE-PEG based polymeric micelles for amphotericin B delivery targeted to the brain. *J. Control. Release* **2010**, *147*, 118–126. [CrossRef] [PubMed]
44. Huile, G.; Shuaiqi, P.; Zhi, Y.; Shijie, C.; Chen, C.; Xinguo, J.; Shun, S.; Zhiqing, P.; Yu, H. A cascade targeting strategy for brain neuroglial cells employing nanoparticles modified with angiopep-2 peptide and EGFP-EGF1 protein. *Biomaterials* **2011**, *32*, 8669–8675. [CrossRef]
45. He, C.; Zhang, Z.; Ding, Y.; Xue, K.; Wang, X.; Yang, R.; An, Y.; Liu, D.; Hu, C.; Tang, Q. LRP1-mediated pH-sensitive polymersomes facilitate combination therapy of glioblastoma in vitro and in vivo. *J. Nanobiotechnol.* **2021**, *19*, 29. [CrossRef]
46. Costagliola di Polidoro, A.; Zambito, G.; Haeck, J.; Mezzanotte, L.; Lamfers, M.; Netti, P.A.; Torino, E. Theranostic Design of Angiopep-2 Conjugated Hyaluronic Acid Nanoparticles (Thera-ANG-cHANPs) for Dual Targeting and Boosted Imaging of Glioma Cells. *Cancers* **2021**, *13*, 503. [CrossRef]
47. Xu, H.; Li, C.; Wei, Y.; Zheng, H.; Zheng, H.; Wang, B.; Piao, J.G.; Li, F. Angiopep-2-modified calcium arsenite-loaded liposomes for targeted and pH-responsive delivery for anti-glioma therapy. *Biochem. Biophys. Res. Commun.* **2021**, *551*, 14–20. [CrossRef]
48. Zhang, W.; Liu, Q.Y.; Haqqani, A.S.; Leclerc, S.; Liu, Z.; Fauteux, F.; Baumann, E.; Delaney, C.E.; Ly, D.; Star, A.T.; et al. Differential expression of receptors mediating receptor-mediated transcytosis (RMT) in brain microvessels, brain parenchyma and peripheral tissues of the mouse and the human. *Fluids Barriers CNS* **2020**, *17*, 47. [CrossRef]

49. Pardridge, W.M.; Kang, Y.S.; Buciak, J.L.; Yang, J. Human insulin receptor monoclonal antibody undergoes high affinity binding to human brain capillaries in vitro and rapid transcytosis through the blood-brain barrier in vivo in the primate. *Pharm. Res.* **1995**, *12*, 807–816. [CrossRef]
50. Boado, R.J.; Pardridge, W.M. Brain and Organ Uptake in the Rhesus Monkey in Vivo of Recombinant Iduronidase Compared to an Insulin Receptor Antibody-Iduronidase Fusion Protein. *Mol. Pharm.* **2017**, *14*, 1271–1277. [CrossRef]
51. Pardridge, W.M.; Boado, R.J.; Giugliani, R.; Schmidt, M. Plasma Pharmacokinetics of Valanafusp Alpha, a Human Insulin Receptor Antibody-Iduronidase Fusion Protein, in Patients with Mucopolysaccharidosis Type I. *BioDrugs* **2018**, *32*, 169–176. [CrossRef] [PubMed]
52. Giugliani, R.; Giugliani, L.; de Oliveira Poswar, F.; Donis, K.C.; Corte, A.D.; Schmidt, M.; Boado, R.J.; Nestrasil, I.; Nguyen, C.; Chen, S.; et al. Neurocognitive and somatic stabilization in pediatric patients with severe Mucopolysaccharidosis Type I after 52 weeks of intravenous brain-penetrating insulin receptor antibody-iduronidase fusion protein (valanafusp alpha): An open label phase 1-2 trial. *Orphanet J. Rare Dis.* **2018**, *13*, 110. [CrossRef] [PubMed]
53. Hemler, M.E.; Strominger, J.L. Characterization of antigen recognized by the monoclonal antibody (4F2): Different molecular forms on human T and B lymphoblastoid cell lines. *J. Immunol.* **1982**, *129*, 623–628.
54. Kubota, H.; Sato, M.; Ogawa, Y.; Iwai, K.; Hattori, M.; Yoshida, T.; Minato, N. Involvement of 4F2 antigen expressed on the MHC-negative target cells in the recognition of murine CD3+CD4-CD8- alpha beta (V alpha 4/V beta 2) T cells. *Int. Immuno.l* **1994**, *6*, 1323–1331. [CrossRef] [PubMed]
55. Matsuo, H.; Tsukada, S.; Nakata, T.; Chairoungdua, A.; Kim, D.K.; Cha, S.H.; Inatomi, J.; Yorifuji, H.; Fukuda, J.; Endou, H.; et al. Expression of a system L neutral amino acid transporter at the blood-brain barrier. *Neuroreport* **2000**, *11*, 3507–3511. [CrossRef] [PubMed]
56. Feral, C.C.; Nishiya, N.; Fenczik, C.A.; Stuhlmann, H.; Slepak, M.; Ginsberg, M.H. CD98hc (SLC3A2) mediates integrin signaling. *Proc. Natl. Acad. Sci. USA* **2005**, *102*, 355–360. [CrossRef] [PubMed]
57. Patching, S.G. Glucose Transporters at the Blood-Brain Barrier: Function, Regulation and Gateways for Drug Delivery. *Mol. Neurobiol.* **2017**, *54*, 1046–1077. [CrossRef]
58. Benarroch, E.E. Brain glucose transporters: Implications for neurologic disease. *Neurology* **2014**, *82*, 1374–1379. [CrossRef]
59. Xie, F.; Yao, N.; Qin, Y.; Zhang, Q.; Chen, H.; Yuan, M.; Tang, J.; Li, X.; Fan, W.; Zhang, Q.; et al. Investigation of glucose-modified liposomes using polyethylene glycols with different chain lengths as the linkers for brain targeting. *Int. J. Nanomed.* **2012**, *7*, 163–175. [CrossRef]
60. Qu, B.; Li, X.; Guan, M.; Li, X.; Hai, L.; Wu, Y. Design, synthesis and biological evaluation of multivalent glucosides with high affinity as ligands for brain targeting liposomes. *Eur. J. Med. Chem.* **2014**, *72*, 110–118. [CrossRef]
61. Hao, Z.F.; Cui, Y.X.; Li, M.H.; Du, D.; Liu, M.F.; Tao, H.Q.; Li, S.; Cao, F.Y.; Chen, Y.L.; Lei, X.H.; et al. Liposomes modified with P-aminophenyl-alpha-D-mannopyranoside: A carrier for targeting cerebral functional regions in mice. *Eur. J. Pharm. Biopharm.* **2013**, *84*, 505–516. [CrossRef] [PubMed]
62. Du, D.; Chang, N.; Sun, S.; Li, M.; Yu, H.; Liu, M.; Liu, X.; Wang, G.; Li, H.; Liu, X.; et al. The role of glucose transporters in the distribution of p-aminophenyl-alpha-d-mannopyranoside modified liposomes within mice brain. *J. Control. Release* **2014**, *182*, 99–110. [CrossRef] [PubMed]
63. Qin, Y.; Fan, W.; Chen, H.; Yao, N.; Tang, W.; Tang, J.; Yuan, W.; Kuai, R.; Zhang, Z.; Wu, Y.; et al. In vitro and in vivo investigation of glucose-mediated brain-targeting liposomes. *J. Drug Target.* **2010**, *18*, 536–549. [CrossRef]
64. Shao, K.; Zhang, Y.; Ding, N.; Huang, S.; Wu, J.; Li, J.; Yang, C.; Leng, Q.; Ye, L.; Lou, J.; et al. Functionalized nanoscale micelles with brain targeting ability and intercellular microenvironment biosensitivity for anti-intracranial infection applications. *Adv. Healthc. Mater.* **2015**, *4*, 291–300. [CrossRef] [PubMed]
65. Guo, Y.; Zhang, Y.; Li, J.; Zhang, Y.; Lu, Y.; Jiang, X.; He, X.; Ma, H.; An, S.; Jiang, C. Cell microenvironment-controlled antitumor drug releasing-nanomicelles for GLUT1-targeting hepatocellular carcinoma therapy. *ACS Appl. Mater. Interfaces* **2015**, *7*, 5444–5453. [CrossRef]
66. Niu, J.; Wang, A.; Ke, Z.; Zheng, Z. Glucose transporter and folic acid receptor-mediated Pluronic P105 polymeric micelles loaded with doxorubicin for brain tumor treating. *J. Drug Target.* **2014**, *22*, 712–723. [CrossRef]
67. Frankel, A.D.; Pabo, C.O. Cellular uptake of the tat protein from human immunodeficiency virus. *Cell* **1988**, *55*, 1189–1193. [CrossRef]
68. Green, M.; Loewenstein, P.M. Autonomous functional domains of chemically synthesized human immunodeficiency virus tat trans-activator protein. *Cell* **1988**, *55*, 1179–1188. [CrossRef]
69. Ando, Y.; Okada, H.; Takemura, G.; Suzuki, K.; Takada, C.; Tomita, H.; Zaikokuji, R.; Hotta, Y.; Miyazaki, N.; Yano, H.; et al. Brain-Specific Ultrastructure of Capillary Endothelial Glycocalyx and Its Possible Contribution for Blood Brain Barrier. *Sci. Rep.* **2018**, *8*, 17523. [CrossRef]
70. Saar, K.; Lindgren, M.; Hansen, M.; Eiriksdottir, E.; Jiang, Y.; Rosenthal-Aizman, K.; Sassian, M.; Langel, U. Cell-penetrating peptides: A comparative membrane toxicity study. *Anal. Biochem.* **2005**, *345*, 55–65. [CrossRef]
71. Moutal, A.; Francois-Moutal, L.; Brittain, J.M.; Khanna, M.; Khanna, R. Differential neuroprotective potential of CRMP2 peptide aptamers conjugated to cationic, hydrophobic, and amphipathic cell penetrating peptides. *Front. Cell Neurosci.* **2014**, *8*, 471. [CrossRef] [PubMed]

72. Wang, Q.; Cheng, S.; Qin, F.; Fu, A.; Fu, C. Application progress of RVG peptides to facilitate the delivery of therapeutic agents into the central nervous system. *RSC Adv.* **2021**, *11*, 8505–8515. [CrossRef]
73. Dos Santos Rodrigues, B.; Arora, S.; Kanekiyo, T.; Singh, J. Efficient neuronal targeting and transfection using RVG and transferrin-conjugated liposomes. *Brain Res.* **2020**, *1734*, 146738. [CrossRef] [PubMed]
74. Chen, W.; Zuo, H.; Zhang, E.; Li, L.; Henrich-Noack, P.; Cooper, H.; Qian, Y.; Xu, Z.P. Brain Targeting Delivery Facilitated by Ligand-Functionalized Layered Double Hydroxide Nanoparticles. *ACS Appl. Mater. Interfaces* **2018**, *10*, 20326–20333. [CrossRef]
75. Kang, J.; Joo, J.; Kwon, E.J.; Skalak, M.; Hussain, S.; She, Z.G.; Ruoslahti, E.; Bhatia, S.N.; Sailor, M.J. Self-Sealing Porous Silicon-Calcium Silicate Core-Shell Nanoparticles for Targeted siRNA Delivery to the Injured Brain. *Adv. Mater.* **2016**, *28*, 7962–7969. [CrossRef]
76. Alvarez-Erviti, L.; Seow, Y.; Yin, H.; Betts, C.; Lakhal, S.; Wood, M.J. Delivery of siRNA to the mouse brain by systemic injection of targeted exosomes. *Nat. Biotechnol.* **2011**, *29*, 341–345. [CrossRef]
77. Wiklander, O.P.; Nordin, J.Z.; O'Loughlin, A.; Gustafsson, Y.; Corso, G.; Mager, I.; Vader, P.; Lee, Y.; Sork, H.; Seow, Y.; et al. Extracellular vesicle in vivo biodistribution is determined by cell source, route of administration and targeting. *J. Extracell. Vesicles* **2015**, *4*, 26316. [CrossRef]
78. Mirzaaghasi, A.; Han, Y.; Ahn, S.H.; Choi, C.; Park, J.H. Biodistribution and Pharmacokinectics of Liposomes and Exosomes in a Mouse Model of Sepsis. *Pharmaceutics* **2021**, *13*, 427. [CrossRef]
79. Sancho-Albero, M.; Navascues, N.; Mendoza, G.; Sebastian, V.; Arruebo, M.; Martin-Duque, P.; Santamaria, J. Exosome origin determines cell targeting and the transfer of therapeutic nanoparticles towards target cells. *J. Nanobiotechnol.* **2019**, *17*, 16. [CrossRef]
80. Qiao, L.; Hu, S.; Huang, K.; Su, T.; Li, Z.; Vandergriff, A.; Cores, J.; Dinh, P.U.; Allen, T.; Shen, D.; et al. Tumor cell-derived exosomes home to their cells of origin and can be used as Trojan horses to deliver cancer drugs. *Theranostics* **2020**, *10*, 3474–3487. [CrossRef]
81. Smyth, T.; Kullberg, M.; Malik, N.; Smith-Jones, P.; Graner, M.W.; Anchordoquy, T.J. Biodistribution and delivery efficiency of unmodified tumor-derived exosomes. *J. Control. Release* **2015**, *199*, 145–155. [CrossRef] [PubMed]
82. Webb, R.L.; Kaiser, E.E.; Scoville, S.L.; Thompson, T.A.; Fatima, S.; Pandya, C.; Sriram, K.; Swetenburg, R.L.; Vaibhav, K.; Arbab, A.S.; et al. Human Neural Stem Cell Extracellular Vesicles Improve Tissue and Functional Recovery in the Murine Thromboembolic Stroke Model. *Transl. Stroke Res.* **2018**, *9*, 530–539. [CrossRef]
83. Yang, T.Z.; Martin, P.; Fogarty, B.; Brown, A.; Schurman, K.; Phipps, R.; Yin, V.P.; Lockman, P.; Bai, S.H. Exosome Delivered Anticancer Drugs Across the Blood-Brain Barrier for Brain Cancer Therapy in Danio Rerio. *Pharm. Res.* **2015**, *32*, 2003–2014. [CrossRef] [PubMed]
84. Yuan, D.; Zhao, Y.; Banks, W.A.; Bullock, K.M.; Haney, M.; Batrakova, E.; Kabanov, A.V. Macrophage exosomes as natural nanocarriers for protein delivery to inflamed brain. *Biomaterials* **2017**, *142*, 1–12. [CrossRef] [PubMed]
85. Chen, C.C.; Liu, L.N.; Ma, F.X.; Wong, C.W.; Guo, X.N.E.; Chacko, J.V.; Farhoodi, H.P.; Zhang, S.X.; Zimak, J.; Segaliny, A.; et al. Elucidation of Exosome Migration Across the Blood-Brain Barrier Model In Vitro. *Cell. Mol. Bioeng.* **2016**, *9*, 509–529. [CrossRef]
86. Kim, G.; Kim, M.; Lee, Y.; Byun, J.W.; Hwang, D.W.; Lee, M. Systemic delivery of microRNA-21 antisense oligonucleotides to the brain using T7-peptide decorated exosomes. *J. Control. Release* **2020**, *317*, 273–281. [CrossRef]
87. Lee, J.H.; Engler, J.A.; Collawn, J.F.; Moore, B.A. Receptor mediated uptake of peptides that bind the human transferrin receptor. *Eur. J. Biochem.* **2001**, *268*, 2004–2012. [CrossRef]
88. Han, L.; Huang, R.; Liu, S.; Huang, S.; Jiang, C. Peptide-conjugated PAMAM for targeted doxorubicin delivery to transferrin receptor overexpressed tumors. *Mol. Pharm.* **2010**, *7*, 2156–2165. [CrossRef]
89. Umeda, R.; Satouh, Y.; Takemoto, M.; Nakada-Nakura, Y.; Liu, K.; Yokoyama, T.; Shirouzu, M.; Iwata, S.; Nomura, N.; Sato, K.; et al. Structural insights into tetraspanin CD9 function. *Nat. Commun.* **2020**, *11*, 1606. [CrossRef]
90. Khan, H.; Pan, J.J.; Li, Y.; Zhang, Z.; Yang, G.Y. Native and Bioengineered Exosomes for Ischemic Stroke Therapy. *Front. Cell Dev. Biol.* **2021**, *9*, 619565. [CrossRef]
91. Jeong, H.; Kim, S.-R.; Kang, Y.; Kim, H.; Kim, S.-Y.; Cho, S.-H.; Kim, K.-N. Real-Time Longitudinal Evaluation of Tumor Blood Vessels Using a Compact Preclinical Fluorescence Imaging System. *Biosensors* **2021**, *11*, 471. [CrossRef] [PubMed]
92. Cooper, J.M.; Wiklander, P.B.; Nordin, J.Z.; Al-Shawi, R.; Wood, M.J.; Vithlani, M.; Schapira, A.H.; Simons, J.P.; El-Andaloussi, S.; Alvarez-Erviti, L. Systemic exosomal siRNA delivery reduced alpha-synuclein aggregates in brains of transgenic mice. *Mov. Disord.* **2014**, *29*, 1476–1485. [CrossRef] [PubMed]
93. Tian, T.; Zhang, H.X.; He, C.P.; Fan, S.; Zhu, Y.L.; Qi, C.; Huang, N.P.; Xiao, Z.D.; Lu, Z.H.; Tannous, B.A.; et al. Surface functionalized exosomes as targeted drug delivery vehicles for cerebral ischemia therapy. *Biomaterials* **2018**, *150*, 137–149. [CrossRef]
94. Smyth, T.; Petrova, K.; Payton, N.M.; Persaud, I.; Redzic, J.S.; Graner, M.W.; Smith-Jones, P.; Anchordoquy, T.J. Surface functionalization of exosomes using click chemistry. *Bioconjug. Chem.* **2014**, *25*, 1777–1784. [CrossRef] [PubMed]
95. Ramasubramanian, L.; Kumar, P.; Wang, A. Engineering Extracellular Vesicles as Nanotherapeutics for Regenerative Medicine. *Biomolecules* **2019**, *10*, 48. [CrossRef] [PubMed]
96. Algar, W.R.; Prasuhn, D.E.; Stewart, M.H.; Jennings, T.L.; Blanco-Canosa, J.B.; Dawson, P.E.; Medintz, I.L. The controlled display of biomolecules on nanoparticles: A challenge suited to bioorthogonal chemistry. *Bioconjug. Chem.* **2011**, *22*, 825–858. [CrossRef] [PubMed]

97. Villata, S.; Canta, M.; Cauda, V. EVs and Bioengineering: From Cellular Products to Engineered Nanomachines. *Int. J. Mol. Sci.* **2020**, *21*, 6048. [CrossRef] [PubMed]
98. Nwe, K.; Brechbiel, M.W. Growing applications of "click chemistry" for bioconjugation in contemporary biomedical research. *Cancer Biother. Radiopharm.* **2009**, *24*, 289–302. [CrossRef]
99. Song, Y.; Kim, Y.; Ha, S.; Sheller-Miller, S.; Yoo, J.; Choi, C.; Park, C.H. The emerging role of exosomes as novel therapeutics: Biology, technologies, clinical applications, and the next. *Am. J. Reprod. Immunol.* **2021**, *85*, e13329. [CrossRef]
100. Herrmann, I.K.; Wood, M.J.A.; Fuhrmann, G. Extracellular vesicles as a next-generation drug delivery platform. *Nat. Nanotechnol.* **2021**, *16*, 748–759. [CrossRef]
101. Choi, H.; Choi, Y.; Yim, H.Y.; Mirzaaghasi, A.; Yoo, J.K.; Choi, C. Biodistribution of Exosomes and Engineering Strategies for Targeted Delivery of Therapeutic Exosomes. *Tissue Eng. Regen. Med.* **2021**, *18*, 499–511. [CrossRef] [PubMed]
102. Yim, N.; Ryu, S.W.; Choi, K.; Lee, K.R.; Lee, S.; Choi, H.; Kim, J.; Shaker, M.R.; Sun, W.; Park, J.H.; et al. Exosome engineering for efficient intracellular delivery of soluble proteins using optically reversible protein-protein interaction module. *Nat. Commun.* **2016**, *7*, 12277. [CrossRef] [PubMed]
103. Stickney, Z.; Losacco, J.; McDevitt, S.; Zhang, Z.; Lu, B. Development of exosome surface display technology in living human cells. *Biochem. Biophys. Res. Commun.* **2016**, *472*, 53–59. [CrossRef] [PubMed]
104. Dooley, K.; McConnell, R.E.; Xu, K.; Lewis, N.D.; Haupt, S.; Youniss, M.R.; Martin, S.; Sia, C.L.; McCoy, C.; Moniz, R.J.; et al. A versatile platform for generating engineered extracellular vesicles with defined therapeutic properties. *Mol. Ther.* **2021**, *29*, 1729–1743. [CrossRef]
105. Skotland, T.; Hessvik, N.P.; Sandvig, K.; Llorente, A. Exosomal lipid composition and the role of ether lipids and phosphoinositides in exosome biology. *J. Lipid Res.* **2019**, *60*, 9–18. [CrossRef]

pharmaceutics

MDPI

Article

Injectable Biodegradable Silica Depot: Two Months of Sustained Release of the Blood Glucose Lowering Peptide, Pramlintide

Puneet Tyagi [1,*], Mika Koskinen [2], Jari Mikkola [2], Sanjay Sarkhel [2], Lasse Leino [2], Asha Seth [3], Shimona Madalli [3], Sarah Will [4], Victor G. Howard [4], Helen Brant [5] and Dominic Corkill [6]

1 Dosage Form Design and Development, BioPharmaceuticals R&D, AstraZeneca, Gaithersburg, MD 20874, USA
2 DelSiTech Ltd., PharmaCity, Itäinen Pitkäkatu 4 B, 20520 Turku, Finland; mika.k.koskinen@delsitech.com (M.K.); jari.mikkola@delsitech.com (J.M.); sanjay.sarkhel@uef.fi (S.S.); lasse.leino@delsitech.com (L.L.)
3 Renal BioScience, Early CVRM, BioPharmaceuticals R&D, AstraZeneca, Cambridge CB21 6GP, UK; asha.seth@astrazeneca.com (A.S.); shimonap7@gmail.com (S.M.)
4 Metabolism BioScience, Early CVRM, BioPharmaceuticals R&D, AstraZeneca, Gaithersburg, MD 20878, USA; sarah.will@astrazeneca.com (S.W.); victor.howard@sparktx.com (V.G.H.)
5 Animal Science & Technologies UK, Clinical Pharmacology & Safety Sciences, AstraZeneca, Cambridge CB21 6GP, UK; helen.brant@kymab.com
6 Early R&I BioPharmaceuticals R&D, AstraZeneca, Cambridge CB21 6GP, UK; dominic.corkill@astrazeneca.com
* Correspondence: puneet.tyagi@astrazeneca.com; Tel.: +1-301-398-5532

Abstract: Diabetes mellitus is a major healthcare challenge. Pramlintide, a peptide analogue of the hormone amylin, is currently used as an adjunct with insulin for patients who fail to achieve glycemic control with only insulin therapy. However, hypoglycemia is the dominant risk factor associated with such approaches and careful dosing of both drugs is needed. To mitigate this risk factor and compliance issues related to multiple dosing of different drugs, sustained delivery of Pramlintide from silica depot administered subcutaneously (SC) was investigated in a rat model. The pramlintide-silica microparticle hydrogel depot was formulated by spray drying of silica sol-gels. In vitro dissolution tests revealed an initial burst of pramlintide followed by controlled release due to the dissolution of the silica matrix. At higher dosing, pramlintide released from subcutaneously administered silica depot in rats showed a steady concentration of 500 pM in serum for 60 days. Released pramlintide retained its pharmacological activity in vivo, as evidenced by loss of weight. The biodegradable silica matrix offers a sustained release of pramlintide for at least two months in the rat model and shows potential for clinical applications.

Keywords: long acting; sustained delivery; biologics; silica microparticles

Citation: Tyagi, P.; Koskinen, M.; Mikkola, J.; Sarkhel, S.; Leino, L.; Seth, A.; Madalli, S.; Will, S.; Howard, V.G.; Brant, H.; et al. Injectable Biodegradable Silica Depot: Two Months of Sustained Release of the Blood Glucose Lowering Peptide, Pramlintide. *Pharmaceutics* **2022**, *14*, 553. https://doi.org/10.3390/pharmaceutics14030553

Academic Editor: Emanuela Fabiola Craparo

Received: 12 October 2021
Accepted: 15 February 2022
Published: 2 March 2022

1. Introduction

Diabetes mellitus poses a major global health challenge, with estimates of the human population affected to touch a staggering 783 million by 2045 [1]. It results from a complete deficiency of insulin (type 1) or impaired insulin secretion (type II) due to β-cell dysfunction. Insulin and related β-cell hormones regulate postprandial glucose regulation by decreasing glucagon secretion [2–4] and slowing gastric emptying. The disease imposes a huge burden on the healthcare system and accounts for more than 10% of its spending [1]. It manifests multiple complications, and an active diabetes care and management program aims at regulating the blood glycemic levels [5]. Therapeutic interventions range from lifestyle changes, drugs, smart delivery technologies, and regenerative medicine [3,5–8]. Although therapeutic drugs have some limitations, they continue to be the main choice in the active management of diabetes care. Currently, the most widely used therapeutic for diabetes control is based on the endogenous hormone, insulin, and its analogues [7,9]. However, due to their complex molecular structure and physicochemical properties, formulation and delivery of these peptides need due consideration [10–14]. Parenteral routes, such as intravenous, intramuscular, and subcutaneous are the most popular routes of delivery for these peptides.

A major challenge in diabetes management concerns regulating the varying amounts of blood glucose during the course of a day. In response to dietary food intake, glucose metabolism is carried out by the pancreas by secreting insulin and the related hormone amylin. Amylin complements insulin in the regulation of postprandial glucose by decreasing glucagon release, slowing gastric emptying, and decreasing food intake [15]. Therapeutic intervention by insulin and amylin-based peptides to regulate blood glucose metabolism in diabetes is thus a logical mimic of the endogenous system. A synthetic analogue of amylin, pramlintide acetate (Mw. = 3951.41) is used as an adjunct to preprandial insulin therapy in diabetic patients who fail to achieve glycemic control with insulin therapy alone [16,17]. The pharmacokinetic (PK) profile of blood glucose-lowering drugs is key in defining their in vivo efficacy. Blood glucose levels vary within a day depending on the timing and nature of food intake. A drug with an inadequate PK profile will lack efficacy in regulating glucose levels and consequently might need multiple dosing. Excessive moderation of glucose levels might result in hypoglycemic conditions and may prove fatal [18]. Engineering the PK profile of a glucose-lowering drug is an area of intense investigation and has resulted in various analogues of insulin designed to be active from short-acting up to long-acting [7]. In this context, reports from clinical studies seem to suggest that maintaining a threshold level of glucose-lowering hormones may better facilitate the management of diabetes [19,20]. Sustained delivery systems such as implants made from a mixture of insulin and micro-recrystallized palmitic acid (marketed as Linbit™ and Linplant™) have shown better therapeutic efficacy as compared to daily insulin injections in rodents [21]. Although insulin implants show promise, they require surgical intervention. This is not only a burden to the healthcare system but also a concern for patient compliance. Sustained injectable drug delivery systems have shown promise and offer the advantage of avoiding the need for repeated dosing to achieve therapeutic effects. Similar to pramlintide activity, GLP-1 peptide elicits insulinotropic effects by binding to the GLP-1 receptor, thereby regulating insulin and glucagon secretion. However, endogenous GLP-1 is rapidly degraded with a 1.5–5 min half-life [22,23]. Nanoparticle-based drug delivery systems have been often employed to enhance the bioavailability of drugs. For example, Choi et al. [24] prepared a copolymer of poly [(dl-lactic acid-co-glycolic acid)-b-ethylene glycol-b-(dl-lactic acid-co-glycolic acid)] that undergoes a temperature-dependent reversible solution–gel transition for in situ depot formation to deliver GLP-1. However, most polymer-based sustained delivery systems lack clinical translation due to limitations issues related to reproducible scale-up of mono-disperse particles [25,26]. In a very recent report, GLP-1 fused recombinantly to elastin-like polypeptide (ELP), has been shown to elicit zero-order release kinetics from a subcutaneous depot and circulation times (also glycemic control) up to 10 days in mice [27].

In this communication, we highlight a sustained delivery strategy for in vivo delivery of the synthetic peptide analogue of amylin, pramlintide acetate. As mentioned earlier, amylin is the endogenous hormone co-secreted with insulin by the pancreas for glucose metabolism in vivo. Clinical investigations seem to suggest that there is an increased risk of severe hypoglycemia (particularly in type I diabetes) when adjunctive therapy is used with insulin and careful dosing is required for patient safety [18]. Such effects can be moderated either by decreasing the single dosing of preprandial insulin/pramlintide or by a sustained long-term slow release of the hormone(s) [19]. Sustained slow delivery of pramlintide might mitigate the need for separate administration of the two drugs by injection each time before a meal and might improve patient compliance. We present here the formulation and in vivo (rat model) release profile of pramlintide from our proprietary silica-based delivery matrix [28–30]. Silica offers numerous advantages as compared to other sustained release systems. It is biodegradable, offers formulation under mild aqueous conditions and its degradation product, silicic acid (weak acid, pKa 9.84) does not acidify the environment and is non-toxic. This presents a significant advantage for formulation (in near-native conditions) and delivery (degraded products do not destabilise protein structure) of biologicals [25,31].

2. Materials and Methods

2.1. Materials

All analytical grade reagents and solvents, including tetraethyl orthosilicate (TEOS) and standard solution for silicon atomic absorption, were purchased from Sigma-Aldrich (St. Louis, MO, USA). Pramlintide acetate was obtained from MedImmune, Inc. (Gaithersburg, MD, USA).

2.2. Preparation of Silica Microparticles

TEOS was hydrolyzed in the presence of deionized water and 0.1 M HCl to prepare the silica sol. TEOS/water/HCl at a molar ratio of 1:15:0.005 was hydrolyzed at room temperature, under vigorous stirring for 25 min. Following hydrolysis, silica sol was stored in an ice bath for 1 h, and the pH adjusted to 2.6. Aqueous solution of pramlintide (10 mg/mL) was mixed with the silica sol to yield 5% *w*/*w* pramlintide load while stirring vigorously. The silica sol–pramlintide mixture was further diluted with water to attain a molar ratio of TEOS/water to 1:150 at pH 4.0. A mini spray dryer (Büchi B-191, Flawil, Switzerland) was used to spray dry the silica sol–pramlintide having inlet and outlet temperatures of 125 °C and 60 °C, respectively, at the feed rate of 4 mL/min.

2.3. Preparation of Pramlintide-Silica Microparticle Silica Hydrogel Depot Formulation

Pramlintide-silica depot was prepared by combining the spray-dried pramlintide-silica microparticles with R400 silica sol. As mentioned earlier, the R400 silica sol was prepared by acid-catalysed (pH 2.0) hydrolysis of TEOS in a molar ratio (TEOS/water) of 1:400. The R400 sol was added to pramlintide-silica microparticles (1 mL/0.5 g) and magnetically stirred to a suspension. The pH of the suspension was adjusted to 6.3 by dropwise addition of 1 M NaOH. Additionally, 1 mL plastic syringes (Becton-Dickinson, Franklin Lake, NJ, USA # 309628) were filled with the homogenous suspension and capped (Sigma-Aldrich, St. Louis, MO, USA, Monoject syringe tip caps). The suspension was allowed to gel at ambient temperature while maintaining homogeneity by placing the syringes on a rotor (Stuart Rotator SB3).

2.4. In Vitro Dissolution Test

To quantify silica dissolution rate, 20 mg of spray-dried pramlintide-silica microparticles were dispersed in 50 mL of 50 mM TRIS buffer (pH 7.4). The microparticle dispersion was kept in a shaking water bath maintained at 37 °C. To quantify pramlintide dissolution rate, pH 7.4 PBS containing 0.01% Tween 80 was used as the dispersing media. Samples were extracted every day and replaced with fresh buffer. Silicon molybdenum blue complex [32] spectrophotometry assay was used to quantify soluble silica. HPLC was used to quantify pramlintide released from the silica depot (described below).

2.5. HPLC Analysis of PRAMLINTIDE

The Agilent Technologies 1260 HPLC system with a Waters XBridge protein BEH C4 3.5 μm, 4.6 × 20 mm column was used to measure pramlintide by a reversed-phase HPLC. Mobile phase A included water and trifluoroacetic acid (1000:1, *v*/*v*) and mobile phase B included acetonitrile and trifluoroacetic acid (1000:0.9 *v*/*v*). Mobile phase gradient was 20% B to 65% B over 3 min followed by a reverse gradient from 65% B to 20% B over 30 s and 2.5 min balancing at the end. A 100 μL sample was injected at a flow rate of 1 mL/min, with a column oven temperature of 80 °C. Absorbance was measured at 204 nm.

2.6. *Total Silica Content Measurement*

Dissolved silica was estimated as a soluble silicon molybdenum blue complex. For this, 20–30 mg of pramlintide-silica depot and 10–15 mg of pramlintide microparticles (in a separate experiment) were completely dissolved in 50 mL of 0.5 M NaOH for 48 h at 37 °C. The relative amount of microparticles in the depot was estimated.

2.7. *Total Pramlintide Content Measurement*

The total content of pramlintide within silica microparticles was estimated by organic elemental analysis (OEA) using a FLASH2000 elemental analyzer instrument (Thermo Fisher Scientific, Waltham, NJ, USA) with a CHNS configuration. Analysis was carried out using 1–2 mg of pramlintide-silica microparticles. By measuring the nitrogen content of the sample (OEA method), the amount of pramlintide within the microparticles could be determined as it is the only source of nitrogen within the sample.

2.8. *Characterization of Pramlintide-silica Microparticles and Depot Formulation*

Scanning electron microscopy (SEM) and particle size distribution (PSD) methods were utilised to characterise the pramlintide-silica microparticles. For SEM analysis, LEO Gemini 153 with a Thermo Scientific UltraDry Silicon Drift Detector (SDD) was used, whereas PSD measurements were carried out with a Sympatec HELOS 2370 laser diffraction instrument. Rheological measurements were made using a single rotational rheometer equipped with a parallel-plate with a HPP20 TC measuring geometry (D = 20 mm). Dynamic viscosity was measured by applying shearing force (0.01 to 1000 1/s at 25 °C). Becton Dickinson pre-filled syringes with a 25-G needle (Fine-Ject, Henke Sass Wolf, Tuttlingen, Germany) were used for injection pressure and force measurements. For this, the syringe was placed in a custom-made fixture device with the needle pointing downwards. The load cell of the compression tester was lowered to the point so that it barely touched the plunger (preload less than 0.2 N) and this was recorded as the zero-point. The plunger was compressed with the load cell at a rate of 60 mm/min. Pressure was calculated as a function of the machine extension and the resulting force (N) was estimated by considering the plunger area (16.04 mm^2) of the Becton Dickinson syringe. NEGYXEN Plus software (Ametek, Largo, FL, USA) was utilised for the measurements.

2.9. *Endotoxin Analysis*

Endotoxin analysis was carried out based on methods outlined in EP 2.6.14/USP<85>.

2.10. *Pharmacokinetic and Pharmacodynamic Study in Rat*

The pharmacokinetic profile was determined in a multidose study in male SD rats weighing approximately 260–290 g. All experiments were conducted at Medimmune, Cambridge, UK, in accordance with the Animals Scientific Procedures Act 1986. Following an acclimatisation period, male SD rats (Charles River, Margate, Kent UK) were assigned to one of two groups, so that bodyweight was equally distributed between the two groups (average weight per group 275 g). Rats were given a single subcutaneous dose of pramlintide microparticle-silica hydrogel depot at a dose of either 5 mg/kg or 15 mg/kg of pramlintide. Pramlintide-silica depot formulation was supplied as a pre-filled syringe, ready to dose. The volume injected was adjusted for each animal to achieve the appropriate mg/kg dose. Serial serum samples obtained from the tail vein were collected from each animal at 6, 24, and 72 h following drug administration. Following this, serum samples were collected at weekly intervals, commencing at one week following dose administration and concluding at eight weeks post-dose. The serum concentration of pramlintide was determined using a human amylin ELISA (Millipore, Darmstadt, Germany EZHA-52K). Graphs and analyses were generated using GraphPad Prism 6.0 (GraphPad Software Inc., La Jolla, CA, USA).

Bodyweight changes were studied in diet-induced obese rats. This experiment was run at AstraZeneca, Gaithersburg, MD, USA according to Institutional Animal Care and Use Committee (IACUC) guidelines. Sprague–Dawley rats arrived at 200–250 g, (Envigo;

Indianapolis, IN, USA) were pair-housed and following acclimation, placed on a condensed milk high-fat diet (D12266B, Research Diets; Brunswick, NJ, USA). Following approximately 10 weeks on a high-fat diet, rats were single housed for 2 weeks prior to study start. Rats were sorted into study groups on body weight (average weight per group 444 g). Rats (n = 8/group) received a single SC injection of pramlintide microparticle-silica hydrogel at a dose of 3.6, 11, or 22 mg/kg. Vehicle rats received an empty matrix SC injection. Bodyweight was monitored over 28 days.

3. Results and Discussion

3.1. *Preparation of Pramlintide Loaded Silica Microparticles*

Acid-catalysed hydrolysis of TEOS resulted in silica sol. The addition of pramlintide solution into the sol encapsulated the peptide within the networked structure of silica. Spray drying yielded pramlintide-loaded non-porous silica microparticles [28,33]. The microparticles were mixed with silica hydrogel (R400) to produce an injectable depot. A load of 3.7% (w/w) of pramlintide with respect to silica was achieved in microparticle formulation (estimated by OEA analysis). Based on the silica content analysis of the depot, the amount of pramlintide in the depot formulation was estimated to be 11 mg/mL.

3.2. *SEM Analysis and Particle Size Distribution of the Microparticles*

A representative SEM image of pramlintide containing microparticles is shown in Figure 1. The SEM images seem to suggest that particle agglomerates are minimal in the microparticle formulation process. Microparticle shapes tend to vary; this could be due to the spray drying process. PSD measurements (mean ± SD, n = 3) were 1.64 ± 0.03 µm, 3.39 ± 0.03 µm, 6.97 ± 0.01, for D10, D50 and D90, respectively. The D value is the diameter at which that % of the sample's mass is comprised of particles with a diameter less than this value.

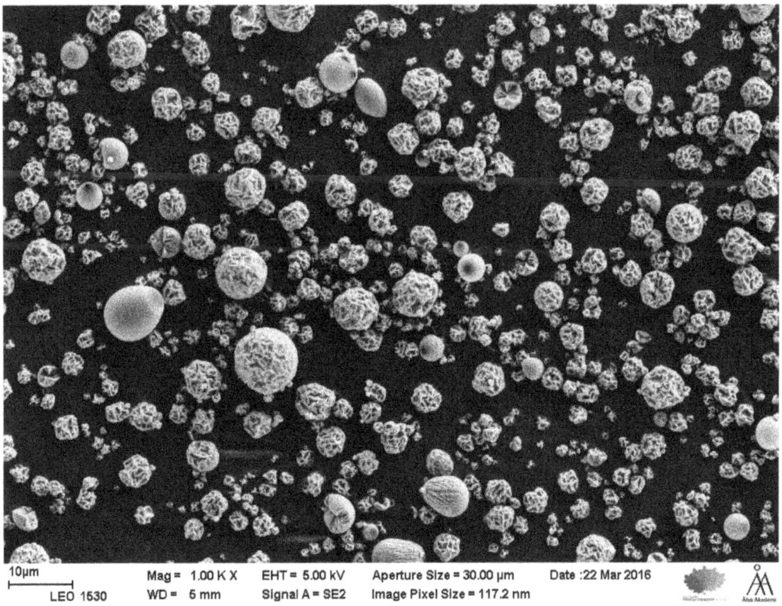

Figure 1. SEM images of pramlintide loaded silica microparticles. Magnification ×1000.

3.3. *Rheology of the Depot Formulation*

Silica hydrogel, R400 (ca. 60 times the silica saturation levels) stabilises the silica microparticles within the aqueous depot and mitigates issues of sedimentation usually associated with particulate-based delivery systems. Rheology measurements (viscosity vs. shear rate) show that the pramlintide-silica depot formulation has shear thinning properties (Figure 2). This helps maintain the homogeneity of the formulation during storage and, importantly, offers a minimally invasive delivery system by reducing injection force and the use of a small-gauge needle [34].

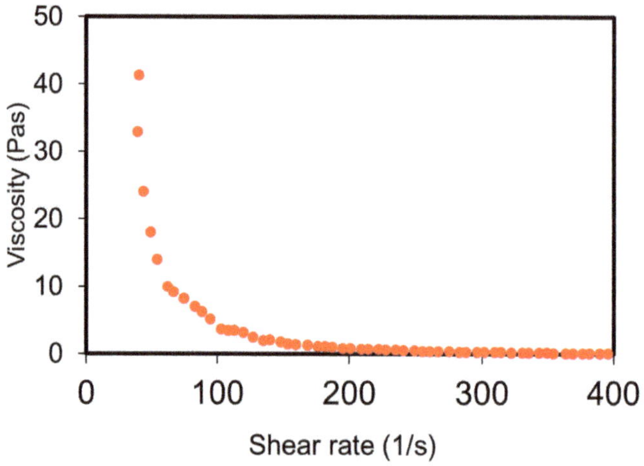

Figure 2. Dynamic viscosity of the pramlintide depot gel formulation in shear rates 0.1 1/s–400 1/s. The data confirm the shear thinning properties of the formulation.

3.4. *Injectability of Depot Formulation*

Injection pressure and force results (Figure 3) show that 100 μL depot formulation could be easily injected with 2–5 N using a 25-G needle. Thus, no significant injection issues are anticipated. On average, the pinch strength of a human hand is about 50 N [35]. The small gauge and the low injection force required to provide a significant advantage as the depot injections are expected to be associated with less pain and incidence of bleeding [36,37].

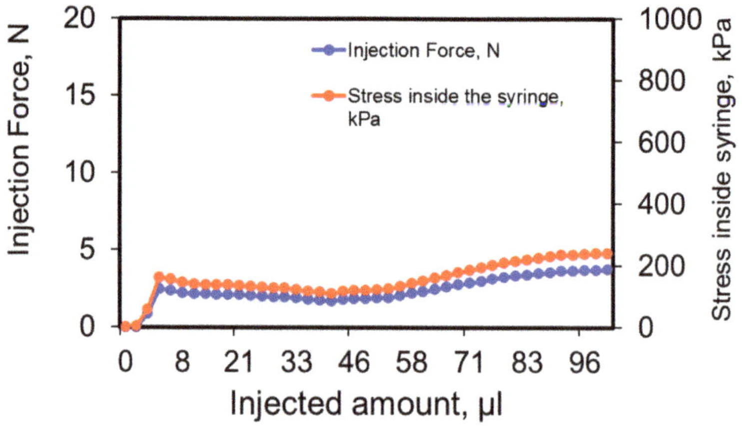

Figure 3. Injection Force and pressure on syringes filled with pramlintide-silica sol-gel system. A 25 G needle was attached to the plunger, and the plunger was pushed at 60 mm/minute.

3.5. In Vitro Dissolution

Results from in vitro dissolution of pramlintide-silica depot under in sink conditions are depicted in Figure 4. Based on an in vitro–in vivo correlation (IVIVC) factor of 10 for subcutaneous administration [29] and linear progression analysis of the release profile from dissolution studies, it is estimated that pramlintide will have an in vivo release profile of approximately 3–3.5 months. The release of pramlintide from the depot was primarily controlled by matrix degradation at later stages. The initial burst release (ca. 18%) seen could be due to the presence of the peptide near the surface of the microparticle.

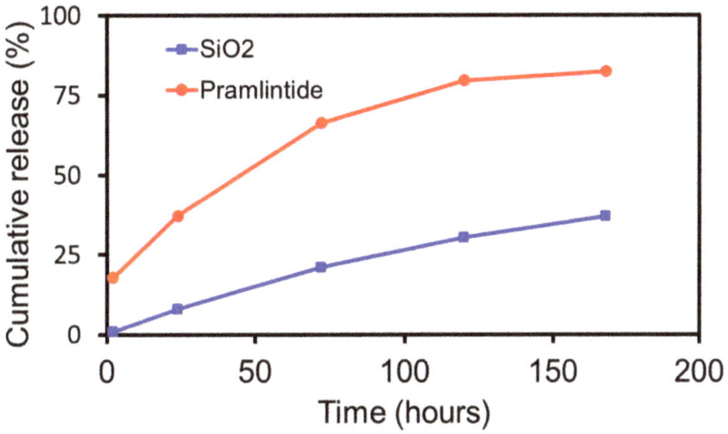

Figure 4. Cumulative estimates of in vitro silica degradation and release of pramlintide from pramlintide-silica depot. Silica dissolution was carried out in 50 mM TRIS–buffer (pH 7.4) and pramlintide release was carried out in PBS (pH 7.4) containing 0.01% Tween 80. Both the studies were carried out at 37 °C under in sink conditions. Data represented as mean for $n = 3$. SD of each data point was less than 2.5%.

3.6. Pharmacokinetic and Pharmcodynamic Study in Rat

After an assessment of endotoxin levels (<0.06 EU/mg of the depot) within the formulation, an in vivo PK study was conducted in rats. The PK profiles of subcutaneously administered pramlintide-silica depot at two dose levels under a single-dose regimen are shown in Figure 5A. With the higher dosing (15 mg/kg), the plasma concentration of pramlintide stayed over 500 pM for close to two months. After the initial burst, pramlintide release from the silica matrix followed zero-order kinetics (Figure 5B) beyond day 10. A steady concentration of the drug could thus be maintained in the plasma for two months. Extended-release profiles have a potential concern for dose dumping. However, drug release from a matrix, such as silica microparticles, depends on the solubility of the drug in the matrix, as well as the release of an encapsulated drug from microparticles is limited to the rate of silica degradation, which occurs from the exterior of the microparticle inward.

Surprisingly, with the lower dose (5 mg/kg), the serum concentrations showed first-order release as the release dropped from about 500 pM (Day 7) to 20 pM levels by the end of the study (Day 56). The lower pramlintide concentration in the silica might be below the concentration needed to represent an "infinite" reservoir and thus shows first-order release, while the higher pramlintide concentration seems to fulfil the requirement and demonstrates zero-order release (Figure 5B) [38].

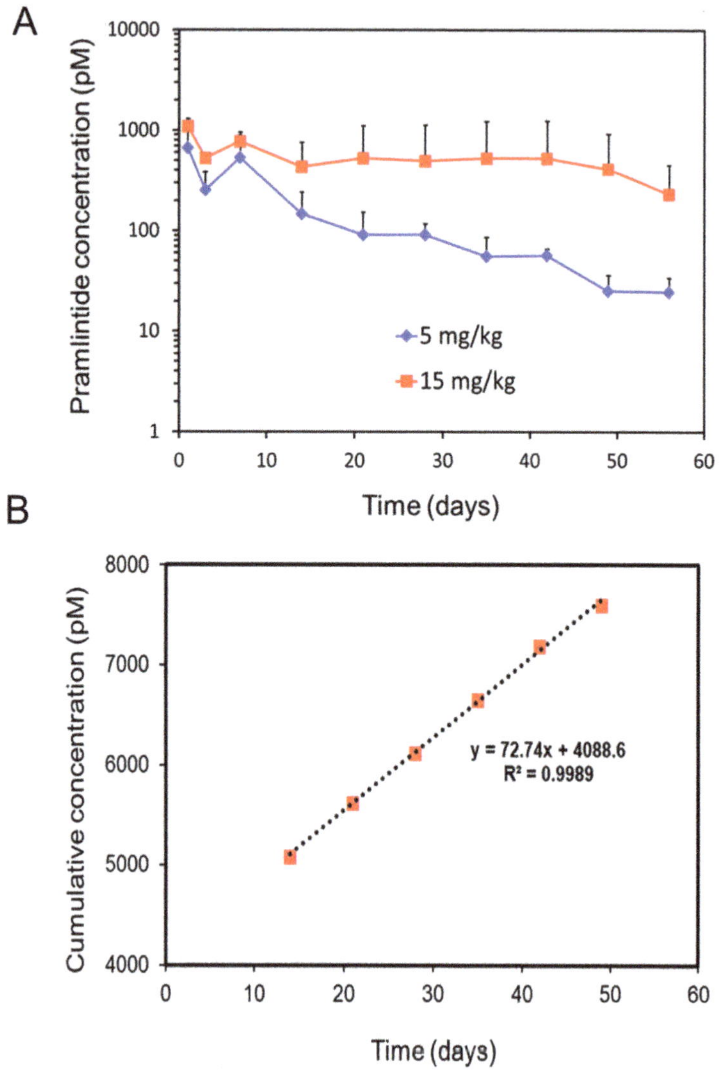

Figure 5. (**A**) Pramlintide plasma concentration in the rat after subcutaneous injection of pramlintide-silica depot at two doses (containing 5 mg/kg and 15 mg/kg pramlintide). Mean and SD, $n = 5$ rats. (**B**) Cumulative concentration vs. time plot depicting the zero-order release of pramlintide from silica depot at higher dosing (15 mg/kg) from 14 to 49 days.

In an earlier preclinical study of pramlintide in rats [39], the peak plasma concentration of pramlintide at 50% maximally effective gastric inhibitory dose was reported to be 15 pM. The lower dose (5 mg/kg) formulation in the present study seems to achieve this concentration level by the end of the study.

The results from our study present an interesting comparison with a very recent report of glycemic control by a recombinant construct of GLP-1 fused to thermosensitive ELP [27]. For a single SC injection of 700 nmol/kg of the GLP-1–ELP construct in mice (ca. equivalent of 2.9 mg/kg of GLP-1 peptide), the investigators found that glycemic control (and circulation time) could be achieved for 10 days. In contrast, the silica-based depot system could easily achieve maintaining serum concentration(s) of pramlintide above the therapeutic level (20 pM) for 60 days at both low and high dosing. This observation points out the efficacy of the silica matrix and thus, its potential towards development for sustained release of anti-glycemic agents for clinical applications.

In agreement with the known pharmacological effect of amylin and its analogues [40], pramlintide depot had a more robust decrease in body weight until about day 9 and then continued to increase throughout the duration of the 29-day study. (Figure 6). This suggests that pramlintide maintains its in vivo activity after release from silica depot. The findings for bodyweight loss mirror very well previously published data in lean rats [41–43]. Roth et al. [41] show body weight returning to baseline levels 8 days after the start of amylin treatment in an experiment assessing the effect of continuous subcutaneous amylin infusion over a period of 24 days. Arnelo et al. [42] also show a dose-dependent reduction in food intake and body weight following subcutaneous infusion of synthetic islet amyloid polypeptide by osmotic minipump over an 8-day period in lean rats. At the lowest dose, the effect on food intake was lost after 5 days and after 8 days, the anorectic effect at the top dose was diminishing towards control levels. In another report, significant effects on food intake were seen for the first 6 days when lean animals were administered amylin by minipump over 14 days. After 6 days, food intake returned to control levels despite the continued administration of the drug [43]. Thus, the time course observed for the weight-reducing actions of the pramlintide depot is consistent with the known pharmacology of amylin. The effect of the depot on food intake and body weight in obese rats has also been observed up to 8 weeks [44]. It would also be worthwhile to point out the complexity of dosing and thus, challenges for delivery systems. In an earlier study, at higher doses of pramlintide administered either subcutaneously or intravenously, plasma glucose levels increased. Such glycemic effects were also observed with the administration of amylin in rats [45]. It appears that the glycemic effects of pramlintide and amylin agonists are more pronounced in the fasting state and the glucose-lowering effects are more pronounced in the postprandial state. The effects seem to be more prominent in rodents and of less significance in humans.

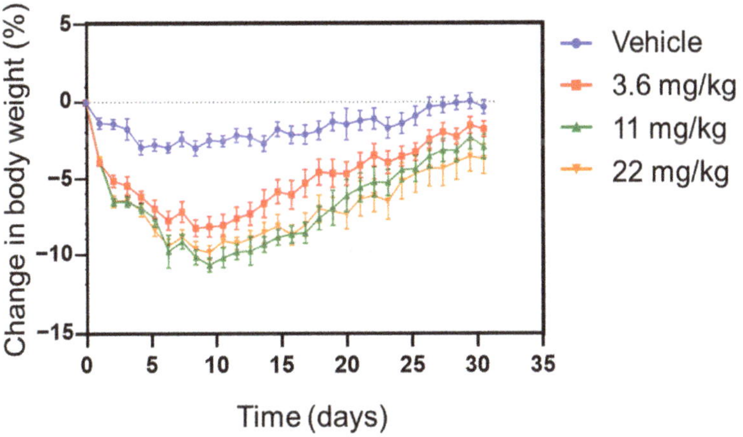

Figure 6. Change in body weight (normalised to % change in body weight in vehicle group) of dietinduced obese rats after a single injection of pramlintide depot containing three different dose strengths. Data is represented as Mean and SEM, $n = 8$ rats.

4. Conclusions

The present study shows the utility of a silica-based matrix for sustained control release of pramlintide in a rat model for two months. The results show that sustained release of pramlintide from silica depot can be achieved to maintain plasma concentration levels of 500 pM. However, optimization of the microparticle formulation is needed to reduce burst release. Further studies are desired to investigate the dosing requirements for achieving therapeutic levels of pramlintide in the serum. This could potentially be achieved by adjusting the drug loading and controlling the rate of silica dissolution. Furthermore, a direct readout of the plasma glucose levels will provide a better estimate of efficacy for the silica-based delivery system. An injectable, scalable, and biodegradable silica-based delivery system has great potential for therapeutic applications in healthcare.

Author Contributions: Conceptualization and methodology, P.T., L.L., J.M. and M.K.; formal analysis, A.S., S.W., S.M., V.G.H., H.B., D.C., J.M. and M.K.; writing—original draft preparation, P.T., A.S., S.W. and S.S.; writing—review and editing, P.T., A.S., S.W., S.M., V.G.H., L.L., J.M., M.K. and S.S.; supervision, P.T. and L.L. All authors have read and agreed to the published version of the manuscript.

Funding: This research received no external funding.

Institutional Review Board Statement: Animal studies were conducted under protocols MI19-0035 (approved Dec. 2019) and PPL 80/2632 (approved April 2016) by the MedImmune Institutional Animal Care and Use Committee.

Informed Consent Statement: Not applicable.

Data Availability Statement: Not applicable.

Conflicts of Interest: The authors declare that they have no conflict of interest. P.T., A.S., S.W. and D.C. are currently employees of AstraZeneca. M.K., J.M. and L.L. are currently employees of Delsitech Ltd. S.M., H.B. and V.G.H., were employees of AstraZeneca when this study was performed. They are no longer employees of AstraZeneca. S.S. was an employee of Delsitech Ltd. when this study was performed. He is no longer an employee of Delsitech Ltd.

References

1. Diabetes Facts & Figures. Available online: http://www.idf.org (accessed on 22 February 2022).
2. National Diabetes Data Group. Classification and Diagnosis of Diabetes Mellitus and Other Categories of Glucose Intolerance. *Diabetes* **1979**, *28*, 1039–1057. [CrossRef] [PubMed]
3. Tripathi, B.K.; Srivastava, A.K. Diabetes mellitus: Complications and therapeutics. *Med. Sci. Monit.* **2006**, *12*, RA130–RA147. [PubMed]
4. American Diabetes Association. Diagnosis and classification of diabetes mellitus. *Diabetes Care* **2014**, *37* (Suppl. 1), S81–S90. [CrossRef] [PubMed]
5. Turner, R.C.; Cull, C.A.; Frighi, V.; Holman, R.R.; for the UK Prospective Diabetes Study (UKPDS) Group. Glycemic Control With Diet, Sulfonylurea, Metformin, or Insulin in Patients With Type 2 Diabetes Mellitus Progressive Requirement for Multiple Therapies (UKPDS 49). *JAMA* **1999**, *281*, 2005–2012. [CrossRef] [PubMed]
6. Groop, L. Bringing diabetes therapeutics to the big screen. *Nat. Biotechnol.* **2003**, *21*, 240–241. [CrossRef]
7. Valla, V. Therapeutics of Diabetes Mellitus: Focus on Insulin Analogues and Insulin Pumps. *Exp. Diabetes Res.* **2010**, *2010*, 178372. [CrossRef]
8. Veiseh, O.; Tang, B.C.; Whitehead, K.A.; Anderson, D.G.; Langer, R. Managing diabetes with nanomedicine: Challenges and opportunities. *Nat. Rev. Drug Discov.* **2015**, *14*, 45–57. [CrossRef]
9. Owens, D.R.; Monnier, L.; Barnett, A.H. Future challenges and therapeutic opportunities in type 2 diabetes: Changing the paradigm of current therapy. *Diabetes Obes. Metab.* **2017**, *19*, 1339–1352. [CrossRef]
10. Walsh, G. Biopharmaceuticals: Recent approvals and likely directions. *Trends Biotechnol.* **2005**, *23*, 553–558. [CrossRef] [PubMed]
11. Wu-Pong, S.; Rojanasakul, Y. (Eds.) *Biopharmaceutical Drug Design and Development*; Springer Science & Business Media: Berlin/Heidelberg, Germany, 2010.
12. Walsh, G. *Biopharmaceuticals: Biochemistry and Biotechnology*; John Wiley & Sons: New York, NY, USA, 2013.
13. Shire, S.J. Formulation and manufacturability of biologics. *Curr. Opin. Biotechnol.* **2009**, *20*, 708–714. [CrossRef]
14. Mitragotri, S.; Burke, P.A.; Langer, R. Overcoming the challenges in administering biopharmaceuticals: Formulation and delivery strategies. *Nat. Rev. Drug Discov.* **2014**, *13*, 655–672. [CrossRef] [PubMed]
15. Schmitz, O.; Brock, B.; Rungby, J. Amylin Agonists: A Novel Approach in the Treatment of Diabetes. *Diabetes* **2004**, *53*, S233–S238. [CrossRef] [PubMed]
16. McQueen, J. Pramlintide acetate. *Am. J. Health-Syst. Pharm.* **2005**, *62*, 2363–2372. [CrossRef] [PubMed]
17. Ryan, G.; Jobe, L.; Briscoe, T. Review of pramlintide as adjunctive therapy in treatment of type 1 and type 2 diabetes. *Drug Des. Dev. Ther.* **2008**, *2*, 203–214. [CrossRef]
18. McCoy, R.G.; Van Houten, H.K.; Ziegenfuss, J.Y.; Shah, N.D.; Wermers, R.A.; Smith, S.A.; Gruden, G.; Barutta, F.; Chaturvedi, N.; Schalkwijk, C.; et al. Increased Mortality of Patients With Diabetes Reporting Severe Hypoglycemia. *Diabetes Care* **2012**, *35*, 1897–1901. [CrossRef]

19. Bode, B.W.; Steed, R.D.; Davidson, P.C. Reduction in Severe Hypoglycemia With Long-Term Continuous Subcutaneous Insulin Infusion in Type I Diabetes. *Diabetes Care* **1996**, *19*, 324–327. [CrossRef]
20. Huffman, D.M.; McLean, G.W.; Seagrove, M.A. Continuous Subcutaneous Pramlintide Infusion Therapy In Patients With Type 1 Diabetes: Observations From A Pilot Study. *Endocr. Pract.* **2009**, *15*, 689–695. [CrossRef]
21. LinBit and Linplant Product Instructions. Available online: http://www.linshincanada.com (accessed on 22 February 2022).
22. Vilsbøll, T.; Agersø, H.; Krarup, T.; Holst, J.J. Similar Elimination Rates of Glucagon-Like Peptide-1 in Obese Type 2 Diabetic Patients and Healthy Subjects. *J. Clin. Endocrinol. Metab.* **2003**, *88*, 220–224. [CrossRef]
23. Hui, H.; Farilla, L.; Merkel, P.; Perfetti, R. The short half-life of glucagon-like peptide-1 in plasma does not reflect its long-lasting beneficial effects. *Eur. J. Endocrinol.* **2002**, *146*, 863–869. [CrossRef]
24. Choi, S.; Baudys, M.; Kim, S.W. Control of blood glucose by novel GLP-1 delivery using biodegradable triblock copolymer of PLGA-PEG-PLGA in type 2 diabetic rats. *Pharm. Res.* **2004**, *21*, 827–831. [CrossRef]
25. Crotts, G.; Park, T.G. Protein delivery from poly(lactic-co-glycolic acid) biodegradable microspheres: Release kinetics and stability issues. *J. Microencapsul.* **1998**, *15*, 699–713. [CrossRef] [PubMed]
26. Paliwal, R.; Babu, R.J.; Palakurthi, S. Nanomedicine Scale-up Technologies: Feasibilities and Challenges. *AAPS PharmSciTech* **2014**, *15*, 1527–1534. [CrossRef] [PubMed]
27. Luginbuhl, K.M.; Schaal, J.; Umstead, B.; Mastria, E.; Li, X.; Banskota, S.; Arnold, S.; Feinglos, M.; D'Alessio, D.; Chilkoti, A. One-week glucose control via zero-order release kinetics from an injectable depot of glucagon-like peptide-1 fused to a thermosensitive biopolymer. *Nat. Biomed. Eng.* **2017**, *1*, 78. [CrossRef] [PubMed]
28. Kortesuo, P.; Ahola, M.; Kangas, M.; Kangasniemi, I.; Yli-Urpo, A.; Kiesvaara, J. In vitro evaluation of sol–gel processed spray dried silica gel microspheres as carrier in controlled drug delivery. *Int. J. Pharm.* **2000**, *200*, 223–229. [CrossRef]
29. Kortesuo, P.; Ahola, M.; Karlsson, S.; Kangasniemi, I.; Yli-Urpo, A.; Kiesvaara, J. Silica xerogel as an implantable carrier for controlled drug delivery—evaluation of drug distribution and tissue effects after implantation. *Biomaterials* **1999**, *21*, 193–198. [CrossRef]
30. Viitala, R.; Jokinen, M.; Tuusa, S.; Rosenholm, J.B.; Jalonen, H. Adjustably biodegradable sol-gel derived SiO_2 matrices for protein release. *J. Sol-Gel Sci. Tech.* **2005**, *36*, 147–156. [CrossRef]
31. Viitala, R.; Jokinen, M.; Maunu, S.L.; Jalonen, H.; Rosenholm, J.B. Chemical characterization of bioresorbable sol–gel derived SiO_2 matrices prepared at protein-compatible pH. *J. Non-Cryst. Solids* **2005**, *351*, 3225–3234. [CrossRef]
32. Coradin, T.; Eglin, D.; Livage, J. The silicomolybdic acid spectrophotometric method and its application to silicate/biopolymer interaction studies. *Spectroscopy* **2004**, *18*, 567–576. [CrossRef]
33. Czuryszkiewicz, T.; Areva, S.; Honkanen, M.; Lindén, M. Synthesis of sol gel silica materials providing a slow release of biphosphonate. *Colloids Surf. A Physicochem. Eng. Asp.* **2005**, *254*, 69–74. [CrossRef]
34. Jokinen, M.; Koskinen, M.; Areva, S. Rationale of Using Conventional Sol-Gel Derived SiO_2 for Delivery of Biologically Active Agents. *Key Eng. Mater.* **2008**, *377*, 195–210. [CrossRef]
35. Nayak, U.; Queiroga, J. Pinch grip, power grip and wrist twisting strengths of healthy older adults. *Gerontechnology* **2004**, *3*, 77–88. [CrossRef]
36. Arendt-Nielsen, L.; Egekvist, H.; Bjerring, P. Pain following controlled cutaneous insertion of needles with different diameters. *Somatosens. Mot. Res.* **2006**, *23*, 37–43. [CrossRef] [PubMed]
37. Rungseevijitprapa, W.; Bodmeier, R. Injectability of biodegradable in situ forming microparticle systems (ISM). *Eur. J. Pharm. Sci.* **2009**, *36*, 524–531. [CrossRef] [PubMed]
38. Siepmann, J.; Siepmann, F. Mathematical modeling of drug delivery. *Int. J. Pharm.* **2008**, *364*, 328–343. [CrossRef]
39. Young, A.A.; Vine, W.; Gedulin, B.R.; Pittner, R.; Janes, S.; Gaeta, L.S.; Percy, A.; Moore, C.X.; Koda, J.E.; Rink, T.J.; et al. Preclinical pharmacology of pramlintide in the rat: Comparisons with human and rat amylin. *Drug Dev. Res.* **1996**, *37*, 231–248. [CrossRef]
40. Dunican, K.C.; Adams, N.M.; Desilets, A.R. The Role of Pramlintide for Weight Loss. *Ann. Pharmacother.* **2010**, *44*, 538–545. [CrossRef]
41. Roth, J.D.; Hughes, H.; Kendall, E.; Baron, A.D.; Anderson, C.M. Antiobesity Effects of the β-Cell Hormone Amylin in Diet-Induced Obese Rats: Effects on Food Intake, Body Weight, Composition, Energy Expenditure, and Gene Expression. *Endocrinology* **2006**, *147*, 5855–5864. [CrossRef]
42. Arnelo, U.; Permert, J.; Adrian, T.E.; Larsson, J.; Westermark, P.; Reidelberger, R.D. Chronic infusion of islet amyloid polypeptide causes anorexia in rats. *Am. J. Physiol. Regul. Integr. Comp. Physiol.* **1996**, *271*, R1654–R1659. [CrossRef]
43. Lutz, T.; Mollet, A.; Rushing, P.; Riediger, T.; Scharrer, E. The anorectic effect of a chronic peripheral infusion of amylin is abolished in area postrema/nucleus of the solitary tract (AP/NTS) lesioned rats. *Int. J. Obes. Relat. Metab. Disord.* **2001**, *25*, 1005–1011. [CrossRef]
44. Mack, C.; Wilson, J.; Athanacio, J.; Reynolds, J.; Laugero, K.; Guss, S.; Vu, C.; Roth, J.; Parkes, D. Pharmacological actions of the peptide hormone amylin in the long-term regulation of food intake, food preference, and body weight. *Am. J. Physiol. Regul. Integr. Comp. Physiol.* **2007**, *293*, R1855–R1863. [CrossRef]
45. Young, A.A.; Cooper, G.J.; Carlo, P.A.; Rink, T.J.; Wang, M.W. Response to intravenous injections of amylin and glucagon in fasted, fed, and hypoglycemic rats. *Am. J. Physiol. Endocrinol. Metab.* **1993**, *264*, E943–E950. [CrossRef] [PubMed]

pharmaceutics

Article

Development and Optimization of Nanolipid-Based Formulation of Diclofenac Sodium: In Vitro Characterization and Preclinical Evaluation

Ameeduzzafar Zafar [1,*], Nabil K Alruwaili [1], Syed Sarim Imam [2,*], Mohd Yasir [3], Omar Awad Alsaidan [1], Ali Alquraini [4], Alenazy Rawaf [5], Bader Alsuwayt [6], Md. Khalid Anwer [7], Sultan Alshehri [2] and Mohammed M. Ghoneim [8]

1 Department of Pharmaceutics, College of Pharmacy, Jouf University, Sakaka 72341, Al-Jouf, Saudi Arabia; nkalruwaili@ju.edu.sa (N.K.A.); osaidan@ju.edu.sa (O.A.A.)
2 Department of Pharmaceutics, College of Pharmacy, King Saud University, Riyadh 11451, Saudi Arabia; salshehri1@ksu.edu.sa
3 Department of Pharmacy, College of Health Science, Arsi University, Asella 396, Ethiopia; mohdyasir31@gmail.com
4 Department of Pharmaceutical Chemistry, Faculty of Clinical Pharmacy, Al Baha University, Al Baha 65779, Saudi Arabia; aalquraini@bu.edu.sa
5 Department of Medical Laboratory, College of Applied Medical Sciences-Shaqra, Shaqra University, Shaqra 11961, Saudi Arabia; ralenazy@su.edu.sa
6 Department of Pharmacy Practice, College of Pharmacy, University of Hafr Al-Batin, Hafr Al-Batin 31991, Saudi Arabia; balsuwayt@uhb.edu.sa
7 Department of Pharmaceutics, College of Pharmacy, Prince Sattam Bin Abdulaziz University, Al-kharj 11942, Saudi Arabia; m.anwer@psau.edu.sa
8 Department of Pharmacy Practice, College of Pharmacy, Almaarefa University, Ad Diriyah 13713, Saudi Arabia; mghoneim@mcst.edu.sa
* Correspondence: azafar@ju.edu.sa (A.Z.); simam@ksu.edu.sa (S.S.I.)

Citation: Zafar, A.; Alruwaili, N.K.; Imam, S.S.; Yasir, M.; Alsaidan, O.A.; Alquraini, A.; Rawaf, A.; Alsuwayt, B.; Anwer, M.K.; Alshehri, S.; et al. Development and Optimization of Nanolipid-Based Formulation of Diclofenac Sodium: In Vitro Characterization and Preclinical Evaluation. *Pharmaceutics* **2022**, *14*, 507. https://doi.org/10.3390/pharmaceutics14030507

Academic Editors: Vibhuti Agrahari and Prashant Kumar

Received: 24 December 2021
Accepted: 17 February 2022
Published: 25 February 2022

Abstract: In the present research study, we formulate bilosomes (BMs) of diclofenac (DC) for oral delivery for enhancement of therapeutic efficacy (anti-inflammatory disease). The BMS were prepared by thin film hydration method and optimized by Box–Behnken design (BBD) using cholesterol (A), lipid (B), surfactant (C), and bile salt (D) as formulation factors. Their effects were evaluated on vesicle size (Y_1) and entrapment efficacy (Y_2). The optimized DC-BMs-opt showed a vesicle size of 270.21 ± 3.76 nm, PDI of 0.265 ± 0.03, and entrapment efficiency of 79.01 ± 2.54%. DSC study result revealed that DC-BMs-opt exhibited complete entrapment of DC in BM matrix. It also depicted significant enhancement ($p < 0.05$) in release (91.82 ± 4.65%) as compared to pure DC (36.32 ± 4.23%) and DC-liposomes (74.54 ± 4.76%). A higher apparent permeability coefficient (2.08×10^{-3} cm/s) was also achieved compared to pure DC (6.6×10^{-4} cm/s) and DC-liposomes (1.33×10^{-3} cm/s). A 5.21-fold and 1.43-fold enhancement in relative bioavailability was found relative to pure DC and DC liposomes (DC-LP). The anti-inflammatory activity result showed a significant ($p < 0.05$) reduction of paw edema swelling compared to pure DC and DC-LP. Our findings revealed that encapsulation of DC in BMs matrix is a good alternative for improvement of therapeutic efficacy.

Keywords: bilosomes; diclofenac; optimization; pharmacokinetic; pharmacodynamic study

1. Introduction

Diclofenac (DC) is a non-steroidal anti-inflammatory (NSAID) agent with anti-inflammatory and antipyretic activity. It is widely used for treatment of acute pain and various anti-inflammatory diseases such as osteoarthritis and rheumatoid arthritis. It has a short half-life of 1–2 h due to extensive first-pass metabolism. It belongs to the BCS-II class drug and reported low solubility [1]. The long exposure to DC inhibits prostaglandin formation which causes gastric irritation, bleeding, and ulcers [2]. These side effects can be minimized by reducing direct contact of drug with GIT [3].

Various studies have been published to overcome complications of gastric irritation and ulcers. Various types of formulation have been reported to increase therapeutic efficacy and side effects of DC. A diclofenac-loaded nanoformulation was prepared and evaluated for different parameters [4]. They reported a nanometric size with high entrapment efficiency. A significant effect was observed on pharmacokinetic and pharmacodynamic activities. The low dose depicted clinical therapeutic levels in blood for up to 120 h, with minimal drug accumulation in organs as well as better efficacy than other controls. Akbari et al. developed transdermal diclofenac niosomal gel for improvement of therapeutic activity. The prepared formulation showed nano-metric size, negative zeta-potential, and high entrapment efficiency. The biological activity result revealed significantly lower licking time than conventional formulation [5]. In another study, diclofenac sodium-loaded nanovesicles were prepared by double solvent displacement method [6]. The prepared liposomes showed nano-metric size, negative zeta potential, and high encapsulation efficiency. The permeation results revealed a higher transdermal passage of drug. Gaur et al. prepared diclofenac sodium-loaded lipid vesicles and analyzed them for physical and biological activity [7]. The prepared formulation depicted more than 90% release with an enhanced pharmacokinetic profile.

The application of lipid-based nanoformulations is rising as an effective method for drug delivery. It can enhance drug solubility as well as bioavailability and reduce side effects. There are various lipid nanoformulations such as solid lipid nanoparticles [8,9], nanostructured lipid carriers [10], liposomes [11], and bilosomes [12]. Among them, bilosomes (BMs) are the new nano-sized lipid vesicular formulation used for different therapeutic agents. They are an elastic vesicular system composed of phospholipid, surfactant, cholesterol, and bile salt [13]. The bile salt enters into the lipid bilayer and lowers the phase transition temperature and builds vesicles deformable under body temperature [14]. They have been reported to enhance bioavailability of many drugs [15,16]. They show less drug leakage and high lymphatic drug transport as compared to niosomes and liposomes. They also prevent the enzymatic degradation in gastrointestinal tract and pass from reticular endothelial system [17]. In the GIT, bile salt that breaks vesicle before reaching to target site [18]. The bile salt acts as a solubilizing and permeation enhancer agent and may improve bioavailability of poorly soluble drugs [19]. Different types of bile salts such as sodium deoxycholate, sodium glycolate, sodium taurocholate, and sodium glycolate are used to prepare BMs. Among them, sodium deoxycholate is commonly used for formulation of BMs due to its nontoxic nature [20]. Shukla et al. formulated a diphtheria toxoid-loaded BM for oral administration. It produced quantifiable anti-diphtheria toxoid response in serum as well as mucosal secretion [21]. In another study, Shukla et al. formulated BM oral delivery of hepatitis B and produced concentration level of systemic and mucosal antibodies [22]. Zakaria et al. formulated piperine-loaded BMs for antiviral and anti-inflammatory activity [23]. Piperine-loaded BMs exhibited significantly reduced oxidant markers and cytokines in MERS-Co-V infected mice compared to pure piperine. El Taweel et al. formulated zolmitriptan-loaded BMs in situ gel for nose brain delivery [24]. BMs in situ gel produced significant bioavailability (1176.9%) compared to BMs dispersion (835.7%).

Up until now, no study has been performed to evaluate efficacy of diclofenac bilosomes (DC-BMs) to improve therapeutic efficacy. The objective of study is to prepare and optimize them using experimental design software (Stat-Ease, Minneapolis, MN, USA). The selected formulation (DC-BMs-opt) was evaluated for physicochemical characterization, in vitro, ex vivo study, and pharmacokinetic and pharmacodynamic study.

2. Experimental

2.1. Materials

Diclofenac potassium, lipid (L-α-Phosphatidylcholine), pluronic F123, cholesterol, and bile salt (sodium deoxycholate) were procured from Sigma Aldrich (St. Louis, MO, USA). Dialysis bag (MWCO 12,000 kDa) was procured from HiMedia laboratory (Mumbai, India). HPLC grade water, acetonitrile, and methanol were obtained from SD-fine chemicals (Mumbai, India).

2.2. Methods

2.2.1. Formulation of Bilosomes

DC-BMs were prepared by slightly modified thin-film hydration method [13]. The lipid, surfactant, and cholesterol with a fixed dose of DC were taken in different ratios and dissolved in organic solvent (methanol: chloroform) as shown in Table 1. The solution was transferred to a round bottom flask and then organic solvent was evaporated at a temperature of 50 °C with reduced pressure using a rotary evaporator (IKA, RV-3V, Staufen, Germany). A thin lipid film was formed on wall of flask and stored in a desiccator for 24 h to remove moisture. The film was hydrated with phosphate buffer (10 mL) containing sodium deoxycholate for 3 h. The dispersion was collected and sonicated for 15 min to reduce size. The prepared formulations were collected and stored at 4 °C for further study.

Table 1. Formulation composition and their effect on vesicle size and entrapment efficiency.

Code	Formulation Factor				Responses	
	CHO (A; %)	Lipid (B; %)	Surfactant (C; %)	Bile Salt (D; %)	Vesicle Size (nm; R_1)	Entrapment Efficiency (%; R_2)
1	0.1	0.5	0.5	1	169.34	50.23
2	0.5	0.5	0.5	1	284.53	88.23
3	0.1	1.5	0.5	1	275.34	75.43
4	0.5	1.5	0.5	1	380.14	92.32
5	0.3	1	0.3	0.5	328.12	65.02
6	0.3	1	0.7	0.5	260.34	84.12
7	0.3	1	0.3	1.5	291.65	76.32
8	0.3	1	0.7	1.5	218.54	81.32
9	0.1	1	0.5	0.5	243.45	58.43
10	0.5	1	0.5	0.5	335.27	85.12
11	0.1	1	0.5	1.5	203.16	72.02
12	0.5	1	0.5	1.5	297.65	94.03
13	0.3	0.5	0.3	1	248.24	57.23
14	0.3	1.5	0.3	1	357.00	75.12
15	0.3	0.5	0.7	1	200.43	77.32
16	0.3	1.5	0.7	1	298.14	93.11
17	0.1	1	0.3	1	256.76	60.23
18	0.5	1	0.3	1	345.65	81.87
19	0.1	1	0.7	1	194.54	70.21
20	0.5	1	0.7	1	290.00	90.24
21	0.3	0.5	0.5	0.5	242.87	57.25
22	0.5	1	0.7	1	341.54	83.51
23	0.3	0.5	0.5	1.5	210.00	77.87
24	0.3	1.5	0.5	1.5	306.23	85.23
25	0.3	1	0.5	1	270.21	79.01
26	0.3	1	0.5	1	270.43	79.09
27	0.3	1	0.5	1	269.36	80.87

2.2.2. Optimization

DC-BMs were optimized by using 4 factors at 3 level Box–Behnken design (BBD). The independent variables cholesterol (A), lipid (B), pluronic F127 (C), and bile salt (D) were taken as independent factors and their effects were assessed on VS (R_1) and EE (R_2).

The design showed twenty-seven formulations with five center points from software. The practical value of dependent variables (VS as R_1 and EE as R_2). The data were fitted into software and evaluated for different models, i.e., linear, 2nd order, and quadratic models to determine best fit model. The regression analysis and ANOVA of best fit model were applied. The three-dimensional plots (3D plots) were plotted to interpret the effect of each factor over each response.

2.2.3. Bilosomes Evaluation

The prepared DC-BMs (F1-F27) vesicle size (VS), PDI, and zeta potential (ZP) were measured by size analyzer (Zeta sizer Nano S90, Malvern, UK) at 25 °C. The diluted DC-BMs were placed in quartz cuvette and their size and PDI were measured. The same samples were evaluated for Zeta potential by using cuvette with an electrode.

2.2.4. Entrapment Efficiency (EE)

EE of DC in prepared BMs was analyzed by indirect method [25]. The prepared DC-BMs (2 mL) were taken in a tube and samples centrifuged at 6000 rpm. The supernatants were collected and diluted and DC content was measured using a UV spectrophotometer. EE in each sample was calculated by using formula:

$$EE = \frac{\text{Total DC} - \text{DC in supernatant}}{\text{Total DC}} \times 100 \quad (1)$$

2.2.5. Surface Morphology

The surface morphology of an optimized bilosomes (DC-BMs-opt) was examined by transmission electron microscopy (TEM, Philips CM 10, Eindhoven, The Netherlands). One drop of diluted sample was placed over grid and stained with phosphotungistic acid. The grid was air-dried and placed into instrument, and image was captured.

2.2.6. Thermal Analysis

DSC analysis of DC, lipid, cholesterol (CHO), Pluronic F127, SC, physical mixture and optimized formulation DC-BMs-opt was analyzed using DSC instrument (Mettler Toledo, South Miami, FL, USA). Each sample (5 mg) was taken, packed into an aluminum pan, and scanned between 25–400 °C under an inert condition. The thermograms were recorded and compared to each other.

2.3. *In Vitro Drug Release*

The release study was performed using a pretreated dialysis bag. The test samples of pure DC, DC-LP and DC-BMs-opt (equivalent to 3 mg DC) were filled into a dialysis bag and tied from both ends. The bag was immersed into release media (500 mL, phosphate buffer pH 6.8) and assembly fixed at a temperature of 37 ± 0.5 °C with stirring speed of 50 rpm. 5 mL of released content was withdrawn at a fixed time and filled with fresh release media to maintain the volume. The absorbance was measured by UV-spectrophotometer (Genesys 10S UV-Vis, Thermo-scientific, Waltham, MA, USA) at 276 nm. The release data fitted to different release kinetic models to find best fit model.

2.4. *Ex Vivo Permeation Study*

The ex vivo permeation study was done using rat intestine. The rats were kept fasted overnight (24 h), then sacrificed and intestines were collected. The intestine was washed with normal saline (0.9% NaCl) and DC-BMs-opt, DC-LP, and pure DC were filled. The intestine was then immersed into a physiological ringer solution (composition NaCl, KCl, KH_2PO_4, $CaCl_2$, glucose) as permeation media and placed over a magnetic stirrer. The system was fixed at 37 ± 0.5 °C with a regular supply of 95% O_2 and 5% CO_2. At specific time, 2 mL sample was collected at a fixed time (0, 30, 60, 90, 120, and 180 min) and analyzed for drug permeation through previously developed HPLC [26]. HPLC system was run using acetonitrile and methanol (7:3) with a flow rate of 0.75 mL/min, injection volume of 20 μL, and UV-detector at 276 nm. The apparent permeability and enhancement ratio was measured.

$$\text{Appearent permeability} = \frac{\text{Flux}}{\text{Area} \times \text{Initial drug concentration}} \quad (2)$$

$$\text{Enhancement ratio} = \frac{\text{Permeability coefficient of DC BLopt}}{\text{Permeability coefficient of the pure DC}} \quad (3)$$

2.5. In Vivo Study

2.5.1. Bioavailability Study

The study protocol was approved by institutional animal ethical committee Jouf University Sakaka, Al-Jouf, Saudi Arabia (Approval Number 04-02-43). The animals (Wistar Albino rats, 200–250 gm, either sex) were procured from an animal house. The animals were provided with free access to food and water and kept at 25 °C/50%RH. The study performed with three animal groups, each group having six rats. Group 1 was administered pure DC, Group 2 and Group 3 were administered with DC-LP and DC-BMs-opt. The samples of pure DC, DC-LP, and DC-BMs (equivalent to 2 mg/kg of DC) were administered orally to rats. At a definite time of 0, 0.5, 1, 2, 3, 6, 12, and 24 h, blood sample was collected from retro-orbital plexus into an EDTA tube. The plasma was separated by centrifuging blood sample at 5000 rpm for 15 min. The plasma was extracted by liquid-phase extraction method. The plasma was mixed with ethyl acetate and acetone (8:2, 0.5 mL), vortexed for 1 min, and then centrifuged to collect supernatant. The supernatant was dried under a stream of nitrogen and dried sample was reconstituted with acetonitrile and filtered through a 0.25 μm membrane filter. The sample (20 μL) was injected into HPLC system to calculate DC concentration in each animal.

2.5.2. Pharmacodynamic Study

The rats were divided into four groups and each group containing six rats (n = 6). Group A was taken as normal control, Group B was used as disease control, Group C was administered with pure DC, group D was treated with DC-LP, and group E was treated with DC-BMs-opt. The carrageenan solution (1%, in saline) was administered to different groups by intra-plantar injection in a right hind paw to induce inflammation. The pure DC, DC-LP, and DC-BMs-opt were administered orally before 30 min of carrageenan injection. The paw volume of each rat was measured by plethysmometer (Ugo Basile, Varese, Italy), before and after carrageenan injection at different time intervals (0, 1, 2, 3, 6, 9, 12, 24 h). The degree of edema induced was assessed by following equation.

$$\%\ \text{Edema inhibition} = \frac{\text{Vt} - \text{V0}}{\text{V0}} \times 100 \quad (4)$$

where Vt and V0, are volume of right hind paw after and before carrageenan treatment.

2.6. Statistical Analysis

Data are represented as average ± SD. Graph Pad software Inc., La Jolla, CA, USA was used for statistical analysis. $p < 0.05$ was taken as statistical significance.

3. Result and Discussion

3.1. Optimization

DC-BMs were optimized by using 4-factor at 3-levels Box–Behnken design. The formulation composition of prepared DC-BMs with their dependent variables VS (R_1) and EE (R_2)are shown in Table 1. The minimum and maximum vesicle size was found in range of 169.34 nm (F1)–380.14 nm (F4). The lowest EE was found for formulation (F1) as 50.23% and highest found for formulation (F12) as 94.03%. The experimental value of all prepared DC-BMs was applied into experimental design model and best fit model was found linear for vesicle size and 2nd order (2F1) model for EE. The adequate precision for VS and EE found >4 and represents model as well fitted [27]. The predicted R^2 values were found to be closer to adjusted R^2 and statistical analysis expressed in Table 2. The ANOVA of both responses were analyzed and sum of square, mean square, F-value, and *p*-value of dependent variable is given in Table 3. 3D-plots were constructed (Figures 1 and 2), and effect of an independent variable over responses were interpreted. The polynomial equation of responses was given below and it explains direct relationship of independent variables to responses. The positive and negative signs denote favorable and unfavorable effect of formulation factors over response.

Table 2. Statistical summary of best fit model for vesicle size (R_1) and entrapment efficiency (R_2).

Source	Vesicle Size (VS)	Entrapment Efficiency (EE)
Model	Linear	2F1
Adjusted R^2	0.9900	0.9318
R^2	0.9915	0.9580
Predicted R^2	0.9867	0.8781
%CV	1.96	4.10
Adequate precision	85.98	21.95
SD	5.37	3.14

Table 3. ANOVA of best fitted designing model for vesicle size (Y_1) and entrapment efficiency (Y_2).

		Vesicle Size (VS)			
Source	**Sum of Squares**	**Mean Square**	**F-Value**	***p*-Value Prob > F**	**Remark**
Model (2nd order)	74,666.22	18,666.55	646.03	<0.0001	Significant
A-CHO	29,058.51	29,058.51	1005.69	<0.0001	–
B-Lipid	30,284.67	30,284.67	1048.13	<0.0001	–
C-Surfactant	11,128.26	11,128.26	385.14	<0.0001	–
D-Bile salt	4194.78	4194.784	145.17	<0.0001	–
Residual	635.66	28.89394	–	–	–
Lack of Fit	631.00	31.55001	13.52	0.0710	NS
Pure Error	4.66	2.333333	–	–	–
Total	75,301.89	–	–	–	–
		Entrapment efficiency (EE)			
Model	3599.88	359.98	36.53	<0.0001	Significant
A-CHO	1779.01	1779.01	180.54	<0.0001	–
B-Lipid	778.43	778.43	79.00	<0.0001	–
C-Surfactant	544.05	544.05	55.21	<0.0001	–
D-Bile salt	239.41	239.41	24.29	0.0002	–
AB	110.25	110.25	11.18	0.0041	–
AC	0.66	0.66	0.06	0.7985	–
AD	6.25	6.25	0.63	0.4374	–
BC	1.22	1.22	0.12	0.7294	–
BD	91.58	91.58	9.29	0.0077	–
CD	49	49	4.97	0.0404	–
Residual	157.65	9.85	–	–	–
Lack of Fit	155.44	11.10	10.04	0.0942	NS
Pure Error	2.21	1.105	–	–	–
Total	3757.54	–	–	–	–

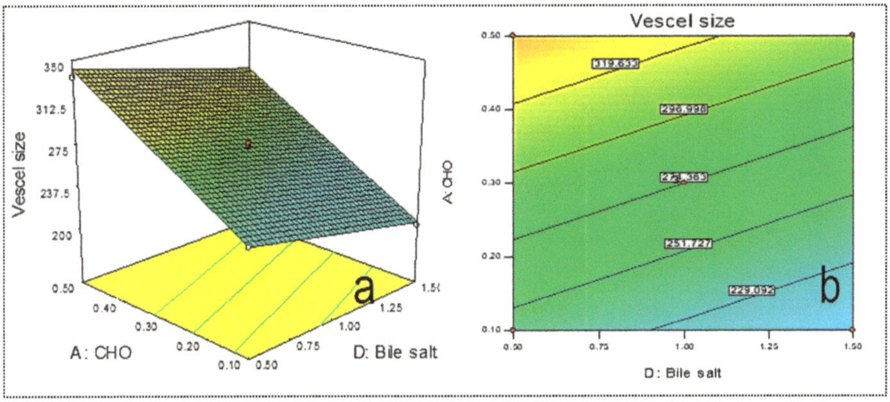

Figure 1. 3D plot showing effect (**a**) of independent variables lipid (A), cholesterol, and bile salt (D) on vesicle size. Contour plot showing effect (**b**) of independent variables lipid (A), cholesterol, and bile salt (D) on vesicle size (R_1).

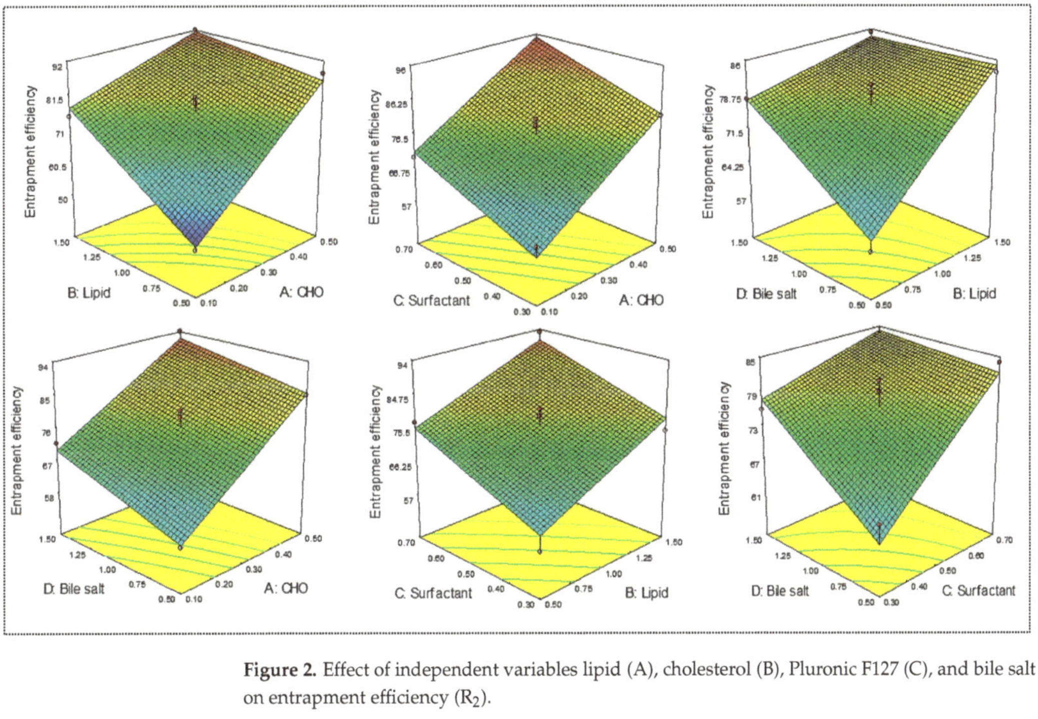

Figure 2. Effect of independent variables lipid (A), cholesterol (B), Pluronic F127 (C), and bile salt (D) on entrapment efficiency (R_2).

3.2. *Effect of Independent Variables over Vesicle Size (R_1)*

The vesicle size of prepared DC-BMs was found in range of 169.34 nm (F1)–380.14 nm (F4). The formulation (F1) prepared with composition cholesterol (A, 0.1%), lipid (B, 0.5%), surfactant (C, 0.5%), and bile salt (D, 1%) showed lowest size and formulation (F4) showed maximum size with composition cholesterol (0.5%), lipid (1.5%), surfactant (0.5%), and bile salt (1%). The difference in size found due to variation in used composition. From the result, it can be observed that used independent variables have shown a significant effect. 3D response surface plot (Figure 1a,b) and polynomial Equation (5) show that increasing a CHO (A) concentration led to an increase in vesicle size due to greater amount of CHO deposited into lipid bilayer [28]. The second factor lipid concentration (B) increases vesicle size due to enhancement in viscosity of dispersion and thickness of lipid bilayers. Similar types of findings reported in reported research of papain liposomes [29], and diclofenac liposome [30]. The surfactant concentration (PP123, C) and bile salt (D) depicted a negative effect on BNs size. The enhancement in surfactant (PP123) gave the reduction in vesicle size because at high concentration of surfactant, interfacial tension reduced between lipid phases and aqueous phase. The bile salt increases flexibility of liposomes by incorporating into lipid bilayer, thereby decreasing vesicle size [31].

$$\text{Vesicle size (nm, } R_1) = 274.36 + 49.20\ A + 50.23\ B - 30.45\ C - 18.69\ D \quad (5)$$

The F-value fitted to linear model and value found to be 646.04 revealed that model was significantly ($p < 0.0001$) fitted. The regression coefficient of best fit model was found to be 0.9915 and it indicates lesser variation between actual and predicted value (Table 2). The ANOVA value showed that model term cholesterol (A), lipid (B), surfactant (C), and bile salt (D) were found to be significant model term ($p < 0.0001$, Table 3). The adequate precision was 85.98 (<4), revealing the close relationship between actual and experimental value [32]. The p-value of lack of fit is >0.05 indicated insignificant which is good for model [33].

3.3. *Effect of Independent Variables (A, B, C, D) on Entrapment Efficiency (R_2)*

EE of DC-BMs was found between 50.23% (F1) and 93.11% (F16). The formulation (F1) prepared with composition cholesterol (A, 0.1%), lipid (B, 0.5%), surfactant (C, 0.5%), and bile salt (D, 1%) showed minimum EE. The maximum EE was shown by formulation (F19) having composition cholesterol (A, 0.5%), lipid (B, 1.5%), surfactant (C, 0.5%), and bile salt (D, 1%). There was a significant ($p < 0.01$) variation in EE was found due to variation in ratio of independent variables. The polynomial Equation (6) and 3D response surface plot (Figure 2) showed the effect of independent variables on EE. The increase in cholesterol (A) leads to enhancement in EE of DC. This effect was found due to deposition of CHO between free spaces of lipid bilayers, which reduces the flexibility, weakens the drug mobility, and reduces diffusion for DC from BMs [34,35]. The second factor lipid (B) also plays an important role on EE. The increase in lipid concentration lead to increase in EE due to enhancement in lipid viscosity. This prevents leaching of DC from lipid bilayer due to increase in hydrophobicity and longer alkyl chain length [36]. However, surfactant (C) showed a positive effect on EE of DC in BMs. The increase in surfactant concentration led to reduction in interfacial tension and increase in viscosity protects leakage of DC from BMs. The fourth variable bile salt (D, SD%) also showed a positive effect on EE. The increases in bile salt led to an increase in EE. It showed a lesser effect than surfactant. It also had surfactant-like properties—it reduced the interfacial tension and then drug easily assimilated into lipid bilayer due to enhanced solubility and flexibility [37].

$$\text{EE } (\%, R_2) = 76.55 + 12.17\ A + 8.054\ B + 6.73\ C + 4.46\ D - 5.25\ AB - 0.40\ AC - 1.25AD - 0.55\ BC - 4.78BD - 3.5\ CD \quad (6)$$

The second order design model (2 F1) was found to be the best fit model for EE. The model F-value 36.53 implies that model was significantly fitted ($p < 0.001$). The lack of fit was found to be non-significant ($p = 0.0942$), and indicates model is well fitted. The regression coefficient of best fit model was found to be 0.958 and it indicates lesser variation between actual and predicted value (Table 2). The polynomial equation (Equation (2)) and ANOVA of best fitted model showed coded terms, i.e., A, B, C, D, AB, BD, CD, are significant ($p < 0.05$) which means these factors had a significant effect on EE of DC in BMs (Table 3).

3.4. *Optimized Formulation (DC-BMs-opt)*

The formulation (DC-BMs-opt) was selected from point prediction of software. The composition CHO (0.3% w/v), lipid (1% w/v), surfactant (0.5% w/v), and bile salt (1% w/v)

depicted an experimental vesicle size of 270.21 ± 3.76 nm and EE of 79.01 ± 2.54%. The software showed a predicted value of vesicle size of 274.36 nm and EE of 76.56%. There was non-significant variation in result observed between experimental and predicted value. The closeness in result revealed that model is valid and reproducible.

3.5. Vesicle Evaluation

The size of prepared DC-BMs (F1-F27) was found between 169.34 nm and 380.14 nm. The optimized composition (DC-BMs-opt) showed VS of 270.21 ± 3.76 nm (Figure 3A). PDI was found to be (0.26 ± 0.03) and revealed homogeneity of BMs-opt [38]. The zeta potential of DC-BMs-opt was of high negative (−36.34 mV) indicating that formulation was highly stable and in disaggregated form. The surface morphology exhibited spherical shape vesicles with a smooth surface without any aggregation (Figure 3B).

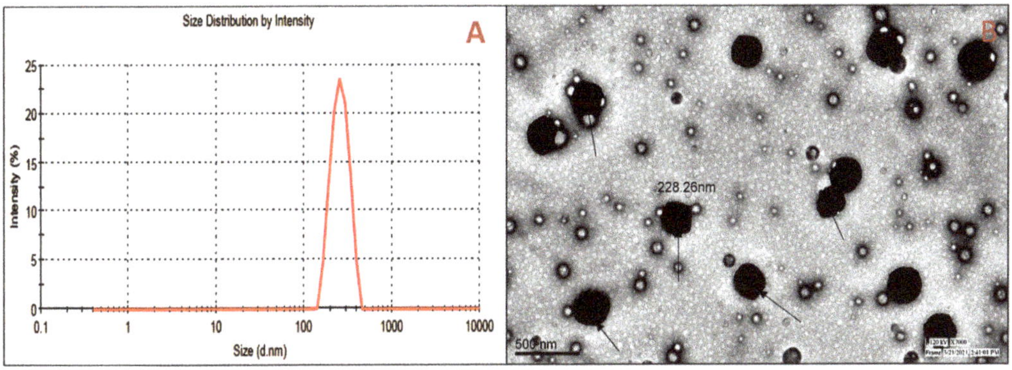

Figure 3. Vesicle size (**A**), and (**B**) TEM image of optimized diclofenac bilosomes (DC-BMs-opt marked with arrow).

3.6. Thermal Analysis

Figure 4 shows DSC spectra of DC, lipid, CHO, Pluronic F127, SC, PM, and DC-BMs-opt. DC showed characteristic endothermic peak at 287.5 °C, which corresponds to its melting point [39]. The lipid, cholesterol, Pluronic F127, and SC exhibited a peak at 180 °C (Figure 4B), at 150 °C (Figure 4C), at 60 °C (Figure 4D), and 190 °C (Figure 4E), respectively. The physical mixture exhibited endothermic peaks at 56 °C (Pluronic F127), an exothermic peak at 180 °C, and a less intense peak of DC at 287.5 °C (Figure 4F). No characteristic endothermic peak of DC was observed in DC-BMs-opt thermogram. The observation revealed complete encapsulation or solubilization of DC into BMs matrix (Figure 4G).

3.7. In Vitro Drug Release

The release of DC-BMs-opt was analyzed and result was compared with DC-LP and pure DC. The data of release study are shown in Figure 5. DC-BMs-opt exhibited 91.82 ± 4.65% release in 24 h of study. The graph showed biphasic release behavior with an initial fast release and later sustained release. The fast release was due to presence of DC on surface of BM-opt and later the sustained release was found due to release of DC from DC-BMs matrix [16]. There was a significantly ($p < 0.001$) lower DC release achieved from DC-LP (74.54 ± 4.76%) and pure DC (36.32 ± 4.23). The liposomes (DC-LP) showed significantly ($p < 0.001$) higher DC release than the pure DC. The pure DC showed poor release due to poor solubility. The significant high release of DC was achieved from the BMs and LP due to enhanced DC solubility in presence of surfactant. There was also a significant difference in release achieved due to presence of bile salt in BMs. Bile salt showed a synergistic effect with used surfactant and can enhance greater solubility.

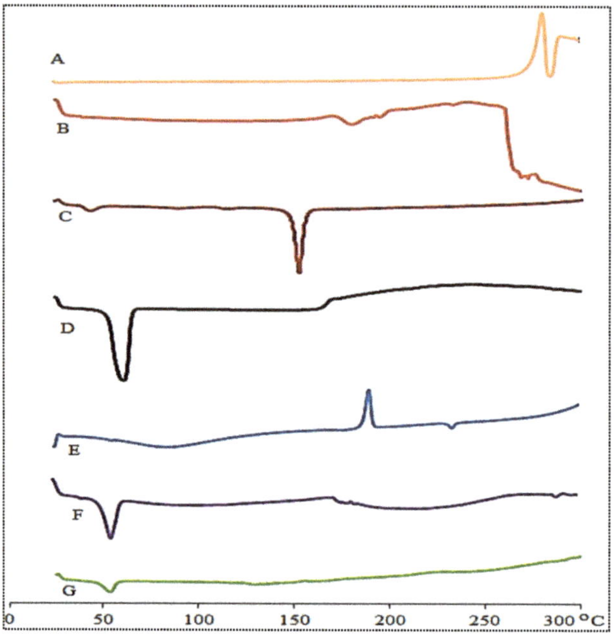

Figure 4. Thermal analysis of (**A**) diclofenac, (**B**) lipid, (**C**) cholesterol, (**D**) Pluronic F127, (**E**) sodium deoxycholate, (**F**), physical mixture, and (**G**) optimized diclofenac bilosomes (DC-BMs-opt).

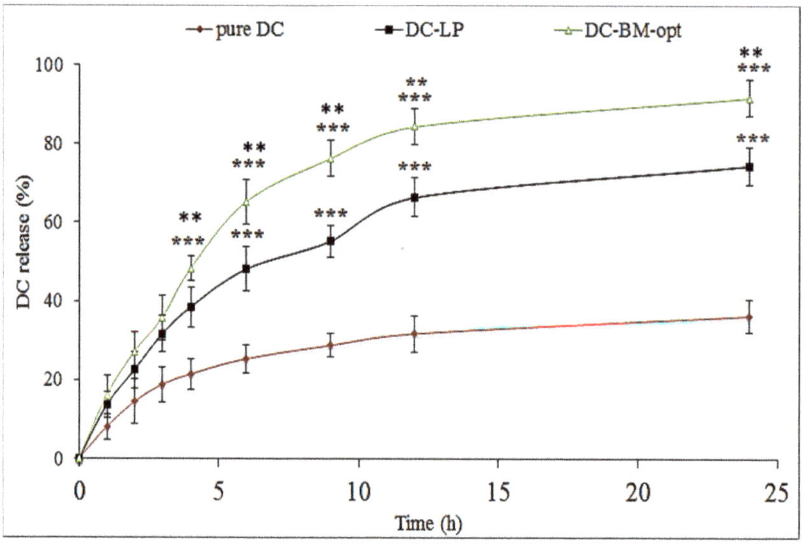

Figure 5. Release study of different treatment groups (pure diclofenac (DC), optimized diclofenac bilosomes (DC-BMs-opt), and diclofenac liposomes (DC-LP)). Study was performed in triplicate and data are shown as mean ± SD. Statistical analysis performed between each group and $p < 0.05$ considered significant. *** highly significant to pure DC; ** significant to pure DC-LP.

The release profile of DC-BMs-opt was fitted into different kinetic models and data showed best fit model as the Korsmeyer–Peppas model (Table 4). The maximum regression value ($R^2 = 0.9354$) confirms best fit. The exponent n-value was 0.58 (0.45 to 0.85) representing non-Fickian mechanism with dual release, i.e., diffusion and swelling release [40].

Table 4. Various kinetic release models and their regression value.

Type of Model	R^2
Zero model	0.7344
First order	0.9257
Higuchi model	0.7744
Korsmeyer–Peppas	0.9354, n = 0.58
Hixon–Crowell model	0.8673

3.8. Ex Vivo Permeation Study

The study of DC-BMs-opt was assessed to compare results with DC-LP and pure DC (Figure 6). The formulation DC-BMs-opt showed significantly ($p < 0.001$) higher permeation (187.59 ± 9.65 μg/cm^2) than DC-LP (119.44 ± 10.06 μg/cm^2) and DC-dispersion (59.52 ± 7.76 μg/cm^2). It also exhibited significant ($p < 0.05$) 3.15-fold (31.26 μg/cm^2/h) higher flux than pure DC (9.92 μg/cm^2/h) and 1.57-fold higher than DC-LP (19.91 μg/cm^2/h). DC-BMs-opt showed the APC of 2.08×10^{-3} cm/s, which was significantly higher ($p < 0.05$) than pure DC (6.6×10^{-4} cm/s) and DC-PL (1.33×10^{-3} cm/s). The pure DC showed lesser permeation due to the poor solubility and not being able to permeate across the biological membrane. The greater amount of DC permeates across the membrane from liposomes due to presence of lipid, cholesterol, and surfactant. The surfactant helps to solubilize drug and due to enhanced solubility, greater effective surface area is available for drug absorption. BMs were prepared with a special component as bile salt which helped to deform the vesicles and also helped to fluidize membrane, possibly because of interaction of phospholipid molecules with membrane layer [41]. Due to this property, it can permeate easily to smaller-sized membrane. The presence of cholesterol helps to extract lipid of membrane and act as a permeation enhancer. The larger amount of drug permeated from BMs. A size of more than 200 nm does not significantly affect permeation of drugs [42].

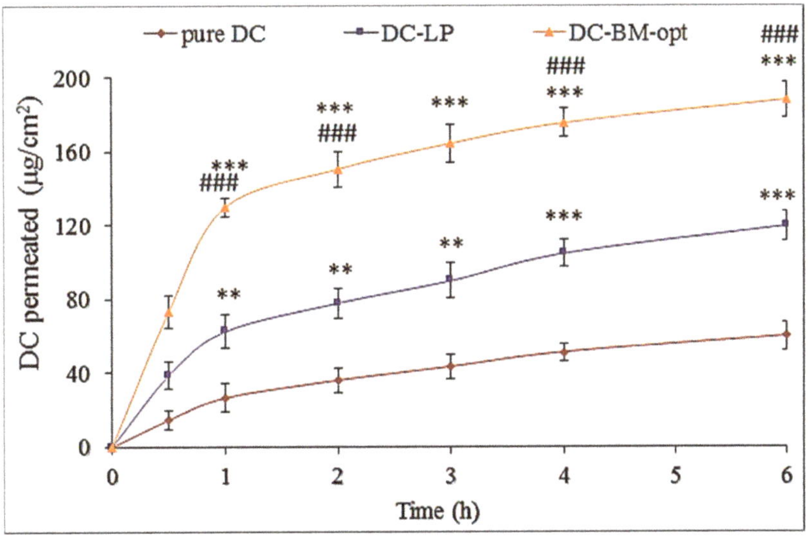

Figure 6. Permeation study of different treatment groups (pure diclofenac (DC), optimized diclofenac bilosomes (DC-BMs-opt), and diclofenac liposomes (DC-LP)). Study was performed in triplicate and result shown as mean ± SD. Statistical analysis performed between each group and $p < 0.05$ considered significant. *** highly significant to pure DC; ### significant to DC-LP; ** significant to pure DC.

3.9. Bioavailability Study

The pharmacokinetic study of pure DC, DC-LP, and DC-BMs-opt was conducted and plasma concentration-time profile is expressed graphically in Figure 7. The result showed significant variation in each tested parameter. DC-BMs-opt showed a C_{max} value of 2654.76 ± ng/mL and was found to be 2.15-fold higher than pure DC (1232.34 ± ng/mL) and 1.29-fold higher than DC-LP (2054 ± ng/mL). The higher C_{max} was achieved due to nano-size of DC-BMs-opt, high permeability, and low first-pass metabolism. The difference was found to be highly significant ($p < 0.001$) compared to pure DC and DC-LP. DC-BMs-opt showed significant ($p < 0.05$) enhancement in AUC_{0-t} (22,340 ng. h/mL) and $AUC_{0-\infty}$ (26,827.92 ng. h/mL) values. It was about 5.2 and 6.2-fold higher than pure DC (AUC_{0-t} of 4288.48 ng. h/mL and $AUC_{0-\infty}$ of 4319.12 ng. h/mL) and 1.43 and 1.56-fold higher than DC-LP (AUC_{0-t} of 15,564, $AUC_{0-\infty}$ of 17,170.09 ng. h/mL). The half-life ($t_{1/2}$) of DC-LP and DC-BMs-opt was found to be higher (6.62 h and 8.39 h) than pure DC (1.95 h), which revealed that DC-BMs-opt was available for a longer time in circulation. DC-BMs-opt exhibited higher T_{max} (1 h) than pure DC dispersion (30 min) due to an increase in solubility of DC in BM as well as LP. The elimination rate constant (Ke) for DC-BMs-opt was found to be significantly ($p < 0.05$) lower (0.08 h^{-1}) than pure DC (0.22 h^{-1}) and DC-LP (0.1 h^{-1}) due to slow and prolonged drug release. The relative bioavailability of DC-BMs-opt showed 5.2-fold enhancement compared to pure DC and 1.43-fold higher compared to DC-LP. The higher bioavailability DC in DC-BMs-opt is due to increased DC solubility, longer circulation, lower first-pass metabolism, and higher uptake of BM by Peyer's patch of M-cell of intestine [43].

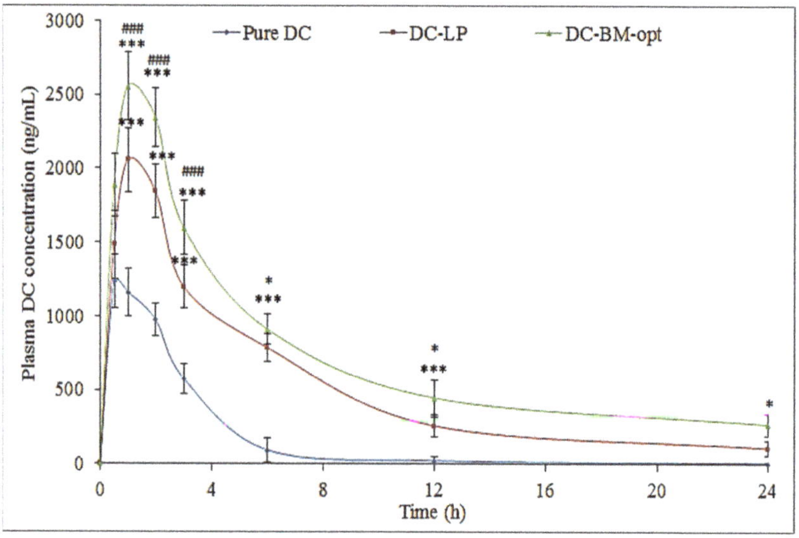

Figure 7. Bioavailability activity of the different treatment groups (pure diclofenac (DC), optimized diclofenac bilosomes (DC-BMs-opt), and diclofenac liposomes (DC-LP)). Study performed with six rats (n = 6) in each group and results shown as mean ± SD. Statistical analysis performed between each group and $p < 0.05$ considered significant. *** highly significant to pure DC; ### significant to DC- LP; * significant to pure DC and DC-LP.

3.10. Pharmacodynamic Study

The anti-inflammatory activity of pure DC, DC-LP, and DC-BMs-opt was evaluated in carrageenan-induced model and results are expressed graphically in Figure 8. The disease control groups showed about 100% swelling. The pure DC, DC-LP, and DC-BMs-opt exhibited a significant effect in lowering paw edema. The pure DC, DC-LP, and DC-BMs-opt showed 26.23 ± 7.83%, 28.43 ± 5.67%, and 31.26 ± 6.13% reduction in paw edema after 2 h carrageenan injection, respectively. The pure DC-treated group showed maximum effect at 2 h, whereas DC-LP and DC-BMs-opt treated group showed a maximum effect up to 6 h and 9 h, respectively. There was a highly significant ($p < 0.001$) effect observed from DC-LP and DC-BMs-opt at 3 h, 6 h, 9 h, and 12 h in comparison to pure DC. At 12 h, maximum reduction was found to be 8.65 ± 3.87%, 23.76 ± 5.92%, and 64.76 ± 11.12% from pure DC, DC-LP, and DC-BMs-opt. At all-time points, a significant effect was observed from tested groups in comparison to disease control. DC-BMs-opt also exhibited a significant ($p < 0.05$) reduction in swelling than DC-LP. This high reduction in swelling was achieved due to high penetration capacity of DC-BMs-opt through intestinal mucosa. The nano-sized vesicle having a greater effective surface area, high circulation time, greater solubility and flexibility in presence of surfactant and bile salt led to greater absorption. Therefore, findings revealed that BMs may increase solubility and circulation of drugs which directly increases anti-inflammatory effect.

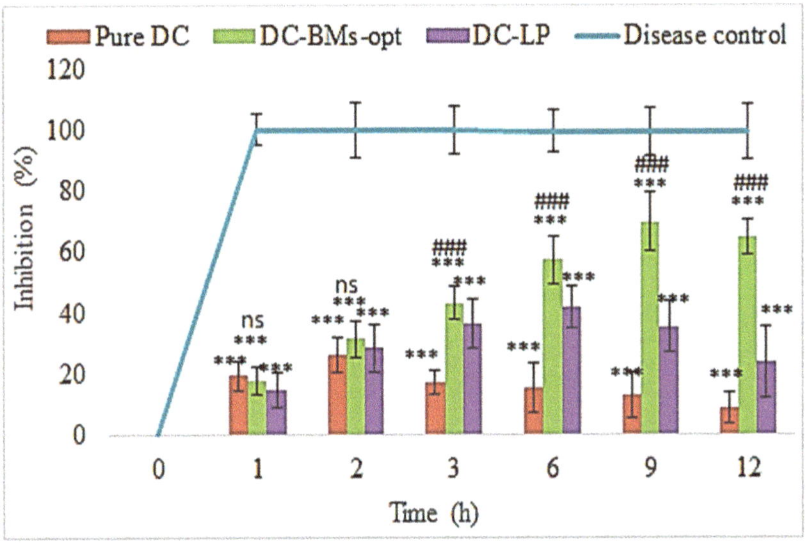

Figure 8. Anti-inflammatory activity of different treatment groups (pure diclofenac (DC), optimized diclofenac bilosomes (DC-BMs-opt), and diclofenac liposomes (DC-LP)) compared with disease control. Study performed with six rats (n = 6) in each group and result shown as mean ± SD. Statistical analysis performed between each group and $p < 0.05$ considered significant. *** highly significant to diabetic control; ### significant to pure DC and DC- LP; ns, non-significant to pure DC and DC-LP.

4. Conclusions

In the present study, DC-BMs were prepared by solvent evaporation method using sodium deoxycholate as bile salt. The formulations were optimized by Box–Behnken design to select optimum composition. The optimized formulation DC-BMs-opt showed a nano vesicle size and high encapsulation efficiency. The in vitro release and ex vivo permeation study showed a prolonged DC release with high permeation flux. The pharmacokinetic and pharmacodynamics study results revealed enhanced bioavailability and anti-inflammatory activity compared to pure DC and DC-LP. Further, prepared formulations need to be evaluated for clinical study. The findings of preclinical data need to be correlated with clinical data for better outcomes. We conclude from our findings that DC-BMs-opt is a promising oral drug delivery for treatment of inflammation.

Author Contributions: Conceptualization and methodology, A.Z. and S.S.I.; software and validation, M.Y., S.S.I. and M.K.A.; resources and investigation, N.K.A., O.A.A. and S.A.; data curation, A.A. and A.R.; writing—original draft preparation, A.Z.; writing—review and editing, B.A. and M.M.G.; visualization and supervision, N.K.A. and O.A.A.; project administration, M.K.A. and M.M.G.; funding acquisition, A.Z. All authors have read and agreed to the published version of the manuscript.

Funding: Deanship of Scientific Research at Jouf University for funding this work through research grant no (DSR-2021-01-0327).

Institutional Review Board Statement: The animal study protocol was approved by the Institutional Review Board (or Ethics Committee) of Jouf University (Approval Number 04-02-43; Approval Date 28 October 2021).

Informed Consent Statement: Not applicable.

Data Availability Statement: Not applicable.

Acknowledgments: The authors extend their appreciation to the Deanship of Scientific Research at Jouf University for funding this work through research grant no (DSR-2021-01-0327).

Conflicts of Interest: The authors declare no conflict of interest.

References

1. Arias, J.L.; Lopez-Viota, M.; López-Viota, J.; Delgado, A.V. Development of iron/ethylcellulose (core/shell) nanoparticles loaded with diclofenac sodium for arthritis treatment. *Int. J. Pharm.* **2009**, *382*, 270–276. [CrossRef] [PubMed]
2. Roth, S.H. Nonsteroidal anti-inflammatory drug gastropathy: New avenues for safety. *Clin. Interv. Aging* **2011**, *6*, 125–131. [CrossRef] [PubMed]
3. Bhatia, N.; Katkar, K.; Ashtekar, S. Formulation and evaluation of co-prodrug of flurbiprofen and methocarbamol. *Asian J. Pharm. Sci.* **2016**, *11*, 449–458. [CrossRef]
4. Narayanan, D.; Pillai, G.J.; Nair, S.V.; Menon, D. Effect of formulation parameters on pharmacokinetics, pharmacodynamics, and safety of diclofenac nanomedicine. *Drug Deliv. Transl. Res.* **2019**, *9*, 867–878. [CrossRef] [PubMed]
5. Akbari, J.; Saeedi, M.; Morteza-Semnani, K.; Hashemi, S.M.H.; Babaei, A.; Eghbali, M.; Mohammadi, M.; Rostamkalaei, S.S.; Asare-Addo, K.; Nokhodchi, A. Innovative topical niosomal gel formulation containing diclofenac sodium (niofenac). *J. Drug Target.* **2022**, *30*, 108–117. [CrossRef] [PubMed]
6. Sala, M.; Locher, F.; Bonvallet, M.; Agusti, G.; Elaissari, A.; Fessi, H. Diclofenac Loaded Lipid Nanovesicles Prepared by Double Solvent Displacement for Skin Drug Delivery. *Pharm. Res.* **2017**, *34*, 1908–1924. [CrossRef] [PubMed]
7. Gaur, P.K.; Purohit, S.; Kumar, Y.; Mishra, S.; Bhandari, A. Preparation, characterization and permeation studies of a nanovesicular system containing diclofenac for transdermal delivery. *Pharm. Dev. Technol.* **2014**, *19*, 48–54. [CrossRef]
8. Dianzani, C.; Foglietta, F.; Ferrara, B.; Rosa, A.C.; Muntoni, E.; Gasco, P.; Della Pepa, C.; Canaparo, R.; Serpe, L. Solid lipid nanoparticles delivering anti-inflammatory drugs to treat inflammatory bowel disease: Effects in an in vivo model. *World J. Gastroenterol.* **2017**, *23*, 4200–4210. [CrossRef]
9. Bhalekar, M.R.; Madgulkar, A.R.; Desale, P.S.; Marium, G. Formulation of piperine solid lipid nanoparticles (SLN) for treatment of rheumatoid arthritis. *Drug Dev. Ind. Pharm.* **2017**, *43*, 1003–1010. [CrossRef]
10. Zewail, M.; Nafee, N.; Helmy, M.W.; Boraie, N. Coated nanostructured lipid carriers targeting the joints–An effective and safe approach for the oral management of rheumatoid arthritis. *Int. J. Pharm.* **2019**, *567*, 118447. [CrossRef]
11. Mohanty, S.; Sahoo, A.K.; Konkimalla, V.B.; Pal, A.; Si, S.C. Naringin in Combination with Isothiocyanates as Liposomal Formulations Potentiates the Anti-inflammatory Activity in Different Acute and Chronic Animal Models of Rheumatoid Arthritis. *ACS Omega* **2020**, *5*, 28319–28332. [CrossRef]
12. Al-Mahallawi, A.M.; Abdelbary, A.A.; Aburahma, M.H. Investigating the potential of employing bilosomes as a novel vesicular carrier for transdermal delivery of tenoxicam. *Int. J. Pharm.* **2015**, *485*, 329–340. [CrossRef]
13. Saifi, Z.; Rizwanullah, M.; Mir, S.R.; Amin, S. Bilosomes nanocarriers for improved oral bioavailability of acyclovir: A complete characterization through in vitro, ex-vivo and in vivo assessment. *J. Drug Deliv. Sci. Technol.* **2020**, *57*, 101634. [CrossRef]
14. Bnyan, R.; Khan, I.; Ehtezazi, T.; Saleem, I.; Gordon, S.; O'Neill, F.; Roberts, M. Surfactant Effects on Lipid-Based Vesicles Properties. *J. Pharm. Sci.* **2018**, *107*, 1237–1246. [CrossRef] [PubMed]
15. Shukla, A.; Mishra, V.; Kesharwani, P. Bilosomes in the context of oral immunization: Development, challenges and opportunities. *Drug Discov. Today* **2016**, *21*, 888–899. [CrossRef] [PubMed]
16. Jain, S.; Indulkar, A.; Harde, H.; Agrawal, A.K. Oral mucosal immunization using glucomannosylated bilosomes. *J. Biomed. Nanotechnol.* **2014**, *10*, 932–947. [CrossRef] [PubMed]

17. Guan, P.; Lu, Y.; Qi, J.; Niu, M.; Lian, R.; Hu, F.; Wu, W. Enhanced oral bioavailability of cyclosporine A by liposomes containing a bile salt. *Int. J. Nanomed.* **2011**, *6*, 965–974.
18. Naguib, M.J.; Kamel, A.M.; Negmeldin, A.T.; Elshafeey, A.H.; Elsayed, I. Molecular docking and statistical optimization of taurocholate-stabilized galactose anchored bilosomes for the enhancement of sofosbuvir absorption and hepatic relative targeting efficiency. *Drug Deliv.* **2020**, *27*, 996–1009. [CrossRef]
19. Deng, F.; Bae, Y.H. Bile acid transporter-mediated oral drug delivery. *J. Control. Release* **2020**, *327*, 100–116. [CrossRef]
20. Niu, M.; Lu, Y.; Hovgaard, L.; Guan, P.; Tan, Y.; Lian, R.; Qi, J.; Wu, W. Hypoglycemic activity and oral bioavailability of insulin-loaded liposomes containing bile salts in rats: The effect of cholate type, particle size and administered dose. *Eur. J. Pharm. Biopharm.* **2012**, *2*, 265–272. [CrossRef]
21. Shukla, A.; Singh, B.; Katare, O.P. Significant systemic and mucosal immune response induced on oral delivery of diphtheria toxoid using nano-bilosomes. *Br. J. Pharmacol.* **2011**, *164*, 820–827. [CrossRef] [PubMed]
22. Shukla, A.; Khatri, K.; Gupta, P.N.; Goyal, A.K.; Mehta, A.; Vyas, S.P. Oral immunization against hepatitis B using bile salt stabilized vesicles (bilosomes). *J. Pharm. Pharm. Sci.* **2008**, *11*, 59–66. [CrossRef] [PubMed]
23. Zakaria, M.Y.; Fayad, E.; Althobaiti, F.; Zaki, I.; Abu Almaaty, A.H. Statistical optimization of bile salt deployed nanovesicles as a potential platform for oral delivery of piperine: Accentuated antiviral and anti-inflammatory activity in MERS-CoV challenged mice. *Drug Deliv.* **2021**, *28*, 1150–1165. [CrossRef]
24. El Taweel, M.M.; Aboul-Einien, M.H.; Kassem, M.A.; Elkasabgy, N.A. Intranasal Zolmitriptan-Loaded Bilosomes with Extended Nasal Mucociliary Transit Time for Direct Nose to Brain Delivery. *Pharmaceutics* **2021**, *13*, 1828. [CrossRef] [PubMed]
25. Ammar, H.; Ghorab, M.; Kamel, R.; Salama, A.H. A trial for the design and optimization of pH-sensitive microparticles for intestinal delivery of cinnarizine. *Drug Deliv. Transl. Res.* **2016**, *6*, 195–209. [CrossRef]
26. Bhattacharya, S.S.; Banerjee, S.; Ghosh, A.K.; Chattopadhyay, P.; Verma, A.; Ghosh, A. A RP-HPLC method for quantification of diclofenac sodium released from biological macromolecules. *Int. J. Biol. Macromol.* **2013**, *58*, 354–359. [CrossRef] [PubMed]
27. Albash, R.; Elmahboub, Y.; Baraka, K.; Abdellatif, M.M.; Alaa-Eldin, A.A. Ultra-deformable liposomes containing terpenes (terpesomes) loaded fenticonazole nitrate for treatment of vaginal candidiasis: Box-Behnken design optimization, comparative ex vivo and in vivo studies. *Drug Deliv.* **2020**, *27*, 1514–1523. [CrossRef]
28. Shaker, S.; Gardouh, A.R.; Ghorab, M.M. Factors affecting liposomes particle size prepared by ethanol injection method. *Res. Pharm. Sci.* **2017**, *12*, 346–352. [CrossRef]
29. Wu, Y.N.; Xu, Y.L.; Sun, W.X. Preparation and particle size controlling of papain nanoliposomes. *J. Shanghai Jiaotong Univ. Agric. Sci.* **2007**, *25*, 105–109.
30. Taghizadeh, S.M.; Bajgholi, S. A new liposomal-drug-in-adhesive patch for transdermal delivery of sodium diclofenac. *J. Biomater. Nanobiotechnol.* **2011**, *2*, 576–581. [CrossRef]
31. Waglewska, E.; Pucek-Kaczmarek, A.; Bazylińska, U. Novel Surface-Modified Bilosomes as Functional and Biocompatible Nanocarriers of Hybrid Compounds. *Nanomaterials* **2020**, *10*, 2472. [CrossRef] [PubMed]
32. Albash, R.; El-Nabarawi, M.A.; Refai, H.; Abdelbary, A.A. Tailoring of PEGylated bilosomes for promoting the transdermal delivery of olmesartan medoxomil: In-vitro characterization, ex-vivo permeation and in-vivo assessment. *Int. J. Nanomed.* **2019**, *14*, 6555–6574. [CrossRef] [PubMed]
33. Fahmy, A.M.; Hassan, M.; El-Setouhy, D.A.; Tayel, S.A.; Al-Mahallawi, A.M. Statistical optimization of hyaluronic acid enriched ultradeformable elastosomes for ocular delivery of voriconazole via Box-Behnken design: In vitro characterization and in vivo evaluation. *Drug Deliv.* **2021**, *28*, 77–86. [CrossRef] [PubMed]
34. Rushmi, Z.T.; Akter, N.; Mow, R.J.; Afroz, M.; Kazi, M.; de Matas, M.; Rahman, M.; Shariare, M.H. The impact of formulation attributes and process parameters on black seed oil loaded liposomes and their performance in animal models of analgesia. *Saudi Pharm. J.* **2017**, *25*, 404–412. [CrossRef] [PubMed]
35. Shivhare, U.D.; Ambulkar, D.U.; Mathur, V.B.; Bhusari, K.P.; Godbole, M.D. Formulation and evaluation of pentoxifylline liposome formulation. *Digest J. Nanomater. Biostruct.* **2009**, *4*, 857–862.
36. Maritim, S.; Boulas, P.; Lin, Y. Comprehensive analysis of liposome formulation parameters and their influence on encapsulation, stability and drug release in glibenclamide liposomes. *Int. J. Pharm.* **2021**, *592*, 120051. [CrossRef]
37. Sun, J.; Deng, Y.; Wang, S.; Cao, J.; Gao, X.; Dong, X. Liposomes incorporating sodium deoxycholate for hexamethylmelamine (HMM) oral delivery: Development, characterization, and in vivo evaluation. *Drug Deliv.* **2010**, *17*, 164–170. [CrossRef]
38. Danaei, M.; Dehghankhold, M.; Ataei, S.; Hasanzadeh Davarani, F.; Javanmard, R.; Dokhani, A.; Khorasani, S.; Mozafari, M.R. Impact of Particle Size and Polydispersity Index on the Clinical Applications of Lipidic Nanocarrier Systems. *Pharmaceutics* **2018**, *10*, 57. [CrossRef]
39. Ozturk, A.A.; Namlı, İ.; Güleç, K.; Kıyan, H.T. Diclofenac sodium loaded PLGA nanoparticles for inflammatory diseases with high anti-inflammatory properties at low dose: Formulation, characterization and in vivo HET-CAM analysis. *Microvasc. Res.* **2020**, *130*, 103991. [CrossRef]
40. Wu, I.Y.; Bala, S.; Basnet, N.S.; Cagno, M.P. Interpreting non-linear drug diffusion data: Utilizing Korsmeyer-Peppas model to study drug release from liposomes. *Eur. J. Pharm. Sci.* **2019**, *138*, 105026. [CrossRef]

41. Shanmugam, S.; Song, C.K.; Sriraman, S.N.; Baskaran, R.; Yong, C.S.; Choi, H.G.; Kim, D.D.; Woo, J.S.; Yoo, B.K. Physicochemical Characterization and Skin Permeation of Liposome Formulations Containing Clindamycin Phosphate. *Arch. Pharm. Res.* **2009**, *32*, 1067–1075. [CrossRef] [PubMed]
42. Lee, S.; Lee, J.; Choi, Y. Skin permeation enhancement of ascorbyl palmitate by liposomal hydrogel (lipogel) formulation and electrical assistance. *Biol. Pharm. Bull.* **2007**, *30*, 393–396. [CrossRef] [PubMed]
43. Elnaggar, Y.S. Multifaceted applications of bile salts in pharmacy: An emphasis on nanomedicine. *Int. J. Nanomed.* **2015**, *10*, 3955–3971. [CrossRef] [PubMed]

pharmaceutics

MDPI

Article

Physicochemical Characterization and Pharmacological Evaluation of Novel Propofol Micelles with Low-Lipid and Low-Free Propofol

Yongchao Chu, Tao Sun *, Zichen Xie, Keyu Sun * and Chen Jiang *

Department of Pharmaceutics, School of Pharmacy, Key Laboratory of Smart Drug Delivery (Ministry of Education), Minhang Hospital, State Key Laboratory of Medical Neurobiology, MOE Frontiers Center for Brain Science, Research Center on Aging and Medicine, Fudan University, Shanghai 201203, China; ytuyongchao@163.com (Y.C.); 18918169503@163.com (Z.X.)

* Correspondence: sunt@fudan.edu.cn (T.S.); sunkeyu@fudan.edu.cn (K.S.); jiangchen@shmu.edu.cn (C.J.)

Abstract: We developed safe and stable mixed polymeric micelles with low lipids and free propofol for intravenous administration, to overcome the biological barrier of the reticuloendothelial system (RES), reduce pain upon injection, and complications of marketed propofol formulation. The propofol-mixed micelles were composed of distearoyl-phosphatidylethanolamine-methoxy-poly (ethylene glycol 2000) (DSPE mPEG2k) and Solutol HS 15 and were optimized using Box Behnken design (BBD). The optimized formulation was evaluated for globule size, zeta potential, loading content, encapsulation efficiency, pain on injection, histological evaluation, hemolysis test, in vivo anesthetic action, and pharmacokinetics, in comparison to the commercialized emulsion Diprivan. The optimized micelle formulation displayed homogenous particle sizes, and the free drug concentration in the micelles was 60.9% lower than that of Diprivan. The paw-lick study demonstrated that propofol-mixed micelles significantly reduced pain symptoms. The anesthetic action of the mixed micelles were similar with the Diprivan. Therefore, we conclude that the novel propofol-mixed micelle reduces injection-site pain and the risk of hyperlipidemia due to the low content of free propofol and low-lipid constituent. It may be a more promising clinical alternative for anesthetic.

Keywords: propofol; micelle; DSPE mPEG2k; Solutol HS 15

Citation: Chu, Y.; Sun, T.; Xie, Z.; Sun, K.; Jiang, C. Physicochemical Characterization and Pharmacological Evaluation of Novel Propofol Micelles with Low-Lipid and Low-Free Propofol. *Pharmaceutics* **2022**, *14*, 414. https://doi.org/10.3390/pharmaceutics14020414

Academic Editor: Patrick J. Sinko

Received: 6 January 2022
Accepted: 4 February 2022
Published: 14 February 2022

1. Introduction

Propofol (2,6-diisopropylphenol) is a short-acting sedative and hypnotic agent that is most frequently administered as an intravenous anesthetic in clinics. It exhibits multiple advantages, e.g., rapid onset and recovery times, and a short duration of action [1,2]. Propofol is a highly lipophilic compound with limited solubility in water (154 μg/mL) [3]. Due to its lipophilic properties, propofol can easily penetrate the blood–brain barrier and lead to rapid anesthetic effects. Moreover, propofol displays a "trend", involving "low accumulation" in the human body, owing to the short half-life in vivo, and rapid clearance [4]. However, due to its poor solubility in water, the development of a novel propofol injectable has become a major challenge with considerable industrial potential and academia significance.

Propofol was initially formulated in a 16% Cremophor EL solvent [5]. However, due to anaphylaxis caused by Cremophor EL, a fat emulsion (Diprivan) was developed by utilizing soybean oil, purified egg lecithin, and glycerol [6]. Despite the considerable success of the present formulation in the market, some defects have been widely reported for the commercial emulsion based on lipids, which limits its clinical application [7]. For instance, intravenous injection of Diprivan often accompanies injection-site pain caused by free propofol. In addition, the fat emulsion of propofol suffers increased chances of hyperlipidemia for prolonged sedation in intensive care unit (ICUs) due to the high lipid content and high risk of external microbial contamination on repeat administration, as a result of high lecithin and soybean oil content [8]. Diprivan containing lecithin is not suitable for vegetarian or religionists. Moreover, due to thermodynamic instability of emulsion, the particle sizes increase significantly during storage. These large droplets might accumulate in the reticuloendothelial system (RES) organs, which could result in increasing oxidative stress and tissue damage to the liver [9].

Researchers have developed multiple approaches to overcome the drawbacks of Diprivan, including use of microemulsions and prodrugs, and complexes with cyclodextrins. Fospropofol, a prodrug of propofol, has been found to reduce pain upon injection compared to propofol. However, the prodrug has a slower onset of efficacy [10]. A novel propofol by complexation with cyclodextrin was also developed, but adverse hemodynamic consequences induced by the complexes limit its further application [11]. Thus, there is an urgent need to develop a novel propofol formulation for-avoiding the undesirable defects of the marketed formulation. In recent years, polymeric micelles have demonstrated enormous potential in improved solubility of poorly water-soluble drugs [12–15]. In 2019, the FDA approved Cequa, the first micelle-based formulation. Generally, when the critical micellization concentration (CMC) is exceeded, amphipathic copolymers self-assemble into core–shell nanostructures in water [16,17]. The copolymer micelle, as a novel carrier, exhibits many unique advantages, such as lessened undesirable effects of drugs, increased drug loading and it is stable during storage [18,19]. Furthermore, they are able to improve drug stability by protecting the molecules from premature degradation due to the core–shell nanostructure [20–22]. Consequently, there has been a need to develop a promising micelle formulation that could effectively resolve the above-mentioned issues.

In order to replace the high level of lipid component and reduce the concentration of free propofol, this study presents a novel micelles formulation based on DSPE mPEG2k and Solutol HS 15. DSPE mPEG2k has emerged as an excellent drug carrier for therapeutics since the initial discovery of its ability to form polymeric micelles in aqueous environments in 1994 [23]. Solutol HS 15 is a potent non-ionic solubilizing agent with low toxicity and a strong solubilization effect [24]. Its relatively bulky hydrophobic compartment possibly facilitates better drug solubilization. The tailored composition of the hydrophobic block can achieve stable encapsulation of lipophilic molecules. A DSPE mPEG2k/Solutol HS 15 mixed micellar structure not only reduces the concentration of free propofol in the aqueous phase, but it also provides a new formulation of propofol with higher safety and efficacy attributes (Figure 1). This study evaluates the new formulation of the propofol-mixed micelle for size distribution, zeta potential, pH, osmolarity, morphology, and the degree of free propofol in the aqueous phase. Moreover, in vivo efficacy and pharmacokinetic studies were conducted in rats.

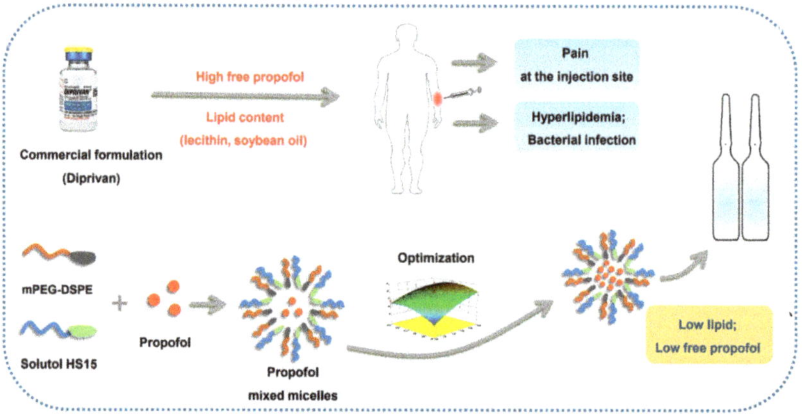

Figure 1. The schematic representation for the propofol mixed micelles.

2. Materials and Methods

2.1. Materials

Propofol was provided from Shanghai Pharmaceuticals Holding Co., Ltd. (Shanghai, China). DSPE mPEG2k copolymers were purchased from AVT Pharmaceutical Tech Co., Ltd. (Shanghai, China). Solutol HS15 was supplied from BASF (Berlin, Germany). Diprivan was obtained by Astra-Zeneca Ltd. (London, UK). Acetonitrile was chromatography-grade and other solvents were of analytical grade.

2.2. Animals

Sprague–Dawley (SD) rats (180–220 g) and BALB/c mice (20–25 g) were supplied from Shanghai SLAC Laboratory Animal Co. Ltd. (Shanghai, China) and All animal handling procedures were approved by Institutional Animal Care and Use Committee of China (2019-03-YJ-JC-01).

2.3. Preparation of Propofol-Mixed Micelles

The propofol-mixed micelle formulation was formulated by a film dispersion method [25]. Briefly, a defined amount of propofol, DSPE-mPEG2k, and Solutol HS 15 was dissolved in a methanol solution and evaporated by rotatory evaporator at 37 °C to ensure the formation of homogeneous film. The thin film was hydrated in saline solution (0.9% sodium chloride) at 37 °C and obtained a uniform spherical micellar solution after filtration through a 0.22 μm filter.

2.4. Determination of Encapsulation Efficiency and Loading Content

The encapsulation efficiency (EE) of mixed micelles was determined as follows. The micelle suspension was added to acetonitrile for demulsification. The propofol concentration in the aqueous phase of the mixed micelles was determined by ultracentrifugation at 3500× g for 40 min by an ultracentrifuge centrifuge tube (Amicon ultracel 3.5 K, Millipore, Billerica, MA, USA). The propofol concentration in micelles was measured by high performance liquid chromatography (HPLC), respectively. Agilent series HPLC system was equipped with a UV detector (Agilent 1260) and C_{18} column (250 mm × 4.6 mm, 5 μm), (Dikma Technologies, Beijing, China). Acetonitrile and water with 0.4% phosphoric acid were applied as the mobile phase. The gradient elution program is shown in Table 1. The flow rate was maintained at 1.0 mL/min with a column temperature of 35 °C. The injection volume was 20 μL and the detection wavelength was 270 nm. The EE of the propofol was calculated using the following formula:

$$EE(\%) = \frac{M_a - M_b}{M_c}$$

where M_a is the total content of propofol in the micellar solution, M_b if the content of free propofol in the micellar solution, and M_c is the initial mass of propofol used in micelles.

Table 1. Gradient program for separation of the propofol.

Time (Min)	Water with 0.4% Phosphoric Acid (%)	Acetonitrile (%)
0	50	50
6	30	70
13	30	70
14	50	50
16	50	50

To determine the drug loading content (LC) of propofol, the mixed micelles were lyophilized and dissolved into acetonitrile. Then, the propofol content was detected by

HPLC analysis according to the above method. The LC of propofol was then calculated using the following formula:

$$LC(\%) = \frac{M_d - M_e}{M_f}$$

where M_d is the total content of propofol in freeze-dried micelles, M_e the content of free propofol in freeze-dried micelles, and M_f the total mass of freeze-dried micelles.

2.5. Particle Size and Zeta Potential

The particle diameter, polymer dispersity index (PDI), and zeta potential of propofol formulation were measured with a dynamic light scattering (DLS) technique (Zetasizer Nano-ZS, Malvern, UK).

2.6. Morphology

The morphologies of propofol-mixed micelles were visualized by a transmission electron microscopy (TEM) (Tecnai^{TM} G2 spirit BioTWIN, Hillsboro). The propofol-mixed micelles were deposited onto the copper net by dropping droplets. Three minutes later, a drop of 1% (*w*/*v*) uranyl acetate was added to the copper grid and diluted negatively stained for three minutes. The samples were air-dried and the grid was observed in the TEM.

2.7. pH and Osmolarity

The pH of the propofol-mixed micelles and Diprivan was detected by a pH meter (PB-10, Sartorius Group, Goettingen, Germany). Their osmolarity was detected by a freezing point osmometer (Osmomat 030, Gonotec GmbH, Berlin, Germany).

2.8. Formulation Optimization

Box–Behnken design (BBD) was used to optimize the formulation. The design is suitable for exploring quadratic response surfaces and constructing second order polynomial models [26]. DSPE mPEG2k concentration, Solutol HS 15 concentration, and propofol concentrations were found to play key roles in affecting the drug LC and EE in the micelles. Therefore, we chose BBD to systemically evaluate the effect of the three key variables on LC and EE of the prepared mixed micelles. The range of each factor was determined according to the results of preliminary experiments and the feasibility of preparing the mixed micelles at the extreme values. The details of the study design are shown in Table 2. The BBD experiments were comprising of three-factors and three-levels designed through Design-Expert Program 8.0.6 software. A total of 17 experiments were performed. The 3D response surface plots were used to determine the importance of the three factors and their interrelationship.

Table 2. Variables employed in BBD.

Independent Variable/Factor	Level		
	−1	0	1
X_1:	5	12.5	20
X_2:	1	10.5	20
X_3:	0.2	2.6	5.0
Dependent variable/response		Constraints	
Y_1:		Maximize	
Y_2:		Maximize	

X_1, X_2, and X_3 represent the concentration of Solutol HS 15, DSPE mPEG2k, and propofol, respectively. Y_1 and Y_2 are EE and LC, respectively.

2.9. Concentration of Free Propofol

The free propofol concentration of the mixed micelles and Diprivan was determined via a reverse dialysis method [26]. In brief, a dialysis tube (Spectrum Laboratories Inc., Piscataway, NJ, USA) (interception molecular weight: 1000 Da) was filled with a 300 μL of glycerol solution (2.5% *w*/*v*) and maintained in 15 mL of mixed micelles or Diprivan for 24 h at room temperature in a thermostatic water bath box. After removal from the propofol formulation, 100 μL of glycerol solution with acetonitrile was diluted to 1 mL of total volume, and then the free propofol concentration was determined by the above-mentioned HPLC analysis.

2.10. Pain on Injection

Pain behavior after injecting propofol formulations was assessed by the SD rat paw-lick test [26]. Rats were randomized in four groups, each consisting of six rats. Each group was treated with either 10 mg/kg of a saline, 0.6% acetic acid solution, Diprivan, or propofol-mixed micelles into the right hind footpad. The onset and duration spent licking the injected hind paw of each rat were recorded for 10 min. The injection site pain is often instantaneous and cannot persist for extended periods of time.

2.11. Histological Evaluation

Twenty male BALB/c mice (20–25 g) were randomized into four groups, and each group was intravenously injected with a saline, 0.6% acetic acid solution, Diprivan or propofol-mixed micelles at a dose of 5 mg/kg. The presence of local inflammation or tissue damage caused by the propofol preparation was evaluated after intraperitoneal administration [27]. The hematoxylin and eosin staining was performed on the peritoneal membranes sections and visualized under a light microscope.

2.12. Hemolysis Test

The hemolytic effect of propofol-mixed micelles in red blood cells (RBC) was investigated by using freshly blood from SD rats. In brief, blood samples were collected via cardiac puncture and immediately transferred to heparin sodium containing tubes. The red blood cells were collected by centrifugation (2000 rpm for 10 min), washed by PBS solution, and then diluted to 1/10 of their volume with PBS for further use. A total of 0.8 mL of different dilution rates (0-, 5-, 10-, 20-fold) of micelles were added to 0.2 mL of RBC suspension and incubated for 2 h at 37 °C in a shaking water bath (50 rpm). The absorbance of supernatants was analyzed at 545 nm after centrifugation at 2500 rpm for 5 min. Purified water and PBS buffer-treated erythrocyte solution were studied as positive (100% lysis) and negative (0% lysis) control, respectively. The hemolysis rate was then calculated using the following formula:

$$\text{Hemolysis rate}(\%) = \frac{\text{Abs}(\text{sample}) - \text{Abs}(\text{negative control})}{\text{Abs}(\text{positive control}) - \text{Abs}(\text{negative control})}$$

2.13. Sleep/Recovery Studies

Male SD rats were injected intravenously with the propofol-mixed micelles or Diprivan at a dose of propofol 10 mg/kg to evaluate recovery from anesthesia. The end of the injection was assigned as time zero. The rats were placed in supine positions, and the loss and recovery time of the righting reflex was monitored.

2.14. Pharmacokinetic Assessment

The SD rats were injected with propofol-mixed micelles and the Diprivan through the tail vein in the dose of 10 mg/kg for the in vivo pharmacokinetic study. A volume of 400 μL blood samples were drawn by retroorbital bleeding at 2, 5, 10, 20, 30, 40, 60, 90, and 120 min after injection, and collected in the heparinized tubes. The plasma samples were separated from blood at 3000 rpm for 10 min, whereafter, the collected blood samples (100 μL) were diluted with 200 μL acetonitrile. The mixtures were vortexed for 3 min and centrifuged with a speed of 13,000 rpm for five min. The supernatants were analyzed by the above-mentioned HPLC method with a sample volume of 20 μL. The pharmacokinetic parameters, including distribution half-life ($t_{1/2\alpha}$), elimination half-life ($t_{1/2\beta}$), T_{max} (the time to reach the C_{max}), C_{max} (maximum plasma concentration), drug clearance (CL), and the area under the curve ($AUC_{(0-120\ min)}$) were analyzed using the Drug and Statistics (DAS) version 2.0 software (Shanghai University of Traditional Chinese Medicine, Shanghai, China).

2.15. Statistical Analysis

All data are presented as mean ± SD. The differences between samples were evaluated using the Student's *t*-test, with $p < 0.05$ considered statistical significance.

3. Results and Discussion

3.1. Optimization of the Preparation Technology

In drug formulation development, high EE and LC were able to ensure that adequate drug delivery to produce therapeutic effects. In the present study, BBD was used to optimize formulations of the propofol-mixed micelles. A total of 17 runs was performed to evaluate the effect of three crucial factors on EE and LC.

A series of single-factor experiments indicated that LC and EE had pronounced changes with varying concentrations of DSPE mPEG2k, Solutol HS 15, and propofol. Therefore, the three factors were conducted as optimization variables through BBD at three experimental levels. The concentration of Solutol HS 15 (labelled as X_1) ranged from 5 to 20 mg/mL, the concentration of DSPE mPEG2k (labelled as X_2) ranged from 1 to 20 mg/mL, and the concentration of propofol (labelled as X_3) ranged from 0.2 to 5.0 mg/mL. EE (Y_1) and LC (Y_2) were used as dependent variables (responses). The experimental design and results are shown in Table 3.

Table 3. Experimental runs and results of responses for BBD.

Formulation Run	Factor 1 X_1	Factor 2 X_2	Factor 3 X_3	Response 1 Y_1	Response 2 Y_2
1	5	1	2.6	51.66	17.94
2	20	1	2.6	77.32	8.52
3	5	20	2.6	67.88	6.5
4	20	20	2.6	82.55	5.24
5	5	10.5	0.2	66.73	1.05
6	20	10.5	0.2	92.45	0.07
7	5	10.5	5.0	73.2	17.96
8	20	10.5	5.0	93.38	12.26
9	12.5	1	0.2	75.46	2.34
10	12.5	20	0.2	87.32	0.63
11	12.5	1	5.0	80.21	22.54
12	12.5	20	5.0	71.52	8.88
13	12.5	10.5	2.6	85.15	8.62
14	12.5	10.5	2.6	78.44	7.98
15	12.5	10.5	2.6	79.52	8.08
16	12.5	10.5	2.6	80.43	7.18
17	12.5	10.5	2.6	79.10	8.04

Table 4 shows the results of the variance analysis for the two responses. According to the regression coefficient significant in the quadratic regression model, factors X_1 ($p < 0.0001$), X_2 ($p < 0.0001$), and X_3 ($p < 0.0001$) were significant terms affecting LC. The interaction terms ($X_{1\times2}$, $X_{1\times3}$, and $X_{2\times3}$) were also significant, whereas the quadratic terms (X_3^2 and X_2^2) were not significant ($p > 0.05$), and X_1^2 was significant for LC responses. For EE, X_1 was the most significant factor ($p < 0.0001$), followed by X_2 ($p < 0.01$). The interaction terms ($X_{1\times2}$, $X_{1\times3}$, and $X_{2\times3}$) were not significant ($p > 0.05$), whereas the quadratic terms (X_3^2 and X_2^2) were significant ($p < 0.05$), and X_1^2 was not significant for EE responses.

Table 4. Analysis of variance for BBD.

Source	Y_1			Y_2		
	F Value	*p*-Value Prob > F	Remarks	F Value	*p*-Value Prob > F	Remarks
Model	9.95	0.0031	Significant	206.69	<0.0001	Significant
X_1	55.62	0.0001		334.44	<0.0001	
X_2	9.95	0.0031		111.32	<0.0001	
X_3	4.53	0.0707		1223.39	<0.0001	
$X_{1 \times 2}$	0.10	0.7615		49.19	0.0002	
$X_{1 \times 3}$	0.46	0.5198		105.50	<0.0001	
$X_{2 \times 3}$	1.81	0.2208		16.46	0.0048	
X_1^2	3.89	0.0890		14.15	0.0071	
X_2^2	6.32	0.0402		1.15	0.3195	
X_3^2	11.46	0.0117		5.24	0.0559	
Lack of Fit	5.91	0.0453	Not significant	10.67	0.0223	Not Significant

The 3D response surface plots were further used to estimate the combined effects of factors on responses (Figure 2). The application of statistical tools of response surfaces allowed determining the optimum experimental conditions for preparation of micelles with high EE and LC: a Solutol HS 15 concentration of 15.8 mg/mL, an DSPE mPEG2k concentration of 1.0 mg/mL, and a propofol concentration of 5.0 mg/mL. The optimized formulation was prepared and the resultant experimental results were compared with predicted values to verify the feasibility of the optimization process. The predicted values of EE and LC in the calculated model were 84.82% and 19.24%, respectively, and the resultant experimental values were close to the predicted values and percentage prediction error was less than 5% (Table 5). Thus, the BBD for optimization of propofol-mixed micelles was validated.

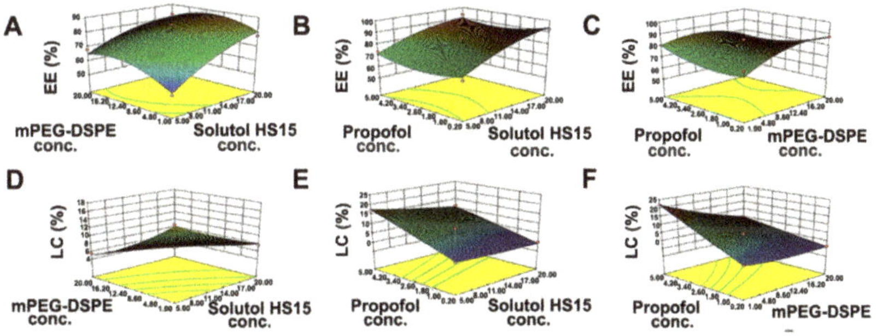

Figure 2. The 3D response surface plots diagrams of EE (**A–C**) and LC (**D–F**). X_1, X_2, and X_3 represent the concentration of Solutol HS 15, DSPE mPEG2k, and propofol, respectively.

Table 5. Predicted and experimental values for the optimized formulation.

Response	Predicted Value	Actual Value	Deviation
EE (%)	84.82	81.73 ± 0.65	3.64%
LC (%)	19.24	18.46 ± 0.82	4.95%

3.2. Particle Size and Zeta Potential

As depicted in Figure 3, the propofol-mixed micelles show that that particle size was 29.9 nm and had a PDI of 0.163 (Figure 3A), which means its suitability for parenteral administration. The zeta potentials of −3.1 mV (Figure 3B) implied good stability of optimized formulation. The TEM image revealed that the propofol-mixed micelle had a spherical appearance (Figure 3C) and the diameters of the micelle particles were consistent with the finding above.

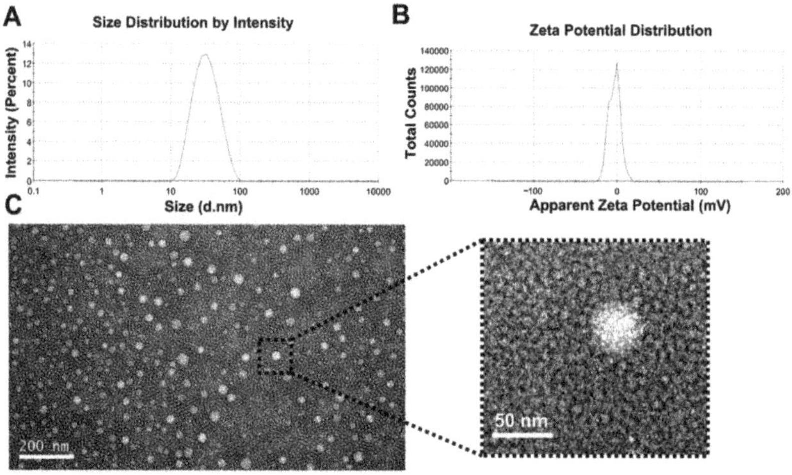

Figure 3. Characterization of the propofol-mixed micelles. (**A**) Size distribution, (**B**) zeta potential, and (**C**) representative TEM image.

3.3. *pH and Osmolarity*

Unphysiological pH is one of key factors likely to induce injection site pain [28]. In our study, the detected pH of propofol-mixed micelles was 7.27 $\pm$ 0.02, which was slightly lower than the Diprivan (7.42 $\pm$ 0.03). However, it was within the suitable range, which was applicable to intravenous use. Similarly, the unphysiological osmotic pressure of the injectable formulation can also result in intravenous injection pain and, thus, it is necessary for determining the appropriate osmotic pressure of the parenteral formulation. The osmolarity of propofol-mixed micelles and Diprivan were 307.0 $\pm$ 1.7 mOsmol/L and 302.5 $\pm$ 1.1 mOsmol/L, respectively. Hence, propofol-mixed micelles showed acceptability for intravenous use.

3.4. *Concentration of Free Propofol*

Many factors induce injection-site pain associated with propofol, including the injection site, the vein size, the injection speed, and concentration of free propofol. However, the leading cause injection pain is related to free propofol concentration in the aqueous phase. Injection pain of propofol can be immediate or lagged reaction [29]. The immediate pain could be due to an irritant effect, while delayed pain possibly contributes to indirect impacts through the kinin cascade that has pain response latency. In clinical anesthesia, propofol is commonly used in combination with several drugs, such as lidocaine and sufentanil. These drugs have been successfully used to minimize propofol-induced pain by inhibiting pain transmission via free nerve endings of vessels, but without decreasing the free propofol concentration [30].

In this study, we found that Diprivan contained a free propofol concentration of 46.2 $\pm$ 2.0 μg/mL in the aqueous phase. In comparison to the Diprivan, optimized propofol-mixed micelles exhibited a marked decrease in the free propofol concentration of 60.9% ($p < 0.001$) (Figure 4A). We speculate that the propofol-mixed micelles could induce less injection pain than marketed Diprivan.

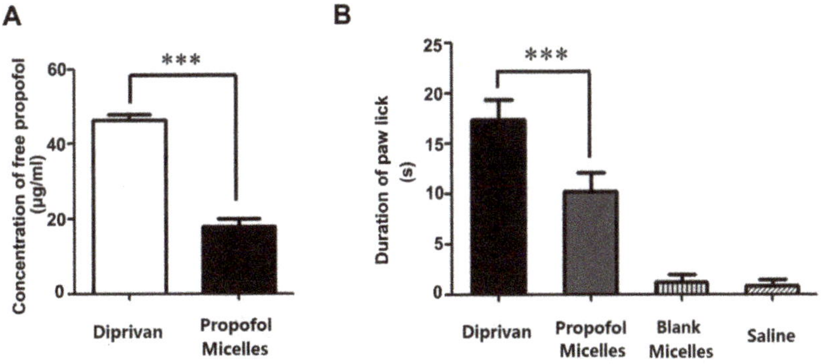

Figure 4. (**A**) Free propofol concentration in the aqueous phase of the mixed micelles and Diprivan (mean ± SD, $n = 6$). (**B**) Duration of rat paw-lick for propofol-mixed micelles and Diprivan ($n = 6$; *** $p < 0.001$).

3.5. Pain on Injection

The rat paw-lick study revealed that the propofol-mixed micelles have significantly less ($p < 0.001$) injection pain (10.17 ± 4.58 s) as compared to the marketed Diprivan (17.33 ± 4.88 s), as shown in Figure 4B. In addition, the results showed a similar effect in the blank mixed-micelles and the saline solution, meaning DSPE mPEG2k and Solutol HS 15 cannot produce any injection pain. Therefore, the less injection pain effect with propofol-mixed micelles could be due to less free propofol in the formulation.

3.6. Histological Evaluation

The micrograph analysis shows no significant peritoneal inflammatory response observed after intraperitoneal injection of either propofol formulations (Figure 5). However, evident congestion of blood vessels is observed after intraperitoneal administration of acetic acid. It indicates that neither propofol formulation resulted in local tissue lesions or inflammation.

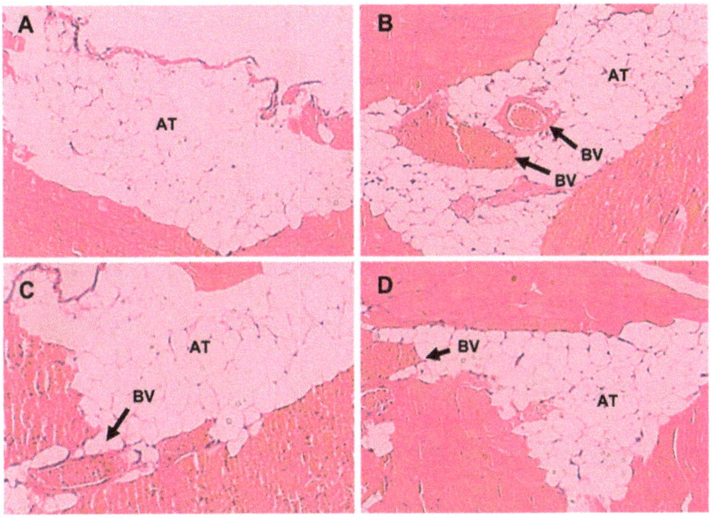

Figure 5. Representative HE-staining micrographs of peritoneal tissues in mice after intraperitoneal administration. Injection with saline (**A**), acetic acid (**B**), Diprivan (**C**), and propofol micelles (**D**). Arrows in the panels indicate AT = adipose tissue and BV = blood vessel.

3.7. Hemolysis Test

It was reported that lipid emulsion Diprivan made with lecithin exhibited potential hemolytic activity, probably associated with the presence of lysophosphatidylcholine and phosphatidyl ethanolamine, which were produced by the hydrolysis of lecithin during preparation and storage of the formations [31]. Thus, to assess the blood compatibility, a hemolysis test of propofol-mixed micelles at different dilution ratios was conducted to confirm the biocompatibility. Figure 6 shows that the hemolysis rate of propofol-mixed micelles was lesser than 5%, indicating the micelles had a non-hemolytic reaction.

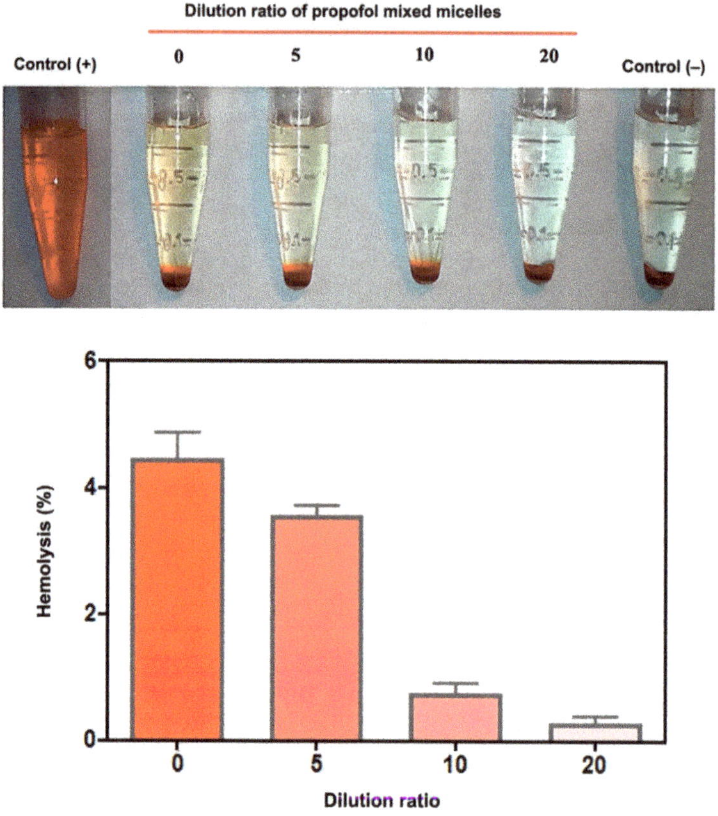

Figure 6. Hemolysis test results of the propofol-mixed micelles at different dilution ratios ($n = 3$).

3.8. Anesthetic Action

The average time for return of the righting reflex was recorded after commercial formulation (Diprivan) and propofol-mixed micelle administration. The time average of loss of the righting reflex of Diprivan and the different doses of micelle are shown in Figure 7. Following administration of the propofol-mixed micelles and Diprivan, animals rapidly lost motility within 20 s. The anesthetic action study of propofol formulation revealed that the propofol-mixed micelle at 10 mg/kg dose had a slightly longer time of anesthesia (8.05 ± 1.84 min) in comparison with the Diprivan (7.51 ± 1.74 min). The duration for the rats to lose and regain motility were not significantly different in both propofol formulations ($p > 0.05$). It could be deduced that the differences of both formulations in drug-release behavior did not substantially change the assignment of propofol in the central nervous systems of the rats. Therefore, similar pharmacological phenomena were presented.

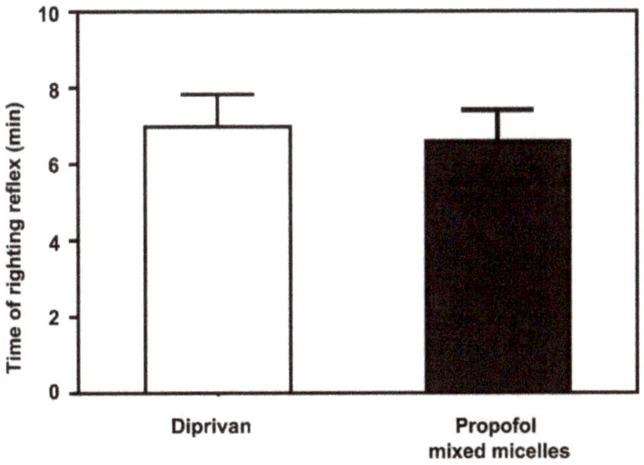

Figure 7. In vivo anesthetic action of propofol-mixed micelles and Diprivan ($n = 9$).

3.9. Pharmacokinetic Study

The average plasma concentration versus time profiles of the propofol-mixed micelles and Diprivan are displayed in Figure 8. The pharmacokinetic parameters were calculated by two-compartment modeling (Table 6). Initial plasma concentration of the propofol for the mixed micelles showed a slight decrease. The distribution half-life ($t_{1/2\alpha}$) of micelles was 6 min, which was approximately 40% shorter than that for Diprivan (10 min). Furthermore, the mixed micelles showed a shorter elimination half-life ($t_{1/2\beta}$) than that of Diprivan. It might be due to the micellar-controlled release property and the drug needs more time to release from the system. In addition, similar results were observed in the apparent volume of CL and $AUC_{(0\text{–}120\ min)}$ between the propofol-mixed micelles and Diprivan, which means that the two formulations have similar absorption and clearance effects after a single dose. Table 6 shows that propofol was absorbed rapidly and eliminated quickly.

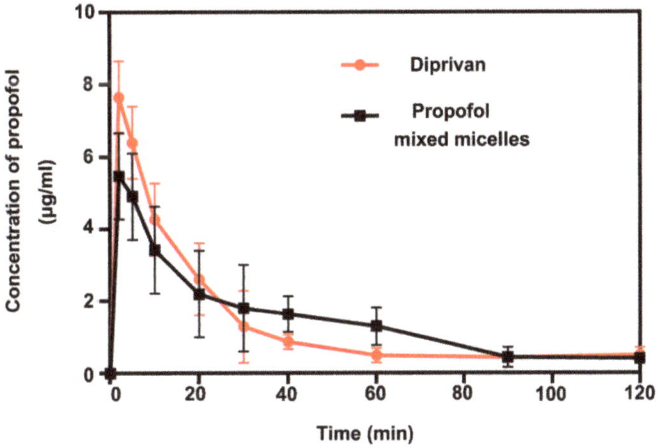

Figure 8. Plasma concentration of propofol vs. time for propofol-mixed micelles and Diprivan following intravenous administration (means ± SD, $n = 5$).

Table 6. Pharmacokinetic parameters of propofol following intravenous injection of propofol-mixed micelles and Diprivan to rats.

Parameter	Unit	Diprivan	Propofol-Mixed Micelles
$t_{1/2\alpha}$	min	10	6
$t_{1/2\beta}$	min	69	384
T_{max}	min	2	2
C_{max}	μg/L	8	5
AUC (0–120 min)	μg·min/L	158	174
CL	L/min/kg	48	48

T_{max}, (the time to reach the C_{max}); C_{max}, (maximum plasma concentration).

4. Conclusions

In summary, we successfully prepared propofol-mixed micelles using DSPE mPEG2k and Solutol HS 15. The mixed micelles showed homogenous particle sizes with diameters maintained at around 30 nm. The micelles were "low lipid", which could diminish the frequency of hyperlipidemia, and the low concentration of free propofol significantly reduced pain in the rat paw-lick study compared to the Diprivan; thus, overcoming the major defect of the commercial formulation. More importantly, the micelle formulation displayed similar anesthetic actions, absorption, and clearance effects after a single dose in comparison with the marketed formulation. In addition, the novel propofol formulation had a non-hemolytic reaction and exhibited a good safety profile. Hence, the novel propofol formulation could act as a commercially viable formulation for parenteral injections of propofol and as a more valid alternative to Diprivan.

Author Contributions: Conceptualization, Y.C., T.S. and C.J.; methodology, Y.C. and T.S.; formal analysis, K.S. and Z.X.; funding acquisition, K.S. and Z.X.; writing—original draft preparation, Y.C., K.S. and Z.X.; supervision, C.J. writing—review and editing, T.S. and C.J. All authors have read and agreed to the published version of the manuscript.

Funding: This work was supported by the National Natural Science Funds of China (92059110/81872808), the Development Fund for Shanghai Talents (2020090), the FDU 2025-Excellence Program Fund, the Program of Shanghai Academic Research Leader (18XD1400500), the Shanghai Municipal Science and Technology Major Projects (2018SHZDZX01) and ZJLab.

Institutional Review Board Statement: Not applicable.

Informed Consent Statement: Not applicable.

Data Availability Statement: Not applicable.

Conflicts of Interest: The authors report no conflict of interest. The authors alone are responsible for the content and writing of this article.

References

1. Gupta, A.; Stierer, T.; Zuckerman, R.; Sakima, N.; Parker, S.D.; Fleisher, L.A. Comparison of recovery profile after ambulatory anesthesia with propofol, isoflurane, sevoflurane and desflurane: A systematic review. *Anesth. Analg.* **2004**, *98*, 632–641. [CrossRef] [PubMed]
2. Trapani, G.; Latrofa, A.; Franco, M.; Lopedota, A.; Sanna, E.; Liso, G. Inclusion complexation of propofol with 2-hydroxypropyl-beta-cyclodextrin. Physicochemical, nuclear magnetic resonance spectroscopic studies, and anesthetic properties in rat. *J. Pharm. Sci.* **1998**, *87*, 514–518. [CrossRef] [PubMed]
3. Thompson, K.A.; Goodale, D.B. The recent development of propofol (DIPRIVAN). *Intensive Care Med.* **2000**, *26* (Suppl. 4), S400–S404. [CrossRef] [PubMed]
4. Langley, M.S.; Heel, R.C. Propofol. A review of its pharmacodynamic and pharmacokinetic properties and use as an intravenous anaesthetic. *Drugs* **1988**, *35*, 334–372. [CrossRef] [PubMed]
5. Baker, M.T.; Naguib, M. Propofol: The challenges of formulation. *Anesthesiology* **2005**, *103*, 860–876. [CrossRef] [PubMed]
6. de Grood, P.M.; Ruys, A.H.; van Egmond, J.; Booij, L.H.; Crul, J.F. Propofol ('Diprivan') emulsion for total intravenous anaesthesia. *Postgrad. Med. J.* **1985**, *61*, 65–69. [PubMed]
7. Park, J.W.; Park, E.S.; Chi, S.C.; Kil, H.Y.; Lee, K.H. The effect of lidocaine on the globule size distribution of propofol emulsions. *Anesth. Analg.* **2003**, *97*, 769–771. [CrossRef]

8. Wolf, A.; Weir, P.; Segar, P.; Stone, J.; Shield, J. Impaired fatty acid oxidation in propofol infusion syndrome. *Lancet* **2001**, *357*, 606–607. [CrossRef]
9. Driscoll, D.F. Lipid injectable emulsions: Pharmacopeial and safety issues. *Pharm. Res.* **2006**, *23*, 1959–1969. [CrossRef]
10. Pergolizzi, J.J.; Gan, T.J.; Plavin, S.; Labhsetwar, S.; Taylor, R. Perspectives on the role of fospropofol in the monitored anesthesia care setting. *Anesth. Res. Pr.* **2011**, *2011*, 458920. [CrossRef]
11. Egan, T.D.; Kern, S.E.; Johnson, K.B.; Pace, N.L. The pharmacokinetics and pharmacodynamics of propofol in a modified cyclodextrin formulation (Captisol) versus propofol in a lipid formulation (Diprivan): An electroencephalographic and hemodynamic study in a porcine model. *Anesth. Analg.* **2003**, *97*, 72–79. [CrossRef]
12. Wang, Y.; Wang, X.; Zhang, J.; Wang, L.; Ou, C.; Shu, Y.; Wu, Q.; Ma, G.; Gong, C. Gambogic acid-encapsulated polymeric micelles improved therapeutic effects on pancreatic cancer. *Chin. Chem. Lett.* **2019**, *30*, 885–888. [CrossRef]
13. Li, H.; Li, J.; He, X.; Zhang, B.; Liu, C.; Li, Q.; Zhu, Y.; Huang, W.; Zhang, W.; Qian, H.; et al. Histology and antitumor activity study of PTX-loaded micelle, a fluorescent drug delivery system prepared by PEG-TPP. *Chin. Chem. Lett.* **2019**, *30*, 1083–1088. [CrossRef]
14. Shi, H.; Zhao, X.; Gao, J.; Liu, Z.; Liu, Z.; Wang, K.; Jiang, J. Acid-resistant ROS-responsive hyperbranched polythioether micelles for ulcerative colitis therapy. *Chin. Chem. Lett.* **2020**, *31*, 3102–3106. [CrossRef]
15. Zhang, X.; Gao, J.; Zhao, X.; Liu, Z.; Liu, Z.; Wang, K.; Lia, G.; Jiang, J. Hyperbranched polymer micelles with triple-stimuli backbone-breakable iminoboronate ester linkages. *Chin. Chem. Lett.* **2020**, *31*, 1822–1826. [CrossRef]
16. Yang, Z.L.; Li, X.R.; Yang, K.W.; Liu, Y. Amphotericin B-loaded poly(ethylene glycol)-poly(lactide) micelles: Preparation, freeze-drying, and in vitro release. *J. Biomed. Mater. Res. A* **2008**, *85*, 539–546. [CrossRef]
17. Li, X.; Yang, Z.; Yang, K.; Zhou, Y.; Chen, X.; Zhang, Y.; Wang, F.; Liu, Y.; Ren, L. Self-assembled polymeric micellar nanoparticles as nanocarriers for poorly soluble anticancer drug ethaselen. *Nanoscale Res. Lett.* **2009**, *4*, 1502–1511. [CrossRef]
18. Li, X.; Li, P.; Zhang, Y.; Zhou, Y.; Chen, X.; Huang, Y.; Liu, Y. Novel mixed polymeric micelles for enhancing delivery of anticancer drug and overcoming multidrug resistance in tumor cell lines simultaneously. *Pharm. Res.* **2010**, *27*, 1498–1511. [CrossRef]
19. Zhang, Y.; Li, X.; Zhou, Y.; Wang, X.; Fan, Y.; Huang, Y.; Liu, Y. Preparation and evaluation of poly(ethylene glycol)-poly(lactide) micelles as nanocarriers for oral delivery of cyclosporine A. *Nanoscale Res. Lett.* **2010**, *5*, 917–925. [CrossRef]
20. Avgoustakis, K. Pegylated poly(lactide) and poly(lactide-co-glycolide) nanoparticles: Preparation, properties and possible applications in drug delivery. *Curr. Drug Deliv.* **2004**, *1*, 321–333. [CrossRef]
21. Shuai, X.; Merdan, T.; Schaper, A.K.; Xi, F.; Kissel, T. Core-cross-linked polymeric micelles as paclitaxel carriers. *Bioconjug. Chem.* **2004**, *15*, 441–448. [CrossRef]
22. Barreiro-Iglesias, R.; Bromberg, L.; Temchenko, M.; Hatton, T.A.; Concheiro, A.; Alvarez-Lorenzo, C. Solubilization and stabilization of camptothecin in micellar solutions of pluronic-g-poly(acrylic acid) copolymers. *J. Control. Release* **2004**, *97*, 537–549. [CrossRef]
23. Torchilin, V.P.; Omelyanenko, V.G.; Papisov, M.I.; Bogdanov, A.J.; Trubetskoy, V.S.; Herron, J.N.; Gentry, C.A. Poly(ethylene glycol) on the liposome surface: On the mechanism of polymer-coated liposome longevity. *Biochim. Biophys. Acta* **1994**, *1195*, 11–20. [CrossRef]
24. Murgia, S.; Fadda, P.; Colafemmina, G.; Angelico, R.; Corrado, L.; Lazzari, P.; Monduzzi, M.; Palazzo, G. Characterization of the Solutol(R) HS15/water phase diagram and the impact of the Delta9-tetrahydrocannabinol solubilization. *J. Colloid Interface Sci.* **2013**, *390*, 129–136. [CrossRef]
25. Zhang, Y.; Li, X.; Zhou, Y.; Fan, Y.; Wang, X.; Huang, Y.; Liu, Y. Cyclosporin A-loaded poly(ethylene glycol)-*b*-poly($_{D,L}$-lactic acid) micelles: Preparation, *in vitro* and *in vivo* characterization and transport mechanism across the intestinal barrier. *Mol. Pharm.* **2010**, *7*, 1169–1182. [CrossRef]
26. Darandale, S.S.; Shevalkar, G.B.; Vavia, P.R. Effect of Lipid Composition in Propofol Formulations: Decisive Component in Reducing the Free Propofol Content and Improving Pharmacodynamic Profiles. *Aaps. Pharmscitech.* **2017**, *18*, 441–450. [CrossRef]
27. Sudo, R.T.; Bonfa, L.; Trachez, M.M.; Debom, R.; Rizzi, M.D.; Zapata-Sudo, G. Anesthetic profile of a non-lipid propofol nanoemulsion. *Rev. Bras. Anestesiol.* **2010**, *60*, 475–483. [CrossRef]
28. Klement, W.; Arndt, J.O. Pain on i.v. injection of some anaesthetic agents is evoked by the unphysiological osmolality or pH of their formulations. *Br. J. Anaesth.* **1991**, *66*, 189–195. [CrossRef]
29. Klement, W.; Arndt, J.O. Pain on injection of propofol: Effects of concentration and diluent. *Br. J. Anaesth.* **1991**, *67*, 281–284. [CrossRef]
30. Yamakage, M.; Iwasaki, S.; Satoh, J.; Namiki, A. Changes in concentrations of free propofol by modification of the solution. *Anesth. Analg.* **2005**, *101*, 385–388. [CrossRef]
31. Li, G.; Fan, Y.; Li, X.; Wang, X.; Li, Y.; Liu, Y.; Li, M. In vitro and in vivo evaluation of a simple microemulsion formulation for propofol. *Int. J. Pharm.* **2012**, *425*, 53–61. [CrossRef] [PubMed]

pharmaceutics

Review

Strategies to Overcome Biological Barriers Associated with Pulmonary Drug Delivery

Adam J. Plaunt *, Tam L. Nguyen, Michel R. Corboz, Vladimir S. Malinin and David C. Cipolla

Insmed Incorporated, Bridgewater, NJ 08807, USA; Tam.nguyen@insmed.com (T.L.N.); Michel.corboz@insmed.com (M.R.C.); Vladimir.malinin@insmed.com (V.S.M.); David.cipolla@insmed.com (D.C.C.)
* Correspondence: Adam.plaunt@insmed.com

Abstract: While the inhalation route has been used for millennia for pharmacologic effect, the biological barriers to treating lung disease created real challenges for the pharmaceutical industry until sophisticated device and formulation technologies emerged over the past fifty years. There are now several inhaled device technologies that enable delivery of therapeutics at high efficiency to the lung and avoid excessive deposition in the oropharyngeal region. Chemistry and formulation technologies have also emerged to prolong retention of drug at the active site by overcoming degradation and clearance mechanisms, or by reducing the rate of systemic absorption. These technologies have also been utilized to improve tolerability or to facilitate uptake within cells when there are intracellular targets. This paper describes the biological barriers and provides recent examples utilizing formulation technologies or drug chemistry modifications to overcome those barriers.

Keywords: inhaled drug delivery; prodrug; liposome formulation

Citation: Plaunt, A.J.; Nguyen, T.L.; Corboz, M.R.; Malinin, V.S.; Cipolla, D.C. Strategies to Overcome Biological Barriers Associated with Pulmonary Drug Delivery. *Pharmaceutics* **2022**, *14*, 302. https://doi.org/10.3390/pharmaceutics14020302

Academic Editors: Vibhuti Agrahari and Prashant Kumar

Received: 23 December 2021
Accepted: 23 January 2022
Published: 27 January 2022

1. Introduction

Pulmonary delivery of therapeutics is now generally accepted as an ideal strategy to deliver an effective amount of drug to the airways to treat diseases including asthma, chronic obstructive pulmonary disease (COPD), cystic fibrosis (CF) and pulmonary arterial hypertension (PAH), among others [1]. Many of the early inhaled therapies were repositioned after initially being administered by the oral or injectable routes [2]. This change in delivery route was initiated in many cases to avoid systemic side effects and improve targeting to the lung allowing delivery of higher doses that improved efficacy. The inhalation route was not the original choice due to the inconvenience, poor efficiency, variability in delivered dose and lack of portability of the early generation of aerosol delivery technologies [3]. However, tremendous innovation has occurred in the past fifty years and product developers can now choose among portable dry powder inhalers (DPIs), metered dose inhalers (MDIs), soft mist inhalers (SMIs) and nebulizers that provide reproducible and efficient delivery to the lung.

The anatomy of the respiratory tract represents the first biological barrier to effective drug delivery to the conducting airways and deeper bronchopulmonary segments. For successful delivery to the lung, the inhaled aerosol must avoid deposition in the oropharyngeal region. As aerosol droplets or particles are inhaled, their momentum can lead to deviation from a bending air flow path, resulting in aerosol impaction on the surfaces of the mouth or throat and a reduction in the dose to the lung [4,5]. Aerosol devices delivering particles with smaller aerodynamic diameters, which can be achieved by a combination of lower density or smaller geometric size, can more easily avoid aerosol impaction in the oropharyngeal region. Additionally, slower patient inhalation flow rates can also reduce oropharyngeal deposition and some device technologies facilitate this paradigm [6]. Furthermore, the aerosol should be delivered in an aerosol volume that can be fully inhaled with each breath, or else delivery efficiency may be compromised. Synchronization of aerosol generation with initiation of inhalation is a feature of some "smart" inhalation systems [7].

In summary, innovations in inhaler device technologies have addressed the first biological hurdle, which is to minimize oropharyngeal deposition, resulting in a reproducible dose of drug to the lung. The criticality of the reproducibility of lung delivery depends on the drug and the indication. Those indications with narrow therapeutic windows may require delivery systems with exceptional control over the emitted dose and how the aerosol is generated and inhaled. While avoiding oropharyngeal deposition is the first biological barrier, there remain other biological barriers summarized below. Each barrier may need to be considered for each new therapeutic opportunity to understand its significance as an impediment to achieving the desired treatment paradigm. In this paper, we provide examples of how these barriers can be overcome using formulation technologies or modifying the chemistry of the compound.

2. Biological Barriers

The major biological barriers to achieving successful inhaled drug therapy have been documented [8], are summarized in Figure 1 and include:

- Avoiding the cough reflex so that the complete aerosol dose can be inhaled and deposited at its pulmonary target site;
- Achieving efficient delivery of the aerosol to the target region within the lung. For example, to ensure that the therapeutic dose reaches the deeper structures of the lung, the aerosol must be able to pass through the trachea-bronchial airways of the respiratory tract with limited deposition;
- Interacting with the airway surface liquid and mucus to access the cellular targets. Upon deposition in the lung fluid, the drug particle may need to be dissolved or released from a matrix, and for prodrugs, may need to be chemically converted to its active form before being able to diffuse to its target site to take effect. Physical barriers can impede that process;
- Overcoming systemic absorption, degradation or clearance of the active molecule to provide drug concentrations that remain within the therapeutic window until the next administration event. When these functions are relatively rapid, therapeutic levels of the drug can be reduced to ineffective levels prior to the next inhalation event;
- Accessing intracellular targets. Many targets may reside within cells including macrophages, and the cellular membrane presents a barrier to delivery of drug within the cells.

2.1. Avoiding the Cough Reflex

Inhaled therapies that result in coughing during the inhalation event may lead not only to incomplete inhalation of the therapeutic, but also to greater upper airway deposition or exhalation of the aerosol that is in transit during inhalation. Cough during an inhalation event may reduce the efficacy of that treatment event and if recurring, would generally lead to non-adherence. Post-inhalation coughing may not physically hinder inhaled drug delivery, but it may be a barrier to patient treatment adherence. Some inhaled drugs or formulations may lead to a coughing bout by triggering two types of afferent nerves: extrapulmonary Widdicombe cough receptors and/or the intrapulmonary bronchopulmonary C-fibers. The former type is sensitive to extreme pH [9–11] and mechanical stimuli while the latter is sensitive to prostaglandin E2, bradykinin, and a variety of environmental irritants [12,13]. Extreme local osmolarity of the airway surface liquid in the vicinity of dissolving inhaled particles can also activate the afferent nerves and generate a coughing reflex [10,14]. Post-inhalation cough frequency varies with sex and age of patients. Sensitivity to chemical stimuli are increased in female and pediatric patients [15,16] while the frequency of cough reflex is significantly lower in elderly patients than in young patients [17,18]. The cough reflex can be overcome by reducing the rate of particle dissolution on the airway surface or by utilizing other formulation strategies that minimize changes in the proton concentration or osmolality of the epithelial lining fluid [19].

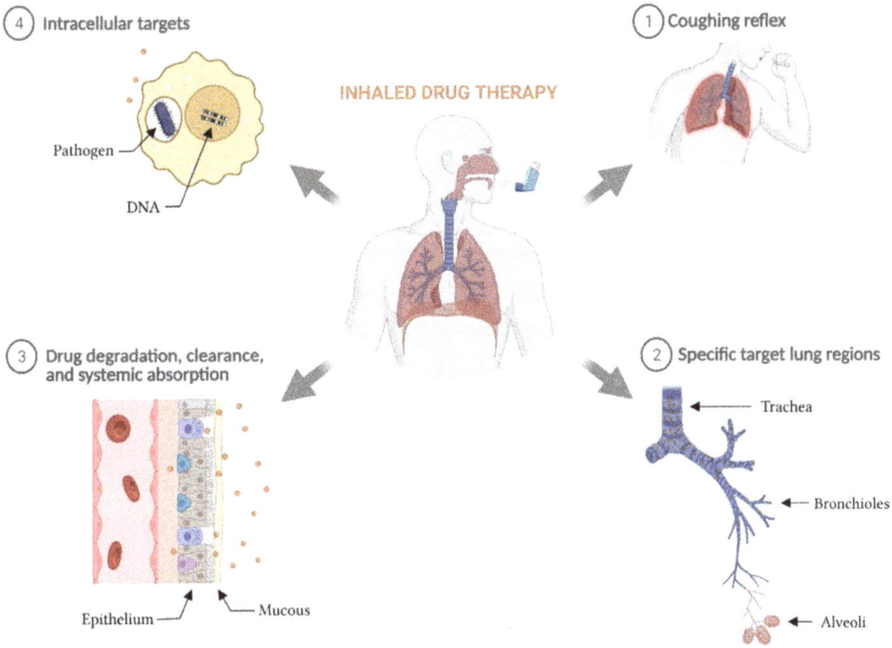

Figure 1. Biological barriers to inhaled drug therapy. The major biological barriers to a successful inhaled drug therapy include: (**1**) post-inhalation coughing reflex, (**2**) low delivery efficiency to specific target lung regions, (**3**) rapid elimination of inhaled active molecules from the lung via degradation, clearance, and/or systemic absorption, and (**4**) the inability for inhaled therapies with intracellular targets to sufficiently penetrate cellular phospholipid membranes and maintain therapeutic concentrations intracellularly.

2.2. Depositing in the Target Region within the Lung

The respiratory tract can be divided into 3 main regions: the upper airways or the oropharyngeal region, the lower airways or the trachea-bronchial region, and the gas exchange or alveolar region [20]. The upper airways consist of the nose, the nasal cavity, the pharynx, and the larynx, while the lower airways comprise the trachea, bronchi, bronchioles and terminal bronchioles. Gas exchange occurs in the alveoli at the end of the terminal bronchioles. From the trachea to the alveoli, there are approximately 23 diverging and asymmetric divisions. As inhaled air travels along the complex respiratory tract, many particles in the airstream are removed by inertial impaction at airway bifurcations [5]. At the end of inhalation, the air flow is reversed. Inhaled particles with smaller size or lower density have limited time to settle to their target sites unless a breath hold maneuver is incorporated at the end of the inhalation. Particles still air-borne at the end of inhalation are then driven out of the lung and some of them land on the respiratory tract walls along the way [5]. Therefore, while employing inhaled air to deliver drugs to the lung is a sensible approach, targeting exclusively the trachea-bronchial or the alveolar regions is extremely difficult [5]. Utilizing more rapid inhalations and larger aerosol particles (e.g., 6 μm) will increase trachea-bronchial deposition over alveolar deposition, although at the expense of greater deposition in the oropharynx. Targeting deposition of inhaled drugs to the alveolar regions can be increased by reducing inhalation flow rate and aerosol size (e.g., to 1–3 μm), and can be further increased by a breath hold to facilitate deposition by sedimentation.

Several studies using radio-labelled particles clearly demonstrated the impact of changes in particle size and inhalation flow rate on drug deposition [21,22]. Moreover, in diseased lungs, the challenge for effective inhaled drug delivery is even more significant due to airway constrictions [23], excessive mucous [24], and/or edema [25].

2.3. Interacting with the Airway Surface Fluid and Overcoming Systemic Absorption, Degradation or Clearance

The surface liquid of the lower airways is composed of 2 layers: a mucous layer with varying thickness [26,27] and a periciliary liquid layer on the airway epithelium. The mucous layer is a gel-like, entangled network of heavily and heterogeneously glycosylated mucins. The diverse carbohydrate chains on mucins allow the mucous layer to interact with and trap a wide range of particles and microorganisms [28] in the inhaled air [29]. The watery periciliary liquid layer is found beneath the mucous layer where the epithelial cilia reside. Synchronized beatings of the epithelial cilia transport mucous and periciliary liquid toward the mouth [30]. Particles trapped by the airway mucus or in the periciliary liquid can be cleared from the lung in a relatively short time frame [31] and thus reduce the active drug concentration, potentially necessitating more frequent dosing. The gas exchange regions are not lined with mucous, making them better target sites for inhaled drugs from that perspective. However, the alveolar epithelial-endothelial layer is thin, and passive transport of small molecular weight drugs into the systemic circulation can be rapid [32] providing only transient drug retaining capacity unless facilitated by a sustained release formulation. In diseased lungs, the mucous of the lower airways can be overexpressed and/or more thickened [26,33], blocking access for inhaled drugs to the target tissues beneath.

The epithelial layer lies immediately beneath the airway surface liquid with its apical surface facing the air space and its basal surface in contact with fluid-filled lung parenchyma. The epithelial layer restricts passages of ions and larger solutes to maintain lung fluid balance. Therefore, crossing the epithelial cell layer can be challenging for inhaled hydrophilic drugs targeting the lung parenchyma. Receptor-mediated transcytosis mechanisms have been identified in lung epithelial cells for some small peptides [34,35]. The efficiency of epithelial active transport depends on the lipophilicity of the molecule, the number of receptors, and the amount of consumed energy. For hydrophilic molecules, slow diffusion through the paracellular tight junction is the only option, and the opening of this tight junction limits the rate of transport for larger molecules [32]. Two distinct pathways through epithelial tight junctions have been identified—the pore pathway mediating passage of small solutes and the leak pathway mediating passage of macromolecules [36–38]. In lung alveolar epithelial cells, the leak pathway depends on the lung-specific tight junction protein claudin 18 [39]. The composition of the leak pathway is still under debate; however, it is known that the "tightness" of the epithelial tight junction varies greatly between the lung regions and is closely regulated by epithelial intracellular activities [38,40].

For people with lung diseases, the epithelial layer is subject to complex structural and functional changes. Infection can cause some component proteins of the tight junction to be upregulated while others are downregulated [41,42]. In asthma, COPD, CF, and idiopathic pulmonary fibrosis, epithelial cells undergo epithelial-to-mesenchymal transition and lose crucial proteins of the tight junctions [43,44]. Epithelial cell damage and massive death are common in *Pseudomonas aeruginosa* infection, acute lung injury, and acute respiratory distress syndrome [45–47].

2.4. Accessing Intracellular Targets

Another barrier for a pharmaceutical molecule to access an intracellular target is the phospholipid bilayer cell membrane. Intracellular treatment targets may include microbiological pathogens, receptors, and attenuation or correction of protein synthesis through the delivery of gene therapy, mRNA and siRNA delivery. Intracellular microbial pathogens often reside within lung alveolar macrophages due to active phagocytotic processes.

As essential components of innate immunity, macrophages play multiple roles in immune surveillance, defense against pathogens, and resolution of inflammation. Airspace macrophages (AMs) are readily retrievable from the airspaces via bronchoalveolar lavage (BAL) and have been well-studied [48]. The healthy human lung contains between 1.4×10^{10} and 2.3×10^{10} AMs, with over 97% present in the alveolar lumen [49,50] A similar number of macrophages are found in the lung interstitium, known as interstitial macrophages (IM), with 78% of all IMs being present in the alveolar septa [49].

Lung resident macrophages further polarize between the M1 state (classically activated macrophages) and the M2 state (alternatively activated macrophages). M1 macrophages play essential roles in host defense through expression of proinflammatory and antimicrobial signals while M2 macrophages help maintain tissue homeostasis and control inflammation through expression of anti-inflammatory cytokines [51,52].

Macrophages have been identified as important sites of infection by both viruses and bacteria for several diseases, including tuberculosis (TB) and non-tuberculous mycobacteria (NTM) lung disease. Microbial pathogens have developed diverse strategies to survive and hide from the host immune response inside the macrophages [53,54], making it difficult to eradicate these pathogens with traditionally formulated antibiotics. Some of these intracellular pathogens reside in the host's cytosol while others reside in intracellular vacuoles. Thus, targeting of the intracellular pathogen populations within the macrophages in the lung presents a particular challenge for developing certain anti-infective lung therapeutics.

Most antibiotics do not easily penetrate cell membranes. Among therapeutics that have been shown to accumulate in macrophages are bedaquiline, oritavancin, and telavancin [55–57]. Novel vancomycin derivatives have also demonstrated the ability to target intracellular infections [58].

The most frequent strategy to improve the penetration of antibiotics into phagocytic cells is the use of carrier systems that deliver these drugs directly to the target cell. Delivery systems such as liposomes, nanoparticles, lipid systems, and conjugates enhance the therapeutic efficacy of antibiotics and antifungal agents in the treatment of infections caused by intracellular microorganisms [54,59,60].

3. Strategies to Overcome Biological Barriers

Through decades of effort, scientists, chemists, and engineers have developed hardware and technology solutions to overcome, and in some cases even capitalize on, the numerous barriers described above. As the relevance of these biological barriers differs by disease, strategies to overcome said barriers is also disease specific. In the context of pulmonary drug delivery, two main strategies are used to overcome these biological barriers: nanoparticle formulation and/or modification of a known active pharmaceutical ingredient (API) using a prodrug strategy. The final choice to use either or both strategies can be nuanced and is dependent on the therapeutic area.

Nanoparticle formulation strategies can be used to alter the way in which active compounds are presented within the body [61–65], including modification of their dissolution profiles [66–70], and some of these strategies have been adapted specifically for pulmonary delivery [71–74]. In some instances, nanoparticles can help overcome specific pharmaceutical development challenges including increased payload delivery, controlled-release kinetics to optimize pharmacokinetic (PK)/pharmacodynamic (PD), improvement of efficacy, and reduction of adverse events [64,75,76]. Similarly, a prodrug modification strategy can be used to alter a compound's PK/PD profile to optimize performance following pulmonary administration. Prodrugs are chemical modifications of an active compound using a labile covalent attachment of a pro-moiety that alters key physical-chemical properties of the active compound, and thus drastically reduces its activity prior to cleavage of the pro-moiety [77,78]. By definition, prodrugs are inactive until the labile covalent bond is cleaved, and the active compound is released. The prodrug strategy carries some extra regulatory burden in that the pro-moiety must be biocompatible and the cleavage mechanism must be robust in all species studied. Furthermore, in the context of pulmonary drug delivery, the decision to use either strategy is impacted by multiple factors including the choice of the delivery device (i.e., DPI, MDI, nebulizer, or soft mist inhaler), the specific disease, and the potency of the active compound.

4. Inhaled Treprostinil Palmitil (TP) for the Treatment of Pulmonary Arterial Hypertension (PAH)

PAH is a progressive, life-threatening disease characterized by the constriction and remodeling of the pulmonary vasculature, leading to increased pulmonary arterial resistance and pulmonary arterial pressure [79–84] that may result in right heart failure and ultimately death [79–87]. Treatment of PAH often involves administration of prostacyclin analogs as pulmonary vasodilating agents. Although these therapies can be effective, most of them are unable to overcome a variety of barriers that make effective treatment difficult to achieve including tolerability issues, rapid absorption, and the requirement for frequent repeat administrations [79,85,86].

One of the most well-known treatments for PAH is a synthetic prostacyclin derivative called treprostinil (TRE). TRE therapies are available as an inhalation solution (Tyvaso), an oral tablet (Orenitram), and as a subcutaneous infusion (Remodulin). TRE acts as a vasodilator with excellent clinical efficacy but its short half-life requires either frequent administration or continuous infusion [87,88]. Frequent administration of TRE results in peak-trough cycles where high levels of TRE shortly after administration may cause patients to experience adverse events, and low levels of TRE prior to the next round of administration may lead to a lack of therapeutic efficacy. Furthermore, inhaled TRE presents tolerability issues with patients often experiencing cough and throat irritation [87,89]. Fortunately, there are ongoing clinical-stage efforts to develop improved, alternative prostacyclin derivative therapies using a variety of pulmonary delivery approaches including liposome encapsulation of iloprost [90–92] and TRE [93,94], nanoparticle formulation [95,96], advanced 3D printing techniques as a way to engineer uniform respirable particles [97,98], and prodrug modification [99].

Development of an inhaled prodrug can be challenging because the associated cleavage mechanism and release of the pro-moiety must be well controlled and not cause any undue toxicities. Therefore, selection of the prodrug chemistry and structure must be well thought out. In the case of TP, a hydrophobic prodrug of TRE, the carboxylic acid functional group from TRE is masked with an ester bond using a 16-carbon hydrophobic chain to form the prodrug. When delivered to the lungs, esterase enzymes that are ubiquitous in the lung microenvironment hydrolyze the ester bond releasing TRE, the active compound, and cetyl alcohol as an inert pro-moiety. Early in vitro experiments confirmed that the rate of hydrolysis for TRE prodrugs can be tuned based on the alkyl chain length of the pro-moiety [99].

Initial formulation efforts using TP focused on a solid lipid nanoparticle formulation, called treprostinil palmitil inhalation solution (TPIS) that was delivered via a nebulizer. This formulation was noteworthy because it relied on three separate strategies to overcome the biological barriers associated with TRE. Firstly, it used a hydrophobic prodrug that allowed for sustained release of TRE. Secondly, it capitalized on the use of solid lipid nanoparticles to aid in solubility (as a technique to deliver a hydrophobic drug in an aqueous media). And thirdly, by delivery of the formulation directly to the lungs using a nebulizer, it targeted the API to the area of interest in the body. Taken together, these strategies resulted in an extended release of TRE that maintains efficacy through 24 h with significantly lower plasma TRE levels, and provides a localized effect specific to the organ of interest, in this case the lungs [100]. More recently, TP has been reformulated for convenient delivery using a DPI using a formulation called Treprostinil Palmitil Inhalation Powder (TPIP), while maintaining the sustained release of TRE. The ability to re-formulate as a DPI is largely due to the high potency of this drug, requiring mere micrograms of material to achieve a therapeutic response.

Indeed, in vivo PK data comparing TRE to TP confirms that administration of the prodrug results in meaningfully reduced peak plasma TRE concentrations and sustained release of TRE over 24 h [101–103]. Clinical studies with both TPIS and TPIP confirmed sustained release profiles of the TP formulation compared to inhaled TRE [100]. TPIS administered at a dose 85 µg (equivalent to TRE dose 54 µg) demonstrated prolonged TRE half-life of 6.4 h, compared to 0.50 h for inhaled TRE solution dosed at 54 µg (Figure 2). The peak plasma TRE concentration following TPIS administration was only 97.6 pg/mL which is roughly 10-fold lower than the peak plasma TRE concentration following a 54 µg dose of TRE (985 pg/mL). TPIS bioavailability was not notably affected, resulting in a systemic plasma TRE exposure (AUC0-24h) of 0.617 ng*h/mL, similar to 0.893 ng*h/mL after TRE inhalation. A similar PK profile was observed following administration of TPIP [manuscript submitted].

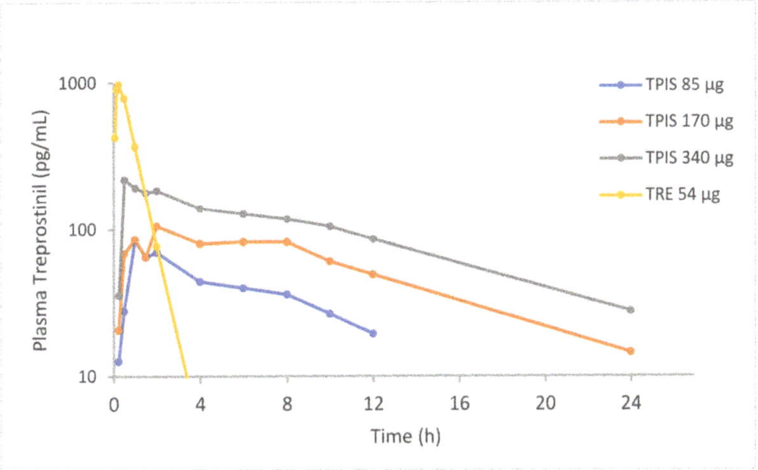

Figure 2. Pharmacokinetics (PK) of Treprostinil (TRE) in healthy volunteers after administration of Treprostinil Palmitil Inhalation Solution (TPIS) or nebulized TRE. Adapted from [104]. European Respiratory Society, 2016.

When tested in a Sugen/Hypoxia (Su/Hx) rat model of PAH, and in comparison with (1) inhaled TRE, (2) intravenous TRE and (3) oral Selexipag, TPIP significantly outperformed the comparator agents [105]. TPIP was associated with a reduction in pulmonary pressure, a reduction in the percentage of muscularized vessels, and a reduction in the percentage of obliterated vessels (Figure 3). Similar results were also observed for the initial nebulizer formulation, TPIS [106]. TPIS demonstrated durable efficacy in vivo, showing a significant reduction in hypoxia-induced right ventricular pressure (RVPP) at plasma TRE concentrations much lower than that observed for infused TRE. In addition to PK/PD advantages, it is worth noting that TP formulations also result in reduced cough and tachyphylaxis relative to TRE in rodent models which could translate to improved patient tolerability via reduction in adverse events in the clinic [107,108]. Thus, for an inhaled prostanoid therapy, the prodrug strategy coupled with an inhaled dry powder format, may enable a once-daily therapy that overcomes the tolerability and rapid absorption barriers, and possibly provide improved efficacy if the remodeling observed in the Su/Hx model translates into the clinic.

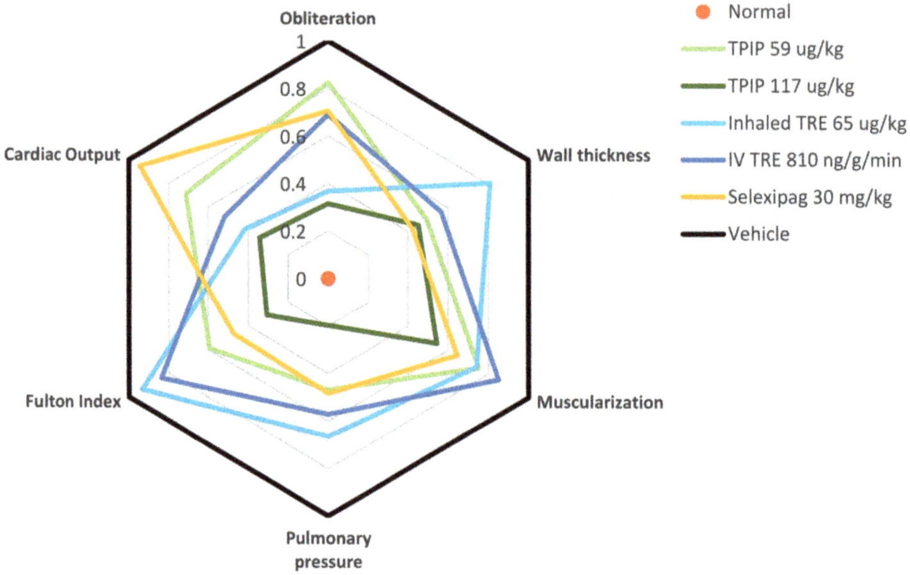

Figure 3. Effect of Treprostinil Palmitil Inhalation Powder (TPIP) in a Sugen/Hypoxia (Su/Hx) rat Pulmonary Arterial Hypertension (PAH) model. This spider graph visually depicts the various readouts from the Su/Hx model including indices of hemodynamics (pulmonary arterial pressure), right ventricular hypertrophy (Fulton index, cardiac output), and vascular remodeling (wall thickness, muscularization and obliteration). In the graph, the individual parameters are represented on separate axes radiating out from the center of the figure. Each parameter is normalized between the normal healthy state (a score of zero, at the center of the figure) and the vehicle control representing the injury after exposure to Su/Hx (a score of 1, at the periphery of the figure). The findings for each compound are depicted in various colors. In this type of figure, the closer that the lines are to the center, the more efficacy they demonstrate. Fulton Index = weight ratio of Right Ventricle/(Left Ventricle + Septum), Pulmonary Pressure = mean Pulmonary Arterial Pressure, Obliteration = percentage (%) of non-obliterated vessels, Wall thickness = Small vessel wall thickness, Muscularization = % of muscularized vessels, Cardiac Output = amount of blood pumped by the heart per minute. Adapted from [105]. American Thoracic Society, 2021.

5. Nebulized CL27c for the Treatment of Pulmonary Fibrosis

Pulmonary fibrosis (PF) is a progressive respiratory condition characterized by chronic fibrosis of the lung interstitial tissues that is associated with diminished lung function and a high mortality rate with limited treatment options [109]. The most common form of PF is idiopathic pulmonary fibrosis (IPF), meaning that the root cause of disease is unknown [110]. During the progression of IPF, alveolar epithelial cells become over-activated which results in accumulation of fibroblasts and myofibroblasts in addition to extensive matrix remodeling [111]. As part of this remodeling, the epithelium becomes scarred and develops a thickened alveolus wall that interferes with gas exchange reducing pulmonary function. Treatment for pulmonary fibrosis typically involves administration of either oral pirfenidone (a pyridine with anti-fibrotic activity) or nintedanib (tyrosine kinase inhibitor), oxygen therapy, pulmonary rehabilitation, or in some instances lung transplant [112]. Recently, prostacyclin analogs [103,113] and phosphoinositide 3-kinase (PI3K) pan inhibitors [114,115] have shown promise in models of PF with examples of both classes of drugs being evaluated via the inhaled route of administration.

The PI3K inhibition strategy is interesting because PI3Ks are involved in a variety of biological processes related to inflammatory conditions such as PF, autoimmune disorders, and certain cancers [116,117]. Recently, Pirali et al. (2017) developed a novel PI3K inhibitor by synthesizing a small library of triazolylquinolones and screening them for PI3K inhibition [118]. Using in vitro PI3K inhibition assays, the authors identified a promising candidate termed CL27e. However, during cell based PI3K activity screening, CL27e failed to affect the PI3K signaling pathway. The authors hypothesized that the ionizable carboxylic acid increased the hydrophilicity of the compound and prevented it from crossing cell membranes and entering the cytoplasm. In other words, the compound could not reach the site of interest and required further modification. To enhance the cell permeation, the authors evaluated a series of ester-based prodrugs, identifying the methyl ester derivative CL27c as the lead candidate that was most effective at inhibiting the PI3K signaling pathway in vitro. The structures of both CL27c and CL27e are shown below in Figure 4.

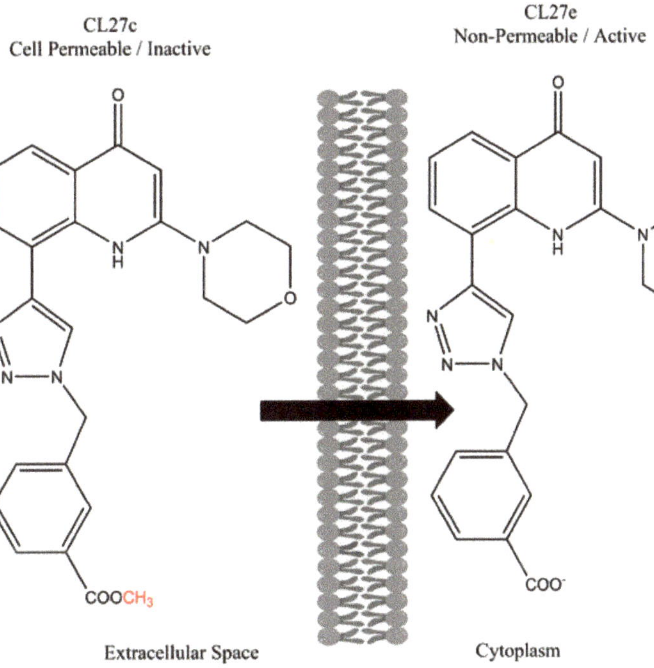

Figure 4. Chemical structures of the active compound CL27e and the corresponding methyl ester prodrug CL27c. Adapted from [119].

In a follow-up publication, Campa et al. (2018) reported on how inhaled delivery of CL27c can improve lung function in rodent models of asthma and fibrosis [120]. Importantly, CL27c was delivered via nebulization to avoid unwanted on-target systemic toxicity observed for other PI3K inhibitors [121–124]. The results indicate that CL27c delivered via inhalation improves lung function in murine models of acute asthma and protects against bleomycin-induced pulmonary fibrosis. Specifically, inhaled CL27c resulted in reduced inflammation and improved survival rate in a bleomycin-induced model of pulmonary fibrosis (Figure 5).

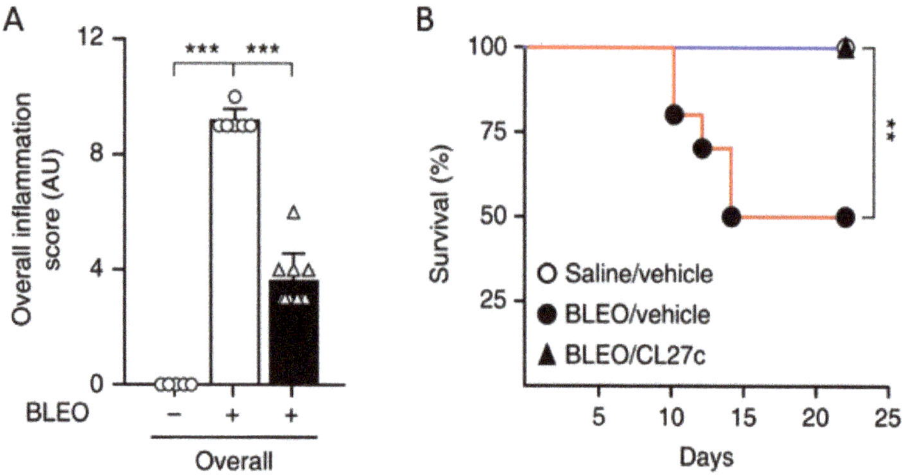

Figure 5. In a bleomycin-induced model of pulmonary fibrosis, treatment with CL27c results in reduced inflammation (**A**) and increased survival (**B**). Histopathologic scoring of inflammatory damage in lung sections derived from control (Bleo−) and Bleo-treated mice (Bleo+) with and without treatment with CL27c (black and white bars, respectively) (n = 5, 6, 10 independent experiments). *** $p < 0.001$ determined using Kruskal–Wallis followed by Dunn's test. ** $p < 0.01$ determined using one-way ANOVA followed by Bonferroni post-hoc test. Adapted from [120]. Nature Communications, 2018.

In summary, if human clinical data replicates these preclinical findings, then the development of CL27c will demonstrate that the combination of prodrug modification that requires intracellular accumulation for release of the active compound, with targeted delivery to the lungs to reduce systemic on-target side effects observed for PI3K inhibitors, can be an effective strategy to overcome biological barriers associated with pulmonary delivery.

6. Inhaled Liposomal Ciprofloxacin for the Treatment of Non-Cystic Fibrosis Bronchiectasis (NCFBE)

NCFBE is characterized by a vicious cycle of infection and inflammation, which leads to structural damage to the airways and deterioration in lung function [125]. NCFBE patients with chronic lung infections have a decreased quality of life and greater morbidity. *Pseudomonas aeruginosa* (PA) lung infections in particular are associated with a seven times greater risk of hospitalization and three times greater mortality compared to NCFBE patients who are uninfected [126]. Thus, an effective inhaled antibiotic targeting PA lung infections in NCFBE patients may reduce the incidence of pulmonary exacerbations and improve morbidity and quality of life. While inhaled antibiotics have become a mainstay of therapy in CF, they have generally been unsuccessful in demonstrating clinical benefit in NCFBE and have been associated with an increased incidence of respiratory adverse events [127,128], bronchospasm [129,130] and drug withdrawals [127–129], compared to placebo. Thus, one of the key barriers to developing an effective inhaled antibiotic in NCFBE is to overcome their poor tolerability [131]. Additionally, most inhaled antibiotics are rapidly absorbed systemically after deposition in the lung, which may necessitate multiple administration events each day to ensure that the antibiotic concentrations remain above the pathogen's minimum inhibitory concentration (MIC) [131,132]. In CF, inhaled tobramycin is labeled for twice-daily administration and aztreonam is administered three times a day. A sustained release formulation of an inhaled antibiotic, which slowly exposes the lung surface to the antibiotic over a 24-h period, thus has the potential to address both the tolerability and residence time barriers.

There are many possible formulation strategies that can provide a sustained release profile in the lung, but liposomes have emerged as a viable strategy for a diverse range of molecules, including antibiotics [69,133]. Robust and reproducible inhaled liposomal formulations can be manufactured utilizing lipids endogenous to the lung including phospholipids and cholesterol [134]. Inhalation and deposition of a biocompatible liposomal formulation on the surface of the airways is unlikely to cause local irritation or sudden perturbations to pH or osmolarity, factors which can lead to cough or bronchospasm [131,132]. A liposomal formulation of ciprofloxacin was thus developed with the goal to provide a sustained release profile in the lung following once-daily inhalation in NCFBE patients with PA lung infections [132].

The development of an inhaled liposomal formulation can be more challenging than the development of traditional inhaled nebulizer solutions and a number of hurdles may need to be addressed: reproducibility of manufacturing each liposome batch, stability of the formulation over its shelf-life, stability of the formulation to the aerosolization process, generation of an appropriate aerosol particle size distribution allowing deposition of an effective dose in the airways, and release of drug from the liposomes at an appropriate rate to maintain drug levels above the MIC until the next administration event [134].

The liposomal ciprofloxacin formulation that was taken into late-stage clinical trials was composed of cholesterol and hydrogenated soy phosphatidylcholine (HSPC) in unilamellar liposomes of 90 nm diameter [132]. This formulation retained its liposome morphology, particle size distribution and in vitro release profile after jet nebulization [132]. The phase 3 trial of inhaled liposomal ciprofloxacin provided PK data that validated the choice of the inhalation route to improve selectivity of the drug for the lung and the choice of the liposome formulation to increase the drug residence time in the lung [135] (Figure 6). Utilization of the inhalation route resulted in a 1700-fold higher peak drug concentration in the sputum compared to oral ciprofloxacin at a similar dose, and a 15-fold lower systemic drug concentration [135]. Consistent with the design thesis, the liposomal component of the formulation provided a sustained presence of drug in the lung over the 24-h period [135].

In the pooled phase 3 trials, inhaled liposomal ciprofloxacin resulted in a delay in the time to first exacerbation of 65 days, which did not reach statistical significance (HR = 0.82 and $p = 0.074$); however, the frequency of moderate to severe pulmonary exacerbations (PE) was significantly ($p = 0.0001$) reduced by 33% and the frequency of severe PEs was significantly ($p = 0.014$) reduced by 42% [136]. The prespecified quality of life metric did not demonstrate improvement in respiratory symptoms at the end of the 48-week trial compared to baseline [137]. However, because liposomal ciprofloxacin was administered in six cycles of 28 days on treatment followed by a 28-day drug holiday, a post-hoc analysis of the on-treatment periods demonstrated significant improvements in respiratory symptoms and declines in CFUs that correlated with improvements in symptoms ($p < 0.0001$) [137]. Following FDA review of clinical trial data, a complete response letter was issued and liposomal ciprofloxacin remains unapproved. While the complete response letter provides a reminder that preclinical success may not always translate to the clinic, the development work and preclinical data surrounding inhaled liposomal ciprofloxacin does validate the use of liposomes as a formulation tool to help overcome biological barriers, specifically in terms of improved patient tolerability and drug residence time in the lung with reduced systemic exposure.

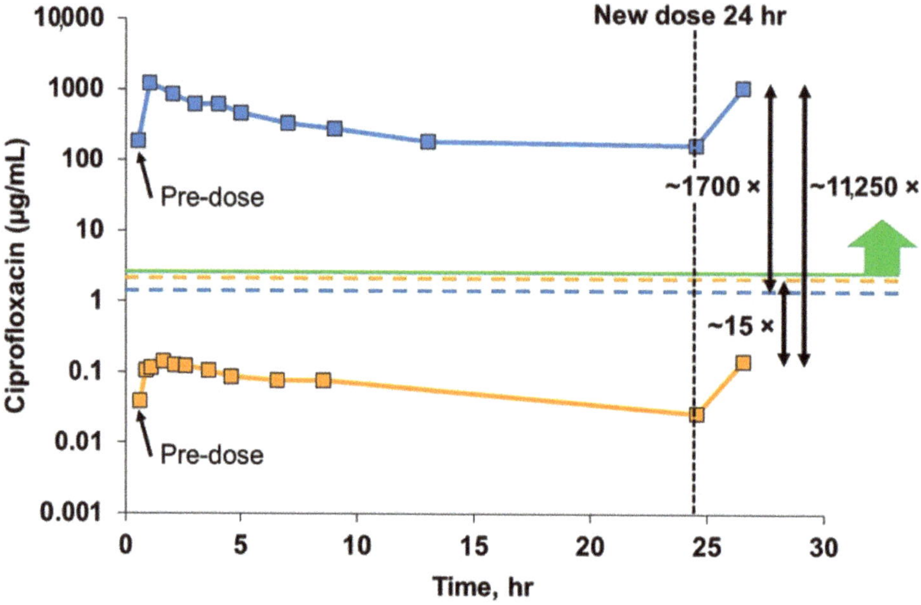

Figure 6. Ciprofloxacin concentrations in blood and sputum samples at steady state. These results cover a single dosing interval over a 24-h period from the Phase 3 open label extension. These data are at steady state achieved after about 4 days of dosing. The solid blue line shows the very high sputum concentrations of ciprofloxacin achieved with inhaled liposomal ciprofloxacin, three orders of magnitude above the MIC for PA (green line) throughout the 24-h dosing interval, and well above the Cmax for oral ciprofloxacin in sputum (dotted blue line). This solid orange line shows a far lower plasma concentration of ciprofloxacin for inhaled liposomal ciprofloxacin, one order of magnitude lower than the Cmax for oral ciprofloxacin (dotted orange line). The peak sputum concentration of ciprofloxacin for inhaled liposomal ciprofloxacin is over 10,000× higher than the peak plasma concentration. Adapted from [135]. World Bronchiectasis Conference, 2017.

7. Inhaled Liposomal Amikacin for the Treatment of Non-Tuberculous Mycobacteria (NTM)

NTM are opportunistic pathogens that are ubiquitous in the environment and can cause pulmonary infections in patients who typically also have underlying respiratory conditions [138,139]. When established, NTM pulmonary infection presents as NTM lung disease. Among mycobacterial species that can cause NTM lung disease, the *Mycobacterium avium* complex (MAC) predominates, while *Mycobacterium abscessus* (Mab) is less common but more pathogenic [138].

NTM can exist extracellularly, in a biofilm form, or intracellularly within macrophages and other cells. NTM biofilms are found in sputum samples and in explanted lungs from CF patients infected with Mab [140]. NTM species can also effectively survive and persist intracellularly evading macrophage's killing mechanisms [141,142] and NTM infections have been found in clinical samples with *M. avium* detected inside peripheral blood leukocytes and bone marrow aspirate [143,144]. Therefore, delivering an effective dose of antibiotic into cells infected with NTM should be an essential component of treatment.

NTM pathogens in planktonic form are sensitive to aminoglycoside antibiotics such as amikacin [145] that demonstrate both inhibitory and bactericidal effects. However, aminoglycoside antibiotics accumulate poorly in cells due to their highly hydrophilic nature. This limits their effectiveness against intracellular infections. By packaging amikacin into liposomes, targeted delivery into the intracellular compartment of macrophages was achieved with improved amikacin activity against intracellular *M. avium* infections [146].

Efficient NTM lung disease treatment requires delivery of high amounts of amikacin to the lung while keeping systemic concentrations low to avoid nephro- and oto-toxicities [147]. Inhalation delivery of liposomal amikacin directly into the lungs may address this problem, but this approach faces three major delivery challenges: (1) efficient delivery of mostly intact liposomes to the lungs; (2) effective distribution of the intact liposomes throughout the lungs; and (3) penetration into biofilms and macrophages to reach the sites of infection. Amikacin liposome inhalation suspension (ALIS), also referred to as Arikayce, or liposomal amikacin for inhalation (LAI), was developed to overcome these challenges and improve the treatment of NTM lung disease.

Liposomal amikacin (ALIS) was tested in in vitro and in vivo preclinical studies to assess whether it was an improvement over amikacin alone with respect to penetration into biofilms and macrophages. In an in vitro study, ALIS liposomes penetrated readily into PA biofilms and through a layer of CF patient mucus in 30 min, that larger (1 μm) fluorescent beads were not able to penetrate [148]. ALIS also penetrated *M. avium* biofilms [149] over a period of 4 h (Figure 7). In this study, mycobacteria biofilm were composed of a dense layer on the slide surface, with more diffuse bacteria and extracellular biofilm components present above. Liposomes could be seen distributed throughout the biofilm, demonstrating that the liposomes penetrated through the extracellular components and reached the cell dense region, suggesting that they may perform well in vivo.

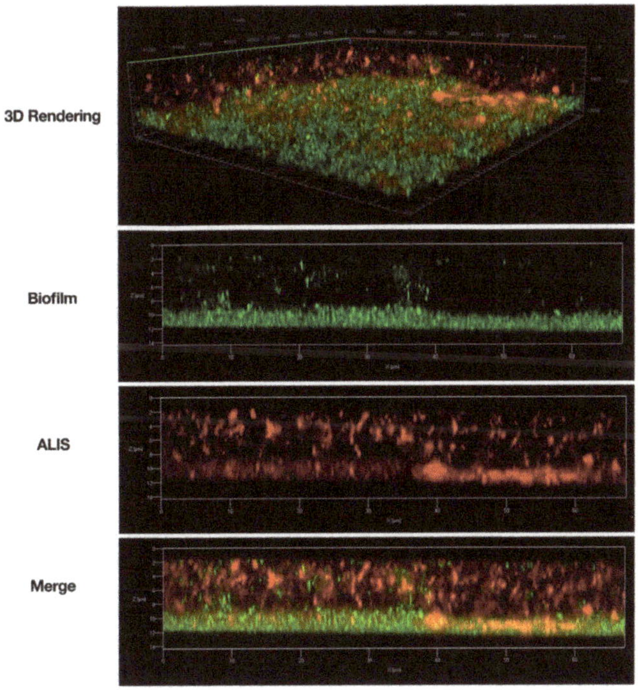

Figure 7. Amikacin liposome inhalation suspension (ALIS) penetrated *Mycobacterium avium* biofilms. Biofilms (strain A5) were established for 7 days in 2-well chamber slides, treated with 512 μg/mL of AF657-labeled ALIS (red) for 4 h, fixed, stained with Syto9 (green), and imaged with a Zeiss LSM 780 confocal scanning microscope (630× magnification). Adapted from [149]. Frontiers, 2018.

The uptake of free or liposomal amikacin into human macrophages was quantified after incubation for 4 or 24 h [149]. Amikacin uptake was time dependent, with cells treated with ALIS containing significantly more amikacin than cells treated with the same concentration of free amikacin (Figure 8A) after 24 h. The amikacin accumulation in macrophages was up to 4-fold higher when treated with ALIS as compared to free amikacin, with meaningful differences between the groups exposed to drug concentrations of 64 and 128 µg/mL. Fluorescence microscopy images taken after 24-h incubation were consistent with the quantitative measurements: macrophages exposed to 32, 64, or 128 µg/mL of ALIS clearly exhibited bright TAMRA fluorescence (yellow) colocalized next to blue DAPI-stained cell nuclei, whereas TAMRA fluorescence was barely visible in cells incubated with free amikacin (Figure 8B).

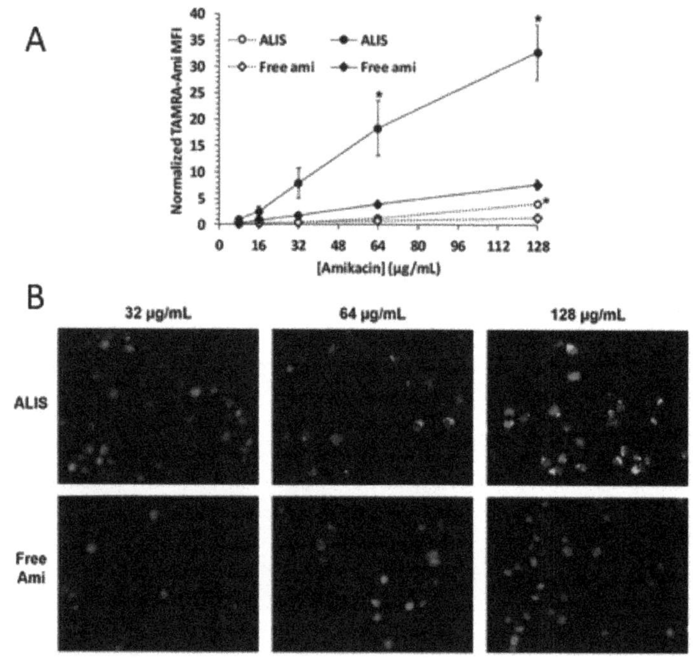

Figure 8. Liposomal and free amikacin uptake into human macrophages. Macrophages were exposed to increasing concentrations of either ALIS or free amikacin (with addition of 0.44% tetramethyl rhodamine (TAMRA) conjugated amikacin) for 4 h (gray symbols) or 24 h (black symbols). (**A**) normalized mean fluorescence intensity (MFI) at each concentration averaged from three independent experiments. (**B**) Visualization of liposomal and free amikacin uptake in human macrophages by fluorescence microscopy. TAMRA fluorescence was visualized by a Zeiss Axio fluorescence microscope (400× magnification) using constant settings for all experimental conditions. Yellow: TAMRA amikacin; Blue: DAPI-stained DNA. * $p < 0.05$ vs. free amikacin at the same concentration and timepoint. Adapted from [149]. Frontiers, 2018. Furthermore, tissue and pulmonary macrophage exposures were compared in vivo after the 96 mg/kg amikacin dose delivered by ALIS nebulization versus the 100 mg/kg amikacin dose given intravenously [149]. In pulmonary macrophages, maximum amikacin concentration (Cmax) after the ALIS dose was nearly 1.0 µg/µg protein and the total macrophage exposure over 24 h (AUC) was 17.8 µg*h/µg protein, 274-fold higher than the exposure following amikacin injection. Similarly, the BAL fluid and lung tissue exposures were 69.5- and 42.7-fold higher, respectively, after inhalation dosing of ALIS compared to intravenous dosing. Simultaneously, the systemic (blood plasma) exposure was 5-fold lower for ALIS than for amikacin injection.

During chronic daily administration of ALIS, lung alveolar macrophages may accumulate significant amounts of liposomal amikacin over time, thus raising the question of their possible effect on macrophage function. Therefore, an in vivo study was conducted to test the effect of continuous treatment of healthy rats by inhalation at a dose of 90 mg/kg over three 30-day treatment periods each followed by a 30-day recovery period [150]. Macrophages demonstrated accumulation of amikacin during treatment periods and nearly complete elimination during recovery periods. The 30-day dosing did not alter macrophage phagocytic activity, yeast killing function, or ability to release inflammatory mediators compared to the control group.

Having established that liposomal amikacin is superior to free amikacin with respect to macrophage uptake, the use of a sophisticated liposomal formulation like ALIS introduced a series of challenges that then had to be addressed, including the ability to nebulize the liposomal amikacin with consistent retention of its liposome properties. To ensure that any batch of liposomal amikacin that satisfied its release specification would provide consistent aerosol performance when used with an intended nebulizer device, in vitro studies were conducted to characterize the product performance [151]. In those studies, nebulized ALIS was shown to maintain a consistent aerosol delivery rate of 0.6 mL/min, aerosol emitted dose of 500 mg amikacin, aerosol fine particle dose of 260 mg amikacin, mean liposome vesicle size between 269–296 nm, and reproducibly generated 35% free amikacin and 65% encapsulated amikacin [151]. Furthermore, in a separate study, aerosol droplets of ALIS were segregated by size and collected in an impactor for subsequent evaluation [152]. In that study, the six aerosol size fractions ranging between 1.1 and 9 μm all maintained equivalent ratios of drug to lipid, percentage of encapsulated and free amikacin, and liposome size [152]. These in vitro experiments provided confidence that nebulized ALIS would perform reproducibly during clinical testing.

In healthy animals dosed with ALIS by inhalation, amikacin was distributed evenly throughout the lungs after single and multiple doses, with equal amikacin concentrations in all lobes of both lungs [150]. In clinical studies, when delivered by inhalation through nebulization, 43% of the ALIS nominal liposome dose was deposited in the lungs of NTM-LD patients [153]. Inhaled ALIS distributed throughout the whole lungs in both healthy volunteers [154] and patients with NTM-LD [153]; the ratio of distribution to central and peripheral lung regions was approximately 1.6–2.0 and more than 50% of the deposited dose was detectable in the lung 24 h post-dose.

Overall, the data demonstrate that nebulization of ALIS results in amikacin delivery to pulmonary macrophages, airways, and lung tissue better than free amikacin given by either inhalation or intravenous administration. This mechanism of improved delivery into pulmonary macrophages and retention within airways and lung tissue has been shown to effectively treat refractory NTM-LD in clinical trials and represents a promising new therapy for patients [155].

ALIS has been shown to effectively target NTM in both preclinical studies and clinical trials. In mice with pulmonary *M. avium* infections, inhalation administration of ALIS lowered viable mycobacteria in the lungs by more than 2 log units [156]. A Phase II trial of patients with refractory NTM-LD demonstrated that ALIS increased the proportion of patients who achieved negative sputum cultures compared with placebo, and the time to first negative sputum culture was shorter with ALIS treatment versus placebo [157]. Based on full results from Phase III studies, ALIS met the primary endpoint by demonstrating that the addition of ALIS to guideline-based therapy eliminated evidence of NTM-LD caused by MAC in sputum by month 6 in a greater proportion of patients than guideline-based therapy alone [155,158,159]. Currently, ALIS is approved in the US, EU, and JPN as ARIKAYCE® and is indicated for the treatment of *Mycobacterium avium* complex (MAC) lung disease as part of a combination antibacterial drug regimen for adult patients who have limited or no alternative treatment options [160].

8. Concluding Remarks

The selection of a prodrug chemistry or nanoparticle formulation, either individually or in combination, can be used to overcome biological barriers related to pulmonary delivery across a wide array of diseases. To develop an improved inhaled prostanoid therapy providing sustained exposure to non-irritating levels of TRE in the lung, a prodrug approach has shown feasibility in either an inhaled dry powder format or when combined with a lipid nanoparticle formulation for nebulization. Two inhaled liposomal products have been utilized to overcome the rapid clearance and subsequent systemic exposure of unencapsulated small molecule drugs. Inhaled liposomal ciprofloxacin was designed to also improve pulmonary tolerability and selectivity for the lung, while liposomal amikacin improved uptake into macrophages at the site of intracellular infection. Looking to the future, while there are many treatments that have been developed for patients with CF, and these have dramatically improved their quality of life and extended survival, a gene therapy that directly corrects the chloride ion channel defect provides the ultimate transformational promise for these patients. To correct the defects in the epithelial cells in the lung may require delivery via the inhalation route. This is also true for other genetic diseases that are manifested primarily in the lung like Primary Ciliary Dyskinesia, and Alpha 1 Antitrypsin Deficiency, where a huge unmet need still exists. Inhaled gene therapy medications will likely require sophisticated formulation strategies to protect and efficiently deliver their genetic cargo to the epithelial cells on the lung surface. The biological barriers become especially challenging to overcome because the genetic cargo is more susceptible to degradation than for traditional small molecular weight drugs and the molecules must remain intact prior to transport into the epithelial cells. The inhaled gene therapy products in development will likely build upon the learnings from the examples described in this review.

Author Contributions: Conceptualization, A.J.P. and D.C.C.; writing—original draft preparation, A.J.P., T.L.N., M.R.C., V.S.M., and D.C.C.; writing—review and editing, A.J.P., T.L.N., M.R.C., V.S.M., and D.C.C.; All authors have read and agreed to the published version of the manuscript.

Funding: The analyses presented in this publication were funded by Insmed Incorporated, Bridgewater, NJ, USA.

Institutional Review Board Statement: Not applicable.

Informed Consent Statement: Not applicable.

Data Availability Statement: All data available are reported in the article.

Conflicts of Interest: All authors are employees of Insmed Incorporated and two of the examples discussed in this review article are part of the Insmed Inc. pipeline. The authors declare no conflict of interest. The funders had no role in the design of the study; in the collection, analyses, or interpretation of data; in the writing of the manuscript, and in the decision to publish the results.

References

1. Anderson, S.; Atkins, P.; Bäckman, P.; Cipolla, D.; Clark, A.; Daviskas, E.; Disse, B.; Entcheva-Dimitrov, P.; Fuller, R.; Gonda, I.; et al. Inhaled Medicines: Past, Present, and Future. *Pharmacol. Rev.* **2022**, *74*, 48–118. [CrossRef] [PubMed]
2. Cipolla, D.; Chan, H.K. Current and Emerging Inhaled Therapies of Repositioned Drugs. *Adv. Drug Deliv. Rev.* **2018**, *133*, 1–4. [CrossRef] [PubMed]
3. Stein, S.W.; Thiel, C.G. The History of Therapeutic Aerosols: A Chronological Review. *J. Aerosol Med. Pulm. Drug Deliv.* **2016**, *30*, 20–41. [CrossRef] [PubMed]
4. Finlay, W.H. 6—Fluid dynamics in the respiratory tract. In *The Mechanics of Inhaled Pharmaceutical Aerosols*; Academic Press: London, UK, 2001; pp. 105–118.
5. Finlay, W.H. 7—Particle deposition in the respiratory tract. In *The Mechanics of Inhaled Pharmaceutical Aerosols*; Academic Press: London, UK, 2001; pp. 119–174.
6. Roche, N.; Scheuch, G.; Pritchard, J.N.; Nopitsch-Mai, C.; Lakhani, D.A.; Saluja, B.; Jamieson, J.; Dundon, A.; Wallace, R.; Holmes, S.; et al. Patient Focus and Regulatory Considerations for Inhalation Device Design: Report from the 2015 IPAC-RS/ISAM Workshop. *J. Aerosol Med. Pulm. Drug Deliv.* **2016**, *30*, 1–13. [CrossRef]
7. Dundon, A.; Cipolla, D.; Mitchell, J.; Lyapustina, S. Reflections on Digital Health Tools for Respiratory Applications. *J. Aerosol Med. Pulm. Drug Deliv.* **2020**, *33*, 127–132. [CrossRef]
8. Patton, J.S.; Brain, J.D.; Davies, L.A.; Fiegel, J.; Gumbleton, M.; Kim, K.-J.; Sakagami, M.; Vanbever, R.; Ehrhardt, C. The Particle has Landed—Characterizing the Fate of Inhaled Pharmaceuticals. *J. Aerosol Med. Pulm. Drug Deliv.* **2010**, *23*, S71–S87. [CrossRef]
9. Canning, B.J.; Farmer, D.G.; Mori, N. Mechanistic studies of acid-evoked coughing in anesthetized guinea pigs. *Am. J. Physiol. Regul. Integr. Comp. Physiol.* **2006**, *291*, R454–R463. [CrossRef]

10. Lowry, R.H.; Wood, A.M.; Higenbottam, T.W. Effects of pH and osmolarity on aerosol-induced cough in normal volunteers. *Clin. Sci.* **1988**, *74*, 373–376. [CrossRef]
11. Higenbottam, T. The mechanism of aerosol-induced bronchoconstriction. *Bull. Eur. Physiopathol. Respir.* **1987**, *23* (Suppl. 10), 77s–80s.
12. Grace, M.; Birrell, M.A.; Dubuis, E.; Maher, S.A.; Belvisi, M.G. Transient receptor potential channels mediate the tussive response to prostaglandin E2 and bradykinin. *Thorax* **2012**, *67*, 891–900. [CrossRef]
13. Birrell, M.A.; Belvisi, M.G.; Grace, M.; Sadofsky, L.; Faruqi, S.; Hele, D.J.; Maher, S.A.; Freund-Michel, V.; Morice, A.H. TRPA1 agonists evoke coughing in guinea pig and human volunteers. *Am. J. Respir. Crit. Care Med.* **2009**, *180*, 1042–1047. [CrossRef]
14. Eschenbacher, W.L.; Boushey, H.A.; Sheppard, D. Alteration in osmolarity of inhaled aerosols cause bronchoconstriction and cough, but absence of a permeant anion causes cough alone. *Am. Rev. Respir. Dis.* **1984**, *129*, 211–215. [PubMed]
15. Geller, D.E.; Nasr, S.Z.; Piggott, S.; He, E.; Angyalosi, G.; Higgins, M. Tobramycin inhalation powder in cystic fibrosis patients: Response by age group. *Respir. Care* **2014**, *59*, 388–398. [CrossRef] [PubMed]
16. Kastelik, J.A.; Thompson, R.H.; Aziz, I.; Ojoo, J.C.; Redington, A.E.; Morice, A.H. Sex-related differences in cough reflex sensitivity in patients with chronic cough. *Am. J. Respir. Crit. Care Med.* **2002**, *166*, 961–964. [CrossRef] [PubMed]
17. Ebihara, S.; Ebihara, T.; Kohzuki, M. Effect of aging on cough and swallowing reflexes: Implications for preventing aspiration pneumonia. *Lung* **2012**, *190*, 29–33. [CrossRef] [PubMed]
18. Newnham, D.M.; Hamilton, S.J. Sensitivity of the cough reflex in young and elderly subjects. *Age Ageing* **1997**, *26*, 185–188. [CrossRef]
19. Sahakijpijarn, S.; Smyth, H.D.C.; Miller, D.P.; Weers, J.G. Post-inhalation cough with therapeutic aerosols: Formulation considerations. *Adv. Drug Deliv. Rev.* **2020**, *165-166*, 127–141. [CrossRef]
20. Winkler, J.; Hochhaus, G.; Derendorf, H. How the lung handles drugs: Pharmacokinetics and pharmacodynamics of inhaled corticosteroids. *Proc. Am. Thorac. Soc.* **2004**, *1*, 356–363. [CrossRef]
21. Biddiscombe, M.; Meah, S.; Barnes, P.; Usmani, O. Drug particle size and lung deposition in COPD. *Eur. Respir. J.* **2016**, *48*, PA313.
22. Sangwan, S.; Agosti, J.M.; Bauer, L.A.; Otulana, B.A.; Morishige, R.J.; Cipolla, D.C.; Blanchard, J.D.; Smaldone, G.C. Aerosolized protein delivery in asthma: Gamma camera analysis of regional deposition and perfusion. *J. Aerosol Med.* **2001**, *14*, 185–195. [CrossRef]
23. Brandsma, C.A.; Van den Berge, M.; Hackett, T.L.; Brusselle, G.; Timens, W. Recent advances in chronic obstructive pulmonary disease pathogenesis: From disease mechanisms to precision medicine. *J. Pathol.* **2020**, *250*, 624–635. [CrossRef] [PubMed]
24. Boucher, R.C. Muco-Obstructive Lung Diseases. *N. Engl. J. Med.* **2019**, *380*, 1941–1953. [CrossRef] [PubMed]
25. Matthay, M.A.; Zemans, R.L.; Zimmerman, G.A.; Arabi, Y.M.; Beitler, J.R.; Mercat, A.; Herridge, M.; Randolph, A.G.; Calfee, C.S. Acute respiratory distress syndrome. *Nat. Rev. Dis. Primers* **2019**, *5*, 18. [CrossRef]
26. Fahy, J.V.; Dickey, B.F. Airway mucus function and dysfunction. *N. Engl. J. Med.* **2010**, *363*, 2233–2247. [CrossRef] [PubMed]
27. Sims, D.E.; Horne, M.M. Heterogeneity of the composition and thickness of tracheal mucus in rats. *Am. J. Physiol.* **1997**, *273*, L1036–L1041. [CrossRef] [PubMed]
28. Duncan, G.A.; Jung, J.; Hanes, J.; Suk, J.S. The Mucus Barrier to Inhaled Gene Therapy. *Mol. Ther.* **2016**, *24*, 2043–2053. [CrossRef]
29. Lamblin, G.; Degroote, S.; Perini, J.M.; Delmotte, P.; Scharfman, A.; Davril, M.; Lo-Guidice, J.M.; Houdret, N.; Dumur, V.; Klein, A.; et al. Human airway mucin glycosylation: A combinatory of carbohydrate determinants which vary in cystic fibrosis. *Glycoconj. J.* **2001**, *18*, 661–684. [CrossRef]
30. Matsui, H.; Randell, S.H.; Peretti, S.W.; Davis, C.W.; Boucher, R.C. Coordinated clearance of periciliary liquid and mucus from airway surfaces. *J. Clin. Investig.* **1998**, *102*, 1125–1131. [CrossRef]
31. Donaldson, S.H.; Corcoran, T.E.; Laube, B.L.; Bennett, W.D. Mucociliary clearance as an outcome measure for cystic fibrosis clinical research. *Proc. Am. Thorac. Soc.* **2007**, *4*, 399–405. [CrossRef]
32. Patton, J.S.; Fishburn, C.S.; Weers, J.G. The lungs as a portal of entry for systemic drug delivery. *Proc. Am. Thorac. Soc.* **2004**, *1*, 338–344. [CrossRef]
33. Serisier, D.J.; Carroll, M.P.; Shute, J.K.; Young, S.A. Macrorheology of cystic fibrosis, chronic obstructive pulmonary disease & normal sputum. *Respir. Res.* **2009**, *10*, 63. [PubMed]
34. Takano, M.; Kawami, M.; Aoki, A.; Yumoto, R. Receptor-mediated endocytosis of macromolecules and strategy to enhance their transport in alveolar epithelial cells. *Exp. Opin. Drug Deliv.* **2015**, *12*, 813–825. [CrossRef] [PubMed]
35. Palaniyandi, S.; Tomei, E.; Li, Z.; Conrad, D.H.; Zhu, X. CD23-Dependent Transcytosis of IgE and Immune Complex across the Polarized Human Respiratory Epithelial Cells. *J. Immunol.* **2011**, *186*, 3484. [CrossRef] [PubMed]
36. Amasheh, S.; Meiri, N.; Gitter, A.H.; Schöneberg, T.; Mankertz, J.; Schulzke, J.D.; Fromm, M. Claudin-2 expression induces cation-selective channels in tight junctions of epithelial cells. *J. Cell. Sci.* **2002**, *115*, 4969–4976. [CrossRef]
37. Watson, C.J.; Rowland, M.; Warhurst, G. Functional modeling of tight junctions in intestinal cell monolayers using polyethylene glycol oligomers. *Am. J. Physiol. Cell Physiol.* **2001**, *281*, C388–C397. [CrossRef]
38. Hasegawa, H.; Fujita, H.; Katoh, H.; Aoki, J.; Nakamura, K.; Ichikawa, A.; Negishi, M. Opposite regulation of transepithelial electrical resistance and paracellular permeability by Rho in Madin-Darby canine kidney cells. *J. Biol. Chem.* **1999**, *274*, 20982–20988. [CrossRef]

39. LaFemina, M.J.; Sutherland, K.M.; Bentley, T.; Gonzales, L.W.; Allen, L.; Chapin, C.J.; Rokkam, D.; Sweerus, K.A.; Dobbs, L.G.; Ballard, P.L.; et al. Claudin-18 deficiency results in alveolar barrier dysfunction and impaired alveologenesis in mice. *Am. J. Respir. Cell Mol. Biol.* **2014**, *51*, 550–558. [CrossRef]
40. Sidhaye, V.K.; Chau, E.; Breysse, P.N.; King, L.S. Septin-2 mediates airway epithelial barrier function in physiologic and pathologic conditions. *Am. J. Respir. Cell Mol. Biol.* **2011**, *45*, 120–126. [CrossRef]
41. Wittekindt, O.H. Tight junctions in pulmonary epithelia during lung inflammation. *Pflug. Arch.* **2017**, *469*, 135–147. [CrossRef] [PubMed]
42. Soini, Y. Claudins in lung diseases. *Respir. Res.* **2011**, *12*, 70. [CrossRef]
43. Yang, Z.C.; Yi, M.J.; Ran, N.; Wang, C.; Fu, P.; Feng, X.Y.; Xu, L.; Qu, Z.H. Transforming growth factor-β1 induces bronchial epithelial cells to mesenchymal transition by activating the Snail pathway and promotes airway remodeling in asthma. *Mol. Med. Rep.* **2013**, *8*, 1663–1668. [CrossRef] [PubMed]
44. Cano, A.; Pérez-Moreno, M.A.; Rodrigo, I.; Locascio, A.; Blanco, M.J.; del Barrio, M.G.; Portillo, F.; Nieto, M.A. The transcription factor snail controls epithelial-mesenchymal transitions by repressing E-cadherin expression. *Nat. Cell Biol.* **2000**, *2*, 76–83. [CrossRef] [PubMed]
45. Deshpande, R.; Zou, C. *Pseudomonas Aeruginosa* Induced Cell Death in Acute Lung Injury and Acute Respiratory Distress Syndrome. *Int. J. Mol. Sci.* **2020**, *21*, 5356. [CrossRef]
46. Guinee, D., Jr.; Brambilla, E.; Fleming, M.; Hayashi, T.; Rahn, M.; Koss, M.; Ferrans, V.; Travis, W. The potential role of BAX and BCL-2 expression in diffuse alveolar damage. *Am. J. Pathol.* **1997**, *151*, 999–1007. [PubMed]
47. Bardales, R.H.; Xie, S.S.; Schaefer, R.F.; Hsu, S.M. Apoptosis is a major pathway responsible for the resolution of type II pneumocytes in acute lung injury. *Am. J. Pathol.* **1996**, *149*, 845–852.
48. Lehnert, B.E.; Valdez, Y.E.; Holland, L.M. Pulmonary macrophages: Alveolar and interstitial populations. *Exp. Lung Res.* **1985**, *9*, 177–190. [CrossRef]
49. Hume, P.S.; Gibbings, S.L.; Jakubzick, C.V.; Tuder, R.M.; Curran-Everett, D.; Henson, P.M.; Smith, B.J.; Janssen, W.J. Localization of Macrophages in the Human Lung via Design-based Stereology. *Am. J. Respir. Crit. Care Med.* **2020**, *201*, 1209–1217. [CrossRef]
50. Crapo, J.D.; Barry, B.E.; Gehr, P.; Bachofen, M.; Weibel, E.R. Cell number and cell characteristics of the normal human lung. *Am. Rev. Respir. Dis.* **1982**, *126*, 332–337.
51. Mosser, D.M.; Edwards, J.P. Exploring the full spectrum of macrophage activation. *Nat. Rev. Immunol.* **2008**, *8*, 958–969. [CrossRef]
52. Martinez, F.O.; Gordon, S. The M1 and M2 paradigm of macrophage activation: Time for reassessment. *F1000Prime Rep.* **2014**, *6*, 13. [CrossRef]
53. Dramé, M.; Buchrieser, C.; Escoll, P. Danger-associated metabolic modifications during bacterial infection of macrophages. *Int. Immunol.* **2020**, *32*, 475–483. [CrossRef] [PubMed]
54. Pizarro-Cerdá, J.; Moreno, E.; Desjardins, M.; Gorvel, J.P. When intracellular pathogens invade the frontiers of cell biology and immunology. *Histol. Histopathol.* **1997**, *12*, 1027–1038. [PubMed]
55. Tanner, L.; Mashabela, G.T.; Omollo, C.C.; de Wet, T.J.; Parkinson, C.J.; Warner, D.F.; Haynes, R.K.; Wiesner, L. Intracellular Accumulation of Novel and Clinically Used TB Drugs Potentiates Intracellular Synergy. *Microbiol. Spectr.* **2021**, *9*, e0043421. [CrossRef] [PubMed]
56. Barcia-Macay, M.; Seral, C.; Mingeot-Leclercq, M.P.; Tulkens, P.M.; Van Bambeke, F. Pharmacodynamic evaluation of the intracellular activities of antibiotics against *Staphylococcus aureus* in a model of THP-1 macrophages. *Antimicrob. Agents Chemother.* **2006**, *50*, 841–851. [CrossRef]
57. Van Bambeke, F.; Carryn, S.; Seral, C.; Chanteux, H.; Tyteca, D.; Mingeot-Leclercq, M.P.; Tulkens, P.M. Cellular pharmacokinetics and pharmacodynamics of the glycopeptide antibiotic oritavancin (LY333328) in a model of J774 mouse macrophages. *Antimicrob. Agents Chemother.* **2004**, *48*, 2853–2860. [CrossRef]
58. Plaunt, A.J.; Rose, S.J.; Kang, J.Y.; Chen, K.J.; LaSala, D.; Heckler, R.P.; Dorfman, A.; Smith, B.T.; Chun, D.; Viramontes, V.; et al. Development and Preclinical Evaluation of New Inhaled Lipoglycopeptides for the Treatment of Persistent Pulmonary Methicillin-Resistant *Staphylococcus aureus* Infections. *Antimicrob. Agents Chemother.* **2021**, *65*, e0031621. [CrossRef]
59. Briones, E.; Colino, C.I.; Lanao, J.M. Delivery systems to increase the selectivity of antibiotics in phagocytic cells. *J. Control. Release* **2008**, *125*, 210–227. [CrossRef]
60. Pinto-Alphandary, H.; Andremont, A.; Couvreur, P. Targeted delivery of antibiotics using liposomes and nanoparticles: Research and applications. *Int. J. Antimicrob. Agents* **2000**, *13*, 155–168. [CrossRef]
61. Deng, Y.; Zhang, X.; Shen, H.; He, Q.; Wu, Z.; Liao, W.; Yuan, M. Application of the Nano-Drug Delivery System in Treatment of Cardiovascular Diseases. *Front. Bioeng. Biotechnol.* **2020**, *7*, 489. [CrossRef]
62. Chenthamara, D.; Subramaniam, S.; Ramakrishnan, S.G.; Krishnaswamy, S.; Essa, M.M.; Lin, F.-H.; Qoronfleh, M.W. Therapeutic efficacy of nanoparticles and routes of administration. *Biomater. Res.* **2019**, *23*, 20. [CrossRef]
63. Wang, A.Z.; Langer, R.; Farokhzad, O.C. Nanoparticle delivery of cancer drugs. *Annu. Rev. Med.* **2012**, *63*, 185–198. [CrossRef] [PubMed]
64. Wilczewska, A.Z.; Niemirowicz, K.; Markiewicz, K.H.; Car, H. Nanoparticles as drug delivery systems. *Pharmacol. Rep.* **2012**, *64*, 1020–1037. [CrossRef]
65. Luo, M.-X.; Hua, S.; Shang, Q.-Y. Application of nanotechnology in drug delivery systems for respiratory diseases (Review). *Mol. Med. Rep.* **2021**, *23*, 325. [CrossRef] [PubMed]

66. Xie, H.; Liu, C.; Gao, J.; Shi, J.; Ni, F.; Luo, X.; He, Y.; Ren, G.; Luo, Z. Fabrication of Zein-Lecithin-EGCG complex nanoparticles: Characterization, controlled release in simulated gastrointestinal digestion. *Food Chem.* **2021**, *365*, 130542. [CrossRef]
67. Franco, P.; Reverchon, E.; De Marco, I. Zein/diclofenac sodium coprecipitation at micrometric and nanometric range by supercritical antisolvent processing. *J. CO_2 Util.* **2018**, *27*, 366–373. [CrossRef]
68. Li, T.; Cipolla, D.; Rades, T.; Boyd, B.J. Drug nanocrystallisation within liposomes. *J. Control. Release* **2018**, *288*, 96–110. [CrossRef]
69. Cipolla, D.; Shekunov, B.; Blanchard, J.; Hickey, A. Lipid-based carriers for pulmonary products: Preclinical development and case studies in humans. *Adv. Drug. Deliv. Rev.* **2014**, *75*, 53–80. [CrossRef]
70. Chan, H.-K.; Kwok, P.C.L. Production methods for nanodrug particles using the bottom-up approach. *Adv. Drug Deliv. Rev.* **2011**, *63*, 406–416. [CrossRef]
71. Khatib, I.; Chow, M.Y.T.; Ruan, J.; Cipolla, D.; Chan, H.-K. Modeling of a spray drying method to produce ciprofloxacin nanocrystals inside the liposomes utilizing a response surface methodology: Box-Behnken experimental design. *Int. J. Pharm.* **2021**, *597*, 120277. [CrossRef]
72. Leung, S.S.Y.; Wong, J.; Guerra, H.V.; Samnick, K.; Prud'homme, R.K.; Chan, H.-K. Porous mannitol carrier for pulmonary delivery of cyclosporine A nanoparticles. *AAPS J.* **2017**, *19*, 578–586. [CrossRef]
73. Cipolla, D.; Wu, H.; Gonda, I.; Chan, H.-K. Aerosol Performance and Long-Term Stability of Surfactant-Associated Liposomal Ciprofloxacin Formulations with Modified Encapsulation and Release Properties. *AAPS PharmSciTech* **2014**, *15*, 1218–1227. [CrossRef] [PubMed]
74. Weers, J.G.; Bell, J.; Chan, H.K.; Cipolla, D.; Dunbar, C.; Hickey, A.J.; Smith, I.J. Pulmonary Formulations: What Remains to be Done? *J. Aerosol Med. Pulm. Drug Deliv.* **2010**, *23*, S-5–S-23. [CrossRef] [PubMed]
75. Abdifetah, O.; Na-Bangchang, K. Pharmacokinetic studies of nanoparticles as a delivery system for conventional drugs and herb-derived compounds for cancer therapy: A systematic review. *Int. J. Nanomed.* **2019**, *14*, 5659–5677. [CrossRef] [PubMed]
76. Pramanik, S.; Mohanto, S.; Manne, R.; Rajendran, R.R.; Deepak, A.; Edapully, S.J.; Patil, T.; Katari, O. Nanoparticle-Based Drug Delivery System: The Magic Bullet for the Treatment of Chronic Pulmonary Diseases. *Mol. Pharm.* **2021**, *18*, 3671–3718. [CrossRef] [PubMed]
77. Rautio, J.; Meanwell, N.A.; Di, L.; Hageman, M.J. The expanding role of prodrugs in contemporary drug design and development. *Nat. Rev. Drug Discov.* **2018**, *17*, 559–587. [CrossRef]
78. Hsieh, P.W.; Hung, C.F.; Fang, J.Y. Current prodrug design for drug discovery. *Curr. Pharm. Des.* **2009**, *15*, 2236–2250. [CrossRef]
79. Chapman, R.W.; Corboz, M.R.; Malinin, V.S.; Plaunt, A.J.; Konicek, D.M.; Li, Z.; Perkins, W.R. An overview of the biology of a long-acting inhaled treprostinil prodrug. *Pulm. Pharmacol. Ther.* **2020**, *65*, 102002. [CrossRef]
80. Gessler, T.; Seeger, W.; Schmehl, T. The potential for inhaled treprostinil in the treatment of pulmonary arterial hypertension. *Ther. Adv. Respir. Dis.* **2011**, *5*, 195–206. [CrossRef]
81. Nadler, S.T.; Edelman, J.D. Inhaled treprostinil and pulmonary arterial hypertension. *Vasc. Health Risk Manag.* **2010**, *6*, 1115–1124. [CrossRef]
82. St Croix, C.M.; Steinhorn, R.H. New Thoughts about the Origin of Plexiform Lesions. *Am. J. Respir. Crit. Care Med.* **2016**, *193*, 484–485. [CrossRef]
83. Vonk Noordegraaf, A.; Galiè, N. The role of the right ventricle in pulmonary arterial hypertension. *Eur. Respir. Rev.* **2011**, *20*, 243–253. [CrossRef] [PubMed]
84. Abe, K.; Toba, M.; Alzoubi, A.; Ito, M.; Fagan, K.A.; Cool, C.D.; Voelkel, N.F.; McMurtry, I.F.; Oka, M. Formation of plexiform lesions in experimental severe pulmonary arterial hypertension. *Circulation* **2010**, *121*, 2747–2754. [CrossRef] [PubMed]
85. Keshavarz, A.; Kadry, H.; Alobaida, A.; Ahsan, F. Newer approaches and novel drugs for inhalational therapy for pulmonary arterial hypertension. *Exp. Opin. Drug Deliv.* **2020**, *17*, 439–461. [CrossRef] [PubMed]
86. Frumkin, L.R. The pharmacological treatment of pulmonary arterial hypertension. *Pharmacol. Rev.* **2012**, *64*, 583–620. [CrossRef] [PubMed]
87. Channick, R.N.; Voswinckel, R.; Rubin, L.J. Inhaled treprostinil: A therapeutic review. *Drug. Des. Devel. Ther.* **2012**, *6*, 19–28. [CrossRef]
88. Ruan, C.-H.; Dixon, R.A.F.; Willerson, J.T.; Ruan, K.-H. Prostacyclin therapy for pulmonary arterial hypertension. *Tex. Heart Inst. J.* **2010**, *37*, 391–399. [PubMed]
89. *Tyvaso®(Treprostinil) [Package Insert]*; United Therapeutics Corporation: Research Triangle Park, NC, USA, 2014. Available online: https://www.tyvasohcp.com/pdf/TYVASO-PI.pdf (accessed on 12 December 2021).
90. Kan, P.; Chen, K.-J.; Hsu, C.-F.; Lin, Y.-F. Inhaled liposomal iloprost shows high drug encapsulation, extended release profile and potentials of improving patient compliance. *Eur. Respir. J.* **2018**, *52*, PA3038.
91. Jain, P.P.; Leber, R.; Nagaraj, C.; Leitinger, G.; Lehofer, B.; Olschewski, H.; Olschewski, A.; Prassl, R.; Marsh, L.M. Liposomal nanoparticles encapsulating iloprost exhibit enhanced vasodilation in pulmonary arteries. *Int. J. Nanomed.* **2014**, *9*, 3249–3261. [CrossRef]
92. Kleemann, E.; Schmehl, T.; Gessler, T.; Bakowsky, U.; Kissel, T.; Seeger, W. Iloprost-containing liposomes for aerosol application in pulmonary arterial hypertension: Formulation aspects and stability. *Pharm. Res.* **2007**, *24*, 277–287. [CrossRef]
93. Kan, P.; Chen, K.-J.; Pan, C. Inhaled liposomal treprostinil (L606) shows extended release in healthy volunteer, as well as prolongs pharmacological effect in hypoxia-induced rat. *Eur. Respir. J.* **2020**, *56*, 1480.

94. Kan, P.; Chen, K.J.; Pan, C. Comparative Pharmacokinetics Between Tyvaso(R) and L606, Extended-Release Formulation of Treprostinil for Inhalation Therapy. In Proceedings of the American Thoracic Society, Virtual, 15 May 2020. Available online: https://www.atsjournals.org/doi/abs/10.1164/ajrccm-conference.2020.201.1_MeetingAbstracts.A3812 (accessed on 12 December 2021).
95. Nakamura, K.; Akagi, S.; Ejiri, K.; Yoshida, M.; Miyoshi, T.; Toh, N.; Nakagawa, K.; Takaya, Y.; Matsubara, H.; Ito, H. Current Treatment Strategies and Nanoparticle-Mediated Drug Delivery Systems for Pulmonary Arterial Hypertension. *Int. J. Mol. Sci.* **2019**, *20*, 5885. [CrossRef] [PubMed]
96. Segura-Ibarra, V.; Wu, S.; Hassan, N.; Moran-Guerrero, J.A.; Ferrari, M.; Guha, A.; Karmouty-Quintana, H.; Blanco, E. Nanotherapeutics for Treatment of Pulmonary Arterial Hypertension. *Front. Physiol.* **2018**, *9*, 890. [CrossRef] [PubMed]
97. Roscigno, R.F.; Vaughn, T.; Parsley, E.; Hunt, T.; Eldon, M.A.; Rubin, L.J. Comparative bioavailability of inhaled treprostinil administered as LIQ861 and Tyvaso® in healthy subjects. *Vascul. Pharmacol.* **2021**, *138*, 106840. [CrossRef]
98. Roscigno, R.; Vaughn, T.; Anderson, S.; Wargin, W.; Hunt, T.; Hill, N.S. Pharmacokinetics and tolerability of LIQ861, a novel dry-powder formulation of treprostinil. *Pulm. Circ.* **2020**, *10*, 2045894020971509. [CrossRef]
99. Leifer, F.G.; Konicek, D.M.; Chen, K.-J.; Plaunt, A.J.; Salvail, D.; Laurent, C.E.; Corboz, M.R.; Li, Z.; Chapman, R.W.; Perkins, W.R.; et al. Inhaled Treprostinil-Prodrug Lipid Nanoparticle Formulations Provide Long-Acting Pulmonary Vasodilation. *Drug Res.* **2018**, *68*, 605–614. [CrossRef] [PubMed]
100. Ismat, F.A.; Usansky, H.; Dhar Murthy, S.; Zou, J.; Teper, A. Safety, tolerability, and pharmacokinetics (PK) of treprostinil palmitil inhalation powder (TPIP): A phase 1, randomised, double-blind, single- and multiple-dose study. *Eur. Heart J.* **2021**, *42*, ehab724-1954. [CrossRef]
101. Corboz, M.R.; Li, Z.; Malinin, V.; Plaunt, A.J.; Konicek, D.M.; Leifer, F.G.; Chen, K.J.; Laurent, C.E.; Yin, H.; Biernat, M.C.; et al. Preclinical Pharmacology and Pharmacokinetics of Inhaled Hexadecyl-Treprostinil (C16TR), a Pulmonary Vasodilator Prodrug. *J. Pharmacol. Exp. Ther.* **2017**, *363*, 348–357. [CrossRef]
102. Chapman, R.W.; Li, Z.; Corboz, M.R.; Gauani, H.; Plaunt, A.J.; Konicek, D.M.; Leifer, F.G.; Laurent, C.E.; Yin, H.; Salvail, D.; et al. Inhaled hexadecyl-treprostinil provides pulmonary vasodilator activity at significantly lower plasma concentrations than infused treprostinil. *Pulm. Pharmacol. Ther.* **2018**, *49*, 104–111. [CrossRef]
103. Corboz, M.R.; Zhang, J.; LaSala, D.; DiPetrillo, K.; Li, Z.; Malinin, V.; Brower, J.; Kuehl, P.J.; Barrett, T.E.; Perkins, W.R.; et al. Therapeutic administration of inhaled INS1009, a treprostinil prodrug formulation, inhibits bleomycin-induced pulmonary fibrosis in rats. *Pulm. Pharmacol. Ther.* **2018**, *49*, 95–103. [CrossRef]
104. Han, D.; Fernandez, C.; Sullivan, E.; Xu, D.; Perkins, W.; Darwish, M.; Rubino, C. Safety and pharmacokinetics study of a single ascending dose of C16TR for inhalation (INS1009). *Eur. Respir. J.* **2016**, *48*, PA2403.
105. Corboz, M.R.; Plaunt, A.J.; Malinin, V.; Li, Z.; Gauani, H.; Chun, D.; Cipolla, D.; Perkins, W.; Chapman, R.W. Beneficial Effects of Treprostinil Palmitil in a Sugen/Hypoxia Rat Model of Pulmonary Arterial Hypertension; A Comparison with Inhaled and Intravenous Treprostinil and Oral Selexipag. In Proceedings of the American Thoracic Society, Online, 15 May 2021. Available online: https://www.atsjournals.org/doi/abs/10.1164/ajrccm-conference.2021.203.1_MeetingAbstracts.A3670 (accessed on 12 December 2021).
106. Corboz, M.R.; Plaunt, A.J.; Malinin, V.; Li, Z.; Gauani, H.; Chun, D.; Cipolla, D.; Perkins, W.R.; Chapman, R.W. Treprostinil palmitil inhibits the hemodynamic and histopathological changes in the pulmonary vasculature and heart in an animal model of pulmonary arterial hypertension. *Eur. J. Pharmacol.* **2021**, *2021*, 174484. [CrossRef] [PubMed]
107. Plaunt, A.J.; Islam, S.; Macaluso, T.; Gauani, H.; Baker, T.; Chun, D.; Viramontes, V.; Chang, C.; Corboz, M.R.; Chapman, R.W.; et al. Development and Characterization of Treprostinil Palmitil Inhalation Aerosol for the Investigational Treatment of Pulmonary Arterial Hypertension. *Int. J. Mol. Sci.* **2021**, *22*, 548. [CrossRef] [PubMed]
108. Chapman, R.W.; Corboz, M.R.; Fernandez, C.; Sullivan, E.; Stautberg, A.; Plaunt, A.J.; Konicek, D.M.; Malinin, V.; Li, Z.; Cipolla, D.; et al. Characterisation of cough evoked by inhaled treprostinil and treprostinil palmitil. *ERJ Open Res.* **2021**, *7*, 00592–02020. [CrossRef] [PubMed]
109. Barratt, S.L.; Creamer, A.; Hayton, C.; Chaudhuri, N. Idiopathic Pulmonary Fibrosis (IPF): An Overview. *J. Clin. Med.* **2018**, *7*, 201. [CrossRef]
110. Lederer, D.J.; Martinez, F.J. Idiopathic Pulmonary Fibrosis. *N. Engl. J. Med.* **2018**, *378*, 1811–1823. [CrossRef]
111. Pardo, A.; Selman, M. Lung Fibroblasts, Aging, and Idiopathic Pulmonary Fibrosis. *Ann. Am. Thorac. Soc.* **2016**, *13* (Suppl. 5), S417–S421. [CrossRef]
112. Laporta Hernandez, R.; Aguilar Perez, M.; Lázaro Carrasco, M.T.; Ussetti Gil, P. Lung Transplantation in Idiopathic Pulmonary Fibrosis. *Med. Sci.* **2018**, *6*, 68. [CrossRef]
113. Nikitopoulou, I.; Manitsopoulos, N.; Kotanidou, A.; Tian, X.; Petrovic, A.; Magkou, C.; Ninou, I.; Aidinis, V.; Schermuly, R.T.; Kosanovic, D.; et al. Orotracheal treprostinil administration attenuates bleomycin-induced lung injury, vascular remodeling, and fibrosis in mice. *Pulm. Circ.* **2019**, *9*, 2045894019881954. [CrossRef]
114. Hettiarachchi, S.U.; Li, Y.H.; Roy, J.; Zhang, F.; Puchulu-Campanella, E.; Lindeman, S.D.; Srinivasarao, M.; Tsoyi, K.; Liang, X.; Ayaub, E.A.; et al. Targeted inhibition of PI3 kinase/mTOR specifically in fibrotic lung fibroblasts suppresses pulmonary fibrosis in experimental models. *Sci. Transl. Med.* **2020**, *12*, eaay3724. [CrossRef]

115. Lukey, P.T.; Harrison, S.A.; Yang, S.; Man, Y.; Holman, B.F.; Rashidnasab, A.; Azzopardi, G.; Grayer, M.; Simpson, J.K.; Bareille, P.; et al. A randomised, placebo-controlled study of omipalisib (PI3K/mTOR) in idiopathic pulmonary fibrosis. *Eur. Respir. J.* **2019**, *53*, 1801992. [CrossRef]
116. Stark, A.-K.; Sriskantharajah, S.; Hessel, E.M.; Okkenhaug, K. PI3K inhibitors in inflammation, autoimmunity and cancer. *Curr. Opin. Pharmacol.* **2015**, *23*, 82–91. [CrossRef] [PubMed]
117. Vanhaesebroeck, B.; Vogt, P.K.; Rommel, C. PI3K: From the bench to the clinic and back. *Curr. Top. Microbiol. Immunol.* **2010**, *347*, 1–19.
118. Pirali, T.; Ciraolo, E.; Aprile, S.; Massarotti, A.; Berndt, A.; Griglio, A.; Serafini, M.; Mercalli, V.; Landoni, C.; Campa, C.C.; et al. Identification of a Potent Phosphoinositide 3-Kinase Pan Inhibitor Displaying a Strategic Carboxylic Acid Group and Development of Its Prodrugs. *ChemMedChem* **2017**, *12*, 1542–1554. [CrossRef] [PubMed]
119. Pesquisadores Sintetizam Fármaco Para Tratamento de Asma e Fibrose Pulmonar. 2018. Available online: https://ufmg.br/comunicacao/noticias/pesquisadores-sintetizam-farmaco-para-tratamento-de-asma-e-fibrose-pulmonar (accessed on 12 December 2021).
120. Campa, C.C.; Silva, R.L.; Margaria, J.P.; Pirali, T.; Mattos, M.S.; Kraemer, L.R.; Reis, D.C.; Grosa, G.; Copperi, F.; Dalmarco, E.M.; et al. Inhalation of the prodrug PI3K inhibitor CL27c improves lung function in asthma and fibrosis. *Nat. Commun.* **2018**, *9*, 5232. [CrossRef]
121. Fruman, D.A.; Chiu, H.; Hopkins, B.D.; Bagrodia, S.; Cantley, L.C.; Abraham, R.T. The PI3K Pathway in Human Disease. *Cell* **2017**, *170*, 605–635. [CrossRef] [PubMed]
122. Kulkarni, S.; Sitaru, C.; Jakus, Z.; Anderson, K.E.; Damoulakis, G.; Davidson, K.; Hirose, M.; Juss, J.; Oxley, D.; Chessa, T.A.; et al. PI3Kβ plays a critical role in neutrophil activation by immune complexes. *Sci. Signal.* **2011**, *4*, ra23. [CrossRef] [PubMed]
123. Condliffe, A.M.; Davidson, K.; Anderson, K.E.; Ellson, C.D.; Crabbe, T.; Okkenhaug, K.; Vanhaesebroeck, B.; Turner, M.; Webb, L.; Wymann, M.P.; et al. Sequential activation of class IB and class IA PI3K is important for the primed respiratory burst of human but not murine neutrophils. *Blood* **2005**, *106*, 1432–1440. [CrossRef] [PubMed]
124. Berghausen, E.M.; Moeller, F.; Vantler, M.; Hirsch, E.; Baldus, S.; Rosenkranz, R. P1938In vitro characterization of a novel PI 3-kinase inhibitor for growth factor-induced effects in pulmonary artery smooth muscle cells. *Eur. Heart J.* **2019**, *40*, ehz748-0685. [CrossRef]
125. McShane, P.J.; Naureckas, E.T.; Tino, G.; Strek, M.E. Non–Cystic Fibrosis Bronchiectasis. *Am. J. Respir. Crit. Care Med.* **2013**, *188*, 647–656. [CrossRef]
126. Finch, S.; McDonnell, M.J.; Abo-Leyah, H.; Aliberti, S.; Chalmers, J.D. A Comprehensive Analysis of the Impact of Pseudomonas aeruginosa Colonization on Prognosis in Adult Bronchiectasis. *Ann. Am. Thorac. Soc.* **2015**, *12*, 1602–1611.
127. Drobnic, M.E.; Suñé, P.; Montoro, J.B.; Ferrer, A.; Orriols, R. Inhaled tobramycin in non-cystic fibrosis patients with bronchiectasis and chronic bronchial infection with *Pseudomonas aeruginosa*. *Ann. Pharmacother.* **2005**, *39*, 39–44. [CrossRef] [PubMed]
128. Barker, A.F.; Couch, L.; Fiel, S.B.; Gotfried, M.H.; Ilowite, J.; Meyer, K.C.; O'Donnell, A.; Sahn, S.A.; Smith, L.J.; Stewart, J.O.; et al. Tobramycin Solution for Inhalation Reduces Sputum *Pseudomonas aeruginosa* Density in Bronchiectasis. *Am. J. Respir. Crit. Care Med.* **2000**, *162*, 481–485. [CrossRef] [PubMed]
129. Bilton, D.; Henig, N.; Morrissey, B.; Gotfried, M. Addition of inhaled tobramycin to ciprofloxacin for acute exacerbations of *Pseudomonas aeruginosa* infection in adult bronchiectasis. *Chest* **2006**, *130*, 1503–1510. [CrossRef] [PubMed]
130. Rubin, B.K. Aerosolized Antibiotics for Non-Cystic Fibrosis Bronchiectasis. *J. Aerosol Med. Pulm. Drug Deliv.* **2008**, *21*, 71–76. [CrossRef] [PubMed]
131. Weers, J. Inhaled antimicrobial therapy—Barriers to effective treatment. *Adv. Drug. Deliv. Rev.* **2015**, *85*, 24–43. [CrossRef]
132. Cipolla, D.; Blanchard, J.; Gonda, I. Development of Liposomal Ciprofloxacin to Treat Lung Infections. *Pharmaceutics* **2016**, *8*, 6. [CrossRef]
133. Cipolla, D.; Gonda, I.; Chan, H.K. Liposomal formulations for inhalation. *Ther. Deliv.* **2013**, *4*, 1047–1072. [CrossRef]
134. Cipolla, D. Inhaled Liposomes. In *Advances in Pulmonary Delivery*; Kwok, P.C.L., Chan, H.K., Eds.; CRC Press: Boca Raton, FL, USA, 2017; Volume 8, pp. 151–173.
135. Froehlich, J.; Cipolla, D.; DeSoyza, A.; Morrish, G.; Gonda, I. Inhaled Liposomal Ciprofloxacin in Patients with Non-Cystic Fibrosis Bronchiectasis and Chronic *Pseudomonas aeruginosa* Infection: Pharmacokinetics of Once-Daily Inhaled ARD-3150. In Proceedings of the 2nd WBE Conference, Milan, Italy, 6–8 July 2017.
136. Haworth, C.S.; Bilton, D.; Chalmers, J.D.; Davis, A.M.; Froehlich, J.; Gonda, I.; Thompson, B.; Wanner, A.; O'Donnell, A.E. Inhaled liposomal ciprofloxacin in patients with non-cystic fibrosis bronchiectasis and chronic lung infection with *Pseudomonas aeruginosa* (ORBIT-3 and ORBIT-4): Two phase 3, randomised controlled trials. *Lancet Respir. Med.* **2019**, *7*, 213–226. [CrossRef]
137. Chalmers, J.D.; Cipolla, D.; Thompson, B.; Davis, A.M.; O'Donnell, A.; Tino, G.; Gonda, I.; Haworth, C.; Froehlich, J. Changes in respiratory symptoms during 48-week treatment with ARD-3150 (inhaled liposomal ciprofloxacin) in bronchiectasis: Results from the ORBIT-3 and -4 studies. *Eru. Respir. J.* **2020**, *56*, 2000110. [CrossRef]
138. Johnson, M.M.; Odell, J.A. Nontuberculous mycobacterial pulmonary infections. *J. Thorac. Dis.* **2014**, *6*, 210–220.
139. Van Ingen, J.; Kuijper, E.J. Drug susceptibility testing of nontuberculous mycobacteria. *Future Microbiol.* **2014**, *9*, 1095–1110. [CrossRef] [PubMed]
140. Qvist, T.; Eickhardt, S.; Kragh, K.N.; Andersen, C.B.; Iversen, M.; Høiby, N.; Bjarnsholt, T. Chronic pulmonary disease with *Mycobacterium abscessus* complex is a biofilm infection. *Eur. Respir. J.* **2015**, *46*, 1823–1826. [CrossRef] [PubMed]

141. Appelberg, R. Pathogenesis of *Mycobacterium avium* infection: Typical responses to an atypical mycobacterium? *Immunol. Res.* **2006**, *35*, 179–190. [CrossRef]
142. Awuh, J.A.; Flo, T.H. Molecular basis of mycobacterial survival in macrophages. *Cell. Mol. Life Sci.* **2017**, *74*, 1625–1648. [CrossRef] [PubMed]
143. Graham, B.S.; Hinson, M.V.; Bennett, S.R.; Gregory, D.W.; Schaffner, W. Acid-fast bacilli on buffy coat smears in the acquired immunodeficiency syndrome: A lesson from Hansen's bacillus. *South. Med. J.* **1984**, *77*, 246–248. [CrossRef]
144. Moffie, B.G.; Krulder, J.W.; de Knijff, J.C. Direct visualization of mycobacteria in blood culture. *N. Engl. J. Med.* **1989**, *320*, 61–62.
145. Cowman, S.; Burns, K.; Benson, S.; Wilson, R.; Loebinger, M.R. The antimicrobial susceptibility of non-tuberculous mycobacteria. *J. Infect.* **2016**, *72*, 324–331. [CrossRef]
146. Kesavalu, L.; Goldstein, J.A.; Debs, R.J.; Düzgünes, N.; Gangadharam, P.R. Differential effects of free and liposome encapsulated amikacin on the survival of *Mycobacterium avium* complex in mouse peritoneal macrophages. *Tubercle* **1990**, *71*, 215–217. [CrossRef]
147. Olivier, K.N.; Shaw, P.A.; Glaser, T.S.; Bhattacharyya, D.; Fleshner, M.; Brewer, C.C.; Zalewski, C.K.; Folio, L.R.; Siegelman, J.R.; Shallom, S.; et al. Inhaled amikacin for treatment of refractory pulmonary nontuberculous mycobacterial disease. *Ann. Am. Thorac. Soc.* **2014**, *11*, 30–35. [CrossRef]
148. Meers, P.; Neville, M.; Malinin, V.; Scotto, A.W.; Sardaryan, G.; Kurumunda, R.; Mackinson, C.; James, G.; Fisher, S.; Perkins, W.R. Biofilm penetration, triggered release and in vivo activity of inhaled liposomal amikacin in chronic *Pseudomonas aeruginosa* lung infections. *J. Antimicrob. Chemother.* **2008**, *61*, 859–868. [CrossRef]
149. Zhang, J.; Leifer, F.; Rose, S.; Chun, D.Y.; Thaisz, J.; Herr, T.; Nashed, M.; Joseph, J.; Perkins, W.R.; DiPetrillo, K. Amikacin Liposome Inhalation Suspension (ALIS) Penetrates Non-tuberculous Mycobacterial Biofilms and Enhances Amikacin Uptake Into Macrophages. *Front. Microbiol.* **2018**, *9*, 915. [CrossRef] [PubMed]
150. Malinin, V.; Neville, M.; Eagle, G.; Gupta, R.; Perkins, W.R. Pulmonary Deposition and Elimination of Liposomal Amikacin for Inhalation and Effect on Macrophage Function after Administration in Rats. *Antimicrob. Agents Chemother.* **2016**, *60*, 6540–6549. [CrossRef] [PubMed]
151. Li, Z.; Perkins, W.; Cipolla, D. Robustness of aerosol delivery of amikacin liposome inhalation suspension using the eFlow® Technology. *Eur. J. Pharm. Biopharm.* **2021**, *166*, 10–18. [CrossRef] [PubMed]
152. Li, Z.; Zhang, Y.; Wurtz, W.; Lee, J.K.; Malinin, V.S.; Durwas-Krishnan, S.; Meers, P.; Perkins, W.R. Characterization of Nebulized Liposomal Amikacin (Arikace™) as a Function of Droplet Size. *J. Aerosol Med. Pulm. Drug Deliv.* **2008**, *21*, 245–254. [CrossRef]
153. Olivier, K.N.; Maas-Moreno, R.; Whatley, M.; Cheng, K.; Lee, J.H.; Fiorentino, C.; Shaffer, R.; Macdonald, S.; Gupta, R.; Corcoran, T.E.; et al. Airway Deposition and Retention of Liposomal Amikacin for Inhalation in Patients with Pulmonary Nontuberculous Mycobacterial Disease. *Am. J. Respir. Crit. Care Med.* **2016**, *193*, A3732. Available online: https://www.atsjournals.org/doi/abs/10.1164/ajrccm-conference.2016.193.1_MeetingAbstracts.A3732 (accessed on 12 December 2021).
154. Weers, J.; Metzheiser, B.; Taylor, G.; Warren, S.; Meers, P.; Perkins, W.R. A gamma scintigraphy study to investigate lung deposition and clearance of inhaled amikacin-loaded liposomes in healthy male volunteers. *J. Aerosol Med. Pulm. Drug Deliv.* **2009**, *22*, 131–138. [CrossRef]
155. Griffith, D.E.; Eagle, G.; Thomson, R.; Aksamit, T.R.; Hasegawa, N.; Morimoto, K.; Addrizzo-Harris, D.J.; O'Donnell, A.E.; Marras, T.K.; Flume, P.A.; et al. Amikacin Liposome Inhalation Suspension for Treatment-Refractory Lung Disease Caused by *Mycobacterium avium* Complex (CONVERT). A Prospective, Open-Label, Randomized Study. *Am. J. Respir. Crit. Care Med.* **2018**, *198*, 1559–1569. [CrossRef]
156. Rose, S.J.; Neville, M.E.; Gupta, R.; Bermudez, L.E. Delivery of aerosolized liposomal amikacin as a novel approach for the treatment of nontuberculous mycobacteria in an experimental model of pulmonary infection. *PLoS ONE* **2014**, *9*, e108703. [CrossRef]
157. Olivier, K.N.; Griffith, D.E.; Eagle, G.; McGinnis, J.P., 2nd; Micioni, L.; Liu, K.; Daley, C.L.; Winthrop, K.L.; Ruoss, S.; Addrizzo-Harris, D.J.; et al. Randomized Trial of Liposomal Amikacin for Inhalation in Nontuberculous Mycobacterial Lung Disease. *Am. J. Respir. Crit. Care Med.* **2017**, *195*, 814–823. [CrossRef]
158. Griffith, D.E.; Thomson, R.; Flume, P.A.; Aksamit, T.R.; Field, S.K.; Addrizzo-Harris, D.J.; Morimoto, K.; Hoefsloot, W.; Mange, K.C.; Yuen, D.W.; et al. Amikacin Liposome Inhalation Suspension for Refractory Mycobacterium avium Complex Lung Disease: Sustainability and Durability of Culture Conversion and Safety of Long-term Exposure. *Chest* **2021**, *160*, 831–842. [CrossRef]
159. Winthrop, K.L.; Flume, P.A.; Thomson, R.; Mange, K.C.; Yuen, D.W.; Ciesielska, M.; Morimoto, K.; Ruoss, S.J.; Codecasa, L.R.; Yim, J.-J.; et al. Amikacin Liposome Inhalation Suspension for Mycobacterium avium Complex Lung Disease: A 12-Month Open-Label Extension Clinical Trial. *Ann. Am. Thorac. Soc.* **2021**, *18*, 1147–1157. [CrossRef] [PubMed]
160. Arikayce® (Amikacin Liposome Inhalation Suspension), for Oral Inhalation Use [Package Insert]. Insmed Incorporated: Bridgewater, NJ, USA. Available online: https://www.arikayce.com/pdf/full_prescribing_information.pdf (accessed on 12 December 2021).

pharmaceutics

MDPI

Article

Quantitative Structure-Activity Relationship of Enhancers of Licochalcone A and Glabridin Release and Permeation Enhancement from Carbomer Hydrogel

Zhuxian Wang †, Yaqi Xue †, Zhaoming Zhu, Yi Hu, Quanfu Zeng, Yufan Wu, Yuan Wang, Chunyan Shen, Cuiping Jiang, Li Liu, Hongxia Zhu * and Qiang Liu *

School of Traditional Chinese Medicine, Southern Medical University, Guangzhou 510515, China; wangzhuxian88@smu.edu.cn (Z.W.); xyq1997@smu.edu.cn (Y.X.); zmnf1988@smu.edu.cn (Z.Z.); huyi12110357@smu.edu.cn (Y.H.); 22020286@smu.edu.cn (Q.Z.); 3161008010@smu.edu.cn (Y.W.); 521wl@smu.edu.cn (Y.W.); shenchunyan@smu.edu.cn (C.S.); jxiaqing126@smu.edu.cn (C.J.); 3188010173@i.smu.edu.cn (L.L.)

* Correspondence: zhuhon@smu.edu.cn (H.Z.); liuqiang@smu.edu.cn (Q.L.); Tel.: + 86-20-6278-9408 (H.Z.); + 86-20-6164-8264 (Q.L.)

† These authors contributed equally to this work.

Abstract: This study aimed to systematically compare licochalcone A (LicA) and glabridin (Gla) (whitening agents) release and permeation from Carbomer 940 (CP) hydrogels with different enhancers, and evaluate the relationship between the quantitative enhancement efficacy and structures of the enhancers. An in vitro release study and an in vitro permeation experiment in solution and hydrogels using porcine skin were performed. We found that the Gla–CP hydrogel showed a higher drug release and skin retention amount than LicA–CP due to the higher solubility in medium and better miscibility with the skin of Gla than that of LicA. Enhancers with a higher molecular weight (MW) and lower polarizability showed a higher release enhancement effect ($ER_{release}$) for both LicA and Gla. The Van der Waals forces in the drug–enhancers–CP system were negatively correlated with the drug release percent. Moreover, enhancers with a higher log P and polarizability displayed a higher retention enhancement effect in solution ($ER_{solution\ retention}$) for LicA and Gla. Enhancers decreased the whole intermolecular forces indrug–enhancers-skin system, which had a linear inhibitory effect on the drug retention. Moreover, C=O of ceramide acted asthe enhancement site for drug permeation. Consequently, Transcutol® P (TP) and propylene glycol (PG), seven enhancers showed a higher retention enhancement effect in hydrogel ($ER_{hydrogel\ retention}$) for LicA and Gla. Taken together, the conclusions provide a strategy for reasonable utilization of enhancers and formulation optimization in topical hydrogel whitening.

Keywords: carbomer hydrogel; whitening agents; enhancers; enhancement site and mechanism; drug release and permeation

Citation: Wang, Z.; Xue, Y.; Zhu, Z.; Hu, Y.; Zeng, Q.; Wu, Y.; Wang, Y.; Shen, C.; Jiang, C.; Liu, L.; et al. Quantitative Structure-Activity Relationship of Enhancers of Licochalcone A and Glabridin Release and Permeation Enhancement from Carbomer Hydrogel. *Pharmaceutics* **2022**, *14*, 262. https://doi.org/10.3390/pharmaceutics14020262

Academic Editors: Giovanna Rassu and Thierry Vandamme

Received: 24 December 2021
Accepted: 19 January 2022
Published: 22 January 2022

1. Introduction

Hydrogels are used extensively in topical and transdermal drug delivery systems, among which carbomer polymers account for a significant proportion. Carbomer 940 (CP) is used in cosmetic formulation benefitting due to its moderate viscosity and good stability [1]. Drug permeation from hydrogel consists of two processes: the first is drug release from the carbomer matrix and the second is skin permeation. Previous literature has described drug–polymers interaction (mainly H–H bond interaction and Van der Waals forces) [2,3], in which the rheological properties, including the viscosity, storage modulus (G'), loss modulus (G''), and phase shift angle (δ) [4], hydration [5], and mesh size [6] of the hydrogels influence drug release. However, the most critical aspects hindering drug permeation are caused by the highly compact structure of the *Stratum corneum* (SC), which limits the efficient delivery of active pharmaceutical ingredients [7,8]. Therefore, a wide range of permeation enhancers are utilized to improve drug release or penetration from the hydrogel system.

Permeation enhancers can enhance drug release from complicated hydrogel systems by reducing the molecular mobility of the systems [9], occupying drug–polymer binding sites [3], etc. Song concluded that permeation enhancers that form hydrogen bonds, such as Span 80 (SP), weaken drug–adhesive interaction, facilitating the release of drug from adhesive [10]. On the other hand, permeation enhancers disrupt the skin lipid arrangement [11,12], change the keratin structure [13], enhance the miscibility of the skin [14], and increase drug partitioning into deeper skin layers [15] to improve the skin permeation of drugs. Plurol® Oleique CC 497 (POCC) showed a preference for occupying sites where skin lipids had interacted with drugs with low PSA and polarizability due to the improved skin–POCC miscibility and stronger interactions [16]. Thus, the physicochemical properties, such as the molecular weight (MW), log P, polar surface area, and polarizability of the enhancers, determine differences in the enhancement effect. Yang systematically evaluated the enhancement action efficacy and sites of different enhancers on drug release and permeation from a patch. It was found that hydrophilic enhancers including Transcutol® P (TP) and propylene glycol (PG) had a better miscibility with matrix carboxyl PSA, indicating their ability to facilitate a higher drug release. In contrast, hydrophobic enhancers including POCC and SP linked with SC lipids more easily, disrupting the lipid arrangement, and thereby improving drug permeation [17]. As a result, demonstrating the molecular interaction of drug–enhancers–CP and drug–enhancers–skin systems is significant, thus shedding new light on the reasonable utilization of enhancers in pharmaceutical and cosmetic preparations.

Licochalcone A (LicA) [18] and glabridin (Gla) [19], flavonoid compounds extracted from the roots of *Glycyrrhiza glabra* L., both have significant anti-melanogenic effects on cellular and animal levels as we previously revealed. However, the poor water solubility and higher log P hinders their transdermal permeation when applied alone, which further influences their practical use. Moreover, it was more difficult for parent LicA to permeate the skin than Gla due to its poorer water solubility and higher log P. Thus, the addition of enhancers represents an effective way to overcome these drawbacks and improve the drug absorption of the two whitening agents. It is expected that higher amounts of Gla and LicA accumulate in the epidermis and dermis rather than in the systemic circulation as melanocytes are located in the basal epidermal layers. The enhancers should firstly accomplish maximum release of the whitening agent from the matrix polymer. Consequently, the ideal enhancers must contribute to the two processes simultaneously. However, to our knowledge, few studies have focused on whitening agents' release and skin delivery behaviors from CP hydrogel based on drug–enhancers–CP (skin) interactions, which has resulted in blindness and uncertainty regarding the utilization of enhancers in whitening formula optimization. Meanwhile, no investigations have systematically compared the enhancing effect of Gla and LicA by different enhancers.

Therefore, for the first time, this study systematically reported the quantitative enhancement efficacy and site of action explaining the drug release and skin absorption of LicA and Gla (whitening agents) from CP hydrogel by different enhancers (Figure 1). Seven enhancers, including POCC, TP, PG, SP, Capryol™ 90 (CP 90), N-methylprolinodone (NMP),and isopropyl myristate (IPM) with different physicochemical parameters (Table 1), were selected. Firstly, Gla–CP and LicA–CP hydrogels with or without enhancers were prepared. The drug release behavior from different CP hydrogels was evaluated by an in vitro drug release experiment. The drug release enhancement effect ($ER_{release}$) and interaction parameters of Gla (LicA)–CP and Gla (LicA)–enhancers–CP hydrogels were demonstrated next. Then, the porcine skin was used to evaluate the enhanced retention and permeation effect of Gla and LicA in solution ($ER_{solution\ retention}$, $ER_{permeation}$) and hydrogel ($ER_{hydrogel\ retention}$, ER_{com}) by enhancers, followed by the enhancement site and mechanisms involved in it. In addition, the correlation between the drug release amount, drug permeation amount, drug retention amount and physicochemical parameters of the enhancers (Table 1), energy of mixing (E_{mix}), and cohesive energy density (CED) were investigated, respectively. These results provide insight into the drug–enhancers–CP and drug–enhancers–skin interactions and the structural characteristics of enhancers, which lays a solid basis for the drug-specific molecular mechanisms of enhancers and pharmaceutical hydrogel design. Moreover, it predicted information for the topical application of enhancers with specific structures for high drug release and skin retention of whitening formulation.

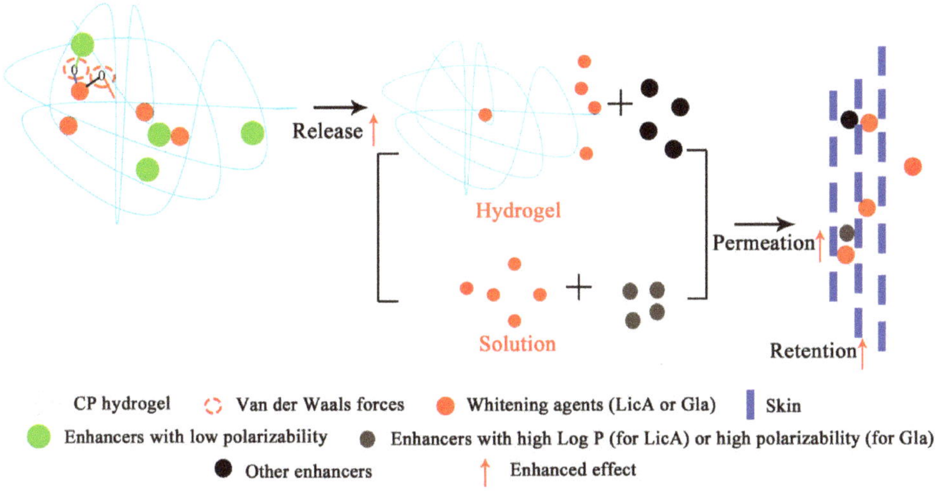

Figure 1. Schematic showing Gla and LicA release and permeation from CP hydrogel with enhancers.

Table 1. The physicochemical parameters of different drugs and enhancers.

Drug/Enhancers	Molecular Weight (Da)	Log P	Solubility in 20% PEG400 (*v*/*v*, µg/mL)	H Bond Donor	H Bond Acceptor	Polarizability	Polar Surface Area (Å)
LicA	338.40	4.95	25.15	2	4	39.8	66.8
Gla	324.40	4.26	121.47	2	4	36.1	58.9
CP 90	203.30	4.97	-	-	-	33.5	47.0
IPM	270.40	4.61	-	-	-	32.7	26.0
NMP	99.10	−0.38	-	-	-	10.6	20.0
PG	76.09	−0.90	-	-	-	7.52	40.5
POCC	726.90	6.21	-	-	-	74.8	269.0
SP	428.60	6.06	-	-	-	47.3	96.0
TP	134.20	−1.08	-	-	-	13.8	39.0

2. Materials and Methods

2.1. Material

Licochalcone A (LicA, purity >98%) and glabridin (Gla, purity >98%) were obtained from Nanjing Spring & Autumn Biological Engineering Co., Ltd. (Nanjing, China). Poly(acrylic acid) (commercial names: Carbomer 940 (CP)), isopropyl myristate (IPM, purity: 98%), diethylene glycol monoethyl ether (commercial names: Transcutol® P (TP), purity: 99%), and 1-methyl-2-pyrrolidinone (NMP, purity >99%) were purchased from Shanghai Macklin Biochemical Co., Ltd. (Shanghai, China). Propylene glycol monocaprylate (commercial names: Capryol™ 90 (CP 90)) and polyglyceryl-3dioleate (commercial names: Plurol® Oleique CC 497 (POCC)) were supplied by Gattefossé (Lyon, France). Polyoxyethylenesorbitan monooleate (commercial names: Span 80 (SP)) and propylene glycol (PG, purity > 99%)

were purchased from Damao Chemical Reagent Factory (Tianjin, China). Polyethylene glycol 400 (PEG 400) and cellophane membranes were purchased from Beijing Solarbio Technology Co., Ltd., Beijing, China. All other reagents were analytical grade.

2.2. Preparation of Hydrogels

The LicA–CP and Gla–CP hydrogels (cargo loading: 5%, *w/w*) were prepared as follows: First, 2 g of CP were dispersed in 100 mL of deionized water and stored at room temperature for 24 h to fully swell the hydrogels. Subsequently, LicA and Gla dissolved in ethanol were added to the CP hydrogels, and the mixture was stirred until it was homogeneous. The pH was to 5 with NaOH solution. Hydrogels with enhancers (drug–enhancers–CP) (cargo loading: 10%, *w/w*) were also fabricated using the same methods. Hydrogels were stored at 4 °C and hydrogel films were prepared using the freeze-dried technique.

2.3. Rheological Properties of Hydrogel

The rheological tests were performed in a MARS iQ Air + P35 rheometer (Thermo Scientific HAAKE, New York, NY, USA).The flow properties of the CP, LicA–CP, and Gla–CP hydrogels were obtained from continuous shear flow tests with shear rates ranging from 0–120 s^{-1} for 120 s. Continuous ramp step were selected for analysis. The elastic and viscous modulus at different frequencies was measured using frequency sweep tests ranging from 0.1 to 100 with a constant %strain of 0.1. The G', G'', and δ values were recorded and the frequency was plotted in a logarithmic scale.

2.4. Determination of the Drug Solubility in the Donor Phase

Briefly, excessive Gla or LicA was added to the PBS/PEG400 (*v/v*, 80/20) and subjected to ultrasound for 30 min at 25 °C. Subsequently, the supernatant of the solution was taken out and filtered with a 0.22 μm microporous membrane for HPLC analysis. The detailed HPLC methods are shown in Methods S1.

2.5. In Vitro Release of Hydrogels

The hydrogels (0.3 g) were added to the cellophane membranes, which were then fixed between the donor and the receptor cells of the Franz diffusion cells (effective diffusional area: 1.77 cm^2; volume: 15 mL; TP-6, China). PBS (pH = 7.4) containing 20% PEG 400 (*v/v*) was chosen as the acceptor medium and stirred at 350 rpm and 32 °C. In total, 1.0 mL of sample was withdrawn after 0.25, 0.5, 1, 2, 3, 4, 6, 8, 10, 12, 24, 36, and 48 h and then replaced by the same volume of fresh medium. The samples were analyzed using HPLC (Agilent 1260, Santa Clara, CA, USA). The detailed HPLC methods are provided in Methods S1.

$R_{hydrogel}$ and $Q_{hydrogel}$ represent the cumulative release percent of drug (%) and cumulative release amount of drug, respectively. The enhancement ratio of drug release in hydrogel ($ER_{release}$) was calculated as follows:

$$ER_{release} = \frac{R_{hydrogel\ with\ enhancer}}{R_{hydrogel\ without\ enhancer}} \quad (1)$$

2.6. Mechanism of Enhancement Drug Release

2.6.1. Attenuated Total Reflection FT-IR (ATR-FT-IR) of the CP Hydrogels

The ATR-FT-IR study was used to confirm the effect of the enhancers on the drug release of the CP systems. The hydrogel films were obtained from the preparation of hydrogels, and the infrared spectra were recorded using a Nicolet iS50 FT-IR spectrometer (Thermos, New York, NY, USA) within the frequency range of 500–4000 cm^{-1} using 32 scans at a resolution of 2.

2.6.2. Raman Spectroscopy

Raman spectra were also used to characterize the potential interactions among the drug, enhancers, and CP by a Raman spectrometer (Renishaw RM2000, London, England). Then, the samples were measured at 25 °C using a 785 nm laser source with 500 mW power.

2.6.3. X-ray Diffraction (XRD)

The proportion of crystalline in different hydrogels was determined by diffracted intensity measurement using an X-ray diffractometer (SmartLab 3KW, Rigaku, Japan) of Cu Kα radiation in the 5–60° 2θ range with a scan rate of 10°/min.

2.6.4. Polarized Light Microscopy (PLM)

PLM measurement was conducted to confirm the results of XRD using a Nikon polarized optical microscope (edipse lv100N pol, Tokyo, Japan). The images were captured using QImaging software (Nis-Elements F) with a first-order compensator at 100× magnification.

2.6.5. Differential Scanning Calorimetry (DSC)

The hydrogel films were placed in the aluminum DSC pans of a thermal analyzer (TA Q2000, TA, New Castle, Lindon, UT, USA), and then heated from 25–250 °C at a rate of 10 °C/min with 3 cycles (to eliminate the thermal history). All samples were performed under a nitrogen atmosphere (40 mL/min). The parameter glass transition temperature (T_g) was recorded at the midpoint of the transition in the curve.

2.6.6. Molecular Interaction Study: Molecular Docking

Molecular docking was conducted to corroborate the results of FT-IR to calculate the intermolecular strength of the Gla (LicA)–CP and Gla (LicA)–enhancers–CP systems using Materials Studio version 8.0 (Accelrys, San Diego, CA, USA). The molecular structures of the CP, Gla, LicA, and seven kinds of enhancers were obtained from the PubChem database and subjected to geometry optimization with Forcite modules in the COMPASS II force field. Next, the mixing energy (E_{mix}) and interaction parameters (χ) were calculated. In addition, the optimized structure of the Gla (LicA)–CP and Gla (LicA)–enhancers–CP associations were obtained.

2.6.7. Molecular Dynamic Simulation

Molecular dynamic simulation was utilized to understand the drug release behaviors of different hydrogels with or without enhancers. The optimized CP, Gla (LicA), and enhancers were placed in the amorphous cell modules according to the proportions of the actual formulation, and the built systems were further optimized by For cite modules. Subsequently, NVT equilibration of 50 ps at 298 K was conducted for each system, after which NPT equilibration of 100 ps was performed at 305 K and 101.325 Kpa with a time step of 1 ps. The CED was calculated for each system. Then, snapshots of the hydrogel systems at the end of the MD were obtained.

2.7. Correlation Analysis 1

First, a linear regression analysis was conducted to investigate the relationship between the drug release amount and physicochemical parameters, including MW, log P, polarizability, and polar surface area, in different hydrogels using SPSS 20.0 software (SPSS, Chicago, IL, USA). On the other hand, the linear regression equation of the drug release amount and E_{mix} and CED were calculated.

2.8. In Vitro Skin Permeation of Drug Solution and Hydrogel

Porcine skin (one-month-old Bama miniature pig, male, 20 kg) was supplied by Aperture Biotech Co., Ltd. (Hong Kong, China) The thickness of porcine skin was maintained at approximately 800 μm and its structural integrity was guaranteed before the experiments. The porcine skin sample was sandwiched between the donors and receptors compartment in Franz diffusion cells with the dermal side facing downwards. Then, different drug aqueous solutions (0.3 g) and 0.3 g of the corresponding hydrogels were added to the donor receptors, and PBS/PEG400 (*v/v*, 80/20) was chosen as the medium to obtain sink conditions. In total, 1 mL of receptor vehicle was withdrawn after1, 2, 4, 6, 8, 10, 12, 24, 36, and 48 h. Others were processed similar to the in vitro release of the hydrogel. All animal experiments were performed in accordance with the "Guiding Principles in the Care and Use of Animals" (China), and approved by the Ethics Committee of Southern Medical University (L2019036, date of approval: 13 April 2019).

$P_{solution}$ and $P_{hydrogel}$ represent the cumulative permeation in the solution and hydrogel, respectively.

The enhancement ratio of the drug skin permeation in the drug solution ($ER_{permeation}$) was calculated as follows:

$$ER_{permeation} = \frac{P_{solution\ with\ enhancer}}{P_{solution\ without\ enhancer}} \quad (2)$$

The enhancement ratio of the drug skin permeation in hydrogel (ER_{com}) was calculated as follows:

$$ER_{com} = \frac{P_{hydrogel\ with\ enhancer}}{P_{hydrogel\ without\ enhancer}} \quad (3)$$

$\beta_{R/P}$ was calculated to evaluate the sites of action of the enhancers [17]:

$$\beta_{R/P} = \frac{ER_{release}}{ER_{permeation}} \quad (4)$$

The rate-limiting step of transdermal drug delivery was assessed using the following equation:

$$F = \frac{P_{hydrogel}}{Q_{hydrogel}} \quad (5)$$

2.9. Drug Retention

After in vitro skin permeation, the treated skin samples were removed from the diffusion cell. Subsequently, the skin at the administration site was wiped to remove the unabsorbed drug, cut into pieces, weighed, and extracted with methanol by ultrasound for 1 h. Then, the supernatant was detected with HPLC to obtain the skin retention amount.

$RE_{solution}$ and $RE_{hydrogel}$ are the cumulative retention amount of drug in the solution and hydrogel, respectively.

The enhancement ratio of the drug skin retention in solution ($ER_{solution\ retention}$) was calculated as follows:

$$ER_{solution\ retention} = \frac{RE_{solution\ with\ enhancer}}{RE_{solution\ without\ enhancer}} \quad (6)$$

The enhancement ratio of the drug skin retention in hydrogel ($ER_{hydrogel\ retention}$) was calculated as follows:

$$ER_{hydrogel\ retention} = \frac{RE_{hydrogel\ with\ enhancer}}{RE_{hydrogel\ without\ enhancer}} \quad (7)$$

2.10. Mechanism of Enhancement Drug Permeation

2.10.1. ATR-FT-IR Spectra of the Porcine Skin

The ATR-FT-IR study was used to investigate the effect of the enhancers on the arrangement variations of the skin lipid and protein region. The skin samples were taken from the in vitro skin permeation of drug solution, and the infrared spectra were recorded as described in Section 2.6.1.

2.10.2. Confocal Laser Microscope (CLSM)

CLSM was used to visualize the LicA and Gla distribution in the skin tissue, and C6 was utilized as a substitute for Gla. Treated skin samples were processed similar to the in vitro skin permeation of drug solution with a permeation time of8 h. The samples were cut longitudinally into 6-μm-thick slices using a Cryostat microtome (Thermo HM525 NX, New York, NY, USA) after fixation. LicA and C6 were emitted at 480 and 485 nm using a confocal laser microscope (CLSM 800, ZEISS, Jena, Germany), respectively.

2.10.3. Molecular Docking and Molecular Dynamic Simulation

Ceramide 2 was used as are presentative of skin lipids for molecular docking and molecular dynamic simulation due to it having the highest proportion in skin lipids [14,20]. The E_{mix}, χ, and CED of Gla (LicA)-skin and Gla (LicA)–enhancers-skin systems and their snapshots were obtained as described.

2.11. Correlation Analysis 2

A multiple linear regression model was also used to detect the correlation between the drug retention, drug permeation amount, and physicochemical parameters of the enhancers as described before. Moreover, the relationships between the drug retention or drug permeation amount and C=O band displacement value in the FT-IR, E_{mix}, and CED were calculated.

2.12. Statistical Analysis

All data were analyzed using SPSS 20.0 software (Chicago, IL, USA). Data were expressed as mean ± SD and subjected to one-way analysis of variance (ANOVA) or two-tailed paired Student's *t*-test. The significance level was set at $p < 0.05$.

3. Results

3.1. Preparation of the CP–Gla and CP–LicA Hydrogel

Lyophilized hydrogels were prepared to investigate the potential interaction between the drugs and CP. First, XRD (Figure 2a) and PLM analyses (Figure 2b) were used to detect the crystals in the hydrogel films, and the results demonstrated that both Gla and LicA almost completely dissolved in the CP hydrogel without the formation of obvious crystals. Moreover, LicA and Gla displayed a similar miscibility to CP. These results indicate that Gla and LicA were molecularly dispersed in the hydrogel, which laid a foundation for the hydrogen bond or the formation of other interactions [21]. The hydroxyl (−OH) and carbonyl group (C=O) of Gla and LicA, and the carboxyl (−COOH) group of CP are the functional groups that may potentially be involved in the drug–CP interaction. In the blank CP, the characteristic band at 2934.05 cm^{-1} was assigned to -OH stretching vibration while the band at 1695.27cm^{-1} was attributed to C=O stretching of the CP (Figure 2c). The band at 2934.05 cm^{-1} shifted to 2933.31 and 2934.24 cm^{-1}, and the C=O band moved to 1696.69 and 1696.22 cm^{-1} for Gla-CP and LicA-CP, respectively, indicating weak interaction in the drug–CP systems. Furthermore, the Gla–CP system showed a stronger interaction strength than LicA-CP. The Raman spectra (Figure 2d) also confirmed the presence of the interaction due to the movement of the −OH band. The values of E_{mix} and χ measured using molecular docking are used to estimate the strength of the intermolecular interactions. The closer E_{mix} and χ are to 0, the greater the miscibility and the stronger the intermolecular interactions. In this case, the Gla–CP system possessed a lower E_{mix} and χ than LicA–CP, further underscoring the stronger interaction between Gla and CP (Table 2). The optimized structures of the Gla (LicA)–CP binary associations are displayed in Figure 2e.

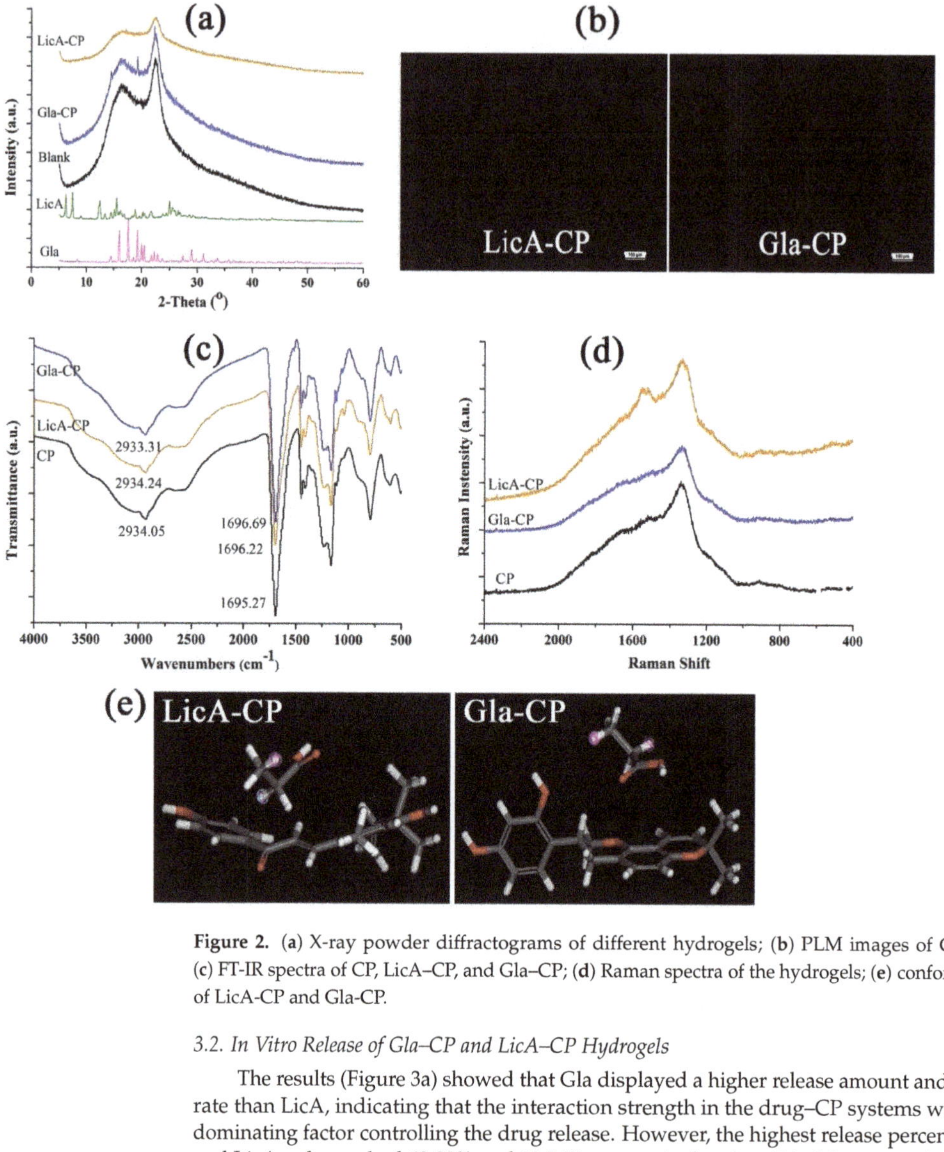

Figure 2. (**a**) X-ray powder diffractograms of different hydrogels; (**b**) PLM images of CP films; (**c**) FT-IR spectra of CP, LicA–CP, and Gla–CP; (**d**) Raman spectra of the hydrogels; (**e**) conformations of LicA-CP and Gla-CP.

3.2. In Vitro Release of Gla–CP and LicA–CP Hydrogels

The results (Figure 3a) showed that Gla displayed a higher release amount and release rate than LicA, indicating that the interaction strength in the drug–CP systems was not a dominating factor controlling the drug release. However, the highest release percent of Gla and LicA only reached 69.08% and 43.56%, respectively, after 48 h. Moreover, the release behaviors of Gla and LicA from CP hydrogel followed the zero-order equation, and the release equations of the release amount percent and time are listed as follows:

$$R_{hydrogel}\ (LicA) = 1.01 \times t + 0.20\ (R^2 = 0.97) \quad (8)$$

$$R_{hydrogel}\ (Gla) = 1.61 \times t + 0.70\ (R^2 = 0.95) \quad (9)$$

Table 2. The E_{mix}, χ, and CED of different Gla (LicA)–enhancers–CP systems.

	χ (kcal/mol)	E_{mix} (kcal/mol)	CED (kcal/mol)
LicA-CP	20.52	12.15	-
Gla-CP	13.00	7.70	-
LicA-CP 90-CP	6.97	4.13	2.57×10^9
LicA-IPM-CP	6.56	3.89	2.38×10^9
LicA-NMP-CP	10.87	6.44	2.21×10^9
LicA-PG-CP	19.48	11.54	2.15×10^9
LicA-POCC-CP	−7.15	−4.23	2.40×10^9
LicA-SP-CP	−1.77	−1.05	2.34×10^9
LicA-TP-CP	9.35	5.54	2.40×10^9
Gla-CP 90-CP	2.45	1.45	2.60×10^9
Gla-IPM-CP	3.01	1.78	2.64×10^9
Gla-NMP-CP	6.50	3.85	2.33×10^9
Gla-PG-CP	8.85	5.24	2.36×10^9
Gla-POCC-CP	2.57	1.52	2.68×10^9
Gla-SP-CP	6.37	3.77	2.38×10^9
Gla-TP-CP	6.34	3.76	2.43×10^9

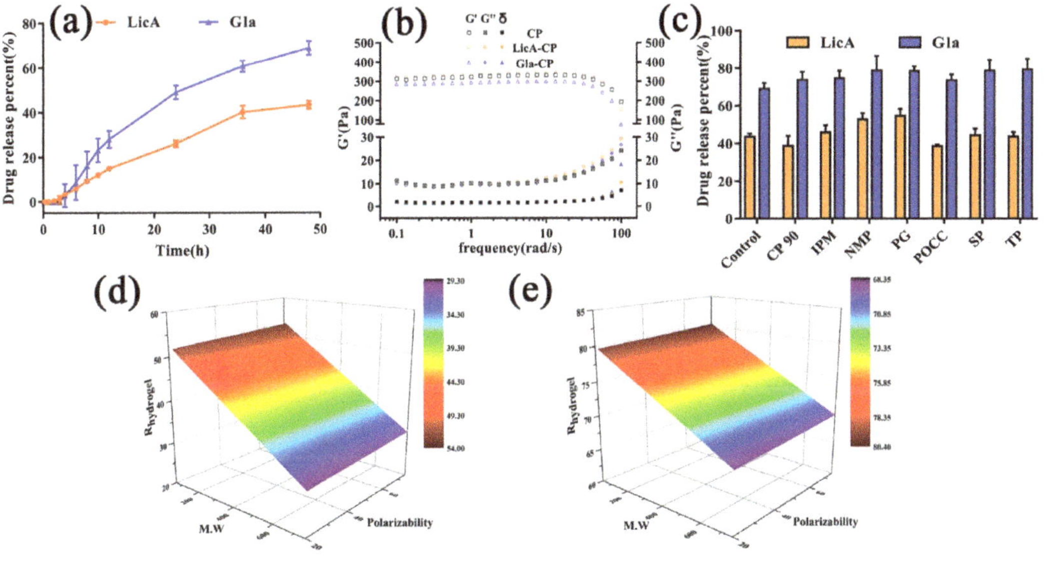

Figure 3. (**a**) In vitro drug release profiles of hydrogel (n = 3); (**b**) frequency sweep (G′, G″, and δ) of the hydrogel (n = 3); (**c**) LicA and Gla release percent after48 h after different enhancers were added (n = 3); (**d**) response surface plot demonstrating the effect of MW and polarizability on the ERrelease of LicA; (**e**) response surface plot demonstrating the effect of MW and polarizability on the $ER_{release}$ of Gla.

To demonstrate the influencing effect on the drug release, DSC study reflecting the free volume and mesh size of the hydrogels was carried out. The results (Figure S1a) demonstrated that Gla–CP showed a similar T_g to LicA–CP, which is indicative of a slight effect of the mesh size on the drug release. In addition, G′ represents the rigidity of hydrogels [22,23], and G″ is a parameter used to demonstrate the friction of a molecular chain and reflect changes in the intermolecular interaction [24]. The rheological study (Figures 3b and S1b) revealed that the zero-shear viscosity, G′, G″, and δ of Gla–CP all showed no significant difference to that of LicA–CP, indicating that the viscoelastic properties of the hydrogel also had no significant influence on the drug release.

3.3. In Vitro Release of Drug in the Presence of Enhancers

To improve the drug release from the hydrogels, different enhancers were added to hydrogels and in vitro release experiments were performed (Figure S1c,d). We found that only PG (highest $ER_{release}$: 1.25) and NMP significantly increased the LicA release percent while TP (highest $ER_{release}$: 1.15), POCC, SP, and IPM all contributed to a significantly higher Gla release percent (Figure 3c and Table 3) after 48 h. Then, multivariate linear regression analysis was conducted to investigate the effect of the physicochemical parameters of the enhancers on $R_{hydrogel}$. The regression equations areexpressed as follows:

$$R_{hydrogel}\ (LicA) = 52.87 + 0.057 \times M.W - 0.74 \times Polarizability \quad (10)$$

$$R_{hydrogel}\ (Gla) = 79.76 + 0.03 \times M.W - 0.36 \times Polarizability \quad (11)$$

Table 3. The enhancement efficacy parameters of enhancers in the drug release and skin penetration process.

	$ER_{release}$	$ER_{permeation}$	ER_{com}	$\beta_{R/P}$	$ER_{solution\ retention}$	$ER_{hydrogel\ retention}$	$F_{P/Q}$
LicA-CP 90	0.89	2.72	1.18	0.33	2.70	1.13	0.015
LicA-IPM	1.05	2.91	0.00	0.36	3.30	0.68	0.00
LicA-NMP	1.21	1.08	0.00	1.12	0.54	0.76	0.00
LicA-PG	1.25	0.55	1.10	2.28	1.23	1.82	0.0099
LicA-POCC	0.89	3.09	1.46	0.29	3.28	0.65	0.018
LicA-SP	1.02	2.77	1.12	0.37	3.78	0.99	0.012
LicA-TP	1.00	1.50	1.92	0.67	1.44	1.23	0.022
Gla-CP 90	1.07	2.93	1.40	0.36	2.11	1.39	0.022
Gla-IPM	1.08	1.15	0.86	0.94	1.49	1.51	0.014
Gla-NMP	1.14	2.20	0.78	0.52	1.47	1.28	0.012
Gla-PG	1.11	0.68	1.28	1.63	1.31	1.11	0.020
Gla-POCC	1.06	2.16	2.05	0.49	1.28	1.79	0.033
Gla-SP	1.14	1.15	1.14	0.99	1.04	1.90	0.017
Gla-TP	1.15	1.38	0.72	0.83	1.51	1.14	0.011

The response surface plot (Figure 3d,e) showed that both $R_{hydrogel}$ of Gla and LicA were negatively correlated with the polarizability, and positively correlated with MW of the enhancers. Moreover, the polarizability dominated the drug release. Polarizability represents the ability of Van der Waals forces to form [25], which are the primary interaction forms in drug–enhancers–CP systems. Enhancers with higher polarizability tended to be linked with drug–CP systems, which is a sign of stronger intermolecular interactions forming in the drug–enhancers–CP ternary systems, thereby decreasing the drug release percent. These results prove the interaction strength in drug–enhancers–CP systems was an important factor determining the drug release.

3.4. Molecular Modeling and Correlation Analysis 1

Then, E_{mix} and χ of different Gla (LicA)–enhancers–CP systems were calculated (Table 2) using Materials Studio version 8.0, and their optimized ternary associations are displayed at Figure S2. For LicA–enhancers–CP, LicA–PG–CP hydrogel showed the highest χ (19.48) and E_{mix} (11.54) while LicA–SP–CP showedthe lowest (−1.77 and −1.05). For Gla–enhancers–CP, the Gla–PG–CP system showed the worst miscibility, with χ of 8.85 and E_{mix} of 5.24, whereas POCC showed the best miscibility with Gla–CP. Linear regression of the drug release percent and E_{mix} was performed to clarify the effect of the interaction strength on $R_{hydrogel}$. The linear regression equation of $R_{hydrogel}$ and E_{mix} is as follows:

$$R_{hydrogel}\ (LicA) = 0.92 \times E_{mix} + 42.10\ (R^2 = 0.57) \quad (12)$$

$$R_{hydrogel}\ (Gla) = 1.64 \times E_{mix} + 71.75\ (R^2 = 0.82) \quad (13)$$

The equations (Figure 4a,b) showed that the better the compatibility between the enhancers and drug–CP binary systems, the lower the release amount. These findings are consistent with the above results. To further corroborate the effect of intermolecular forces on the drug release, molecular dynamics simulation was carried out to calculate the CED values to reflect the interactions among the drugs, enhancers, and CP. The results are displayed in Table 2 and snapshots of the hydrogels systems at the end of the MD are shown in Figures 4e and S3. A higher CED value means a stronger interaction [3]. Similarly, linear regression of the drug release percent and CED was also conducted, and the linear regression equations are expressed as follows:

$$R_{hydrogel}\ (LicA) = -42.21 \times CED + 144.75\ (R^2 = 0.85) \quad (14)$$

$$R_{hydrogel}\ (Gla) = -17.01 \times CED + 119.09\ (R^2 = 0.89) \quad (15)$$

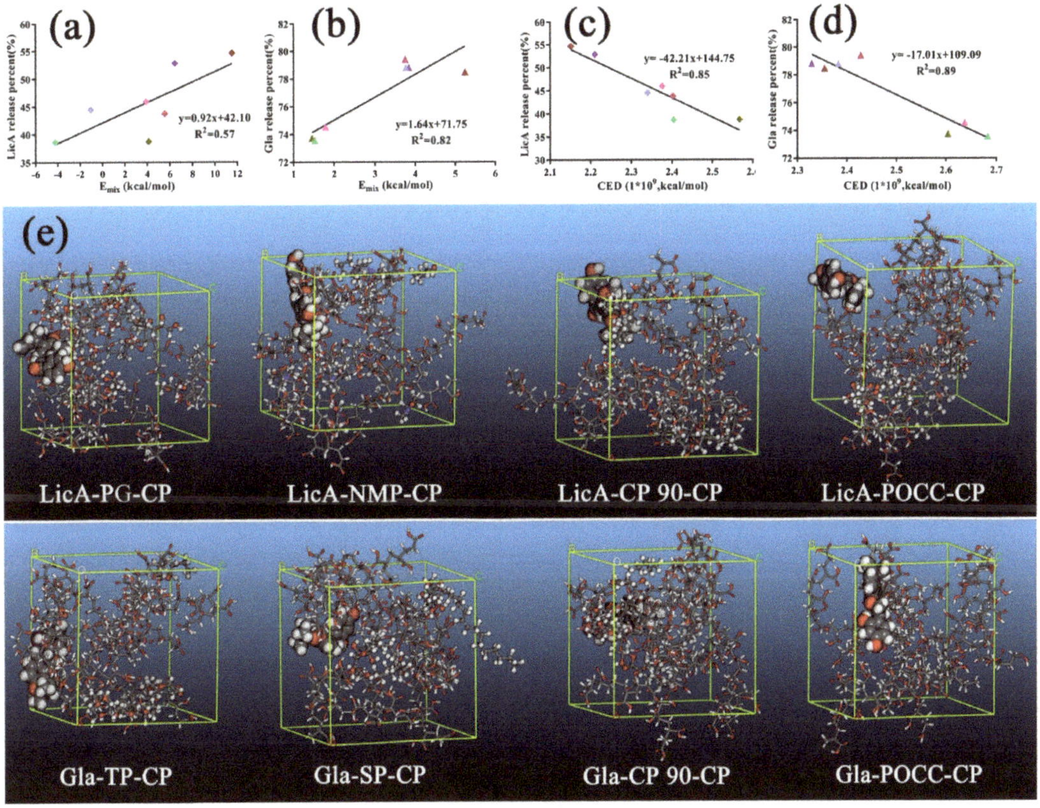

Figure 4. (**a**) The correlation relationship between the LicA release percent and E_{mix} of ternary systems; (**b**) linear analysis of the Gla release percent and E_{mix} of ternary systems; (**c**) the correlation relationship between the LicA release percent and CED of ternary systems; (**d**) linear analysis of the Gla release percent and CED of ternary systems; (**e**) snapshots of the LicA (Gla)–enhancers–CP systems at the end of the MD (drug: ball and stick model; enhancers: CPK model).

The results (Figure 4c,d) further emphasize the decreasing effect of Van der Waals forces on the drug release. The stronger the interaction strength in the compound systems, the lower the drug release percent.

3.5. The Release Mechanism of the Drug from the Drug–Enhancers–CP System

To demonstrate the drug release mechanism of the ternary systems, FT-IR and PLM were conducted. LicA–CP was used as the control group, and CP showed a typical band at 2931.5 cm^{-1} representing the -OH group (Figure 5a,b), while the band at 1696.21 cm^{-1} belonged to the C=O band (Figures S4a and 4b). Upon mixing SP or POCC with CP, the −OH bands showed a red shift to 2925.14 and 2924.66 cm^{-1}, respectively (Figure 5a), attributing to a strong interaction between SP or POCC and CP. However, the position of the −OH band did not show any significant difference when mixing CP 90 or NMP with CP. Moreover, only NMP and POCC induced a weak movement of the C=O band for LicA–CP (Figure S4a). For the Gla–CP binary systems, the bands appearing at 2932.12 and 1696.6 cm^{-1} also represented the −OH and C=O groups, respectively. The addition of SP or POCC also led to significant movement of the−OH band (Figure 5b), which was similar to LicA–CP. In contrast, upon loading with NMP and IPM, the −OH band showed no significant difference with the control group. The bands of the C=O groups did not show significant movement except for the addition of NMP (Figure S4b). The results revealed that the -OH of CP was not the enhancement site for LicA and Gla release.

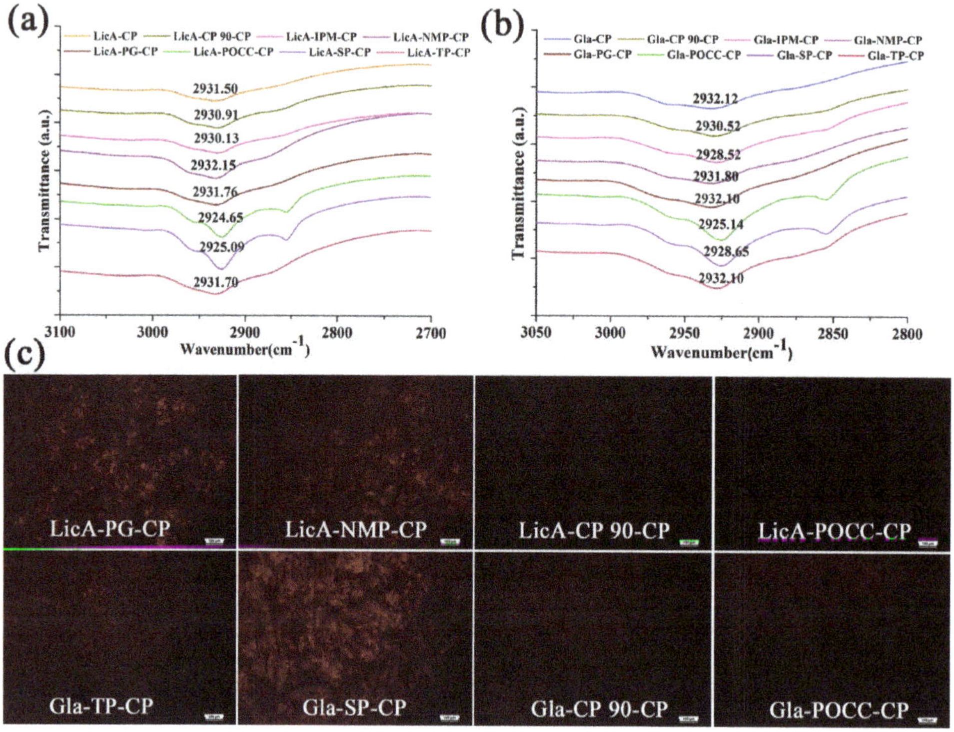

Figure 5. (**a**) FT-IR spectra (−OH group) of LicA–enhancers–CP systems; (**b**) FT-IR spectra (−OH group) of Gla–enhancers–CP systems; (**c**) PLM images of drug–CP films after different enhancers were added.

PLM was used to observe the re-crystallization of the drug after the addition of enhancers. Higher drug re-crystallization indicates weaker enhancers–CP interactions and a better drug release ability. After mixing with SP, CP 90, IPM, NMP, or POCC, no significant LicA crystals were detected in the drug–enhancers–CP films (Figures 5c and S4c). However, a significantly larger amount of LicA crystals were observed in the film system after PG or

NMP addition. These results indicated that the enhancers, such as PG or NMP, occupied the LicA–CP binding site, enabling LicA release from the hydrogel. For the Gla–CP system, upon adding NMP, PG, SP, or TP, a significantly larger amount of Gla crystals appeared in the hydrogel film. In contrast, IPM, CP 90, and POCC showed better miscibility with the Gla–CP systems; therefore, no Gla was detected in these ternary systems. These results are consistent with the in vitro release study.

3.6. In Vitro Skin Permeation and Drug Retention of Drug Solution

A comparison of the enhancement of LicA and Gla skin retention after 48 h is shown in Figure 6. The results demonstrated that the amount of Gla that accumulated in the skin within 48 h was 5.63 times higher than that of LicA (Figure 6a). Furthermore, approximately a 7.02 times increase in the amount of Gla permeating into the receptor fluids was observed when compared with LicA (Figure 6b). The addition of CP 90, POCC, SP, and IPM significantly enhanced the retention of LicAin the skin, and the enhancement effect was rank ordered as SP ($ER_{solution\ retention}$: 3.78) > POCC ≈ IPM > CP 90 > TP > PG > NMP (Figure 6a and Table 3). CP 90, POCC, SP, and IPM also significantly facilitated LicA's permeation across the skin and POCC showed the highest $ER_{permeation}$ value (Figure 6b and Table 3). However, the seven enhancers all significantly improved Gla's disposition into the skin, and the enhancement effect followed the order of CP 90 ($ER_{solution\ retention}$: 2.11) >TP ≈ IPM≈ NPM >PG > POCC > SP (Figure 6a and Table 3). However, only POCC, CP 90, and NMP significantly facilitated Gla's permeation and CP 90 showed the highest $ER_{permeation}$value (Figure 6b and Table 3). In addition, it was observed that the permeation amount of LicA and Gla showed a positive linear relation with the LicA and Gla retention amount (R^2 = 0.85 and R^2 = 0.47), respectively, indicating that the seven enhancers all demonstrated a similar contributory effect on the drug retention and drug permeation.

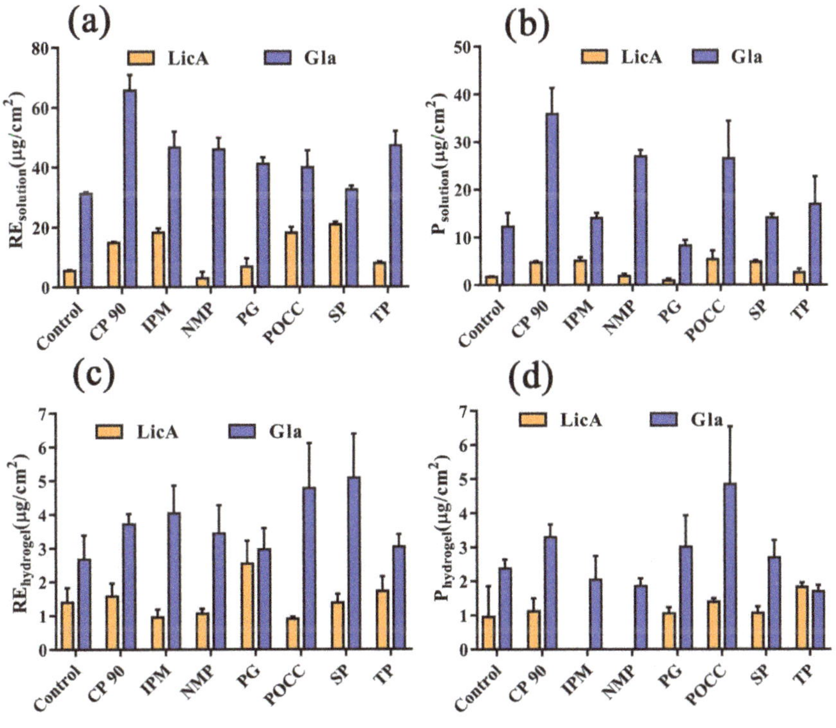

Figure 6. (**a**) $RE_{solution}$ of LicA and Gla after 48 h (*n* = 4); (**b**) $P_{solution}$ of LicA and Gla after 48 h (*n* = 4); (**c**) $RE_{hydrogel}$ of LicA and Gla after 48 h (*n* = 4); (**d**) $P_{hydrogel}$ of LicA and Gla after 48 h (*n* = 4).

3.7. *The Enhancement Mechanism of the LicA and Gla*

3.7.1. ATR-FT-IR of the Skin

ATR–FT-IR was conducted to elucidate the effects of the enhancers on the lipid and keratin arrangement of the porcine skin, and to further characterize drug–enhancers–skin interactions. The characteristic infrared absorption bands at 2918.02 and 2850.44 cm^{-1} represent the asymmetric $V_{as}CH_2$ and symmetric V_sCH_2 stretching vibrations of SC lipid (Figure S5a,b), and the bands at 1647.97 and 1538.07 cm^{-1} correspond to Amide I and Amide II of keratin (Figure 7a,b). In the LicA–skin control group, when POCC was added, the $V_{as}CH_2$, V_sCH_2, and Amide II moved to 2920.05, 2851.60, and 1538.65 cm^{-1}, respectively (Figure S5a). SP also caused a blueshift of the Amide I and Amide II bands to 1648.41 and 1539.55 cm^{-1}, respectively (Figure 7a). The results indicate that POCC and SP interacted with keratin of SC and disrupted the protein structure for enhanced drug permeation and retention. However, PG and NMP did not induce any changes in the lipids and keratin bands, suggesting an insignificant enhancement of LicA retention. When Gla–skin was considered as an entirety, the seven enhancers all changed the Amide I and Amide II bands to a higher position (blueshift) to different degrees (Figure 7b), indicating that the enhancers promoted Gla deposition by changing the secondary structures of the proteins. However, no linear correlation between the drug retention amount and the Amide I and Amide II bands' displacement values was observed. These results prove that the C=O group of porcine skin was the main enhancement site for LicA and Gla permeation.

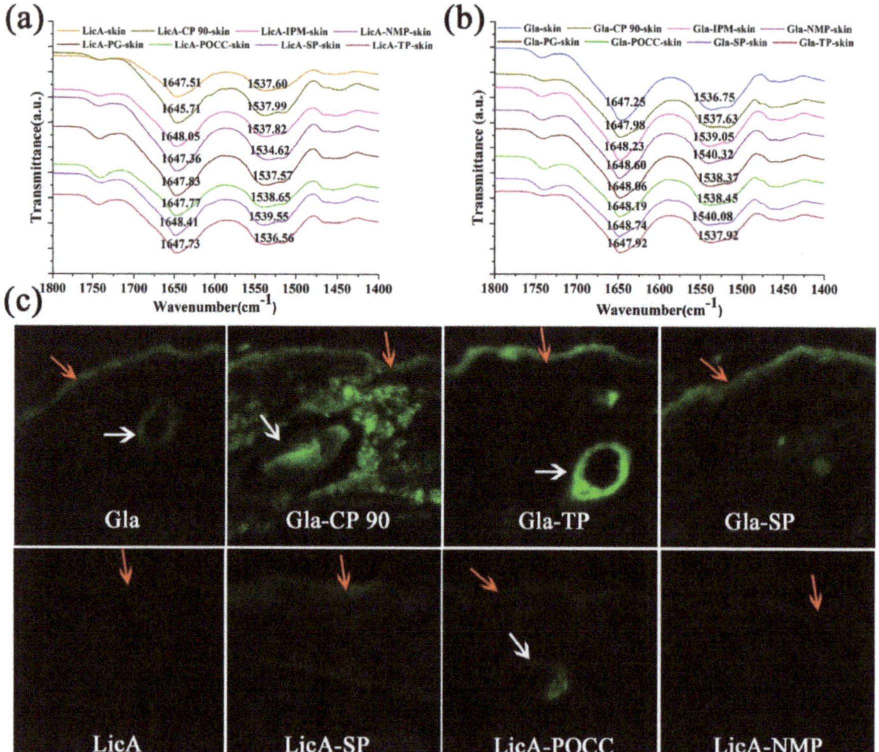

Figure 7. (**a**) FT-IR spectra (C=O group) of LicA–enhancers–skin systems; (**b**) FT-IR spectra (C=O group) of Gla–enhancers–skin systems; (**c**) CLSM images of the penetration depth and fluorescence intensity LicA and C6 in porcine skin treated with enhancers (Bar = 100 μm, the red arrows and white arrows represent the SC and hair follicles of the skin, respectively).

3.7.2. CLSM

The results of CLSM are shown in Figures 7c and S5c. Coumarin 6 was used as a probe as a substitute for Gla in this study. It was observed that LicA permeated to a deeper skin layer in the presence of CP 90, POCC, SP, and IPM, and significantly stronger LicA fluorescence was distributed in the epidermis and dermis when compared with the parent LicA. However, PG, TP, and NMP did not facilitate drug permeation into deeper skin layers. For Gla, the seven enhancers all improved the drug retention amount and drug fluorescence intensity, and CP 90 and TP had the most significant improvement effect. The results are in accordance with the in vitro skin permeation and retention study. Interestingly, we found that hair follicles were the main permeation routes for LicA and Gla, and most fluorescence was located in the hair follicles.

3.7.3. Molecular Modeling and Correlation Analysis 2

Gla showed a higher E_{mix} (12.24) with skin than that of LicA (9.96), indicating that LicA showed better miscibility with skin than that of Gla. However, CED of Gla–skin was similar to LicA–skin. Then, the E_{mix}, χ and CED values of different drug–enhancers–skin ternary systems were calculated as before (Table 4).The optimized ternary associations are displayed in Figures 8d, S6 and S7. After enhancers were added, they could occupy the site of drug–skin interaction and link with the skin, leading to better compatibility between the enhancers and skin. Thus, a lower E_{mix} value is indicative of better enhancers–skin interaction and higher drug permeation [17].

Table 4. Molecular docking and molecular dynamics (MD) simulation results of Gla (LicA)–enhancers–skin systems.

	χ (kcal/mol)	E_{mix} (kcal/mol)	CED (kcal/mol)
LicA-CP 90-Skin	27.54	16.31	1.49×10^9
LicA-IPM-Skin	24.82	14.70	1.37×10^9
LicA-NMP-Skin	39.04	23.12	1.59×10^9
LicA-PG-Skin	48.50	28.72	1.62×10^9
LicA-POCC-Skin	17.13	10.14	1.41×10^9
LicA-SP-Skin	16.74	9.92	1.35×10^9
LicA-TP-Skin	42.52	25.18	1.49×10^9
Gla-CP 90-Skin	10.82	6.41	1.30×10^9
Gla-IPM-Skin	6.97	4.13	1.39×10^9
Gla-NMP-Skin	28.00	16.58	1.46×10^9
Gla-PG-Skin	31.06	18.40	1.54×10^9
Gla-POCC-Skin	14.07	8.33	1.45×10^9
Gla-SP-Skin	1.44	0.86	1.54×10^9
Gla-TP-Skin	21.41	12.68	1.47×10^9

Next, multivariate linear regression analysis was conducted to confirm the correlation between the $P_{solution}$, $RE_{solution}$, and physicochemical parameters of enhancers and the regression equations are expressed as follows:

$$P_{solution}\ (\text{LicA}) = 1.90 + 7.59 \times \log P\ (R^2 = 0.88) \quad (16)$$

$$RE_{solution}\ (\text{LicA}) = -2.26 + 0.49 \times \log P\ (R^2 = 0.89) \quad (17)$$

$$P_{solution}\ (\text{Gla}) = -1.57 + 3.84 \times \text{Polarizability} - 9.12 \times \log P \quad (18)$$

$$RE_{solution}\ (\text{Gla}) = 34.90 - 0.34 \times \text{M.W} + 3.85 \times \text{Polarizability} \quad (19)$$

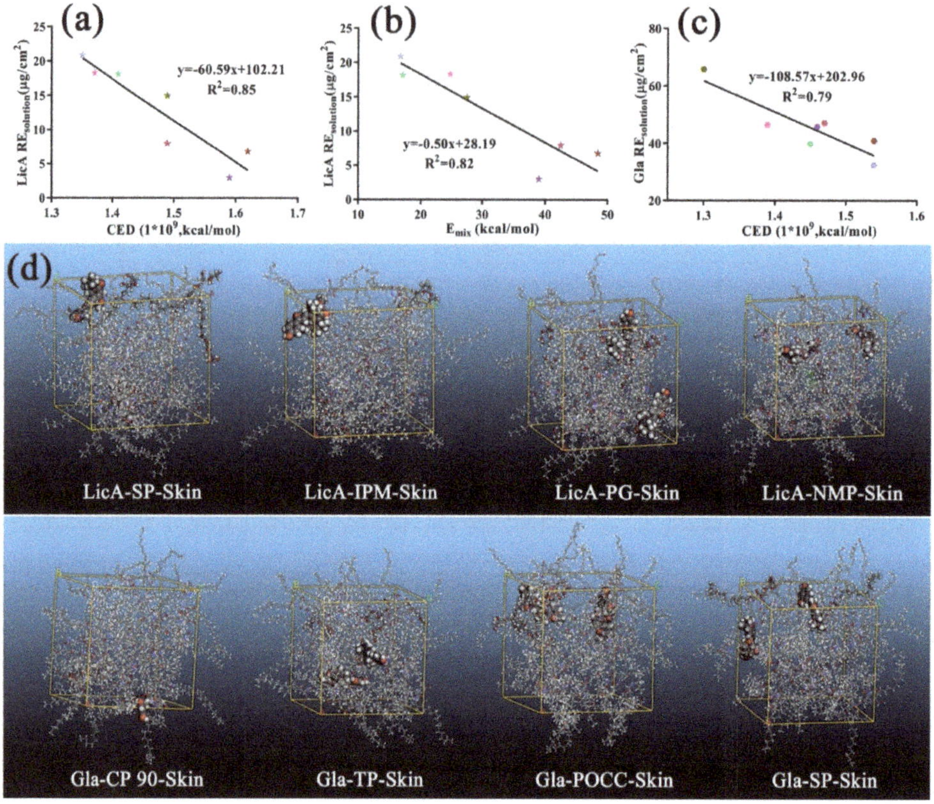

Figure 8. (**a**) Correlation analysis between LicA$RE_{solution}$ and CED of ternary systems; (**b**) correlation analysis between LicA$RE_{solution}$ and E_{mix} of ternary systems; (**c**) the correlation relationship between Gla$RE_{solution}$ and CED of ternary systems; (**d**) snapshots of LicA(Gla)–enhancers–skin systems at the end of the MD (drug: ball and stick model; enhancers: CPK model).

The results (Figure 9a,b) showed that both $RE_{solution}$ and $P_{solution}$ of LicA were positively correlated with log P of the enhancers. The response surface plots (Figure 9c,d) showed that $RE_{solution}$ and $P_{solution}$ of Gla increased as the polarizability increased. A linear regression of the drug retention amount and E_{mix} or CED was also carried out to explain the interaction force on drug retention, respectively, and the linear regression equations are expressed as follows:

$$RE_{solution}\ (LicA) = -60.59 \times CED + 102.21\ (R^2 = 0.85) \tag{20}$$

$$RE_{solution}\ (LicA) = -0.50 \times E_{mix} + 28.19\ (R^2 = 0.82) \tag{21}$$

$$RE_{solution}\ (Gla) = -108.57 \times CED + 202.96\ (R^2 = 0.79) \tag{22}$$

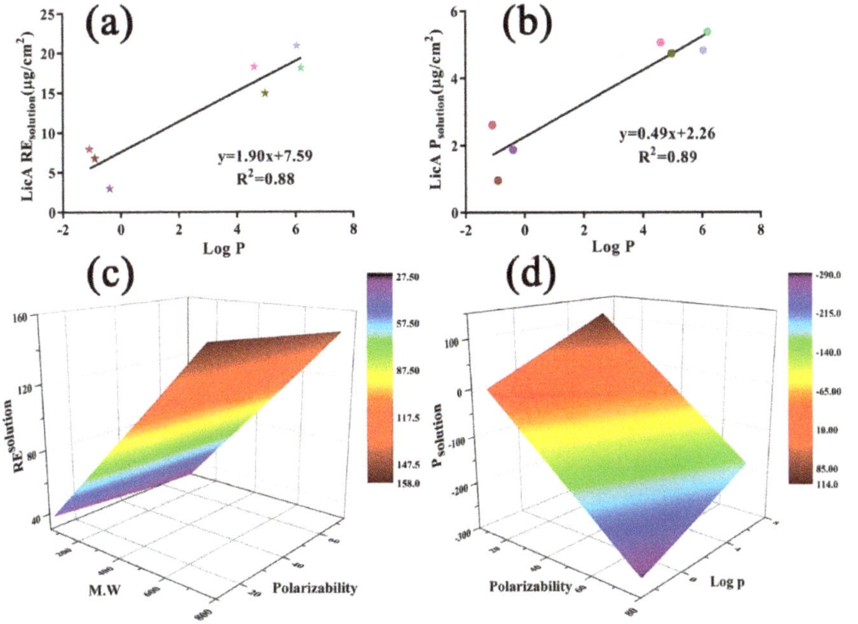

Figure 9. (**a**) The correlation relationship between LicARE$_{solution}$ and log P of enhancers; (**b**) linear analysis of LicAP$_{solution}$ and log P of enhancers; (**c**) response surface plot demonstrating the effect of MW and polarizability on RE$_{solution}$ of Gla; (**d**) response surface plot demonstrating the effect of log P and polarizability on P$_{solution}$ of Gla.

The results (Figure 8a,b) indicated that both the retention of LicA and Gla increased as the CED or E_{mix} value decreased, revealing the inhibitory effect of the intermolecular force on the drug retention. Taken together, for LicA–skin, enhancers with a higher log P showed better miscibility with skin, which resulted in increased LicA retention in the skin. For the Gla–skin binary system (Figure 8c), enhancers with a higher polarizability tended to occupy the site of the skin, thereby facilitating greater Gla deposition on the skin.

3.8. In Vitro Skin Permeation and Drug Retention of Drug Hydrogel

For the hydrogel system, only PG and TP could facilitate a significantly higher amount of LicA accumulation in the skin, and PG possessed the highest $ER_{hydrogel\ retention}$ value. The seven enhancers all improved Gla retention in the CP systems, and the $ER_{hydrogel\ retention}$ value was ranked as SP > POCC > IPM > CP > NMP > TP > PG (Figure 6c and Table 3). Moreover, a significantly higher amount of LicA was detected in the diffusion cells from hydrogel after the intervention of TP and POCC. Furthermore, only CP 90 and POCC could significantly disrupt the skin barrier for Gla penetration from the hydrogel (Figure 6d). $\beta_{R/P}$ values >1 indicate that the enhancers mainly facilitated the drug release process while $\beta_{R/P}$ values <1 indicate that the enhancement action site was mainly skin [17]. The results (Table 3) showed that the $\beta_{R/P}$ values of PG were 2.28 and 1.63 for the LicA–CP and Gla–CP systems, respectively, which proves that the site of action of the enhancement was mainly the CP matrix for PG. For LicA, the $\beta_{R/P}$ values of POCC, SP, IPM, and CP were all less than 0.5, demonstrating that skin was the main site of action of the enhancement.

4. Discussion

Although we observed an ascending trend for the utilization of enhancers in whitening products for anti-pigmentation, the interaction of whitening compounds, enhancers, and CP or skin in the drug release or permeation process has been neglected, which has resulted in the unreasonable utilization of enhancers and unscientific design of cosmetic formulations. This study systematically demonstrated the quantitative enhancement efficacy of the release and permeation of Gla and LicA by enhancers with different physicochemical parameters, providing a comprehensive understanding of the interaction of drugs, enhancers, and polymer or skin. More importantly, we provided strategies for reasonable selection of enhancers in hydrogel formulations to obtain high drug release and permeation.

Both LicA and Gla showed an anti-melanogenic effect in our previous studies; however, their poor solubility and high partition coefficient affected their formulation design and storage stability. In this work, to ensure the complete dispersion of drug in the CP system, 5% Gla and LicA (*w/w*) were added, respectively, and the XRD and PLM study confirmed this. FT-IR and Raman studies together indicated weak Van der Waals forces interactions present in the Gla–CP and LicA–CP systems. Moreover, the interaction of Gla–CP was significantly higher than that of the LicA–CP binary system due to the better compatibility between the drug and CP. Correspondingly, LicA–CP was expected to possess a higher release percent than that of the Gla–CP due to its easier escape from the hydrogel network. However, the result was contrary to this. Previous studies concluded that the intermolecular force, viscoelasticity, and mesh size of the drug-loaded hydrogels jointly influenced the drug release from hydrogel [4]. The mesh size can be tested by thermal analysis, which was performed to reflect the molecular mobility of the hydrogel and is described by T_g. A lower T_g is indicative of good molecular flexibility and a larger mesh size [26]. Next, the study confirmed that the G', G'', and mesh size of the hydrogel did not significantly contribute to the drug release percent supported by rheological studies and DSC. In fact, drug release from hydrogel is due to the two processes of hydrogel relaxation and drug diffusion while intermolecular force, viscoelasticity, and the mesh size mainly influence the hydrogel relaxation process [27–29]. When diffusion dominates drug release, the drug release percent is primarily inhibited by the drug solubility in receptor fluids. In this work, it was found that Gla had a significantly higher solubility in PEG 400/PBS (20/80, *v/v*) (Table 1), thereby facilitating a higher Gla release percent.

To obtain a higher drug release percent, hydrophilic and hydrophobic enhancers were added. Moreover, the proportion of enhancers was chosen to be 10% to acquire an apparent release and penetration enhancement effect, and to obtain a stronger drug–enhancers–CP or drug–enhancers–skin interaction. Both the LicA and Gla release amount promoted an increase in the MW of the enhancers, which is attributed to the enhanced mesh size induced by the increasing MW. This conclusion is supported by the results showing that molecules with high MW can form a larger pore size in the hydrogel network, leading to a higher drug release amount [3,30]. More importantly, we found that enhancers with high polarizability (α) had higher $ER_{release}$ for both LicA and Gla. The higher polarizability suggests that the drug was more easily polarized by polar molecules, which indicates stronger Van der Waals forces [16]. As a result, enhancers, which had higher polarizability, could link with the drug–CP binary systems to form drug–enhancers–CP ternary systems, or occupied drug–CP sites to form enhancers–CP binary systems. The detailed explanation is discussed below. To further confirm these results, we calculated the E_{mix} and χ values of different drug–enhancers–CP systems and CED of the built amorphous cell systems. Interestingly, th eLicA and Gla release percent showed a good positive correlation with E_{mix} and a negative relationship with CED. Thus, the key intermolecular interaction (Van der Waals forces) was theoretically consistent with the results of the correlation analysis, underscoring the dominant role of interaction forces in hindering drug release.

Next, FT-IR was used to demonstrate the enhancement site of the different enhancers and the enhancement efficacy can be reflected by the displacement degree of –OH and C=O groups. In this work, dry CP rather than aqueous CP was utilized to measure the whole system's energy. Previous studies revealed that the C=O group show a redshift in CP systems from a dry to a hydrated state, leading to a discrepancy in the interaction between drugs and CP in the two systems. The presence of water reduces the ionic interaction force and increases the H-bonding between the drug and polymers [31,32]. In this work, Van der

Waals forces were the dominating forces that controlled the drug release; therefore, dry CP is suitable as an alternative to hydrated CP to measure the interaction in different hydrogel systems. For LicA–CP and Gla–CP systems, POCC and SP generated stronger Van der Waals forces with CP by linking with the –OH group, which inhibited the drug release. However, the addition of CP 90 or NMP did not cause movement of the –OH group. These results proved that –OH of CP was not the enhancement site of drug release, which was different from the –OH enhancement site for loxoprofen release from the PSA matrix in a previous study [17]. The re-crystallization of the drug after the addition of enhancers was also necessary to assess the enhancement mechanism and higher drug re-crystallization indicates a better drug release ability. It was seen that a significantly larger amount of LicA crystals were re-crystallized in the film after the addition of PG or NMP while CP 90 and TP contributed to Gla re-crystallization. This result was consistent with the in vitro release study. It further proved that the drug–CP interaction was destroyed by the enhancers and enhancers–CP interactions occurred.

From the $F_{P/Q}$ value (Table 3), the skin barrier is still the dominating rate-limiting step for Gla and LicA permeation. The amount of Gla retention was significantly higher than LicA retention due to the higher log P of LicA, resulting in better miscibility with skin, which hindered LicA molecules' penetration into the skin. This result was consistent with previous reports. Usually, permeation enhancers improve the permeation of drug into the skin by disordering the arrangement of lipids and improving the lipid flexibility of SC [11,33]. Moreover, this process is dependent on the physicochemical properties of the enhancers rather than the amount of enhancers [34]. In this work, more LicA and Gla molecules were expected to accumulate in the skin to exert a remarkable anti-melanogenic effect. The seven enhancers chosen could all improve the LicA permeation and retention proportionally. For LicA, enhancers with high log P showed the highest $ER_{permeation}$ and $ER_{solution\ retention}$, whereas enhancers with high polarizability facilitated a higher amount of Gla retention. Enhancers with high log P, such as POCC, weakened the LicA–skin interaction and then decreased the interaction forces of the whole LicA–enhancers–skin ternary systems, thereby improving the diffusion of LicA into the skin. Thus, a good linear relation was observed between $Q_{retention}$ (LicA) and CED or E_{mix} after different enhancers were used. However, Gla–skin interaction, which was weaker than LicA–skin, was easier to be destroyed by enhancers with higher polarizability. Enhancers with higher polarizability could also occupy the Gla–skin binding sites to decrease the intermolecular force of the whole system. Taken together, the addition of enhancers disrupted the drug–skin interaction and then reduced the interaction forces of the whole systems, resulting in an improvement of the drug retention or permeation.

FT-IR is an analytical tool used to measure the disorder degree of proteins and lipids in the skin. Porcine skin was used for in vitro skin penetration studies because it possesses a similar epidermal thickness, lipid composition, low frequency impedance, and more importantly, permeability with human skin. Therefore, the $V_{as}CH_2$, V_sCH_2 and Amide I, Amide II displacement values were not as significant as rat skin [35,36]. A slight movement of the CH_2 or amide groups results in disarrangement of lipids or distortion of the protein structure. POCC and SP enhanced LicA retention by interacting with the C=O group of the ceramide, thereby a blueshift of the Amide I and Amide II bands was observed. Similarly, C=O was also the main enhancement site for Gla retention by the seven enhancers, indicating enhancers decreased the barrier's resistance by distorting the protein structure for enhanced LicA and Gla retention. Since Gla showed weaker interaction forces with skin than that of LicA, the seven enhancers all occupied the Gla–skin binding sites and improved Gla accumulation in the skin. CLSM is another tool that was used to confirm the effect of the enhancers on LicA and Gla retention. Higher fluorescence intensity and deeper skin location were indicative of a stronger penetration enhancement effect. This result was also consistent with the in vitro permeation study. Interestingly, the enhancers mainly facilitated drug retention via hair follicle pathways, which was mainly attributed to large hair follicles and a high number of hair follicles in porcine skin [37].

CP hydrogel is a complicated system including CP, water, and drug. Thus, the drug permeation and retention behaviors of hydrogel are not simply a combination of drug release and skin penetration. For LicA, the seven enhancers all improved LicA accumulation in the skin from the solution; however, PG showed the highest $ER_{hydrogel\ retention}$ and $ER_{release}$ for LicA, indicating that both the drug release and skin permeation processes limited LicA's permeability. Interestingly, the seven enhancers all showed a significant enhancement effect on Gla retention from hydrogel, which was different from the enhanced effect of Gla retention by CP, POCC, and PG in solution. These results further indicate that the main rate-limiting of Gla's penetration is its skin permeability.

5. Conclusions

In this work, a systematic approach was established to evaluate the enhanced release and retention of whitening agents from CP hydrogel in the presence of enhancers based on interactions among the drug, enhancers, and CP or skin. $ER_{release}$, $ER_{permeation}$, ER_{com}, $ER_{solution\ retention}$, and $ER_{hydrogel\ retention}$ were utilized to evaluate the quantitative enhanced effect, and $\beta_{R/P}$ was calculated to evaluate the enhancement action sites of the enhancers. We found that the release and retention enhancement effect were closely related to the structures of the enhancers. Gla–CP hydrogel showed higher drug release and retention ability than LicA–CP, which was attributed to the higher solubility in medium and better miscibility with skin of Gla than that of LicA. Enhancers with higher MW and lower polarizability showed a higher $ER_{release}$ for both LicA and Gla, whereas enhancers with higher log P and polarizability displayed a higher $ER_{solution\ retention}$ for LicA and Gla. More importantly, Van der Waals forces among the drug, enhancers and CP showed a negative correlation with the drug release percent, and intermolecular interaction between the drug, enhancers, and skin also showed a linear decreasing effect on drug retention. Additionally, the C=O group of the ceramide was the enhancement site for drug permeation by the enhancers. Consequently, TP and PG, and the seven enhancers showed a higher $ER_{hydrogel\ retention}$ for LicA–CP and Gla–CP respectively. Taken together, the conclusions provide a strategy for reasonable utilization of enhancers and formulation optimization in whitening topical hydrogels.

Supplementary Materials: The following are available online at https://www.mdpi.com/article/10.3390/pharmaceutics14020262/s1, Methods S1: The HPLC methods of LicA and Gla, Figure S1: (a) DSC curves of different hydrogels; (b) Flow characterization of the hydrogels (n = 3); (c) In vitro drug release profiles of LicA-CP hydrogel when enhancers were added (n = 3); (d) In vitro drug release profiles of LicA-CP hydrogel when enhancers were added (n = 3), Figure S2: Conformation of LicA-enhancers-CP and Gla-enhancers-CP ternary systems, Figure S3: The snapshots of LicA (Gla)-enhancers-CP systems at the end of the MD. (Drug: Ball and stick model; Enhancers: CPK model), Figure S4: (a) FT-IR spectra (C=O group) of LicA-enhancers-CP systems; (b) FT-IR spectra (C=O group) of Gla-enhancers-CP systems; (c) PLM images of drug-CP films after different enhancers were added, Figure S5: (a) FT-IR spectra (CH_2- group) of LicA-enhancers-skin systems; (b) FT-IR spectra (CH2-group) of Gla-enhancers-skin systems; (c) CLSM images of penetration depth and fluorescence intensity LicA and C6 in porcine skin treated by enhancers (bar = 100 μm), Figure S6: Conformations of LicA-enhancers-skin and Gla-enhancers-skin ternary systems, Figure S7: The snapshots of LicA (Gla)-enhancers-skin systems at the end of the MD. (Drug: Ball and stick model; Enhancers: CPK model).

Author Contributions: Conceptualization, Z.W. and Q.L.; methodology, Z.Z.; software, Y.H.; validation, Y.W. (Yufan Wu), Q.Z. and Z.Z.; formal analysis, Y.W. (Yuan Wang); investigation, Z.W. and Y.X.; resources, Q.L.; data curation, Y.X. and C.J.; writing—original draft preparation, Z.W. and Y.X.; writing—review and editing, C.J. and C.S.; visualization, L.L. and H.Z.; supervision, Q.L.; project administration, H.Z. and Q.L.; funding acquisition, Q.L. All authors have read and agreed to the published version of the manuscript.

Funding: This research was funded by National Natural Science Foundation of China, grant number 82074023, 81874346.

Institutional Review Board Statement: All animal experiments were performed in accordance with the "Guiding Principles in the Care and Use of Animals" (China), and approved by the Ethics Committee of Southern Medical University (L2019036, date of approval: 13 April 2019).

Informed Consent Statement: Not applicable.

Data Availability Statement: Not applicable.

Acknowledgments: The authors would like to send their gratitude to the National Natural Science Foundation of China.

Conflicts of Interest: The authors declare no conflict of interest. The funders had no role in the design of the study; in the collection, analyses, or interpretation of data; in the writing of the manuscript, or in the decision to publish the results.

References

1. Xiao, Q.; Chen, G.; Zhang, Y.-H.; Chen, F.-Q.; Weng, H.-F.; Xiao, A.-F. Agarose Stearate-Carbomer$_{940}$ as Stabilizer and Rheology Modifier for Surfactant-Free Cosmetic Formulations. *Mar. Drugs* **2021**, *19*, 344. [CrossRef] [PubMed]
2. Zhang, S.; Liu, C.; Yang, D.G.; Ruan, J.H.; Luo, Z.; Quan, P.; Fang, L. Mechanism insight on drug skin delivery from polyurethane hydrogels: Roles of molecular mobility and intermolecular interaction. *Eur. J. Pharm. Sci.* **2021**, *161*, 105783. [CrossRef] [PubMed]
3. Luo, Z.; Liu, C.; Quan, P.; Yang, D.G.; Zhao, H.Q.; Wan, X.C.; Fang, L. Mechanistic insights of the controlled release capacity of polar functional group in transdermal drug delivery system: The relationship of hydrogen bonding strength and controlled release capacity. *Acta Pharm. Sin. B* **2020**, *10*, 928–945. [CrossRef] [PubMed]
4. Li, J.Y.; Mooney, D.J. Designing hydrogels for controlled drug delivery. *Nat. Rev. Mater.* **2016**, *1*, 16071. [CrossRef]
5. Meacham, R.; Liu, M.; Guo, J.; Zehnder, A.T.; Hui, C.Y. Effect of Hydration on Tensile Response of a Dual Cross-linked PVA Hydrogel. *Exp. Mech.* **2020**, *60*, 1161–1165. [CrossRef]
6. Censi, R.; Vermonden, T.; van Steenbergen, M.J.; Deschout, H.; Braeckmans, K.; De Smedt, S.C.; van Nostrum, C.F.; di Martino, P.; Hennink, W.E. Photopolymerized thermosensitive hydrogels for tailorable diffusion-controlled protein delivery. *J. Control. Release* **2009**, *140*, 230–236. [CrossRef]
7. Wang, E.; Klauda, J.B. Models for the *Stratum corneum* Lipid Matrix: Effects of Ceramide Concentration, Ceramide Hydroxylation, and Free Fatty Acid Protonation. *J. Phys. Chem. B* **2018**, *122*, 11996–12008. [CrossRef]
8. Wang, Z.X.; Liu, L.; Xiang, S.J.; Jiang, C.P.; Wu, W.F.; Ruan, S.F.; Du, Q.Q.; Chen, T.T.; Xue, Y.Q.; Chen, H.J.; et al. Formulation and Characterization of a 3D-Printed Cryptotanshinone-Loaded Niosomal Hydrogel for Topical Therapy of Acne. *AAPS Pharm.* **2020**, *21*, 159. [CrossRef]
9. Wang, W.; Liu, C.; Luo, Z.; Wan, X.C.; Fang, L. Investigation of molecular mobility of pressure-sensitive-adhesive in oxybutynin patch in vitro and in vivo: Effect of sorbitan monooleate on drug release and patch mechanical property. *Eur. J. Pharm. Sci.* **2018**, *122*, 116–124. [CrossRef]
10. Song, W.T.; Quan, P.; Li, S.S.; Liu, C.; Lv, S.; Zhao, Y.S.; Fang, L. Probing the role of chemical enhancers in facilitating drug release from patches: Mechanistic insights based on FT-IR spectroscopy, molecular modeling and thermal analysis. *J. Control. Release* **2016**, *227*, 13–22. [CrossRef]
11. Ruan, S.F.; Wang, Z.X.; Xiang, S.J.; Chen, H.J.; Liu, Q. Mechanisms of white mustard seed (*Sinapis alba* L.) volatile oils as transdermal penetration enhancers. *Fitoterapia* **2019**, *138*, 104195. [CrossRef] [PubMed]
12. Liu, X.C.; Quan, P.; Li, S.S.; Liu, C.; Zhao, Y.; Zhao, Y.S.; Fang, L. Time dependence of the enhancement effect of chemical enhancers: Molecular mechanisms of enhancing kinetics. *J. Control. Release* **2017**, *248*, 33–44. [CrossRef] [PubMed]
13. Witting, M.; Boreham, A.; Brodwolf, R.; Vavrova, K.; Alexiev, U.; Friess, W.; Hedtrich, S. Interactions of Hyaluronic Acid with the Skin and Implications for the Dermal Delivery of Biomacromolecules. *Mol. Pharm.* **2015**, *12*, 1391–1401. [CrossRef] [PubMed]
14. Nan, L.Y.; Liu, C.; Li, Q.Y.; Wan, X.C.; Guo, J.P.; Quan, P.; Fang, L. Investigation of the enhancement effect of the natural transdermal permeation enhancers from *Ledum palustre* L. var. angustum N. Busch: Mechanistic insight based on interaction among drug, enhancers and skin. *Eur. J. Pharm. Sci.* **2018**, *124*, 105–113. [CrossRef]
15. Calatayud-Pascual, M.A.; Sebastian-Morelló, M.; Balaguer-Fernández, C.; Delgado-Charro, M.B.; López-Castellano, A.; Merino, V. Influence of Chemical Enhancers and Iontophoresis on the In Vitro Transdermal Permeation of Propranolol: Evaluation by Dermatopharmacokinetics. *Pharmaceutics* **2018**, *10*, 265. [CrossRef]
16. Xu, W.W.; Liu, C.; Zhang, Y.; Quan, P.; Yang, D.G.; Fang, L. An investigation on the effect of drug physicochemical properties on the enhancement strength of enhancer: The role of drug-skin-enhancer interactions. *In. J. Pharm.* **2021**, *607*, 120945. [CrossRef]
17. Yang, D.G.; Liu, C.; Quan, P.; Fang, L. A systematic approach to determination of permeation enhancer action efficacy and sites: Molecular mechanism investigated by quantitative. *J. Control. Release* **2020**, *322*, 1–12. [CrossRef] [PubMed]
18. Wang, Z.; Xue, Y.; Chen, T.; Du, Q.; Zhu, Z.; Wang, Y.; Wu, Y.; Zeng, Q.; Shen, C.; Jiang, C.; et al. Glycyrrhiza acid micelles loaded with licochalcone A for topical delivery: Co-penetration and anti-melanogenic effect. *Eur. J. Pharm. Sci.* **2021**, *68*, 106029. [CrossRef]
19. Du, Q.Q.; Liu, Q. ROS-responsive hollow mesoporous silica nanoparticles loaded with Glabridin for anti-pigmentation properties. *Microporous Mesoporous Mater.* **2021**, *327*, 111429. [CrossRef]

20. Masukawa, Y.; Narita, H.; Shimizu, E.; Kondo, N.; Sugai, Y.; Oba, T.; Homma, R.; Ishikawa, J.; Takagi, Y.; Kitahara, T.; et al. Characterization of overall ceramide species in human *Stratum corneum*. *J. Lipid Res.* **2008**, *49*, 1466–1476. [CrossRef]
21. Quan, P.; Wan, X.C.; Tian, Q.; Liu, C.; Fang, L. Dicarboxylic acid as a linker to improve the content of amorphous drug in drug-in-polymer film: Effects of molecular mobility, electrical conductivity and intermolecular interactions. *J. Control. Release* **2020**, *317*, 142–153. [CrossRef]
22. Zhang, R.Q.; Tao, Y.Z.; Xu, W.L.; Xiao, S.L.; Du, S.M.; Zhou, Y.S.; Hasan, A. Rheological and controlled release properties of hydrogels based on mushroom hyperbranched polysaccharide and xanthan gum. *Int. J. Biol. Macromol.* **2018**, *120*, 2399–2409. [CrossRef]
23. Islam, A.; Riaz, M.; Yasin, T. Structural and viscoelastic properties of chitosan-based hydrogel and its drug delivery application. *Int. J. Biol. Macromol.* **2013**, *59*, 119–124. [CrossRef]
24. Tanriverdi, S.T.; Cheaburu-Yilmaz, C.N.; Carbone, S.; Ozer, O. Preparation and in vitro evaluation of melatonin-loaded HA/PVA gel formulations. *Pharm. Dev. Technol.* **2018**, *23*, 815–825. [CrossRef]
25. Kothari, K.; Ragoonanan, V.; Suryanarayanan, R. The Role of Polymer Concentration on the Molecular Mobility and Physical Stability of Nifedipine Solid Dispersions. *Mol. Pharm.* **2015**, *12*, 1477–1484. [CrossRef]
26. Liu, C.; Quan, P.; Li, S.S.; Zhao, Y.S.; Fang, L. A systemic evaluation of drug in acrylic pressure sensitive adhesive patch in vitro and in vivo: The roles of intermolecular interaction and adhesive mobility variation in drug controlled release. *J. Control. Release* **2017**, *252*, 83–94. [CrossRef]
27. Das, D.; Das, R.; Ghosh, P.; Dhara, S.; Panda, A.B.; Pal, S. Dextrin cross linked with poly(HEMA): A novel hydrogel for colon specific delivery of ornidazole. *RSC Adv.* **2013**, *3*, 25340–25350. [CrossRef]
28. Wang, Y.M.; Wang, J.; Yuan, Z.Y.; Han, H.Y.; Li, T.; Li, L.; Guo, X.H. Chitosan cross-linked poly(acrylic acid) hydrogels: Drug release control and mechanism. *Coll. Surfaces B Biointerfaces* **2017**, *152*, 252–259. [CrossRef] [PubMed]
29. Zhao, C.Y.; Quan, P.; Liu, C.; Li, Q.Y.; Fang, L. Effect of isopropyl myristate on the viscoelasticity and drug release of a drug-in-adhesive transdermal patch containing blonanserin. *Acta Pharm. Sin. B* **2016**, *6*, 623–628. [CrossRef] [PubMed]
30. Browning, M.B.; Wilems, T.; Hahn, M.; Cosgriff-Hernandez, E. Compositional control of poly(ethylene glycol) hydrogel modulus independent of mesh size. *J. Biomed. Mater. Res. Part A* **2011**, *98A*, 268–273. [CrossRef]
31. Islam, M.T.; Rodríguez-Hornedo, N.; Ciotti, S.; Ackermann, C. Fourier transform infrared spectroscopy for the analysis of neutralizer-carbomer and surfactant-carbomer interactions in aqueous, hydroalcoholic, and anhydrous gel formulations. *AAPS J.* **2004**, *6*, 61–67. [CrossRef]
32. Kim, S.M.; Lee, S.M.; Bae, Y.C. Influence of hydroxyl group for thermoresponsive poly(N-isopropylacrylamide) gel particles in water/co-solvent (1,3-propanediol, glycerol) systems. *Eur. Polym. J.* **2014**, *54*, 151–159. [CrossRef]
33. Williams, A.C.; Barry, B.W. Penetration enhancers. *Adv. Drug Deliv. Rev.* **2012**, *64*, 128–137. [CrossRef]
34. Liu, X.; Liu, M.; Liu, C.; Quan, P.; Zhao, Y.; Fang, L. An insight into the molecular mechanism of the temporary enhancement effect of isopulegol decanoate on the skin. *Int. J. Pharm.* **2017**, *529*, 161–167. [CrossRef]
35. Smejkalova, D.; Muthny, T.; Nesporova, K.; Hermannova, M.; Achbergerova, E.; Huerta-Angeles, G.; Svoboda, M.; Cepa, M.; Machalova, V.; Luptakova, D.; et al. Hyaluronan polymeric micelles for topical drug delivery. *Carbohydr. Polym.* **2017**, *156*, 86–96. [CrossRef] [PubMed]
36. Tian, Q.; Quan, P.; Fang, L.; Xu, H.; Liu, C. A molecular mechanism investigation of the transdermal/topical absorption classification system on the basis of drug skin permeation and skin retention. *Int. J. Pharm.* **2021**, *608*, 121082. [CrossRef]
37. Jacobi, U.; Kaiser, M.; Toll, R.; Mangelsdorf, S.; Audring, H.; Otberg, N.; Sterry, W.; Lademann, J. Porcine ear skin: An in vitro model for human skin. *Skin Res. Technol.* **2007**, *13*, 19–24. [CrossRef]

pharmaceutics MDPI

Review

The Monoterpenoid Perillyl Alcohol: Anticancer Agent and Medium to Overcome Biological Barriers

Thomas C. Chen [1,*], Clovis O. da Fonseca [2], Daniel Levin [3] and Axel H. Schönthal [4,*]

1 Department of Neurological Surgery, Keck School of Medicine, University of Southern California, Los Angeles, CA 90089, USA
2 Department of Neurological Surgery, Federal Hospital of Ipanema, Rio de Janeiro 22411-020, Brazil; clovis.orlando@uol.com.br
3 Norac Pharma, Azusa, CA 91702, USA; dlevin@noracpharma.com
4 Department of Molecular Microbiology & Immunology, Keck School of Medicine, University of Southern California, Los Angeles, CA 90089, USA
* Correspondence: Thomas.Chen@med.usc.edu (T.C.C.); schontha@usc.edu (A.H.S.)

Abstract: Perillyl alcohol (POH) is a naturally occurring monoterpenoid related to limonene that is present in the essential oils of various plants. It has diverse applications and can be found in household items, including foods, cosmetics, and cleaning supplies. Over the past three decades, it has also been investigated for its potential anticancer activity. Clinical trials with an oral POH formulation administered to cancer patients failed to realize therapeutic expectations, although an intra-nasal POH formulation yielded encouraging results in malignant glioma patients. Based on its amphipathic nature, POH revealed the ability to overcome biological barriers, primarily the blood–brain barrier (BBB), but also the cytoplasmic membrane and the skin, which appear to be characteristics that critically contribute to POH's value for drug development and delivery. In this review, we present the physicochemical properties of POH that underlie its ability to overcome the obstacles placed by different types of biological barriers and consequently shape its multifaceted promise for cancer therapy and applications in drug development. We summarized and appraised the great variety of preclinical and clinical studies that investigated the use of POH for intranasal delivery and nose-to-brain drug transport, its intra-arterial delivery for BBB opening, and its permeation-enhancing function in hybrid molecules, where POH is combined with or conjugated to other therapeutic pharmacologic agents, yielding new chemical entities with novel mechanisms of action and applications.

Keywords: blood–brain barrier; drug formulation; drug hybrids; intra-arterial delivery; intracranial malignancies; intranasal delivery; monoterpene; monoterpenoid; NEO100

Citation: Chen, T.C.; da Fonseca, C.O.; Levin, D.; Schönthal, A.H. The Monoterpenoid Perillyl Alcohol: Anticancer Agent and Medium to Overcome Biological Barriers. *Pharmaceutics* **2021**, *13*, 2167. https://doi.org/10.3390/pharmaceutics13122167

Academic Editors: Vibhuti Agrahari and Prashant Kumar

Received: 10 October 2021
Accepted: 11 December 2021
Published: 16 December 2021

1. Introduction

The blood–brain barrier (BBB) is a highly selective semipermeable interface between the bloodstream and the brain parenchyma that acts as a gatekeeper to control the entry of substances from the systemic circulation into the brain. It not only manages the brain entry of endogenous substances present in the circulation, such as neuroactive solutes, nutrients, hormones, and antibodies, but also provides protection by restricting brain access by potentially harmful agents, such as metals and toxins. The influx and efflux of molecules are actively regulated with the prime objective to maintain brain homeostasis and protect this organ from harm [1,2]. For a detailed description of these mechanisms and their underlying anatomical elements, the interested reader is referred to excellent recent reviews [3,4].

By allowing necessary nutrients and other beneficial materials to enter the brain whilst allowing waste products to exit and preventing harmful substances from entering the brain, the BBB provides great benefit in protecting and ensuring optimal brain function. At the same time, however, this armor-like role of the BBB represents a double-edged sword because it can also block brain access by a large number of pharmacological agents that may be needed within the brain in order to effect their therapeutic action against brain-localized diseases. In fact, within the context of brain-metastatic spread from peripheral tumors of the lung, breast, melanoma, and some others, effective exclusion of therapeutic agents from the brain has resulted in the well-recognized paradox of an increasing incidence of brain metastases despite improvements in general clinical care and substantial progress in developing novel therapeutic agents [5–7]. For example, in the case of breast cancer subtypes that overexpress epidermal growth factor receptor 2 (EGFR2/HER2/Neu; generally called HER2+), the introduction of the humanized monoclonal antibody trastuzumab (Herceptin®) and other HER2-targeted agents resulted in significantly improved treatment outcomes for the peripheral disease. However, HER2+ breast cancer has a propensity to metastasize to the brain and these brain seeds cannot effectively be reached by therapeutic antibodies. As a result, while extracranial malignancy generally responds well to intravenous trastuzumab (and other HER2-targeted therapeutics), cancerous seeds in the brain are, for the most part, isolated from this systemic therapeutic intervention. Whilst treatment success in the periphery enables patients to live longer, cancer cells residing in the sanctuary of the brain consequently have more time to develop sizable metastases and eventually trigger cancer recurrence and a grim prognosis [5–8].

Secondary brain cancer as a result of metastatic spread from peripheral cancer types represents the most frequent intracranial malignancy. Primary brain cancers, malignant gliomas in particular, present with no better prognosis and their effective management also remains an inadequately met clinical need. For instance, glioblastoma (GBM, formerly known as glioblastoma multiforme; IDH wildtype, grade IV) is the most aggressive cancer that originates in the brain, with a median overall survival of 8–10 months from the time of diagnosis [9–11]. Patients with higher performance scores (based on functional impairment [12]) and overall greater physical robustness at the time of diagnosis are better predisposed to withstand the rigors of extensive and taxing therapies and, therefore, are more likely to experience an extended average survival of another 6–12 months. However, even with patients demonstrating higher Karnofsky performance scores (KPS), recurrence of GBM is nearly universal and the vast majority of patients eventually die from this insidious disease within just a few years at best.

The current standard of care for GBM consists of surgery (if possible), followed by chemoradiation, which consists of oral temozolomide (TMZ; Temodar®) combined with ionizing radiation. TMZ is a prodrug that releases diazomethane, which is an alkylating agent. The clinical use of TMZ for GBM was cemented by a landmark clinical study by Stupp et al. [13], showing that the combination of radiation therapy (RT) with TMZ for 6 weeks, followed by 6 months of TMZ alone, resulted in greater patient survival duration than was achieved by the use of radiation alone. It was, however, noted that the median survival benefit was small: inclusion of TMZ with the RT regime extended the average survival from 12.1 months (RT alone) to 14.6 months, i.e., a life expectancy increase of only 2.5 months. The fraction of patients surviving 5 years also showed an increase, from 1.9% for RT alone to 10.9% for the combination treatment [13,14]. While these improvements were validated by subsequent studies, it remains noteworthy that clinical trials generally harbor selection bias, usually favoring patients with higher performance scores and, therefore, patients in ordinary clinical practice may not always be able to receive or tolerate the full spectrum of therapeutic interventions. As such, the publicized survival data derived from most clinical trials represent a somewhat skewed picture as compared to the entire cohort of GBM patients, and improved therapies are still urgently needed [15].

Similar to the above example of trastuzumab, where the BBB severely limits access of this therapeutic antibody to its intracranial HER2+ targets, the BBB significantly interferes with TMZ brain entry as well. Although TMZ is generally considered BBB permeable, neuropharmacokinetic measurements in patients with primary or metastatic brain tumors established a brain-to-plasma TMZ concentration ratio of only 0.2 [16,17], indicating that in practice, only a small fraction of systemically available TMZ enters the brain. This low amount entering the brain is not entirely surprising because TMZ was not specifically developed as a brain-targeting agent.

Within malignant brain lesions, the organization and function of the BBB can be altered due to pathological changes caused by tumor cells, including extensive neo-angiogenesis, which is particularly prominent in GBM tissue. Such structural alterations are generally referred to as the blood–tumor barrier (BTB), which is located between brain tumor tissue and adjacent capillary vessels [18,19]. It was observed that the barrier function of a BTB is compromised and not as effective as a normal BBB, a phenomenon called leakiness. This may explain why some chemotherapeutic drugs, such as etoposide, cisplatin, methotrexate, or cyclophosphamide, which are known to not effectively penetrate the BBB, can achieve occasional therapeutic responses in the brain when given at higher dosages [20,21]. The severity of barrier breakdown is, however, highly heterogeneous, both in primary and secondary brain malignancies. For example, a detailed preclinical analysis [22] of 2000 individual lesions of breast–brain metastases in mice demonstrated large differences between individual lesions—and even within the same lesion—with regard to BBB/BTB permeability. Although 90% of these lesions showed barrier compromise, their uptake of different clinically used chemotherapeutic drugs was less than 15% of that of other tissues or peripheral metastases. Clinical studies in GBM patients that used contrast-enhanced magnetic resonance imaging (MRI), positron emission tomography (PET) imaging, and analysis of surgically removed tissues also established significant heterogeneity: while some tumor regions present with deteriorated BTB, others display an intact barrier [23,24]. Therefore, despite being partially compromised within brain tumor lesions, the BTB is still operational enough to substantially impede effective drug delivery and prevent therapeutic activity. Despite the presence of more or less "leaky" sections of the BTB, effective drug delivery requires consideration of the intact BBB for reliable and more broadly applicable therapeutic benefit.

Several diverse strategies are being explored to increase drug penetration of the BBB and achieve efficient brain entry of therapeutic agents. Some of these are highly invasive procedures that may require surgery and hospitalization of patients, such as intrathecal and intraventricular injection, convection-enhanced delivery by direct injection, or implantation of gels, wafers, and microchips for localized release, all of which seek to circumvent the BBB and place therapeutic agents directly into the brain or tumor tissue. Transient opening of the BBB by intracarotid infusion of mannitol or chemical disruptors (e.g., leukotrienes, bradykinins) represents another invasive method that can facilitate brain access for drugs present in the systemic circulation. All of these procedures are, however, associated with significant risks, such as vasogenic brain edema, embolism, seizures, and neurological deficits, as well as high costs [19,25,26].

There is a great need then for less invasive procedures that allow for effective drug access to brain-localized malignancies. Among the strategies that are being pursued to achieve this goal are novel interventions that reversibly open the BBB, drug modifications that enable more efficient penetration of the BBB, or intranasal delivery with the goal to achieve direct nose-to-brain drug transport to circumvent the BBB altogether. In the discussion that follows, we review progress in this field that was achieved with the use of perillyl alcohol (POH), a naturally occurring monoterpenoid related to limonene [27], and with NEO100, an engineered version of this monoterpenoid that features ultra-high purity and is being produced under Current Good Manufacturing Practice (CGMP) regulations. NEO100 has revealed multifaceted applicability and uses that include intranasal delivery (either alone in monotherapy fashion or as a facilitator of enhanced permeability for other drugs), intra-arterial delivery to reversibly open the BBB, and as a covalently attached modifier for other drugs to achieve superior penetration, not only of the BBB but also of other critical barriers, the cell membranes (cytoplasmic and nuclear), and the skin. Below, we provide a detailed description of the physicochemical properties of POH and NEO100, followed by a review of their versatile applications to overcome biological barriers and allow for improved therapeutic access to malignant lesions.

2. The Monoterpenoid Perillyl Alcohol (POH)

2.1. Biochemical Description of POH

POH was first extracted from herbs of the genus *Perilla* [28], from which it derived its name, and to various extents is a constituent of essential oils from a variety of botanicals, including peppermint, spearmint, lavender, bergamot, lemongrass, sage, caraway, thyme, rosemary, celery seeds, cherries, and cranberries [27,29]. Common synonyms of POH are perilla alcohol, perillol, and p-mentha-1,8-dien-7-ol, among others. Its IUPAC name is (4-prop-1-en-2-ylcyclohexen-1-yl)methanol. It is a terpene (or, more accurately, a terpenoid, as it is a terpene modified by derivatization through the addition of a hydroxyl group). The terpenes were so-named in 1866 by the German chemist August Kekulé from the name of the pine-oil extract turpentine [30], which is primarily comprised of terpenes, a classification expanded to include tens of thousands of chemical substances made up of repeating 5-carbon isoprenyl subunits (see Scheme 1 for an overview of some terpene biosynthetic pathways) [31].

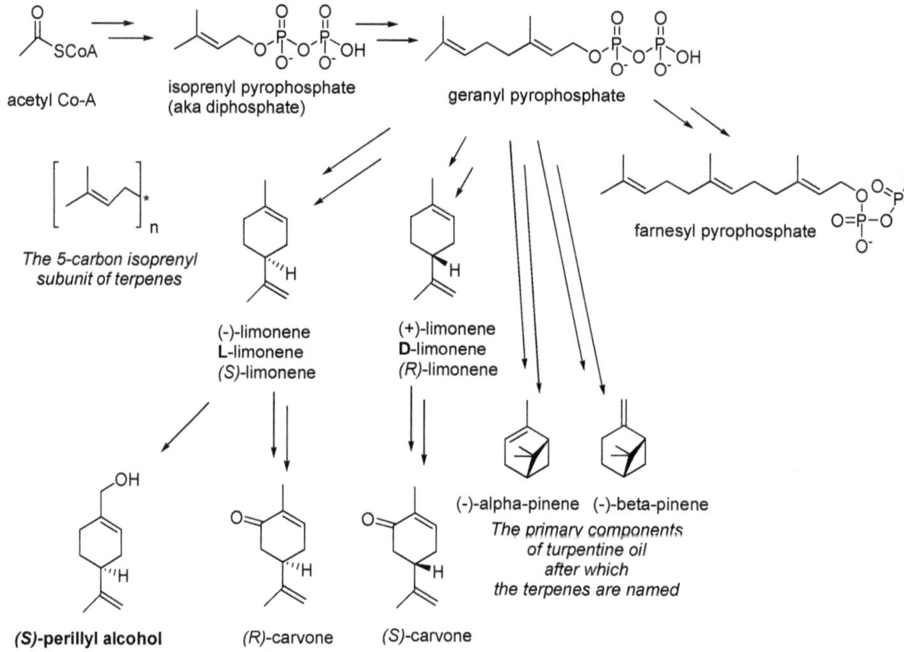

Scheme 1. Biosynthesis of some terpenes and terpenoids. The biosynthesis of terpenes proceeds via the isoprenyl building block to assemble higher-order geranyl (2× isoprenyl moieties), farnesyl (3× isoprenyl moieties), and other intermediates en route to terpenes, such as limonenes (in citrus oils) and pinenes (in pine oils), and further functionalized (e.g., oxidized) terpenoids, such as carvones and (S)-perillyl alcohol.

POH itself is a fragrant oil with a somewhat heavy, floral, lavender-like fragrance that is used in perfumes, cosmetics, and some cleaning products. Other reported uses are as an ingredient in baked goods, frozen dairy, gelatine, puddings, beverages, and candies [32]. It is, however, now also of increasing interest as a therapeutic agent in the prevention and treatment of cancers (details below). POH is a chiral compound (i.e., one whose 3-D shape is not superimposable on its mirror image "enantiomer"). The naturally occurring form of POH is primarily the enantiomer with (S)-stereochemistry at the chiral center (which is the carbon atom having the substituents that are non-superimposable on their mirror image) (Scheme 1). Although the biological activity of the other mirror image (R)-enantiomer is, as yet, untested, most biological components and most biochemical processes involve single enantiomer stereochemistry such that it is likely that different enantiomers will interact differently with biological receptors and pathways. This is evident, for example (Scheme 1), with the terpenoid (R)-carvone (from spearmint oil), which, unsurprisingly, smells of spearmint, whilst its enantiomer (S)-carvone (from caraway or dill seed oil) exhibits the totally different odor of rye bread (which is flavored by caraway seeds) due to the carvones' stereochemically differentiated interactions with the chiral olfactory receptors in our nasal cavities [33,34].

Scheme 1 shows the biosynthesis and chemical structures of these aforementioned terpenoid materials. Note that the stereochemistry in this reaction scheme (for example illustrated by the limonene enantiomer intermediates in the biosynthesis of POH and carvones) may be designated by (+)/(−), D/L, or (R)/(S), which can be confusing. (R) and (S) are determined from the 3-D chemical structure, where (R) denotes the enantiomer with the hydrogen (H) substituent on the chiral carbon atom oriented to lie backward away from the viewer and the other substituents arranged clockwise in descending order of priority (atomic weight), whilst the (S) enantiomer is the mirror image of the (R) enantiomer. The D designation refers to the stereochemistry derived by chemical synthesis from D-glyceraldehyde and vice versa for L. Meanwhile, the (+) or (−) refer to the direction of rotation of plane-polarized light by a solution of the material where (+) implies clockwise rotation of plane-polarized light and (−) denotes the opposite. Suffice to say that there is no reliable general rule to predict the correlation of (R) vs. (S) with D or L and with (+) or (−) [35].

POH is classified as a cyclic monoterpenoid (where the monoterpene designation refers to its biosynthesis from a single geranyl pyrophosphate moiety, shown in Scheme 1, followed by oxidation of the terpene backbone while catalyzed by cytochrome P450 enzyme to achieve the terminal hydroxylation; hence, the designation "terpenoid" rather than "terpene"). Its molecular weight is 152.2 g/mol, which is about 2.5 times the molecular weight of, for example, acetic acid in vinegar; therefore, it is a lot less volatile than acetic acid (boiling point 118–119 °C at atmospheric pressure), with a consequently higher boiling temperature of 244 °C at atmospheric pressure, but it still exerts sufficient vapor pressure and active interaction with our olfactory biochemistry to be easily detected by smell. The polar hydroxyl functionality makes the molecule more hydrophilic (i.e., water miscible) than non-hydroxylated equivalent terpenes, such as pinenes, which are water immiscible, such that POH does demonstrate some limited solubility in water (around 1.9 mg/mL) and a mix of lipophilic (fat solubility) and hydrophilic (water solubility) properties. It is this biphilic (or amphiphilic) nature (both fat and water affinity) that perhaps explains the remarkable properties of POH in achieving essentially free passage throughout the body, across the blood–brain barrier, and across cell membranes to realize its therapeutic potential and to potentiate the therapeutic potential of other materials with which it is partnered.

Whilst nature does an astonishingly efficient job at converting carbon dioxide, water, sunlight, and air to POH via biosynthesis in plants, the POH so generated is present in a cocktail with other products; as such, this POH is unsuitable for pharmaceutical use without costly and extensive purification. This is because regulatory approval for pharmaceutical use requires consistent high-purity composition to verify safety and efficacy, without risk of any changes in composition that could introduce toxicity risks or variation in therapeutic efficacy that may imply potential risks to patients. Industrial manufacturing of POH therefore generally relies upon a combination of biosynthetically produced high-purity, low-cost (-)-beta-pinene, with subsequent industrial manufacturing conversion of this to POH, i.e., utilizing a "semi-synthetic" preparation. An example is outlined in Scheme 2 [36]. Chemistry along these lines is used for the industrial manufacture of POH at around 95% purity for perfume and antimicrobial purposes. Furthermore, the ability of bacterial enzymes to modify the monoterpene backbone has been exploited for the production of "natural" aromas for the flavor and fragrance industries, where suitably genetically engineered bacterial strains are used as a source of POH and other known and novel monoterpene derivatives [37–39]. For pharmaceutical use, however, even higher purity and consistency of composition are ideally required so that derivatization of POH is developed to generate a crystalline dinitrobenzoate ester intermediate (which is more easily purifiable by crystallization), followed by hydrolysis to release the purified POH (Scheme 3) [40]. The POH manufactured in this way was named NEO100 and is undergoing clinical trials for the treatment of glioblastoma (see details in sections below).

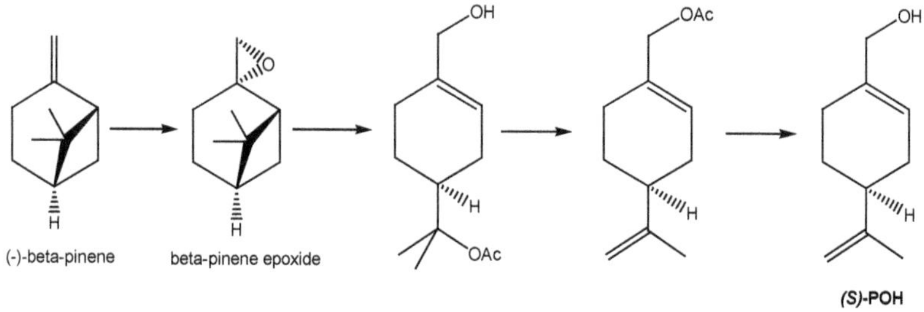

Scheme 2. Semi-synthetic manufacture of POH. An example of semi-synthetic industrial manufacture of POH from pine oil, whereby (-)-beta pinene is epoxidized by treatment with peracetic acid; the beta-pinene epoxide is then rearranged with sodium acetate in acetic acid to give POH with acetic acid added across the isopropylene substituent, and acetic acid is subsequently eliminated via pyrolysis. A final hydrolysis step gives (S)-POH.

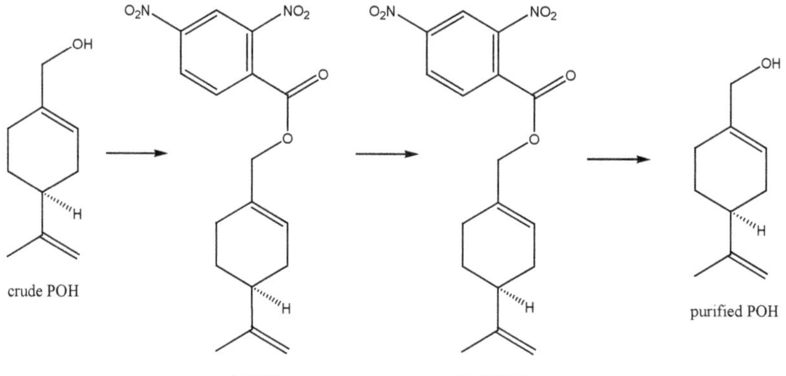

Scheme 3. Purification of POH for pharmaceutical use. Commercial or industrial POH can be further purified from contaminating related substances for pharmaceutical use by converting the POH to a solid dinitrobenzoate ester derivative, which can be purified via recrystallization and isolation from the impurities left in recrystallization mother liquors before the purified nitrobenzoate ester is then hydrolyzed to give purified POH, from which the unwanted dinitrobenzoic acid is removed via aqueous extraction under alkaline conditions. This extra purification step leads to the synthesis of NEO100 (NeOnc Technologies, Los Angeles, CA, USA).

2.2. Recognizing POH's Potential for Anticancer Purposes

The earliest studies that explored the potential of POH for anticancer purposes were spearheaded by the team of Michael Gould, Jill Haag, Pamela Crowell, and others at the University of Wisconsin–Madison in Madison, Wisconsin [41–43]. Using a rat carcinogenesis model with 7,12-dimethylbenz(a)anthrazene (DMBA)-initiated mammary tumors, it was shown that 2% POH mixed with a daily diet (*w*/*w*) over 10 weeks resulted in regression of the majority of small and advanced mammary carcinomas [43]. Of note, the authors compared the activity of POH side by side to that of limonene and observed greater activity of the former, which they ascribed, at least in part, to differences in metabolic pharmacokinetics, where an acute dose of 2% POH achieved 2–3 times higher levels of terpene metabolites (primarily perillic acid and dihydroperillic acid) in the plasma of the treated rats as compared to rats fed 10% limonene. Similarly, when POH and limonene were dosed chronically at the same levels, the terpene metabolites were measured at >10-fold higher plasma levels in the case of POH. In parallel studies that compared the inhibitory activity of POH and limonene on the isoprenylation of small G proteins (details below), it was found that POH was greater than fivefold more potent than limonene [42]. Therefore, despite numerous earlier reports on the oncotherapeutic properties of limonene [44–47], these newer studies favored POH for further development and clinical trials (details below).

2.3. Mechanisms of POH Anticancer Function

The first cellular target of POH to be identified was the process of isoprenylation of small G proteins, where POH and, to a lesser extent, limonene were found to inhibit small G protein isoprenylation, along with restricted cell proliferation [41,42,48,49]. In particular, the inhibition of farnesylation of p21-Ras generated excitement in view of the recognized critical role of this proto-oncoprotein in cell growth regulation and carcinogenesis [50–52]. A critical step during the activation process of Ras is its posttranslational modification via farnesylation, providing an anchor for attachment of the protein to the inner leaflet of the cytoplasmic membrane, which is critically required for the protein's mitogenic and oncogenic activity [53]. The discovery that this process could be inhibited by POH provided early insight into how this monoterpenoid might interfere with tumor cell growth [48,51,54]. Besides Ras, however, numerous additional targets were recognized over the years that followed and it appears that the anticancer function of POH might be derived from its influence over a variety of different targets and processes in cancer cells.

Several studies reported on the ability of POH to restrict the cell cycle progression of tumor cells through its effects on components of the cell cycle machinery. For instance, treatment of cells with POH in vitro results in the downregulation of various cyclin proteins, which represent the regulatory subunits of cyclin-dependent kinases (CDKs) whose activity is essential for cell cycle progression. Conversely, POH stimulates the expression of CDK-inhibitory proteins p15 (INK4b, *CDKN2B*), p21 (WAF/Cip1, *CDKN1A*), and p27 (Kip1, *CDKN1B*), all of which are able to block CDK activity [55–58]. The ensuing cell cycle arrest prevents tumor cell proliferation in vitro, translating to the inhibition of tumor growth in vivo.

A host of other cellular targets of POH were identified, including immediate-early genes c-Fos and c-Jun (which heterodimerize to form transcription factor AP1) [55,59]; telomerase reverse transcriptase (hTERT) [60,61]; eukaryotic translation initiation factors eIF4E and eIF4G, along with their binding partner 4E-BP1 (key components of the translational cap-binding complex) [62,63]; sodium/potassium adenosine triphosphatase (Na/K-ATPase) [64,65]; Notch (which plays a role in tumor cell invasion and metastasis) [66]; nuclear factor kappa B (NF-κB) [67–69]; mammalian target of rapamycin complex (mTORC) [61,70]; and transforming growth factor beta (TGFβ) [55]. Furthermore, POH was characterized as an effective trigger of endoplasmic reticulum (ER) stress, which was revealed through its ability to stimulate the expression of two ER stress markers, CCAAT/enhancer-binding protein homologous protein (CHOP, also known as GADD153) and glucose-regulated protein of molecular weight 78 kDa (GRP78, also known as BiP) [71]. CHOP represents the key pro-apoptotic effector of ER stress [72], and its prominently increased expression in response to the treatment of tumor cells with POH is consistent with resulting cell death. The tumor-selective impact of POH (and of other agents that are able to aggravate cellular stress levels) via the ER stress response was conjectured to be based on pre-existing, chronic stress levels in tumor cells, which are lacking in normal cells. In tumor cells, aggravated stress reaches the maximum tolerated threshold quicker, whereas normal cells have more leeway to accommodate and therefore tolerate these increased levels [73,74].

While a plethora of cellular POH targets was identified, the decisive contribution of each one has not yet been clearly established. It is likely that some targets are more critical than others, and cell-type-specific availability of some targets might factor in as well. Furthermore, in view of multiple alterations that are generally acquired during the carcinogenic process of tumor cell development, a pleiotropic impact on tumor cell functions might in fact be desirable and beneficial to achieve improved therapeutic outcomes.

3. Clinical Evaluation of Oral POH

Based on the well-documented, highly promising anticancer functions of POH that were characterized in a variety of preclinical in vitro and in vivo models, the agent was moved forward to clinical trials in humans. In the first of these trials [75], 18 patients with advanced malignancies received POH that was formulated in soft gelatin capsules containing 250 mg POH mixed with 250 mg soybean oil. Dosing was by mouth three times a day, every day, at escalating doses of up 2400 $mg/m^2/dose$ (approximately 4 g POH in 16 capsules per dose for a 60 kg patient; 12 g total per day). POH was generally tolerated, with gastrointestinal (GI) toxicities as the most frequent events, presenting as nausea, belching, vomiting, unpleasant taste, and early satiety, which were correlated with increasing dose levels and proved dose-limiting. Pharmacokinetic plasma measurements were able to quantify the major metabolites perillic acid and dihydro-perillic acid [75] but did not detect the parent compound POH, consistent with earlier studies in POH-fed rats that easily detected the terpene metabolites but not POH itself [43]. The metabolite half-lives were approximately 2 h and there was no evidence of drug or metabolite accumulation [75], which spawned the rationale to spread drug administration more evenly in the hopes of achieving greater exposure by increasing the dosing frequency. Therefore, in a subsequent Phase I trial, the dosing frequency was increased to four times a day at up to 1600 $mg/m^2/dose$ [76]. Similar GI toxicities as before were noted, and the maximum tolerated dose of POH was determined as 1200 $mg/m^2/dose$ (approximately 8 g total per patient per day from 32 capsules per day), which was recommended as the starting dose for Phase II studies.

Several Phase II trials with oral POH followed in cohorts of patients with advanced ovarian cancer [77], metastatic prostate cancer [78], metastatic breast cancer [79], metastatic androgen-independent pancreatic cancer [80], and metastatic colorectal cancer [81]. Dosing was four times each day for an initially planned 6-month period. As in the previous Phase I studies, the toxicity was mild to moderate and primarily limited to GI effects and fatigue, although there was significant variability in patient responses. Overall, however, the therapeutic activity of POH was unimpressive and mostly disappointing. Furthermore, while GI toxicity was not unacceptably severe based on common clinical criteria, the chronic and unrelenting nature of these effects caused problems with patient tolerance and compliance to the point where some patients discontinued their participation in these trials [77,78,81]. These results dampened the enthusiasm that was generated by the highly promising preclinical studies of POH and, so far, no Phase III clinical trials of orally administered POH have been initiated [82]. A newer route of administration, dosing POH intranasally rather than orally (so as to avoid the GI-related side effects), has revived some of the lost excitement and has sparked new hope that POH might still find its place among new and improved clinically used cancer therapeutics. The efforts to establish intranasal POH as a beneficial cancer treatment, in particular for cancer types in the brain that are protected by the BBB, are described below.

4. Intranasal Perillyl Alcohol

Intranasal drug delivery represents a non-invasive route of administration with several advantages over oral drug delivery. Although the extent of these advantages may differ significantly, based on the specifics of the delivery methods, drug formulation, and physicochemical properties of the active pharmacological ingredient (API), they usually include quicker biological availability, avoidance of hepatic first-pass metabolism, and potentially less systemic side effects. Moreover, the potential for direct nose-to-brain transport offers the prospect of increased central nervous system (CNS) drug availability by side-stepping the BBB [83–85].

As outlined in Figure 1, after drugs have entered the nasal cavity, there are four main routes by which such drugs may reach the brain [83,86–88]: (#1) Direct nose-to-brain transport is offered through drug absorption by the olfactory bulb and through drug uptake by branches of the trigeminal nerve. This pathway is of particular interest for purposes of delivering drugs aimed at the brain, because it does not involve the drawbacks of having to overcome the BBB. (#2) Extensive vascularization of the nasal epithelium and a rich lymphatic network are conducive to effective drug uptake that will deliver the drug into the systemic circulation. However, subsequent brain uptake by this path will be subjected to the limitations of having to cross the BBB. (#3) Intranasally delivered drugs may also be inhaled or aspirated into the lungs, in particular when APIs are formulated as aerosols. From here, they effectively enter the bloodstream, only to again encounter the BBB as an obstacle on their way to the brain. (#4) Postnasal drip and mucociliary clearance result in drug transport to the GI tract. Depending on the lipophilicity of the drug and other properties, the API may continue through the portal vein and liver, or via intestinal lymphatic transport. The route via the portal vein poses the additional challenge of substantial drug metabolism, which may result in effective drug inactivation. In both these cases, the drug ends up in the systemic circulation and encounters the BBB.

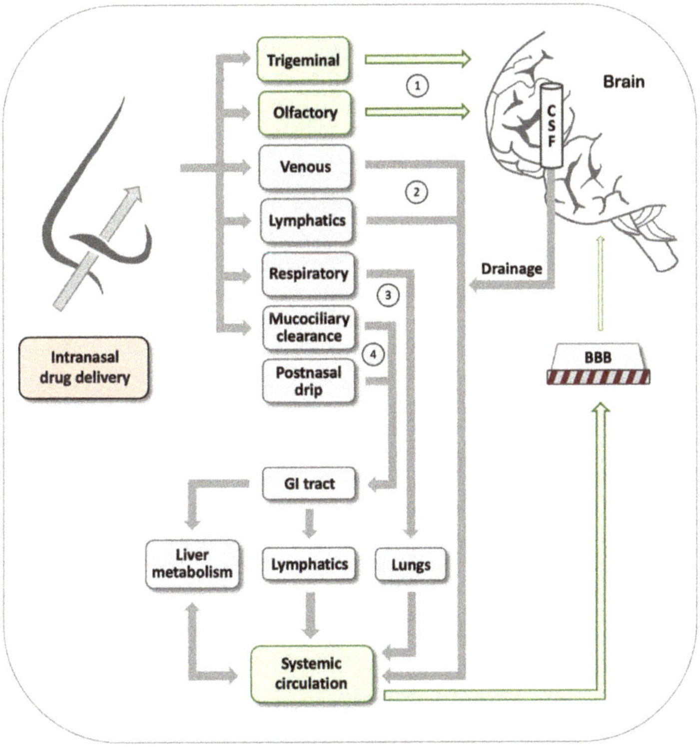

Figure 1. Available routes for intranasal drug delivery. After intranasal delivery, drugs can potentially reach the brain through several quite distinct routes: either through direct nose-to-brain transport via the trigeminal and olfactory nerves (labeled as 1), or indirectly via first entering the bloodstream through the mechanisms labeled as 2–4. In the latter routes, however, drugs will encounter the BBB, which prevents efficient brain entry of the vast majority of pharmaceutical agents. See the text for further details.

Comparing the above four pathways illustrates the potential advantages of intranasal drug delivery. Only the first one, i.e., direct nose-to-brain transport, has the potential for direct delivery to the brain without encountering the obstacle placed by the BBB. While the efficiency of this route is very low in general and can be as low as 0.01–1% of the oral dosage [83] (depending in large part on biopharmaceutical formulation and physicochemical properties of the API [88,89]), this small amount can nevertheless prove advantageous over oral delivery due to avoidance of potentially inefficient absorption and elimination in the GI tract, hepatic first-pass metabolism, and dilution and protein binding in the bloodstream. Furthermore, several oral CNS drugs barely penetrate the BBB and, therefore, must be given at increased dosages that raise the risk for adverse effects in the periphery. This latter consideration applies to parenteral injections of drugs as well, further emphasizing the potential advantages of intranasal delivery. For further reading, see the following excellent reviews: [83,84,90,91].

4.1. *Intranasal POH as Monotherapy*

While several Phase I and II clinical trials of oral POH, as described above, yielded disappointing results and never moved into Phase III [92], a case report published in 2006 [93] stimulated renewed interest in POH by way of intranasal delivery. This report described a 62-year-old woman in Brazil with histologically confirmed anaplastic oligodendroglioma, a malignant grade III glioma. Despite standard combination therapy with surgery, radiotherapy, and chemotherapy, she presented with a second recurrency, at which time, intranasal POH (obtained from Sigma-Aldrich/MilliporeSigma, St. Louis, Missouri, USA) was initiated at 0.3% concentration and four times daily dosing. After 5 months of treatment, a follow-up MRI revealed regression of the tumor [93].

Based on this positive outcome, intranasal POH delivery was further investigated in additional relapsed glioma patients. A follow-up study reported on a small cohort of 37 patients with recurrent high-grade glioma, where the same four-times-daily POH regimen was administered intranasally (55 mg per dose for 220 mg total per day) [94]. Here as well, it was reported that this novel treatment strategy resulted in encouraging outcomes, with decreased tumor size (Figure 2) and increased survival in several patients. Further expansion of these studies included several hundred recurrent patients with malignant glioma, including GBM, and dosing was further increased to 133 mg per dose (533 mg/day) [95,96]. Overall, these Phase I/II studies further indicated the encouraging therapeutic activity of intranasal POH, with numerous patients remaining under clinical remission even after several years of exclusive POH treatment. Of note, despite the four-times-daily dosing, this regimen was very well tolerated and adverse events were almost non-existent, contributing to very high patient compliance [96].

The above studies were performed in Brazil and are in part still ongoing. Despite the inclusion of hundreds of patients and numerous encouraging observations, limitations include the absence of an independent Contract Research Organization (CRO) for external clinical data management and trial monitoring. Inspired by the promising Brazilian experience, a Phase I/IIa study with recurrent GBM patients was initiated in the United States (ClinicalTrials.gov identifier: NCT02704858) and the results from the Phase I part were published in early 2021 [97]. For this trial, POH had to be produced for pharmaceutical use under CGMP regulations, which yielded a highly pure (>99%) product that was labeled NEO100 (see Scheme 3). The dose finding in Phase I used four cohorts of three patients each and escalated the four-times-daily dose up to a maximum of 288 mg, for a total of 1152 mg/day, which represented roughly double the dosage used in the Brazilian trials.

This new study [97] found that intranasal NEO100 was very well tolerated, consistent with the earlier Brazilian trials' findings. Among the 12 patients in Phase I, there were no grade 3 or 4 adverse events (based on NCI Common Terminology Criteria for Adverse Events [98]). Among the few lower-grade events defined as "definitely treatment-related" were rhinorrhea, skin irritation around the nose, nasal pruritus, and cough, which were observed in a minority of patients. Intriguingly, the frequency of these events did not correlate with increased dosages and, in fact, most of them were observed at the lowest dosage. It was concluded that intranasal delivery of NEO100 to recurrent GBM patients is safe [97] and free from the problematic side effects suffered from oral dosing.

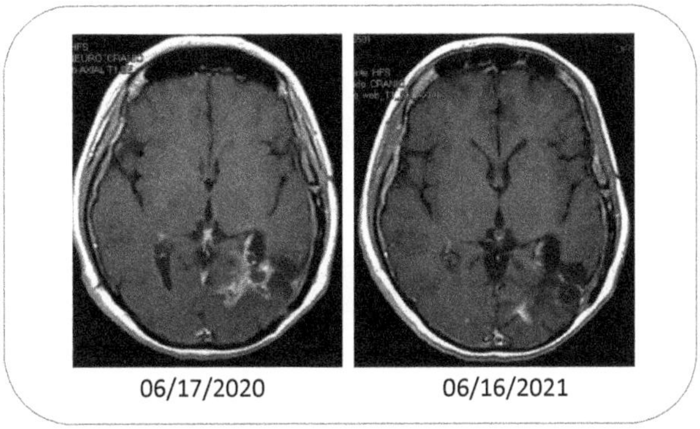

Figure 2. MRIs showing the effect of inhaling POH in a patient with relapsed GBM. Note the tumor tissue in the initial MRI on 06/17/2020, as indicated by intense non-homogeneous enhancement. One year later (06/16/2021), the lesions presented with reduced dimensions and a marked reduction in contrast enhancement, suggesting a response to the POH treatment. While these MRIs present an illustrative example derived from the group of patients who responded favorably to intranasal POH and achieved stable disease status, not all patients responded similarly well, with some patients progressing after the initial response, despite continuous treatment.

Although Phase IIa of this trial is still ongoing, further analysis of Phase I data sought to provide preliminary insight into the activity of intranasal NEO100, which was determined based on radiographic responses, i.e., magnetic resonance imaging (MRI) performed every two months. Despite the small cohort of only 12 patients, there were intriguing signs of therapeutic benefit. Overall survival at 12 months (OS-12) was 55%, median OS was 15 months, and two-year survival was 37%. These results compared favorably with historical controls and other recent trials with cohorts of recurrent GBM patients (Figure 3) [99–102]. For example, a 2018 retrospective [102] reviewed the clinical experience with bevacizumab, an anti-angiogenic monoclonal antibody that is approved for recurrent malignant glioma [103]. This analysis showed that therapy with bevacizumab yielded an OS-12 of 49%, median OS of 11 months, and two-year survival of 15%. A randomized Phase III trial with 65 recurrent GBM patients who received lomustine (also known as CCNU, a nitrosourea-based DNA alkylating agent commonly used in the recurrent GBM setting [104]), yielded an OS-12 of 30% and 2-year survival of below 4% [100]. Among such comparisons, it remains noteworthy to emphasize the lack of serious adverse events with the use of intranasal POH/NEO100, which is not the case for the majority of other commonly used therapies applied to recurrent GBM. Thus, even if there are only relatively small increments in survival in comparison to other regimens, quality of life (QoL) issues need to be factored into treatment decisions as well. Furthermore, maintenance of QoL for longer periods may increase the chances that further salvage therapies could be considered subsequent to a later recurrence (given enhanced patient strength and robustness for additional therapies compared with the outcomes after more debilitating conventional cytotoxic treatments).

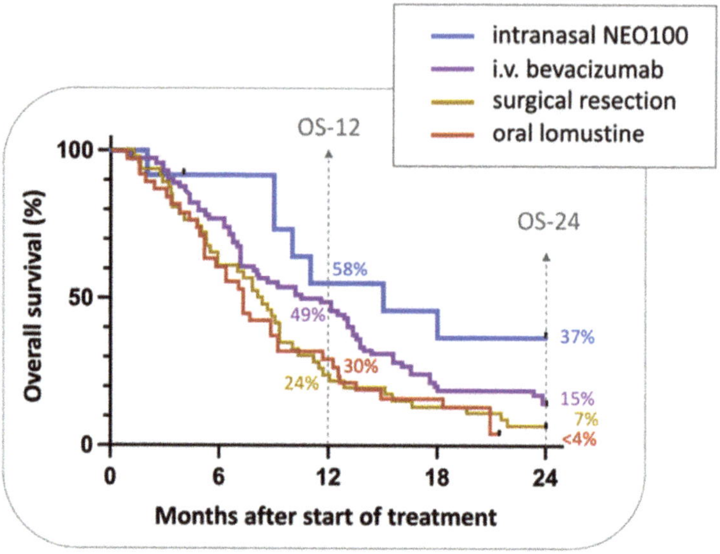

Figure 3. Comparison of the overall survival of recurrent GBM patients. Shown are the Kaplan–Meier curves representing the probability of survival of recurrent GBM patients undergoing different treatment regimens. The blue line indicates results for intranasal POH/NEO100 treatment (n = 12) obtained from a Phase I study [97]. The purple line represents a single-institution retrospective of the clinical real-world experience with bevacizumab (n = 74) [102]. The gold line is a historical comparison from 1998 that monitored the survival of patients after surgical resection of recurrent tumors (n = 46) [99]. The red line represents data from a randomized Phase III trial published in 2013 [100], where patients (n = 65) received lomustine. Percentages shown in the graph refer to the OS-12 and 2-year survival (OS-24) of the different treatment regimens after diagnosis of recurrence.

As with most cancer therapies, efforts are underway to establish predictors of response to intranasal therapy with POH. One such study indicated that patients with recurrent GBM and treated with intranasal POH survived significantly longer when tumors were located deep in the basal ganglia as compared to lobar localization [105]. Another study provided preliminary evidence that those recurrent GBM patients harboring a hypermethylated tumor phenotype and preferential concurrent polymorphism for the thymidine-thymidine (TT) variant of *rs1801133* of the methylene-tetrahydrofolate reductase (MTHFR) gene appeared to respond more favorably to intranasal POH, as indicated by prolonged survival [106]. Furthermore, isocitrate dehydrogenase 1 (IDH1) and IDH2 are emerging as potentially useful markers [107]. Specific mutations in either of these genes result in a neomorphic phenotype of the encoded protein, where enzymatic activity switches from the production of alpha-ketoglutarate to the synthesis of D-2-hydroxyglutarate [108]. In the case of newly diagnosed malignant glioma, such mutations in either IDH1 or IDH2 result in a better prognosis irrespective of the selected treatment approach [109], although this has not yet been firmly established for recurrent GBM [110]. Data from the above-described Phase I trial of NEO100 were separated into IDH-wild type and IDH-mutant cases, which revealed pronounced survival advantage for those intranasal NEO100-treated patients that harbored IDH-mutant tumors [97]. Due to the small cohort in this study, it remains to be established whether this survival advantage is primarily based on IDH status (and possibly enhanced by NEO100) or whether intranasal NEO100 contributes the decisive benefit. The currently ongoing Phase IIa part of this study is expected to provide clarification.

In the meantime, other ongoing studies are building on the highly promising results obtained with intranasal POH by exploring respective combination approaches. For instance, a case study [111] reported a 51-year-old woman with inoperable GBM who had recurred after standard treatment with TMZ-based chemoradiotherapy and subsequently was enrolled in a clinical trial of intranasal POH concomitant with oral TMZ. After initiation of POH + TMZ, MRI scans revealed a marked reduction of the initially enhanced lesion, and no recurrences were noted over the following two years. This provided an encouraging example where the combination approach appeared to demonstrate benefit in this case of non-resected recurrent GBM. Other efforts sought to explore the combination of intranasal POH with dietary interventions. In one such study [112], 32 recurrent GBM patients were enrolled and divided into two groups, one where intranasal POH was combined with a ketogenic diet (KD) and one where intranasal POH was given without any specific dietary intervention. After 90 days of treatment, the average tumor area in the combination group showed greater reduction as compared to baseline at time 0, suggesting more effective therapeutic activity. A similar approach, this time with 29 recurrent GBM patients and combined with a low carbohydrate diet (LCD) also showed a trend for the greater activity of intranasal POH when combined with an LCD [113].

Collectively, the above studies established POH as the best-studied intranasally delivered anticancer agent. As of 2021, there are patients who have been using this regimen uninterrupted for many years, indicating the prospect that this form of circumventing the BBB might be able to convert a deadly disease to a chronic one, at least in some of the patients.

Among the challenges of studying brain-targeted delivery of POH has been the difficulty of performing neuro-pharmacokinetic measurements of this compound. As mentioned above in the context of clinical trials with oral POH, PK measurements of blood levels relied on the quantification of the stable metabolite perillic acid because POH was not detectable with the analytical methods used. However, more sensitive and optimized approaches have become available. For instance, Zhang et al. reported on their detection of intact POH and perillic acid in plasma from a patient after oral delivery of POH using gas chromatographic–mass spectrometry (GC-MS) [114]. In studies with mice or rats, other groups applied ultra-performance liquid chromatography/tandem mass spectrometry (UPLC-MS/MS) [115] or high-performance liquid chromatography (HPLC)–ultraviolet (UV)-based approaches [116] to quantitate POH (and perillic acid) in the plasma and lungs of animals after intranasal delivery of POH. In a very recent study that investigated the impact of intranasal POH in a mouse model of cerebral malaria, the authors succeeded in quantifying POH in brain tissue using GC-MS [117]. Using a rat model, Nehra et al. quantitated POH (and perillic acid) levels in plasma and cerebrospinal fluid (CSF) after intranasal and intravascular POH delivery [118]. Very interestingly, this group was able to demonstrate that intranasal administration of POH resulted in tenfold higher CSF-to-plasma ratios for POH and perillic acid as compared to what was achieved after an equal dose of POH was administered intravascularly. While neuro-PK data are not yet available from patients, the results from these preclinical studies further indicate that intranasal administration of POH results in direct nose-to-brain delivery, further underscoring the potential value of this mode of drug delivery for brain cancer therapy.

4.2. Intranasal POH as a Co-Delivery System

Co-delivery systems for drug delivery come in many designs. They may comprise carriers, where one or more drugs are packaged into liposomes, nanoparticles, hydrogels, dendrimers, or other vehicles [119,120], and some of these are being developed specifically for the purpose of intranasal delivery to reach the brain via the nose-to-brain route [121,122]. Studies with POH have also revealed characteristics that make this monoterpenoid suitable for the purpose of transporting other drugs directly to the brain via the nose-to-brain route.

For instance, the intranasal delivery of NEO100, in combination with bortezomib, was investigated in rodent models of GBM [123]. Bortezomib (Velcade®) is a proteasome inhibitor that was approved to treat multiple myeloma and mantle cell lymphoma [124]. Its penetration of the BBB is extremely poor [125], which is consistent with its demonstrated lack of therapeutic effect in mouse GBM models [126,127] or when tested in the clinic with recurrent glioma patients [128–130] after intravenous delivery. In stark contrast, bortezomib showed high activity in mouse models of orthotopic GBM when it was delivered directly into the tumor using an Alzet pump [127], and at low nanomolar concentrations against glioma cells in vitro [131–133]. Collectively, these observations indicate that, in principle, bortezomib can be highly effective against GBM, but in reality, this benefit cannot be realized due to the agent's inability to penetrate the BBB. In an attempt to circumvent this obstacle, bortezomib was mixed with NEO100 and delivered intranasally to mice harboring xenografted human GBM cells in their brains. Results from this study [123] demonstrated that the co-delivery of bortezomib with NEO100 significantly prolonged the survival of tumor-bearing animals as compared to untreated mice, mice receiving intranasal bortezomib in the absence of NEO100, or mice receiving bortezomib via intravenous infusion. Furthermore, the authors were able to demonstrate substantially greater amounts of bortezomib in the cerebrospinal fluid (CSF) of rats after treatment with the bortezomib/NEO100 combination than after treatment with bortezomib alone. Together, these studies provided proof of principle that a pharmacologic agent with very poor BBB penetration can effectively be delivered to the brain by using a NEO100-based formulation and intranasal delivery, where the amphiphilic physicochemical properties of NEO100 serve to increase permeation of both components through the BBB and cell membranes.

5. Intra-Arterial Perillyl Alcohol

While intranasal applications of POH and NEO100 exploit direct nose-to-brain access routes and thereby circumvent the obstacle placed by the BBB, an intra-arterial path of administering NEO100 has provided evidence that it also can directly confront the BBB and "open" it, i.e., diminish its barrier function to enable mostly unrestricted permeation of otherwise BBB-impermeable compounds. This procedure is being explored and characterized in preclinical models and might have certain advantages over the currently established clinical method of opening the BBB with mannitol.

Intracarotid injection of mannitol has been used for the past three decades as a means to reversibly open the BBB. Its disruptive mechanism is based on the contraction of endothelial cells and the resulting widening of tight junctions as a result of the hyperosmotic impact of high concentrations of this sugar alcohol. However, this procedure has led to variable responses in BBB breakdown, seizures, risk of brain embolism, and catastrophic bleeds [134,135]. As a result, the use of this procedure is restricted to specialized centers, has not found widespread acceptance, and does not lend itself to use in general clinical practice. Similarly, the effects of radiation on BBB permeability have long been recognized [136] and are thought to impact BBB integrity through the killing of endothelial cells and resulting neuro-inflammatory reactions [137]. However, many details, including the time course and magnitude of increased opening, remain to be established [138]. A more recently introduced BBB disruption technique is transcranial-focused ultrasound coupled with intravenously delivered microbubbles [139], which has advanced to clinical trials [140,141]. This procedure disrupts the BBB through cavitation and acoustic forces, leading to reduced expression of tight junction proteins, along with an inflammatory response. However, it represents a rather invasive procedure because the skull needs to be opened in order to introduce the ultrasound probe that triggers BBB permeation. Overall, despite progress in the development of new procedures, the need for safer, more efficient, and reversible BBB-opening methods persists [142].

Based on the use of preclinical models, intra-arterial injection of NEO100 was very recently presented as a novel BBB-disruptive method [143,144]. In these studies, intra-arterial injections of NEO100 were accomplished via ultrasound-guided intracardiac injections in mouse models, which resulted in rapid BBB opening that lasted up to four hours. During this window of opportunity, intravenously delivered agents were able to effectively enter the brain. For instance, Evans blue present in the systemic circulation was shown to prominently stain mouse brains blue after NEO100-induced BBB opening. This effect was not achieved via intra-arterial injection of a vehicle without NEO100, nor in cases where NEO100 was injected intravenously instead of intra-arterially (possibly due to dilution by the circulatory system and surrounding tissue). The mechanism of action of NEO100-induced BBB opening was demonstrated to be secondary to transient downregulation of specific gap junction proteins, resulting in short-term, fully reversible breakdown of barrier function [143,144]. Similar outcomes were seen with the non-BBB-permeable anticancer drug methotrexate, which accumulated to high levels in brain tissue and CSF after NEO100-induced BBB opening. Intriguingly, increased brain entry was not limited to small therapeutic molecules, such as methotrexate, but could also be documented for therapeutic antibodies, e.g., a checkpoint-inhibitory anti-PD1 antibody and the anti-HER2 antibody trastuzumab, and even for whole cells, using chimeric antigen receptor (CAR) T cells as a model [144]. Furthermore, these authors provided proof of principle that NEO100-based BBB opening is able to achieve therapeutic benefit in mouse models of intracranially implanted HER2+ breast cancer cells [143]. Mice harboring such tumors were subjected to a single round of intra-arterial injection of NEO100, along with intravenous delivery of trastuzumab or the trastuzumab-drug conjugate ado-trastuzumab emtansine (T-DM1; Kadcyla®). There was a tumor-selective accumulation of these therapeutic antibodies in the brain and significantly prolonged survival of mice receiving this treatment.

With regard to translating the above preclinical results to patient applications, it was proposed [143] that patients with intracranial malignancies would be subjected to standard interventional neuroradiology that would allow for selective delivery of NEO100 to tumor-feeding intracranial arteries. Intra-arterial injections would be performed via cannulation of the femoral artery with selective threading toward one of the cerebral arteries. This transfemoral approach [145–147] represents a common, straightforward procedure in a variety of clinical settings and is generally considered a safe procedure [148–150]. It is routinely performed by endovascular neurosurgeons in the context of cerebral angiograms, aneurysm coiling, tumor embolization, and thrombectomies [151]. Combining this transfemoral approach with NEO100 as the injectate has not yet been tested in the clinic. However, if the safety of transient BBB opening with this approach could be confirmed, it would have far-reaching implications. It would provide a significantly safer alternative to intracarotid mannitol, its use would not be restricted to specialized medical centers, and its application would expand to include the treatment of many neurological diseases beyond intracranial malignancies.

6. Perillyl Alcohol Derivatives, Analogs, and Conjugates

Based on the recognition of POH's suitable physicochemical properties in combination with its anticancer activity, numerous studies have explored whether alterations and modifications of this molecule might result in enhanced therapeutic activity. For instance, the glycosylation of drugs can often significantly alter their pharmacological properties and ADMET (absorption, distribution, metabolism, excretion, and toxicity) [152]. Glycosides of POH exist in nature and some of them were initially characterized as aldose reductase inhibitors [153]. Additional unnatural POH derivatives were synthesized and tested for their potential anticancer activity [154–156]. For instance, Nandurkar et al. [155] generated a group of 34 POH glycosides that were tested for their antiproliferative activity against two established cancer cell lines in vitro. This group identified several new compounds that exerted greater in vitro cytotoxicity than POH, with POH 4′-azido-D-glucoside as the most potent POH adduct. Similarly, a series of cyclodiprenyl phenols were synthesized from perillyl alcohol and synthetic phenols, and some of these meroterpenes showed strong antiproliferative and apoptosis-inducing activity against three different cancer cell lines in vitro [157]. POH was also complexed with β-cyclodextrin, which resulted in improved anticancer potency in vitro and in a sarcoma S180-induced mouse model in vivo [158]. Beyond these selected examples, several more reports on modified POH (or perillic acid) molecules exist, and the interested reader is referred to excellent recent reviews [159,160] for additional information and detailed references.

Some hybrid drugs are generated as multifunctional compounds, where two or more molecules with already well-characterized pharmacologic activity are conjugated through a stable or metabolizable linker. The central rationale of associating these pharmacophores is to increase their potency, to possibly enable overall dosing at lower levels to minimize toxic side effects, and to reduce the likelihood of emerging drug resistance [161,162]. For example, it was investigated [163] whether linking POH to dihydropyrimidinones would generate increased anticancer impact. Dihydropyrimidinones are important heterocyclic compounds and, like POH, have revealed a large scope of pharmacological activities, including anticancer properties [164]. Fifteen novel perillyl–dihydropyrimidinone compounds were generated and some of them were found to effectively kill established ovarian cancer, melanoma, and glioblastoma cell lines, but spared a normal keratinocyte cell line [163]. The cytotoxic IC_{50} ratio between the keratinocyte cell line and the glioblastoma cell line was about 50, meaning that 50-fold higher drug concentrations were required to kill the normal cells as compared to the tumor cells, indicating promising cancer cell-selectivity of some of these novel compounds.

6.1. Conjugation with POH to Enhance Permeability

In a different approach toward generating POH-based multifunctional compounds, the group of Thomas Chen at the University of Southern California sought to exploit the amphipathic nature of POH to modify existing drugs toward increased penetration of biological barriers, in particular the BBB. Using software from Advanced Chemistry Development, Inc. (ACD Labs, Toronto, ON, Canada), to predict BBB penetration and brain entry of a given molecule, they performed in silico characterization of novel molecules, where POH was conjugated to pharmacologic agents of interest with the objective to identify therapeutics with superior ability to enter the brain.

6.1.1. POH Conjugated to Temozolomide (NEO212)

The so-far best-characterized hybrid molecule emerging from in silico studies of BBB penetration is NEO212 (Figure 4), consisting of POH covalently conjugated via a carbamate bond to TMZ, the alkylating agent in clinical use for GBM. NEO212 has been investigated in over a dozen studies that used a variety of preclinical in vitro and in vivo tumor models and consistently established the robust anticancer activity of this novel molecule, along with low toxicity [165–168] and superior ability to penetrate the BBB [169].

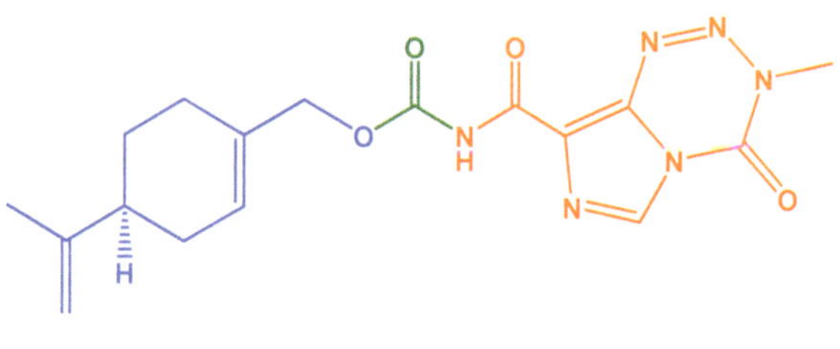

Figure 4. Chemical structure of a TMZ–POH conjugate (NEO212). NEO212 was generated by covalent conjugation of POH (perillyl alcohol; blue) to TMZ (temozolomide; orange) via a carbamate linkage (green).

Among the remarkable results was the finding that the NEO212 hybrid molecule exerted greater anticancer activity than an equimolar mix of its individual constituents, i.e., combining POH with TMZ—akin to the conventional combination therapy mode—was unable to achieve the same tumoricidal potency in vitro or in vivo as the conjugated molecule, indicating that the activity of the conjugated compound was greater than the sum of its parts [165–168,170]. For example, the effects of NEO212 were investigated in mouse brain tumor models of GBM [170,171] or intracranial breast cancer (to mimic brain-metastatic conditions) [165]. It was demonstrated that oral treatment with NEO212 exerted greater therapeutic activity than equivalent doses of TMZ or POH, either individually or when combined. When compared side by side and given at equal doses, the amount of NEO212 measured in brain tissue was threefold higher than the amount of TMZ [169], confirming the in silico results, where NEO212 was predicted to cross the BBB more efficiently than TMZ.

NEO212's superior penetration ability was not restricted to having the BBB as the target. Cellular membranes present important biological barriers too, and here, NEO212 revealed beneficial characteristics as well. In a key in vitro experiment, it was measured how much TMZ was present inside cells after treatment of cells with equal concentrations of either NEO212 or TMZ [169]. The results showed >10-fold higher intracellular TMZ levels when cells were treated with NEO212 as compared to treatment of cells with TMZ [169]. Similarly, the expected metabolite of TMZ breakdown, the relatively stable 5-aminoimidazole-4-carboxamide (AIC), was correspondingly elevated as well, indicating that NEO212-treated cells generated substantially more of the active, DNA-alkylating species than TMZ-treated cells. Overall, these observations are consistent with a model where the conjugation of POH to TMZ enables superior barrier penetration and consequential enhancement of the anticancer impact of the TMZ partner molecule, qualifying POH as a potent permeation enhancer.

Based on the highly efficient cellular uptake of NEO212, it was hypothesized [167] that NEO212 might also exert a beneficial impact on leukemic cancer types, where the encounter between drug and tumor cells might be more immediate and most conducive to optimal drug uptake. The veracity of this conjecture was tested in acute myeloid leukemia (AML) cells in vitro and in vivo, which included AML cell lines that were strongly resistant to cytosine arabinoside (AraC), the most commonly used chemotherapeutic agent for this disease [172]. The in vitro experiments showed potent cytotoxic activity of NEO212 at low micromolar concentrations, along with confirmation that TMZ and its breakdown product AIC were present at high levels inside NEO212-treated AML cells. The most striking results were generated when AML cells were implanted into immunocompromised mice, followed by short cycles of NEO212 treatment. In these in vivo experiments, the majority of NEO212-treated animals survived until the end of the observation period (300 days), while all vehicle-treated control animals succumbed to disease within a few weeks [167]. The same outcome was achieved with AraC-resistant AML cell lines. Although the authors did not verify whether the NEO212 treatment was eradicative, i.e., whether residual, potentially dormant tumor cells were still present after 300 days, they concluded that treatment was curative, because the long-term survivors continued to thrive in the absence of any signs of disease.

The strikingly impressive therapeutic activity of NEO212 in this preclinical leukemia model is consistent with the above-stated assessment of POH as a permeation enhancer, in this case, for conjugated TMZ as the partner. However, it raises the question of tumor specificity and toxic side effects because normal cells—bone marrow cells and white blood cells (WBC) in particular—might be as susceptible as tumor cells. In the case of TMZ, for example, myelosuppression is a well-recognized, dose-limiting side effect of treatment [173]. Surprisingly, however, detailed analysis of complete blood counts (CBC) from NEO212-treated mice, together with histopathology of bone marrow and several other organs, failed to reveal signs of toxicity in these compartments [165–168]. Instead, NEO212 appeared to be very well tolerated, even during extended treatment periods and escalated dosages [167]. While this wide therapeutic window observed in these preclinical studies bodes well for future clinical applications, the underlying determinants of tumor selectivity of NEO212 remain to be established.

6.1.2. POH Conjugated to Rolipram or 3-Bromopyruvate or Valproic Acid

Beyond NEO212, other POH-based conjugates emerged from in silico analysis using ACD Lab's software that predicted greater BBB penetration and possibly increased membrane permeation. NEO214 is a conjugate of POH and rolipram, a selective phosphodiesterase 4 (PDE4) inhibitor that was in clinical development as an anti-depressant in the 1990s. Although rolipram was never approved for marketing [174], it was considered for repurposing as an anticancer agent based on its recognized beneficial activity in preclinical cancer models [175,176]. In mouse models of intracranial glioblastoma, NEO214 revealed significant therapeutic activity [177], indicating that it was indeed able to effectively cross the BBB, as was predicted from the in silico analysis. Intriguingly, as was observed with NEO212, combination therapy with the individual components, i.e., POH mixed with rolipram, was unable to mimic the much stronger anticancer effects of the conjugated NEO214 molecule [177,178].

Another interesting observation was made with NEO218, a conjugate of POH and 3-bromopyruvate (3BP), a synthetic halogenated derivative of pyruvate that was also investigated as an anticancer agent [179]. Cellular uptake of 3BP is strictly dependent on the presence of a transmembrane transport protein mono-carboxylate transporter 1 (MCT-1), where cells lacking MCT-1 are resistant to the toxic impact of 3BP [180]. It was demonstrated that applying selective pressure to MCT-1-positive HCT116 colon carcinoma cells by exposing them to 3BP in vitro resulted in the elimination of transporter-positive cells, with the simultaneous emergence of an MCT-1-negative sub-population that displayed resistance to 3BP [181]. In comparison, NEO218 exerts its cytotoxic impact in the absence of MCT-1, i.e., the conjugation of POH to 3BP enabled cellular 3BP import across the cytoplasmic membrane without the need for an active transport mechanism. Consequently, treatment of HCT116 cells with NEO218 did not result in emergent resistant clones, because the loss of MCT-1 expression could not provide a survival advantage [181], providing an example of POH's applicability to minimize the emergence of cancer cell drug resistance during therapy.

Yet another conjugate, NEO216, which is POH covalently linked to valproic acid (VPA), was preliminarily characterized. Compared to VPA, a well-known inhibitor of histone deacetylase (HDAC) activity [182], NEO216 showed reduced HDAC inhibition properties but revealed an ability to inhibit 4-aminobutyrate aminotransferase (ABAT), a key enzyme responsible for the catabolism of the neurotransmitter gamma-aminobutyric acid (GABA) [183]. This novel function has made NEO216 useful for a recent study that established the role of GABA metabolism in leptomeningeal dissemination of medulloblastoma [183] and more applications of this novel conjugate are anticipated.

6.2. POH and Penetration of the Skin

Similar to intranasal delivery, transdermal drug delivery (TDD) is being explored as an alternative route to other modes of drug administration, as it too has certain advantages that include the avoidance of hepatic first-pass drug metabolism, reduced GI side effects, and good patient compliance. The key barrier to efficient TDD is presented by the stratum corneum, the outermost layer of the epidermis that can severely limit percutaneous drug absorption [184,185]. To overcome this barrier, a great variety of chemical compounds have been investigated for their use as potential skin penetration enhancers, i.e., as promoters or accelerants to enable and increase the transdermal flux of topically applied pharmacologic agents (see details and further references in excellent reviews [186,187]). While many terpenes were identified as potential skin penetration enhancers [188,189], POH stands out among them because it also appears to exert beneficial transdermal activity on its own, i.e., without the need for other co-transported therapeutic agents.

For instance, when applied topically to the skin, POH was able to inhibit tumor development in the skin of mice exposed to the carcinogen DMBA [190,191] or to ultraviolet B radiation [192]. These preclinical observations prompted clinical studies to investigate whether topical application of POH might prove effective as a skin cancer chemoprevention strategy. A Phase I study enrolled participants with normal, healthy skin who applied POH, formulated as a cream [193], to their forearms twice daily for 30 days. The results showed that the POH cream was well tolerated and no cutaneous or systemic toxicities were observed [194]. In a subsequent Phase IIa study with POH cream and twice-daily applications to the forearms of participants over three months, it was investigated whether this treatment could reverse actinic (sun) damage. Modest effects of POH in sun-damaged skin could be documented, but the overall outcome was unimpressive [195], and no follow-up studies have been reported since. In other investigations, the authors used two murine models of dermatitis (induced by 12-O-tetradecanoylphorbol-13-acetate (TPA)) and of mechanical skin lesions (induced by epidermal incisions) that received daily treatments with topical POH prepared in sunflower oil. These studies showed that POH exerted significant anti-inflammatory effects along with improved tissue repair and wound healing [196]. Related observations were made with a mouse model of neuronal injury (although, in these cases, POH was given orally), where POH reduced gliosis and improved sensory and motor function recovery [197].

Among the above-introduced POH hybrid molecules, NEO412 was designed as a topical treatment for melanoma in situ (MIS). Although MIS has a better prognosis than metastatic melanoma, its effective treatment is complicated by ill-defined margins during surgical removal of the lesions, potentially leading to invasive melanoma [198]. Therefore, a topical treatment that would target unrecognized malignant components that might remain after surgery could be of great benefit to minimize the risk of recurrence. NEO412 is a tripartite agent consisting of three bioactive agents: POH, TMZ, and linoleic acid, with the latter representing a well-established transdermal penetration enhancer [199,200]. In vitro studies confirmed that NEO412 was able to effectively kill melanoma cells through the alkylation effect of TMZ [201]. In a mouse model of subcutaneous melanoma, topical application of NEO412 increased tumor cell death, along with decreased neo-angiogenesis in tumor tissue. Intriguingly, these effects could also be observed in tumors that were located distant from the skin treatment site, indicating that topical NEO412 was able to enter the circulation and reach tumor cells that might have metastasized already [201]. Although it remains to be established how much each penetration enhancer, i.e., POH vs. linoleic acid, contributed to transdermal migration of the tripartite molecule, the significant anti-melanoma effect that was achieved clearly indicates the benefit of this combination.

7. Conclusions and Outlook

POH is a monoterpenoid with an amphipathic character that appears to provide the physicochemical basis for its multifaceted applicability to overcome biological barriers. By means of further purification and CGMP manufacture, an effective pharmaceutical agent, namely, NEO100, was realized from POH that demonstrates good therapeutic prospects from in vitro, in vivo, and clinical testing. It can circumvent the BBB when administered via the intranasal route or physically open the BBB when given intra-arterially. It easily penetrates the cytoplasmic membrane without the need for cell surface transport proteins to facilitate its cell entry. In addition, it appears to harbor skin-penetrating potency. While much research has focused on characterizing the anticancer activity of the POH molecule, other avenues of investigation have further established its ability to enhance the therapeutic impact of different pharmacologic agents, either through enabling the transport of BBB-impermeable drugs via the intranasal route directly into the brain or through its covalent conjugation to specific drugs that results in overall increased penetration of the above-described biological barriers by the conjugated molecule.

The general principles attributed to the use of POH for increasing permeability across various biological barriers represent platform technologies that could be applicable to multiple clinical needs and situations. Although the bulk of applications is currently outlined for the treatment of primary and metastatic brain tumors, these POH-based concepts are adaptable for use in therapies aimed at neurodegenerative and infectious conditions of the brain. Moreover, the variety of molecules that could be delivered to the brain with the use of these platforms is not restricted to established drugs, but may include nucleic acids, i.e., siRNA, miRNA, and mRNA, as well as therapeutic proteins and antibodies, and possibly even intact cells and stem cells.

Author Contributions: A.H.S. assembled an outline of this review. T.C.C., C.O.d.F. and D.L. contributed to the writing and revising of the manuscript. All authors have read and agreed to the published version of the manuscript.

Funding: Studies in the authors' labs were supported in part through generous funding provided by the Hale Family Research Fund, Garza Foundation, and Sounder Foundation (to T.C.C.), and by the California Breast Cancer Research Program and METAvivor (to A.H.S.). The funding sources had no role in the design of the studies and collection, analysis, or interpretation of the data.

Institutional Review Board Statement: Not applicable.

Informed Consent Statement: Not applicable.

Data Availability Statement: Not applicable.

Acknowledgments: We thank all current and previous members of our laboratories for their valuable contributions.

Conflicts of Interest: T.C.C. and C.O.d.F. are founders and stakeholders of NeOnc Technologies, Inc., Los Angeles, California, USA. D.L. is a shareholder and member of the science advisory board of NeOnc. A.H.S. declares no potential conflict of interest.

Abbreviations

API	Active pharmacologic ingredient
BBB	Blood–brain barrier
CGMP	Current Good Manufacturing Practices
CNS	Central nervous system
GBM	Glioblastoma
IDH	Isocitrate dehydrogenase
MRI	Magnetic resonance imaging
POH	Perillyl alcohol
RT	Radiation therapy
TMZ	Temozolomide

References

1. Smith, Q.R. A Review of Blood–Brain Barrier Transport Techniques. *Methods Mol. Med.* **2003**, *89*, 193–208. [CrossRef] [PubMed]
2. Obermeier, B.; Daneman, R.; Ransohoff, R.M. Development, maintenance and disruption of the blood-brain barrier. *Nat. Med.* **2013**, *19*, 1584–1596. [CrossRef]
3. Langen, U.H.; Ayloo, S.; Gu, C. Development and Cell Biology of the Blood-Brain Barrier. *Annu. Rev. Cell Dev. Biol.* **2019**, *35*, 591–613. [CrossRef] [PubMed]
4. Sharif, Y.; Jumah, F.; Coplan, L.; Krosser, A.; Sharif, K.; Tubbs, R.S. Blood brain barrier: A review of its anatomy and physiology in health and disease. *Clin. Anat.* **2018**, *31*, 812–823. [CrossRef] [PubMed]
5. Frisk, G.; Svensson, T.; Bäcklund, L.M.; Lidbrink, E.; Blomqvist, P.; E Smedby, K. Incidence and time trends of brain metastases admissions among breast cancer patients in Sweden. *Br. J. Cancer* **2012**, *106*, 1850–1853. [CrossRef] [PubMed]
6. Kim, Y.-J.; Kim, J.-S.; Kim, I.A. Molecular subtype predicts incidence and prognosis of brain metastasis from breast cancer in SEER database. *J. Cancer Res. Clin. Oncol.* **2018**, *144*, 1803–1816. [CrossRef] [PubMed]
7. Krishnan, M.; Krishnamurthy, J.; Shonka, N. Targeting the Sanctuary Site: Options when Breast Cancer Metastasizes to the Brain. *Oncology* **2019**, *33*, 683730. [PubMed]
8. Garcia-Alvarez, A.; Papakonstantinou, A.; Oliveira, M. Brain Metastases in HER2-Positive Breast Cancer: Current and Novel Treatment Strategies. *Cancers* **2021**, *13*, 2927. [CrossRef]
9. Aulakh, S.; DeDeo, M.R.; Free, J.; Rosenfeld, S.S.; Quinones-Hinojosa, A.; Paulus, A.; Manna, A.; Manochakian, R.; Chanan-Khan, A.A.; Ailawadhi, S. Survival trends in glioblastoma and association with treating facility volume. *J. Clin. Neurosci.* **2019**, *68*, 271–274. [CrossRef]
10. Efremov, L.; Abera, S.F.; Bedir, A.; Vordermark, D.; Medenwald, D. Patterns of glioblastoma treatment and survival over a 16-years period: Pooled data from the german cancer registries. *J. Cancer Res. Clin. Oncol.* **2021**, *147*, 3381–3390. [PubMed]
11. Louis, D.N.; Perry, A.; Wesseling, P.; Brat, D.J.; A Cree, I.; Figarella-Branger, D.; Hawkins, C.; Ng, H.K.; Pfister, S.M.; Reifenberger, G.; et al. The 2021 WHO Classification of Tumors of the Central Nervous System: A summary. *Neuro-Oncology* **2021**, *23*, 1231–1251. [CrossRef] [PubMed]

12. Frappaz, D.; Bonneville-Levard, A.; Ricard, D.; Carrie, S.; Schiffler, C.; Xuan, K.H.; Weller, M. Assessment of Karnofsky (KPS) and WHO (WHO-PS) performance scores in brain tumour patients: The role of clinician bias. *Support. Care Cancer* **2021**, *29*, 1883–1891. [CrossRef]
13. Stupp, R.; Mason, W.P.; van den Bent, M.J.; Weller, M.; Fisher, B.; Taphoorn, M.J.; Belanger, K.; Brandes, A.A.; Marosi, C.; Bogdahn, U.; et al. Radiotherapy plus Concomitant and Adjuvant Temozolomide for Glioblastoma. *N. Engl. J. Med.* **2005**, *352*, 987–996. [CrossRef] [PubMed]
14. Stupp, R.; Hegi, M.E.; Mason, W.P.; van den Bent, M.J.; Taphoorn, M.J.B.; Janzer, R.C.; Ludwin, S.K.; Allgeier, A.; Fisher, B.; Belanger, K.; et al. Effects of radiotherapy with concomitant and adjuvant temozolomide versus radiotherapy alone on survival in glioblastoma in a randomised phase III study: 5-year analysis of the EORTC-NCIC trial. *Lancet Oncol.* **2009**, *10*, 459–466. [CrossRef]
15. Kazda, T.; Dziacky, A.; Burkon, P.; Pospisil, P.; Slavik, M.; Řehák, Z.; Jancalek, R.; Slampa, P.; Slaby, O.; Lakomy, R. Radiotherapy of glioblastoma 15 years after the landmark Stupp's trial: More controversies than standards? *Radiol. Oncol.* **2018**, *52*, 121–128. [CrossRef]
16. Ostermann, S.; Csajka, C.; Buclin, T.; Leyvraz, S.; Lejeune, F.; Decosterd, L.; Stupp, R. Plasma and Cerebrospinal Fluid Population Pharmacokinetics of Temozolomide in Malignant Glioma Patients. *Clin. Cancer Res.* **2004**, *10*, 3728–3736. [CrossRef] [PubMed]
17. Portnow, J.; Badie, B.; Chen, M.; Liu, A.; Blanchard, S.; Synold, T. The Neuropharmacokinetics of Temozolomide in Patients with Resectable Brain Tumors: Potential Implications for the Current Approach to Chemoradiation. *Clin. Cancer Res.* **2009**, *15*, 7092–7098. [CrossRef] [PubMed]
18. Guyon, J.; Chapouly, C.; Andrique, L.; Bikfalvi, A.; Daubon, T. The Normal and Brain Tumor Vasculature: Morphological and Functional Characteristics and Therapeutic Targeting. *Front. Physiol.* **2021**, *12*, 622615. [CrossRef] [PubMed]
19. Wang, D.; Wang, C.; Wang, L.; Chen, Y. A comprehensive review in improving delivery of small-molecule chemotherapeutic agents overcoming the blood-brain/brain tumor barriers for glioblastoma treatment. *Drug Deliv.* **2019**, *26*, 551–565. [CrossRef]
20. Boogerd, W.; Groenveld, F.; Linn, S.; Baars, J.W.; Brandsma, D.; Van Tinteren, H. Chemotherapy as primary treatment for brain metastases from breast cancer: Analysis of 115 one-year survivors. *J. Cancer Res. Clin. Oncol.* **2012**, *138*, 1395–1403. [CrossRef] [PubMed]
21. Franciosi, V.; Cocconi, G.; Michiara, M.; Di Costanzo, F.; Fosser, V.; Tonato, M.; Carlini, P.; Boni, C.; Di Sarra, S. Front-line chemotherapy with cisplatin and etoposide for patients with brain metastases from breast carcinoma, nonsmall cell lung carcinoma, or malignant melanoma: A prospective study. *Cancer* **1999**, *85*, 1599–1605. [CrossRef]
22. Lockman, P.; Mittapalli, R.K.; Taskar, K.S.; Rudraraju, V.; Gril, B.; Bohn, K.A.; Adkins, C.E.; Roberts, A.; Thorsheim, H.R.; Gaasch, J.A.; et al. Heterogeneous Blood–Tumor Barrier Permeability Determines Drug Efficacy in Experimental Brain Metastases of Breast Cancer. *Clin. Cancer Res.* **2010**, *16*, 5664–5678. [CrossRef] [PubMed]
23. Sarkaria, J.N.; Hu, L.S.; Parney, I.F.; Pafundi, D.H.; Brinkmann, D.H.; Laack, N.N.; Giannini, C.; Burns, T.C.; Kizilbash, S.; Laramy, J.K.; et al. Is the blood–brain barrier really disrupted in all glioblastomas? A critical assessment of existing clinical data. *Neuro-Oncology* **2018**, *20*, 184–191. [CrossRef] [PubMed]
24. Pitz, M.W.; Desai, A.; Grossman, S.A.; Blakeley, J.O. Tissue concentration of systemically administered antineoplastic agents in human brain tumors. *J. Neuro-Oncol.* **2011**, *104*, 629–638. [CrossRef] [PubMed]
25. Arvanitis, C.D.; Ferraro, G.B.; Jain, R.K. The blood–brain barrier and blood–tumour barrier in brain tumours and metastases. *Nat. Rev. Cancer* **2020**, *20*, 26–41. [CrossRef] [PubMed]
26. Marcucci, F.; Corti, A.; Ferreri, A. Breaching the Blood–Brain Tumor Barrier for Tumor Therapy. *Cancers* **2021**, *13*, 2391. [CrossRef] [PubMed]
27. Crowell, P.L.; Elson, C.E. Isoprenoids, health and disease. In *Neutraceuticals and Functional Foods*; Wildman, R.E.C., Ed.; CRC Press: Boca Raton, FL, USA, 2001.
28. Pan, J.; Xu, Z.; Ji, L.; Zhao, Z.; Tang, X. Constituents of Essential Oils from Leaves, Stems, and Fruits of *Perilla frutescens* (L.) britt. *Zhongguo Zhong Yao Za Zhi* **1992**, *17*, 164–165, 192. [PubMed]
29. Shojaei, S.; Kiumarsi, A.; Moghadam, A.R.; Alizadeh, J.; Marzban, H.; Ghavami, S. Perillyl Alcohol (Monoterpene Alcohol), Limonene. *Struct. Funct. Regul. Tor Complexes Yeasts Mamm. Part B* **2014**, *36*, 7–32. [CrossRef]
30. Kekulé, A. *Lehrbuch der Organischen Chemie*; Verlag von Ferdinand Enke: Erlangen, Germany, 1866; Volume 2.
31. Newman, A.A. *Chemistry of Terpenes and Terpenoids*; Academic Press: Cambridge, MA, USA, 1972; p. 449.
32. Dionísio, A.P.; Molina, G.; de Carvalho, D.S.; dos Santos, R.; Bicas, J.; Pastore, G. Natural flavourings from biotechnology for foods and beverages. In *Natural Food Additives, Ingredients and Flavourings*; Elsevier: Amsterdam, The Netherlands, 2012; pp. 231–259.
33. Leitereg, T.J.; Guadagni, D.G.; Harris, J.; Mon, T.R.; Teranishi, R. Evidence for the Difference between the Odours of the Optical Isomers (+)- and (−)-Carvone. *Nat. Cell Biol.* **1971**, *230*, 455–456. [CrossRef]
34. Sato, T.; Kobayakawa, R.; Kobayakawa, K.; Emura, M.; Itohara, S.; Kizumi, M.; Hamana, H.; Tsuboi, A.; Hirono, J. Supersensitive detection and discrimination of enantiomers by dorsal olfactory receptors: Evidence for hierarchical odour coding. *Sci. Rep.* **2015**, *5*, 14073. [CrossRef] [PubMed]
35. Moss, G.P. Basic terminology of stereochemistry (IUPAC Recommendations 1996). *Pure Appl. Chem.* **1996**, *68*, 2193–2222. [CrossRef]
36. Chastain, D.E.; Mody, N.; Majetich, G. Method of preparing perillyl alcohol and perillyl acetate. United. U.S. Patent US5994598, 30 November 1999.

37. Alonso-Gutierrez, J.; Chan, R.; Batth, T.S.; Adams, P.; Keasling, J.; Petzold, C.; Lee, T.S. Metabolic engineering of *Escherichia coli* for limonene and perillyl alcohol production. *Metab. Eng.* **2013**, *19*, 33–41. [CrossRef] [PubMed]
38. Ren, Y.; Liu, S.; Jin, G.; Yang, X.; Zhou, Y.J. Microbial production of limonene and its derivatives: Achievements and perspectives. *Biotechnol. Adv.* **2020**, *44*, 107628. [CrossRef] [PubMed]
39. Soares-Castro, P.; Soares, F.; Santos, P.M. Current Advances in the Bacterial Toolbox for the Biotechnological Production of Monoterpene-Based Aroma Compounds. *Molecules* **2020**, *26*, 91. [CrossRef] [PubMed]
40. Chen, T.; Levin, D.; Puppali, S. Pharmaceutical compositions comprising monoterpenes. United. U.S. Patent US9700524B2, 11 July 2017.
41. Crowell, P.L.; Lin, S.; Vedejs, E.; Gould, M.N. Identification of metabolites of the antitumor agent d-limonene capable of inhibiting protein isoprenylation and cell growth. *Cancer Chemother. Pharmacol.* **1992**, *31*, 205–212. [CrossRef] [PubMed]
42. Crowell, P.L.; Ren, Z.; Lin, S.; Vedejs, E.; Gould, M.N. Structure-activity relationships among monoterpene inhibitors of protein isoprenylation and cell proliferation. *Biochem. Pharmacol.* **1994**, *47*, 1405–1415. [CrossRef]
43. Haag, J.D.; Gould, M.N. Mammary carcinoma regression induced by perillyl alcohol, a hydroxylated analog of limonene. *Cancer Chemother. Pharmacol.* **1994**, *34*, 477–483. [CrossRef] [PubMed]
44. Elegbede, J.; Elson, C.; Qureshi, A.; Tanner, M.; Gould, M. Inhibition of DMBA-induced mammary cancer by the monoterpene d-limonene. *Carcinogenesis* **1984**, *5*, 661–664. [CrossRef] [PubMed]
45. Elegbede, J.A.; Elson, C.E.; Qureshi, A.; Tanner, M.A.; Gould, M.N. Regression of Rat Primary Mammary Tumors Following Dietary d-Limonene2. *J. Natl. Cancer Inst.* **1986**, *76*, 323–325. [CrossRef] [PubMed]
46. Homburger, F.; Treger, A.; Boger, E. Inhibition of Murine Subcutaneous and Intravenous Benzo(rst)pentaphene Carcinogenesis by Sweet Orange Oils and d-Limonene. *Oncology* **1971**, *25*, 1–10. [CrossRef] [PubMed]
47. Wattenberg, L.W.; Coccia, J.B. Inhibition of 4-(methylnitrosamino)-1-(3-pyridyl)-1-butanone carcinogenesis in mice by D-limonene and citrus fruit oils. *Carcinogenesis* **1991**, *12*, 115–117. [CrossRef] [PubMed]
48. Gelb, M.H.; Tamanoi, F.; Yokoyama, K.; Ghomashchi, F.; Esson, K.; Gould, M.N. The inhibition of protein prenyltransferases by oxygenated metabolites of limonene and perillyl alcohol. *Cancer Lett.* **1995**, *91*, 169–175. [CrossRef]
49. Crowell, P.; Chang, R.; Ren, Z.; Elson, C.; Gould, M. Selective inhibition of isoprenylation of 21-26-kDa proteins by the anticarcinogen d-limonene and its metabolites. *J. Biol. Chem.* **1991**, *266*, 17679–17685. [CrossRef]
50. Da Fonseca, C.O.; Linden, R.; Futuro, D.; Gattass, C.R.; Quirico-Santos, T. Ras pathway activation in gliomas: A strategic target for intranasal administration of perillyl alcohol. *Arch. Immunol. Ther. Exp.* **2008**, *56*, 267–276. [CrossRef]
51. Gould, M.N. Prevention and therapy of mammary cancer by monoterpenes. *J. Cell. Biochem.* **1995**, *59*, 139–144. [CrossRef]
52. Holstein, S.A.; Hohl, R.J. Monoterpene regulation of Ras and Ras-related protein expression. *J. Lipid Res.* **2003**, *44*, 1209–1215. [CrossRef]
53. Rowinsky, E.K.; Windle, J.J.; Von Hoff, D.D. Ras Protein Farnesyltransferase: A Strategic Target for Anticancer Therapeutic Development. *J. Clin. Oncol.* **1999**, *17*, 3631–3652. [CrossRef] [PubMed]
54. Ren, Z.; Elson, C.E.; Gould, M.N. Inhibition of type I and type II geranylgeranyl-protein transferases by the monoterpene perillyl alcohol in NIH3T3 cells. *Biochem. Pharmacol.* **1997**, *54*, 113–120. [CrossRef]
55. A Ariazi, E.; Satomi, Y.; Ellis, M.J.; Haag, J.D.; Shi, W.; A Sattler, C.; Gould, M.N. Activation of the transforming growth factor beta signaling pathway and induction of cytostasis and apoptosis in mammary carcinomas treated with the anticancer agent perillyl alcohol. *Cancer Res.* **1999**, *59*, 1917–1928.
56. Koyama, M.; Sowa, Y.; Hitomi, T.; Iizumi, Y.; Watanabe, M.; Taniguchi, T.; Ichikawa, M.; Sakai, T. Perillyl alcohol causes g1 arrest through p15(ink4b) and p21(waf1/cip1) induction. *Oncol. Rep.* **2013**, *29*, 779–784. [CrossRef]
57. Wiseman, D.; Werner, S.R.; Crowell, P.L. Cell Cycle Arrest by the Isoprenoids Perillyl Alcohol, Geraniol, and Farnesol Is Mediated by p21Cip1and p27Kip1in Human Pancreatic Adenocarcinoma Cells. *J. Pharmacol. Exp. Ther.* **2006**, *320*, 1163–1170. [CrossRef] [PubMed]
58. Yuri, T.; Danbara, N.; Tsujita-Kyutoku, M.; Kiyozuka, Y.; Senzaki, H.; Shikata, N.; Kanzaki, H.; Tsubura, A. Perillyl Alcohol Inhibits Human Breast Cancer Cell Growth in vitro and in vivo. *Breast Cancer Res. Treat.* **2004**, *84*, 251–260. [CrossRef] [PubMed]
59. Satomi, Y.; Miyamoto, S.; Gould, M.N. Induction of AP-1 activity by perillyl alcohol in breast cancer cells. *Carcinogenesis* **1999**, *20*, 1957–1961. [CrossRef]
60. Sundin, T.; Peffley, D.M.; Gauthier, D.; Hentosh, P. The isoprenoid perillyl alcohol inhibits telomerase activity in prostate cancer cells. *Biochimie* **2012**, *94*, 2639–2648. [CrossRef]
61. Sundin, T.; Peffley, D.M.; Hentosh, P. Disruption of an htert-mtor-raptor protein complex by a phytochemical perillyl alcohol and rapamycin. *Mol. Cell. Biochem.* **2013**, *375*, 97–104. [CrossRef] [PubMed]
62. Peffley, D.M.; Sharma, C.; Hentosh, P.; Buechler, R.D. Perillyl alcohol and genistein differentially regulate PKB/Akt and 4E-BP1 phosphorylation as well as eIF4E/eIF4G interactions in human tumor cells. *Arch. Biochem. Biophys.* **2007**, *465*, 266–273. [CrossRef] [PubMed]
63. Sundin, T.; Peffley, D.; Hentosh, P. eIF4E-Overexpression imparts perillyl alcohol and rapamycin-mediated regulation of telomerase reverse transcriptase. *Exp. Cell Res.* **2013**, *319*, 2103–2112. [CrossRef] [PubMed]
64. Garcia, D.G.; Amorim, L.M.F.; Faria, M.V.D.C.; Freire, A.S.; Santelli, R.E.; Da Fonseca, C.O.; Quirico-Santos, T.; Burth, P. The anticancer drug perillyl alcohol is a Na/K-ATPase inhibitor. *Mol. Cell. Biochem.* **2010**, *345*, 29–34. [CrossRef] [PubMed]

65. Garcia, D.G.; de Castro-Faria-Neto, H.C.; da Silva, C.I.; Souza, K.F.C.D.S.E.; Gonçalves-De-Albuquerque, C.F.; Silva, A.R.; Amorim, L.M.D.F.D.; Freire, A.S.; Santelli, R.E.; Diniz, L.P.; et al. Na/K-ATPase as a target for anticancer drugs: Studies with perillyl alcohol. *Mol. Cancer* **2015**, *14*, 1–14. [CrossRef] [PubMed]
66. Ma, Y.; Bian, J.; Zhang, F. Inhibition of perillyl alcohol on cell invasion and migration depends on the Notch signaling pathway in hepatoma cells. *Mol. Cell. Biochem.* **2015**, *411*, 307–315. [CrossRef] [PubMed]
67. Berchtold, C.M.; Chen, K.S.; Miyamoto, S.; Gould, M.N. Perillyl alcohol inhibits a calcium-dependent constitutive nuclear factor-kappab pathway. *Cancer Res.* **2005**, *65*, 8558–8566. [CrossRef] [PubMed]
68. Khan, A.Q.; Nafees, S.; Sultana, S. Perillyl alcohol protects against ethanol induced acute liver injury in Wistar rats by inhibiting oxidative stress, NFκ-B activation and proinflammatory cytokine production. *Toxicology* **2011**, *279*, 108–114. [CrossRef]
69. Tabassum, R.; Vaibhav, K.; Shrivastava, P.; Khan, A.; Ahmed, M.E.; Ashafaq, M.; Khan, M.B.; Islam, F.; Safhi, M.M.; Islam, F. Perillyl alcohol improves functional and histological outcomes against ischemia-reperfusion injury by attenuation of oxidative stress and repression of cox-2, nos-2 and nf-kappab in middle cerebral artery occlusion rats. *Eur. J. Pharmacol.* **2015**, *747*, 190–199. [CrossRef] [PubMed]
70. Ma, J.; Li, J.; Wang, K.S.; Mi, C.; Piao, L.X.; Xu, G.H.; Li, X.; Lee, J.J.; Jin, X. Perillyl alcohol efficiently scavenges activity of cellular ROS and inhibits the translational expression of hypoxia-inducible factor-1α via mTOR/4E-BP1 signaling pathways. *Int. Immunopharmacol.* **2016**, *39*, 1–9. [CrossRef] [PubMed]
71. Cho, H.-Y.; Wang, W.; Jhaveri, N.; Torres, S.; Tseng, J.; Leong, M.N.; Lee, D.J.; Goldkorn, A.; Xu, T.; Petasis, N.; et al. Perillyl Alcohol for the Treatment of Temozolomide-Resistant Gliomas. *Mol. Cancer Ther.* **2012**, *11*, 2462–2472. [CrossRef] [PubMed]
72. Nishitoh, H. CHOP is a multifunctional transcription factor in the ER stress response. *J. Biochem.* **2012**, *151*, 217–219. [CrossRef]
73. Schönthal, A.H. Endoplasmic Reticulum Stress: Its Role in Disease and Novel Prospects for Therapy. *Scientifica* **2012**, *2012*, 1–26. [CrossRef] [PubMed]
74. Schönthal, A.H. Pharmacological targeting of endoplasmic reticulum stress signaling in cancer. *Biochem. Pharmacol.* **2013**, *85*, 653–666. [CrossRef] [PubMed]
75. Ripple, G.H.; Gould, M.N.; A Stewart, J.; Tutsch, K.D.; Arzoomanian, R.Z.; Alberti, D.; Feierabend, C.; Pomplun, M.; Wilding, G.; Bailey, H.H. Phase I clinical trial of perillyl alcohol administered daily. *Clin. Cancer Res.* **1998**, *4*, 1159–1164.
76. Ripple, G.H.; Gould, M.N.; Arzoomanian, R.Z.; Alberti, D.; Feierabend, C.; Simon, K.; Binger, K.; Tutsch, K.D.; Pomplun, M.; Wahamaki, A.; et al. Phase I clinical and pharmacokinetic study of perillyl alcohol administered four times a day. *Clin. Cancer Res.* **2000**, *6*, 390–396. [PubMed]
77. Bailey, H.H.; Levy, D.; Harris, L.S.; Schink, J.C.; Foss, F.; Beatty, P.; Wadler, S. A Phase II Trial of Daily Perillyl Alcohol in Patients with Advanced Ovarian Cancer: Eastern Cooperative Oncology Group Study E2E96. *Gynecol. Oncol.* **2002**, *85*, 464–468. [CrossRef] [PubMed]
78. Liu, G.; Oettel, K.; Bailey, H.; Van Ummersen, L.; Tutsch, K.; Staab, M.J.; Horvath, D.; Alberti, N.; Arzoomanian, R.; Rezazadeh, H.; et al. Phase II trial of perillyl alcohol (NSC 641066) administered daily in patients with metastatic androgen independent prostate cancer. *Investig. New Drugs* **2003**, *21*, 367–372. [CrossRef] [PubMed]
79. Bailey, H.H.; Attia, S.; Love, R.R.; Fass, T.; Chappell, R.; Tutsch, K.; Harris, L.; Jumonville, A.; Hansen, R.; Shapiro, G.R.; et al. Phase II trial of daily oral perillyl alcohol (NSC 641066) in treatment-refractory metastatic breast cancer. *Cancer Chemother. Pharmacol.* **2007**, *62*, 149–157. [CrossRef] [PubMed]
80. Matos, J.M.; Schmidt, C.M.; Thomas, H.J.; Cummings, O.W.; Wiebke, E.A.; Madura, J.A.; Patrick, L.J.; Crowell, P. A Pilot Study of Perillyl Alcohol in Pancreatic Cancer. *J. Surg. Res.* **2008**, *147*, 194–199. [CrossRef] [PubMed]
81. Meadows, S.M.; Mulkerin, D.; Berlin, J.; Bailey, H.; Kolesar, J.; Warren, D.; Thomas, J.P. Phase II Trial of Perillyl Alcohol in Patients with Metastatic Colorectal Cancer. *Int. J. Pancreatol.* **2002**, *32*, 125–128. [CrossRef]
82. Durço, A.O.; Conceição, L.S.R.; de Souza, D.S.; Lima, C.A.; Quintans, J.D.S.S.; dos Santos, M.R.V. Perillyl alcohol as a treatment for cancer: A systematic review. *Phytomedicine Plus* **2021**, *1*, 100090. [CrossRef]
83. Erdő, F.; Bors, L.A.; Farkas, D.; Bajza, Á.; Gizurarson, S. Evaluation of intranasal delivery route of drug administration for brain targeting. *Brain Res. Bull.* **2018**, *143*, 155–170. [CrossRef]
84. Keller, L.-A.; Merkel, O.; Popp, A. Intranasal drug delivery: Opportunities and toxicologic challenges during drug development. *Drug Deliv. Transl. Res.* **2021**, 1–23. [CrossRef]
85. Pardeshi, C.V.; Belgamwar, V.S. Direct nose to brain drug delivery via integrated nerve pathways bypassing the blood-brain barrier: An excellent platform for brain targeting. *Epert Opin. Drug Deliv.* **2013**, *10*, 957–972. [CrossRef] [PubMed]
86. Dhas, N.; Yadav, D.; Singh, A.; Garkal, A.; Kudarha, R.; Bangar, P.; Savjani, J.; Pardeshi, C.V.; Garg, N.; Mehta, T. Direct transport theory: From the nose to the brain. In *Direct Nose-to-Brain Drug Delivery*; Pardeshi, C.V., Souto, E.B., Eds.; Academic Press: San Diego, CA, USA; Cambridge, MA, USA; Oxford, UK; London, UK, 2021; pp. 15–38.
87. Khunt, D.; Misra, M. Basic considerations of anatomical and physiological aspects of the nose and the brain. In *Direct Nose-to-Brain Drug Delivery*; Pardeshi, C.V., Souto, E.B., Eds.; Academic Press: San Diego, CA, USA; Cambridge, MA, USA; Oxford, UK; London, UK, 2021; pp. 3–14.
88. Laddha, U.D.; Tagalpallewar, A.A. Physicochemical, biopharmaceutical, and practical considerations for efficient nose-to-brain drug delivery. In *Direct Nose-to-Brain Drug Delivery*; Pardeshi, C.V., Souto, E.B., Eds.; Academic Press: San Diego, CA, USA; Cambridge, MA, USA; Oxford, UK; London, UK, 2021; pp. 39–56.

89. Gänger, S.; Schindowski, K. Tailoring Formulations for Intranasal Nose-to-Brain Delivery: A Review on Architecture, Physico-Chemical Characteristics and Mucociliary Clearance of the Nasal Olfactory Mucosa. *Pharmaceutics* **2018**, *10*, 116. [CrossRef] [PubMed]
90. Crowe, T.; Greenlee, M.H.W.; Kanthasamy, A.; Hsu, W.H. Mechanism of intranasal drug delivery directly to the brain. *Life Sci.* **2018**, *195*, 44–52. [CrossRef] [PubMed]
91. Djupesland, P.G.; Messina, J.C.; A Mahmoud, R. The nasal approach to delivering treatment for brain diseases: An anatomic, physiologic, and delivery technology overview. *Ther. Deliv.* **2014**, *5*, 709–733. [CrossRef] [PubMed]
92. Chen, T.C.; Da Fonseca, C.O.; Schönthal, A.H. Preclinical development and clinical use of perillyl alcohol for chemoprevention and cancer therapy. *Am. J. Cancer Res.* **2015**, *5*, 1580–1593.
93. Da Fonseca, C.O.; Masini, M.; Futuro, D.; Caetano, R.; Gattass, C.R.; Quirico-Santos, T. Anaplastic oligodendroglioma responding favorably to intranasal delivery of perillyl alcohol: A case report and literature review. *Surg. Neurol.* **2006**, *66*, 611–615. [CrossRef] [PubMed]
94. da Fonseca, C.O.; Schwartsmann, G.; Fischer, J.; Nagel, J.; Futuro, D.; Quirico-Santos, T.; Gattass, C.R. Preliminary results from a phase I/II study of perillyl alcohol intranasal administration in adults with recurrent malignant gliomas. *Surg. Neurol.* **2008**, *70*, 259–266. [CrossRef]
95. Da Fonseca, C.O.; Simão, M.; Lins, I.R.; Caetano, R.O.; Futuro, D.; Quirico-Santos, T. Efficacy of monoterpene perillyl alcohol upon survival rate of patients with recurrent glioblastoma. *J. Cancer Res. Clin. Oncol.* **2010**, *137*, 287–293. [CrossRef] [PubMed]
96. Da Fonseca, C.O.; Teixeira, R.M.; Silva, J.C.T.; Fischer, J.D.S.D.G.; Meirelles, O.C.; Landeiro, J.A.; Quirico-Santos, T. Long-term outcome in patients with recurrent malignant glioma treated with Perillyl alcohol inhalation. *Anticancer Res.* **2013**, *33*, 5625–5631.
97. Schönthal, A.H.; Peereboom, D.M.; Wagle, N.; Lai, R.; Mathew, A.J.; Hurth, K.M.; Simmon, V.F.; Howard, S.P.; Taylor, L.P.; Chow, F.; et al. Phase I trial of intranasal NEO100, highly purified perillyl alcohol, in adult patients with recurrent glioblastoma. *Neuro-Oncol. Adv.* **2021**, *3*, vdab005. [CrossRef]
98. National Cancer Institute. Common Terminology Criteria for Adverse Events (CTCAE) Version 5.0. Available online: https://ctep.cancer.gov/protocoldevelopment/electronic_applications/ctc.htm#ctc_50 (accessed on 15 July 2021).
99. Barker, F.G., II; Chang, S.M.; Gutin, P.H.; Malec, M.K.; McDermott, M.W.; Prados, M.D.; Wilson, C.B. Survival and functional status after resection of recurrent glioblastoma multiforme. *Neurosurgery* **1998**, *42*, 709–720, discussion 720–703. [CrossRef]
100. Batchelor, T.T.; Mulholland, P.; Neyns, B.; Nabors, L.B.; Campone, M.; Wick, A.; Mason, W.; Mikkelsen, T.; Phuphanich, S.; Ashby, L.S.; et al. Phase III Randomized Trial Comparing the Efficacy of Cediranib As Monotherapy, and in Combination With Lomustine, Versus Lomustine Alone in Patients With Recurrent Glioblastoma. *J. Clin. Oncol.* **2013**, *31*, 3212–3218. [CrossRef]
101. Brandes, A.A.; Finocchiaro, G.; Zagonel, V.; Reni, M.; Caserta, C.; Fabi, A.; Clavarezza, M.; Maiello, E.; Eoli, M.; Lombardi, G.; et al. AVAREG: A phase II, randomized, noncomparative study of fotemustine or bevacizumab for patients with recurrent glioblastoma. *Neuro-Oncology* **2016**, *18*, 1304–1312. [CrossRef]
102. Desjardins, A.; Herndon, J.E., II; McSherry, F.; Ravelo, A.; Lipp, E.S.; Healy, P.; Peters, K.B.; Sampson, J.H.; Randazzo, D.; Sommer, N.; et al. Single-institution retrospective review of patients with recurrent glioblastoma treated with bevacizumab in clinical practice. *Health Sci. Rep.* **2019**, *2*, e114. [CrossRef] [PubMed]
103. Ghiaseddin, A.; Peters, K.B. Use of bevacizumab in recurrent glioblastoma. *CNS Oncol.* **2015**, *4*, 157–169. [CrossRef]
104. Weller, M.; Le Rhun, E. How did lomustine become standard of care in recurrent glioblastoma? *Cancer Treat. Rev.* **2020**, *87*, 102029. [CrossRef] [PubMed]
105. Da Fonseca, C.O.; Silva, J.T.; Lins, I.R.; Simão, M.; Arnobio, A.; Futuro, D.; Quirico-Santos, T. Correlation of tumor topography and peritumoral edema of recurrent malignant gliomas with therapeutic response to intranasal administration of perillyl alcohol. *Investig. New Drugs* **2009**, *27*, 557–564. [CrossRef] [PubMed]
106. Faria, G.M.; Soares, I.D.P.; D'Alincourt Salazar, M.; Amorim, M.R.; Pessoa, B.L.; da Fonseca, C.O.; Quirico-Santos, T. Intranasal perillyl alcohol therapy improves survival of patients with recurrent glioblastoma harboring mutant variant for mthfr rs1801133 polymorphism. *BMC Cancer* **2020**, *20*, 294. [CrossRef] [PubMed]
107. Waitkus, M.S.; Diplas, B.H.; Yan, H. Biological Role and Therapeutic Potential of IDH Mutations in Cancer. *Cancer Cell* **2018**, *34*, 186–195. [CrossRef] [PubMed]
108. Yang, H.; Ye, D.; Guan, K.-L.; Xiong, Y. IDH1 and IDH2 Mutations in Tumorigenesis: Mechanistic Insights and Clinical Perspectives. *Clin. Cancer Res.* **2012**, *18*, 5562–5571. [CrossRef]
109. Huang, L.E. Friend or foe—IDH1 mutations in glioma 10 years on. *Carcinogenesis* **2019**, *40*, 1299–1307. [CrossRef] [PubMed]
110. Tabei, Y.; Kobayashi, K.; Saito, K.; Shimizu, S.; Suzuki, K.; Sasaki, N.; Shiokawa, Y.; Nagane, M. Survival in patients with glioblastoma at a first progression does not correlate with isocitrate dehydrogenase (IDH)1 gene mutation status. *Jpn. J. Clin. Oncol.* **2021**, *51*, 45–53. [CrossRef]
111. Da Fonseca, C.; Soares, I.P.; Clemençon, D.S.; Rochlin, S.; Cardeman, L.; Quirico-Santos, T. Perillyl alcohol inhalation concomitant with oral temozolomide halts progression of recurrent inoperable glioblastoma: A case report. *J. Histol. Histopathol.* **2015**, *2*, 12. [CrossRef]
112. Santos, J.G.; Da Cruz, W.M.S.; Schönthal, A.H.; Salazar, M.D.; Fontes, C.A.P.; Quirico-Santos, T.; Da Fonseca, C.O. Efficacy of a ketogenic diet with concomitant intranasal perillyl alcohol as a novel strategy for the therapy of recurrent glioblastoma. *Oncol. Lett.* **2017**, *15*, 1263–1270. [CrossRef] [PubMed]

113. Santos, J.G.; Faria, G.; Cruz, W.D.C.S.D.; Fontes, C.A.; Schönthal, A.H.; Quirico-Santos, T.; Da Fonseca, C.O. Adjuvant effect of low-carbohydrate diet on outcomes of patients with recurrent glioblastoma under intranasal perillyl alcohol therapy. *Surg. Neurol. Int.* **2020**, *11*, 389. [CrossRef] [PubMed]
114. Zhang, Z.; Chen, H.; Chan, K.K.; Budd, T.; Ganapathi, R. Gas chromatographic–mass spectrometric analysis of perillyl alcohol and metabolites in plasma. *J. Chromatogr. B Biomed. Sci. Appl.* **1999**, *728*, 85–95. [CrossRef]
115. Santos, J.D.S.; Diedrich, C.; Machado, C.S.; da Fonseca, C.O.; Khalil, N.M.; Mainardes, R.M. Intranasal administration of perillyl alcohol–loaded nanoemulsion and pharmacokinetic study of its metabolite perillic acid in plasma and brain of rats using ultra-performance liquid chromatography/tandem mass spectrometry. *Biomed. Chromatogr.* **2021**, *35*, e5037. [CrossRef] [PubMed]
116. De Lima, D.C.; Rodrigues, S.V.; Boaventura, G.T.; Cho, H.; Chen, T.C.; Schönthal, A.H.; Da Fonseca, C.O. Simultaneous measurement of perillyl alcohol and its metabolite perillic acid in plasma and lung after inhalational administration in Wistar rats. *Drug Test. Anal.* **2019**, *12*, 268–279. [CrossRef] [PubMed]
117. Marin, A.A.; Murillo, O.; Sussmann, R.A.; Ortolan, L.S.; Battagello, D.S.; Quirino, T.D.C.; Bittencourt, J.C.; Epiphanio, S.; Katzin, A.M.; Carvalho, L.J.M. Perillyl Alcohol Reduces Parasite Sequestration and Cerebrovascular Dysfunction during Experimental Cerebral Malaria. *Antimicrob. Agents Chemother.* **2021**, *65*. [CrossRef] [PubMed]
118. Nehra, G.; Andrews, S.; Rettig, J.; Gould, M.N.; Haag, J.D.; Howard, S.P.; Thorne, R.G. Intranasal administration of the chemotherapeutic perillyl alcohol results in selective delivery to the cerebrospinal fluid in rats. *Sci. Rep.* **2021**, *11*, 1–11. [CrossRef]
119. Eftekhari, R.B.; Maghsoudnia, N.; Samimi, S.; Zamzami, A.; Dorkoosh, F.A. Co-Delivery Nanosystems for Cancer Treatment: A Review. *Pharm. Nanotechnol.* **2019**, *7*, 90–112. [CrossRef]
120. Guo, P.; He, Y.; Xu, T.; Pi, C.; Jiang, Q.; Wei, Y.; Zhao, L. Co-delivery system of chemotherapy drugs and active ingredients from natural plants: A brief overview of preclinical research for cancer treatment. *Expert Opin. Drug Deliv.* **2020**, *17*, 665–675. [CrossRef] [PubMed]
121. Ferreira, N.N.; Junior, E.D.O.; Granja, S.; Boni, F.I.; Ferreira, L.M.; Cury, B.S.; Santos, L.C.; Reis, R.M.; Lima, E.M.; Baltazar, F.; et al. Nose-to-brain co-delivery of drugs for glioblastoma treatment using nanostructured system. *Int. J. Pharm.* **2021**, *603*, 120714. [CrossRef] [PubMed]
122. Mignani, S.; Shi, X.; Karpus, A.; Majoral, J.-P. Non-invasive intranasal administration route directly to the brain using dendrimer nanoplatforms: An opportunity to develop new CNS drugs. *Eur. J. Med. Chem.* **2021**, *209*, 112905. [CrossRef] [PubMed]
123. Wang, W.; Swenson, S.; Cho, H.-Y.; Hofman, F.M.; Schönthal, A.H.; Chen, T.C. Efficient brain targeting and therapeutic intracranial activity of bortezomib through intranasal co-delivery with NEO100 in rodent glioblastoma models. *J. Neurosurg.* **2020**, *132*, 959–967. [CrossRef] [PubMed]
124. Scott, K.; Hayden, P.J.; Will, A.; Wheatley, K.; Coyne, I. Bortezomib for the treatment of multiple myeloma. *Cochrane Database Syst. Rev.* **2016**, *4*, CD010816. [CrossRef]
125. Hemeryck, A.; Geerts, R.; Monbaliu, J.; Hassler, S.; Verhaeghe, T.; Diels, L.; Verluyten, W.; Van Beijsterveldt, L.; Mamidi, R.N.V.S.; Janssen, C.; et al. Tissue distribution and depletion kinetics of bortezomib and bortezomib-related radioactivity in male rats after single and repeated intravenous injection of 14C-bortezomib. *Cancer Chemother. Pharmacol.* **2007**, *60*, 777–787. [CrossRef] [PubMed]
126. Pinel, S.; Labussiere, M.; Delfortrie, S.; Plenat, F.; Chastagner, P. Proteasome inhibition by bortezomib does not translate into efficacy on two malignant glioma xenografts. *Oncol. Rep.* **1994**, *20*, 1283–1287. [CrossRef]
127. Wang, W.; Cho, H.-Y.; Rosenstein-Sisson, R.; Ramos, N.I.M.; Price, R.; Hurth, K.; Schönthal, A.H.; Hofman, F.M.; Chen, T.C. Intratumoral delivery of bortezomib: Impact on survival in an intracranial glioma tumor model. *J. Neurosurg.* **2018**, *128*, 695–700. [CrossRef]
128. Friday, B.B.; Anderson, S.K.; Buckner, J.; Yu, C.; Giannini, C.; Geoffroy, F.; Schwerkoske, J.; Mazurczak, M.; Gross, H.; Pajon, E.; et al. Phase II trial of vorinostat in combination with bortezomib in recurrent glioblastoma: A north central cancer treatment group study. *Neuro-Oncology* **2011**, *14*, 215–221. [CrossRef]
129. Odia, Y.; Kreisl, T.N.; Aregawi, D.; Innis, E.K.; Fine, H.A. A phase II trial of tamoxifen and bortezomib in patients with recurrent malignant gliomas. *J. Neuro-Oncol.* **2015**, *125*, 191–195. [CrossRef] [PubMed]
130. Raizer, J.J.; Chandler, J.P.; Ferrarese, R.; Grimm, S.A.; Levy, R.M.; Muro, K.; Rosenow, J.; Helenowski, I.; Rademaker, A.; Paton, M.; et al. A phase II trial evaluating the effects and intra-tumoral penetration of bortezomib in patients with recurrent malignant gliomas. *J. Neuro-Oncol.* **2016**, *129*, 139–146. [CrossRef] [PubMed]
131. Bota, D.A.; Alexandru, D.; Keir, S.T.; Bigner, D.; Vredenburgh, J.; Friedman, H.S. Proteasome inhibition with bortezomib induces cell death in GBM stem-like cells and temozolomide-resistant glioma cell lines, but stimulates GBM stem-like cells' VEGF production and angiogenesis. *J. Neurosurg.* **2013**, *119*, 1415–1423. [CrossRef]
132. Kardosh, A.; Golden, E.B.; Pyrko, P.; Uddin, J.; Hofman, F.M.; Chen, T.C.; Louie, S.G.; Petasis, N.; Schönthal, A.H. Aggravated Endoplasmic Reticulum Stress as a Basis for Enhanced Glioblastoma Cell Killing by Bortezomib in Combination with Celecoxib or Its Non-Coxib Analogue, 2,5-Dimethyl-Celecoxib. *Cancer Res.* **2008**, *68*, 843–851. [CrossRef]
133. Styczynski, J.; Olszewska-Slonina, D.; Kolodziej, B.; Napieraj, M.; Wysocki, M. Activity of bortezomib in glioblastoma. *Anticancer. Res.* **2007**, *26*, 4499–4503.
134. Joshi, S.; Ergin, A.; Wang, M.; Reif, R.; Zhang, J.; Bruce, J.N.; Bigio, I.J. Inconsistent blood brain barrier disruption by intraarterial mannitol in rabbits: Implications for chemotherapy. *J. Neuro-Oncol.* **2010**, *104*, 11–19. [CrossRef] [PubMed]

135. Joshi, S.; Meyers, P.M.; Ornstein, E. Intracarotid delivery of drugs: The potential and the pitfalls. *Anesthesiology* **2008**, *109*, 543–564. [CrossRef] [PubMed]
136. Lundqvist, H.; Rosander, K.; Lomanov, M.; Lukjashin, V.; Shimchuk, G.; Zolotov, V.; Minakova, E. Permeability of the Blood-Brain Barrier in the Rat after Local Proton Irradiation. *Acta Radiol. Oncol.* **1982**, *21*, 267–271. [CrossRef] [PubMed]
137. A Peña, L.; Fuks, Z.; Kolesnick, R.N. Radiation-induced apoptosis of endothelial cells in the murine central nervous system: Protection by fibroblast growth factor and sphingomyelinase deficiency. *Cancer Res.* **2000**, *60*, 321–327. [PubMed]
138. Sprowls, S.A.; Arsiwala, T.; Bumgarner, J.; Shah, N.; Lateef, S.S.; Kielkowski, B.N.; Lockman, P.R. Improving CNS Delivery to Brain Metastases by Blood–Tumor Barrier Disruption. *Trends Cancer* **2019**, *5*, 495–505. [CrossRef] [PubMed]
139. Dasgupta, A.; Liu, M.; Ojha, T.; Storm, G.; Kiessling, F.; Lammers, T. Ultrasound-mediated drug delivery to the brain: Principles, progress and prospects. *Drug Discov. Today Technol.* **2016**, *20*, 41–48. [CrossRef] [PubMed]
140. Abrahao, A.; Meng, Y.; Llinas, M.; Huang, Y.; Hamani, C.; Mainprize, T.; Aubert, I.; Heyn, C.; Black, S.E.; Hynynen, K.; et al. First-in-human trial of blood–brain barrier opening in amyotrophic lateral sclerosis using MR-guided focused ultrasound. *Nat. Commun.* **2019**, *10*, 1–9. [CrossRef]
141. Carpentier, A.; Canney, M.; Vignot, A.; Reina, V.; Beccaria, K.; Horodyckid, C.; Karachi, C.; Leclercq, D.; Lafon, C.; Chapelon, J.-Y.; et al. Clinical trial of blood-brain barrier disruption by pulsed ultrasound. *Sci. Transl. Med.* **2016**, *8*, 343re2. [CrossRef] [PubMed]
142. Arvanitis, C.D.; Askoxylakis, V.; Guo, Y.; Datta, M.; Kloepper, J.; Ferraro, G.B.; Bernabeu, M.O.; Fukumura, D.; McDannold, N.; Jain, R.K. Mechanisms of enhanced drug delivery in brain metastases with focused ultrasound-induced blood–tumor barrier disruption. *Proc. Natl. Acad. Sci. USA* **2018**, *115*, E8717–E8726. [CrossRef] [PubMed]
143. Wang, W.; He, H.; Marín-Ramos, N.I.; Zeng, S.; Swenson, S.; Cho, H.-Y.; Fu, J.; Beringer, P.M.; Neman, J.; Chen, L.; et al. Enhanced brain delivery and therapeutic activity of trastuzumab after blood-brain barrier opening by neo100 in mouse models of brain-metastatic breast cancer. *Neuro Oncol.* **2021**, e-pub ahead of print. [CrossRef] [PubMed]
144. Wang, W.; I Marín-Ramos, N.; He, H.; Zeng, S.; Cho, H.-Y.; Swenson, S.D.; Zheng, L.; Epstein, A.L.; Schönthal, A.H.; Hofman, F.M.; et al. NEO100 enables brain delivery of blood–brain barrier impermeable therapeutics. *Neuro-Oncology* **2021**, *23*, 63–75. [CrossRef]
145. Aouad-Maroun, M.; Raphael, C.K.; Sayyid, S.K.; Farah, F.; Akl, E.A. Ultrasound-guided arterial cannulation for paediatrics. *Cochrane Database Syst. Rev.* **2016**, *9*, CD011364. [CrossRef] [PubMed]
146. Hou, X.-T.; Sun, Y.-Q.; Zhang, H.-J.; Zheng, S.-H.; Liu, Y.-Y.; Wang, J.-G. Femoral Artery Cannulation in Stanford Type a Aortic Dissection Operations. *Asian Cardiovasc. Thorac. Ann.* **2006**, *14*, 35–37. [CrossRef]
147. Saadat, S.; Schultheis, M.; Azzolini, A.; Romero, J.; Dombrovskiy, V.; Odroniec, K.; Scholz, P.; Lemaire, A.; Batsides, G.; Lee, L. Femoral cannulation: A safe vascular access option for cardiopulmonary bypass in minimally invasive cardiac surgery. *Perfusion* **2016**, *31*, 131–134. [CrossRef]
148. Bangalore, S.; Bhatt, D.L. Femoral Arterial Access and Closure. *Circulation* **2011**, *124*, e147–e156. [CrossRef]
149. Scheer, B.V.; Perel, A.; Pfeiffer, U.J. Clinical review: Complications and risk factors of peripheral arterial catheters used for haemodynamic monitoring in anaesthesia and intensive care medicine. *Crit. Care* **2002**, *6*, 199–204. [CrossRef] [PubMed]
150. Fusco, D.S.; Shaw, R.K.; Tranquilli, M.; Kopf, G.S.; Elefteriades, J.A. Femoral Cannulation is Safe for Type A Dissection Repair. *Ann. Thorac. Surg.* **2004**, *78*, 1285–1289. [CrossRef] [PubMed]
151. Sattenberg, R.J.; Meckler, J.; Saver, J.L.; Gobin, Y.P.; Liebeskind, D.S. Cerebral angiography. In *Stroke: Pathophysiology, Diagnosis, and Management*, 6th ed.; Grotta, J.C., Ed.; Elsevier Inc.: Amsterdam, The Netherlands, 2016; pp. 790–805.
152. Gantt, R.W.; Peltier-Pain, P.; Thorson, J.S. Enzymatic methods for glyco(diversification/randomization) of drugs and small molecules. *Nat. Prod. Rep.* **2011**, *28*, 1811–1853. [CrossRef] [PubMed]
153. Fujita, T.; Ohira, K.; Miyatake, K.; Nakano, Y.; Nakayama, M. Inhibitory Effect of Perillosides A and C, and Related Monoterpene Glucosides on Aldose Reductase and Their Structure-Activity Relationships. *Chem. Pharm. Bull.* **1995**, *43*, 920–926. [CrossRef] [PubMed]
154. Arafa, H.M. Possible contribution of beta-glycosidases and caspases in the cytotoxicity of novel glycoconjugates in colon cancer cells. *Invest New Drugs* **2010**, *28*, 306–317. [CrossRef]
155. Nandurkar, N.S.; Zhang, J.; Ye, Q.; Ponomareva, L.V.; She, Q.-B.; Thorson, J.S. The Identification of Perillyl Alcohol Glycosides with Improved Antiproliferative Activity. *J. Med. Chem.* **2014**, *57*, 7478–7484. [CrossRef] [PubMed]
156. Xanthakis, E.; Magkouta, S.; Loutrari, H.; Stamatis, H.; Roussos, C.; Kolisis, F.N. Enzymatic synthesis of perillyl alcohol derivatives and investigation of their antiproliferative activity. *Biocatal. Biotransformation* **2009**, *27*, 170–178. [CrossRef]
157. Said, B.; Montenegro, I.; Valenzuela, M.; Olguín, Y.; Caro, N.; Werner, E.; Godoy, P.; Villena, J.; Madrid, A. Synthesis and Antiproliferative Activity of New Cyclodiprenyl Phenols against Select Cancer Cell Lines. *Molecules* **2018**, *23*, 2323. [CrossRef] [PubMed]
158. Rezende, A.A.; Santos, R.S.; Andrade, L.N.; Amaral, R.G.; Pereira, M.M.; Bani, C.; Chen, M.; Priefer, R.; da Silva, C.F.; de Albuquerque Junior, R.L.C.; et al. Anti-tumor efficiency of perillylalcohol/beta-cyclodextrin inclusion complexes in a sarcoma s180-induced mice model. *Pharmaceutics* **2021**, *13*, 245. [CrossRef]
159. Da Silva, C.E.H.; Gosmann, G.; de Andrade, S.F. Limonene and perillyl alcohol derivatives: Synthesis and anticancer activity. *Mini Rev. Med. Chem.* **2021**, *21*, 1813–1829. [CrossRef] [PubMed]

160. Zielińska-Błajet, M.; Pietrusiak, P.; Feder-Kubis, J. Selected Monocyclic Monoterpenes and Their Derivatives as Effective Anticancer Therapeutic Agents. *Int. J. Mol. Sci.* **2021**, *22*, 4763. [CrossRef] [PubMed]
161. Hopkins, A.L. Network pharmacology: The next paradigm in drug discovery. *Nat. Chem. Biol.* **2008**, *4*, 682–690. [CrossRef] [PubMed]
162. Szumilak, M.; Wiktorowska-Owczarek, A.; Stanczak, A. Hybrid Drugs—A Strategy for Overcoming Anticancer Drug Resistance? *Molecules* **2021**, *26*, 2601. [CrossRef] [PubMed]
163. Vendrusculo, V.; de Souza, V.P.; LA, M.F.; MG, M.D.O.; Banzato, T.P.; Monteiro, P.A.; Pilli, R.A.; de Carvalho, J.E.; Russowsky, D. Synthesis of novel perillyl-dihydropyrimidinone hybrids designed for antiproliferative activity. *Medchemcomm* **2018**, *9*, 1553–1564. [CrossRef] [PubMed]
164. Mohammadi, B.; Behbahani, F.K. Recent developments in the synthesis and applications of dihydropyrimidin-2(1H)-ones and thiones. *Mol. Divers.* **2018**, *22*, 405–446. [CrossRef]
165. Chen, T.C.; Cho, H.-Y.; Wang, W.; Barath, M.; Sharma, N.; Hofman, F.M.; Schönthal, A.H. A Novel Temozolomide–Perillyl Alcohol Conjugate Exhibits Superior Activity against Breast Cancer Cells In Vitro and Intracranial Triple-Negative Tumor Growth In Vivo. *Mol. Cancer Ther.* **2014**, *13*, 1181–1193. [CrossRef] [PubMed]
166. Chen, T.C.; Cho, H.-Y.; Wang, W.; Wetzel, S.J.; Singh, A.; Nguyen, J.; Hofman, F.M.; Schönthal, A.H. Chemotherapeutic effect of a novel temozolomide analog on nasopharyngeal carcinoma in vitro and in vivo. *J. Biomed. Sci.* **2015**, *22*, 71–80. [CrossRef] [PubMed]
167. Schönthal, A.; Swenson, S.; Minea, R.; Kim, H.; Cho, H.; Mohseni, N.; Kim, Y.-M.; Chen, T. Potentially Curative Therapeutic Activity of NEO212, a Perillyl Alcohol-Temozolomide Conjugate, in Preclinical Cytarabine-Resistant Models of Acute Myeloid Leukemia. *Cancers* **2021**, *13*, 3385. [CrossRef] [PubMed]
168. Chen, T.C.; Cho, H.-Y.; Wang, W.; Nguyen, J.; Jhaveri, N.; Rosenstein-Sisson, R.; Hofman, F.M.; Schönthal, A.H. A novel temozolomide analog, NEO212, with enhanced activity against MGMT-positive melanoma in vitro and in vivo. *Cancer Lett.* **2015**, *358*, 144–151. [CrossRef] [PubMed]
169. Cho, H.-Y.; Swenson, S.; Thein, T.Z.; Wang, W.; Wijeratne, N.R.; I Marín-Ramos, N.; E Katz, J.; Hofman, F.M.; Schönthal, A.H.; Chen, T.C. Pharmacokinetic properties of the temozolomide perillyl alcohol conjugate (NEO212) in mice. *Neuro-Oncol. Adv.* **2020**, *2*, vdaa160. [CrossRef] [PubMed]
170. Cho, H.-Y.; Wang, W.; Jhaveri, N.; Lee, D.J.; Sharma, N.; Dubeau, L.; Schönthal, A.H.; Hofman, F.M.; Chen, T.C. NEO212, Temozolomide Conjugated to Perillyl Alcohol, Is a Novel Drug for Effective Treatment of a Broad Range of Temozolomide-Resistant Gliomas. *Mol. Cancer Ther.* **2014**, *13*, 2004–2017. [CrossRef] [PubMed]
171. Jhaveri, N.; Agasse, F.; Armstrong, D.; Peng, L.; Commins, D.; Wang, W.; Rosenstein-Sisson, R.; Vaikari, V.P.; Santiago, S.V.; Santos, T.; et al. A novel drug conjugate, NEO212, targeting proneural and mesenchymal subtypes of patient-derived glioma cancer stem cells. *Cancer Lett.* **2016**, *371*, 240–250. [CrossRef] [PubMed]
172. Di Francia, R.; Crisci, S.; De Monaco, A.; Cafiero, C.; Re, A.; Iaccarino, G.; De Filippi, R.; Frigeri, F.; Corazzelli, G.; Micera, A.; et al. Response and Toxicity to Cytarabine Therapy in Leukemia and Lymphoma: From Dose Puzzle to Pharmacogenomic Biomarkers. *Cancers* **2021**, *13*, 966. [CrossRef]
173. Zhang, J.; Stevens, M.F.; Bradshaw, T.D. Temozolomide: Mechanisms of action, repair and resistance. *Curr. Mol. Pharmacol.* **2012**, *5*, 102–114. [CrossRef]
174. Zhu, J.; Mix, E.; Winblad, B. The Antidepressant and Antiinflammatory Effects of Rolipram in the Central Nervous System. *CNS Drug Rev.* **2001**, *7*, 387–398. [CrossRef] [PubMed]
175. Chen, T.C.; Wadsten, P.; Su, S.; Rawlinson, N.; Hofman, F.M.; Hill, C.K.; Schonthal, A.H. The type iv phosphodiesterase inhibitor rolipram induces expression of the cell cycle inhibitors p21(cip1) and p27(kip1), resulting in growth inhibition, increased differentiation, and subsequent apoptosis of malignant a-172 glioma cells. *Cancer Biol. Ther.* **2002**, *1*, 268–276. [CrossRef] [PubMed]
176. Goldhoff, P.; Warrington, N.M.; Limbrick, D.D., Jr.; Hope, A.; Woerner, B.M.; Jackson, E.; Perry, A.; Piwnica-Worms, D.; Rubin, J.B. Targeted Inhibition of Cyclic AMP Phosphodiesterase-4 Promotes Brain Tumor Regression. *Clin. Cancer Res.* **2008**, *14*, 7717–7725. [CrossRef] [PubMed]
177. Cho, H.-Y.; Thein, T.Z.; Wang, W.; Swenson, S.D.; Fayngor, R.A.; Ou, M.; Marín-Ramos, N.I.; Schönthal, A.H.; Hofman, F.M.; Chen, T.C. The Rolipram–Perillyl Alcohol Conjugate (NEO214) Is A Mediator of Cell Death through the Death Receptor Pathway. *Mol. Cancer Ther.* **2019**, *18*, 517–530. [CrossRef] [PubMed]
178. Chen, T.C.; Chan, N.; Labib, S.; Yu, J.; Cho, H.-Y.; Hofman, F.M.; Schönthal, A.H. Induction of Pro-Apoptotic Endoplasmic Reticulum Stress in Multiple Myeloma Cells by NEO214, Perillyl Alcohol Conjugated to Rolipram. *Int. J. Mol. Sci.* **2018**, *19*, 277. [CrossRef] [PubMed]
179. Fan, T.; Sun, G.; Sun, X.; Zhao, L.; Zhong, R.; Peng, Y. Tumor Energy Metabolism and Potential of 3-Bromopyruvate as an Inhibitor of Aerobic Glycolysis: Implications in Tumor Treatment. *Cancers* **2019**, *11*, 317. [CrossRef] [PubMed]
180. Birsoy, K.; Wang, T.; Possemato, R.; Yilmaz, O.H.; E Koch, C.; Chen, W.; Hutchins, A.W.; Gultekin, Y.; Peterson, T.R.; Carette, J.; et al. MCT1-mediated transport of a toxic molecule is an effective strategy for targeting glycolytic tumors. *Nat. Genet.* **2013**, *45*, 104–108. [CrossRef]
181. Chen, T.C.; Yu, J.; Nigjeh, E.N.; Wang, W.; Myint, P.T.; Zandi, E.; Hofman, F.M.; Schönthal, A.H. A perillyl alcohol-conjugated analog of 3-bromopyruvate without cellular uptake dependency on monocarboxylate transporter 1 and with activity in 3-BP-resistant tumor cells. *Cancer Lett.* **2017**, *400*, 161–174. [CrossRef] [PubMed]

182. Göttlicher, M. Valproic acid: An old drug newly discovered as inhibitor of histone deacetylases. *Ann. Hematol.* **2004**, *83* (Suppl. 1), S91–S92. [PubMed]
183. Martirosian, V.; Deshpande, K.; Zhou, H.; Shen, K.; Smith, K.; Northcott, P.; Lin, M.; Stepanosyan, V.; Das, D.; Remsik, J.; et al. Medulloblastoma uses GABA transaminase to survive in the cerebrospinal fluid microenvironment and promote leptomeningeal dissemination. *Cell Rep.* **2021**, *36*, 109475. [CrossRef] [PubMed]
184. Haque, T.; Talukder, M.U. Chemical Enhancer: A Simplistic Way to Modulate Barrier Function of the Stratum Corneum. *Adv. Pharm. Bull.* **2018**, *8*, 169–179. [CrossRef]
185. Li, B.S.; Cary, J.H.; Maibach, H.I. Stratum corneum substantivity: Drug development implications. *Arch. Dermatol. Res.* **2018**, *310*, 537–549. [CrossRef]
186. Kováčik, A.; Kopečná, M.; Vávrová, K. Permeation enhancers in transdermal drug delivery: Benefits and limitations. *Expert Opin. Drug Deliv.* **2020**, *17*, 145–155. [CrossRef]
187. Lopes, L.B.; Garcia, M.T.J.; Bentley, M.V.L. Chemical penetration enhancers. *Ther. Deliv.* **2015**, *6*, 1053–1061. [CrossRef] [PubMed]
188. Chen, J.; Jiang, Q.-D.; Chai, Y.-P.; Zhang, H.; Peng, P.; Yang, X.-X. Natural Terpenes as Penetration Enhancers for Transdermal Drug Delivery. *Molecules* **2016**, *21*, 1709. [CrossRef] [PubMed]
189. Kopečná, M.; Macháček, M.; Nováčková, A.; Paraskevopoulos, G.; Roh, J.; Vávrová, K. Esters of terpene alcohols as highly potent, reversible, and low toxic skin penetration enhancers. *Sci. Rep.* **2019**, *9*, 1–12. [CrossRef]
190. Lluria-Prevatt, M.; Morreale, J.; Gregus, J.; Alberts, D.S.; Kaper, F.; Giaccia, A.; Powell, M.B. Effects of perillyl alcohol on melanoma in the TPras mouse model. *Cancer Epidemiol. Biomark. Prev.* **2002**, *11*, 573–579.
191. Chaudhary, S.C.; Alam, M.S.; Siddiqui, M.; Athar, M. Perillyl alcohol attenuates Ras-ERK signaling to inhibit murine skin inflammation and tumorigenesis. *Chem.-Biol. Interact.* **2009**, *179*, 145–153. [CrossRef] [PubMed]
192. Barthelman, M.; Chen, W.; Gensler, H.L.; Huang, C.; Dong, Z.; Bowden, G.T. Inhibitory effects of perillyl alcohol on UVB-induced murine skin cancer and AP-1 transactivation. *Cancer Res.* **1998**, *58*, 711–716. [PubMed]
193. Gupta, A.; Myrdal, P.B. Development of a perillyl alcohol topical cream formulation. *Int. J. Pharm.* **2004**, *269*, 373–383. [CrossRef] [PubMed]
194. Stratton, S.P.; Saboda, K.L.; Myrdal, P.B.; Gupta, A.; McKenzie, N.E.; Brooks, C.; Salasche, S.J.; Warneke, J.A.; Ranger-Moore, J.; Bozzo, P.D.; et al. Phase 1 Study of Topical Perillyl Alcohol Cream for Chemoprevention of Skin Cancer. *Nutr. Cancer* **2008**, *60*, 325–330. [CrossRef] [PubMed]
195. Stratton, S.P.; Alberts, D.S.; Einspahr, J.G.; Sagerman, P.M.; Warneke, J.A.; Curiel-Lewandrowski, C.; Myrdal, P.B.; Karlage, K.L.; Nickoloff, B.J.; Brooks, C.; et al. A Phase 2a Study of Topical Perillyl Alcohol Cream for Chemoprevention of Skin Cancer. *Cancer Prev. Res.* **2010**, *3*, 160–169. [CrossRef]
196. D'Alessio, P.; Mirshahi, M.; Bisson, J.-F.; Bene, M. Skin Repair Properties of d-Limonene and Perillyl Alcohol in Murine Models. *Anti-Inflamm. Anti-Allergy Agents Med. Chem.* **2014**, *13*, 29–35. [CrossRef] [PubMed]
197. Araujo-Filho, H.G.; Pereira, E.W.M.; Heimfarth, L.; Souza Monteiro, B.; Santos Passos, F.R.; Siqueira-Lima, P.; Gandhi, S.R.; Viana Dos Santos, M.R.; Guedes da Silva Almeida, J.R.; Picot, L.; et al. Limonene, a food additive, and its active metabolite perillyl alcohol improve regeneration and attenuate neuropathic pain after peripheral nerve injury: Evidence for il-1beta, tnf-alpha, gap, ngf and erk involvement. *Int. Immunopharmacol.* **2020**, *86*, 106766. [CrossRef] [PubMed]
198. Erickson, C.; Miller, S.J. Treatment options in melanoma in situ: Topical and radiation therapy, excision and Mohs surgery. *Int. J. Dermatol.* **2010**, *49*, 482–491. [CrossRef] [PubMed]
199. Van Zyl, L.; du Preez, J.; Gerber, M.; du Plessis, J.; Viljoen, J. Essential Fatty Acids as Transdermal Penetration Enhancers. *J. Pharm. Sci.* **2016**, *105*, 188–193. [CrossRef] [PubMed]
200. Viljoen, J.; Cowley, A.; du Preez, J.; Gerber, M.; Du Plessis, J. Penetration enhancing effects of selected natural oils utilized in topical dosage forms. *Drug Dev. Ind. Pharm.* **2015**, *41*, 2045–2054. [CrossRef] [PubMed]
201. Swenson, S.; Silva-Hirschberg, C.; Wang, W.; Singh, A.; Hofman, F.M.; Chen, K.L.; Schönthal, A.H.; Chen, T.C. NEO412: A temozolomide analog with transdermal activity in melanoma in vitro and in vivo. *Oncotarget* **2018**, *9*, 37026–37041. [CrossRef] [PubMed]

pharmaceutics

MDPI

Article

Intranasal Zolmitriptan-Loaded Bilosomes with Extended Nasal Mucociliary Transit Time for Direct Nose to Brain Delivery

Mai M. El Taweel *, Mona H. Aboul-Einien, Mohammed A. Kassem and Nermeen A. Elkasabgy

Department of Pharmaceutics and Industrial Pharmacy, Faculty of Pharmacy, Cairo University, Kasr El-Aini Street, Cairo 11562, Egypt; mona.abouleinien@pharma.cu.edu.eg (M.H.A.-E.); mohamed.kassem@pharma.cu.edu.eg (M.A.K.); nermeen.ahmed.elkasabgy@pharma.cu.edu.eg (N.A.E.)
* Correspondence: mai.eltaweel@pharma.cu.edu.eg

Abstract: This study aimed at delivering intranasal zolmitriptan directly to the brain through preparation of bilosomes incorporated into a mucoadhesive in situ gel with extended nasal mucociliary transit time. Zolmitriptan-loaded bilosomes were constructed through a thin film hydration method applying Box–Behnken design. The independent variables were amount of sodium deoxycholate and the amount and molar ratio of cholesterol/Span® 40 mixture. Bilosomes were assessed for their entrapment efficiency, particle size and in vitro release. The optimal bilosomes were loaded into mucoadhesive in situ gel consisting of poloxamer 407 and hydroxypropyl methylcellulose. The systemic and brain kinetics of Zolmitriptan were evaluated in rats by comparing intranasal administration of prepared gel to an IV solution. Statistical analysis suggested an optimized bilosomal formulation composition of sodium deoxycholate (5 mg) with an amount and molar ratio of cholesterol/Span® 40 mixture of 255 mg and 1:7.7, respectively. The mucoadhesive in situ gel containing bilosomal formulation had a sol-gel temperature of 34.03 °C and an extended mucociliary transit time of 22.36 min. The gelling system possessed enhanced brain bioavailability compared to bilosomal dispersion (1176.98 vs. 835.77%, respectively) following intranasal administration. The gel revealed successful brain targeting with improved drug targeting efficiency and direct transport percentage indices. The intranasal delivery of mucoadhesive in situ gel containing zolmitriptan-loaded bilosomes offered direct nose-to-brain drug targeting with enhanced brain bioavailability.

Keywords: zolmitriptan; intranasal; bilosomes; sodium deoxycholate; mucoadhesive gel; brain targeting

Citation: El Taweel, M.M.; Aboul-Einien, M.H.; Kassem, M.A.; Elkasabgy, N.A. Intranasal Zolmitriptan-Loaded Bilosomes with Extended Nasal Mucociliary Transit Time for Direct Nose to Brain Delivery. *Pharmaceutics* **2021**, *13*, 1828. https://doi.org/10.3390/pharmaceutics13111828

Academic Editors: Vibhuti Agrahari, Prashant Kumar and Roberta Cavalli

Received: 23 August 2021
Accepted: 22 October 2021
Published: 1 November 2021

1. Introduction

Migraine is the most abundant type of neurological disorder; coupled with atypical serotonergic activity [1,2], it is considered the second major cause of disability, especially among young people [3]. A migraine is a special kind of headache, consisting of a throbbing and severe headache in one side of the head [4]. Migraine can be associated with aura or not, with the latter being the most common type. Any of these symptoms can be associated with different etiologies [5]. Migraine with aura causes the patient to see strange colors and lights, which is sometimes scary and in some cases can also, be associated with ischemic stroke [6].

Zolmitriptan is a potent second generation triptan which acts as a selective serotonin receptor agonist [2]. It is used as pain terminator in migraine and cluster headache treatment and is given to patients with migraine attacks, with or without an aura. Although the oral administration of zolmitriptan is the most common route of administration, it is associated with poor bioavailability (≈40%) owing to severe hepatic first pass effect, slow onset of action [7,8] and systemic side effects such as nausea, dizziness, paraesthesia, neck pain and tightness [9]. Generally, the oral administration of anti-migraine drugs can be inconvenient, especially in patients with associated with nausea and vomiting.

For these reasons, attempts have been made to deliver zolmitriptan through other routes in order to bypass the hepatic metabolism and provide fast onset of action with enhanced bioavailability [7,8]. Among those routes, nose to brain drug delivery is of pronounced interest. Nasal delivery is an easy and non-invasive route for controlling migraine attacks, and is considered to be an attractive route of administration. There are six branches of arteries serving the nasal cavity which can enhance the systemic absorption of drugs; additionally, the presence of the olfactory region can provide a means of direct brain targeting [10]. All of these factors, as well as the increased surface area of the nasal cavity, can aid in enhanced drug absorption.

In 2003, the first zolmitriptan nasal spray was approved by FDA. Nevertheless, the approved aqueous solution provided only similar bioavailability to oral tablets, due to the first pass effect the drug is subjected to after systemic absorption [11]. Therefore, the fabrication of efficient nasal formulations capable of delivering the drug in sufficient amounts to the brain while avoiding rapid mucociliary clearance and poor membrane penetration is highly necessary.

Bilosomes (bile salts containing niosomes) are nanovesicular carriers composed of a non-ionic surfactant bilayer along with bile salts [12]. The literature includes several studies reporting the use of bilosomes in the efficient oral delivery of drugs and vaccines [13,14] thanks to their ability to resist gastrointestinal enzymes and consequent conferring of protection to the loaded active ingredient [14,15]. Additionally, the nature of the vesicular wall is considered a major point of difference between bilosomes and niosomes; the structure of niosomes lacks the additional edge activators of like bile salts. Edge activators act by lowering the surface tension of the vesicular bilayer, resulting in its destabilization and the formation of deformable vesicles [16] with enhanced tissue penetration [17].

Bilosomes have been applied for transdermal [18], topical [19] and ocular drug delivery [20]. However, to the authors' knowledge, no published research has studied the influence of intranasal application of drug-loaded bilosomes on drug absorption and brain targeting. Although bilosomes have not yet been explored for intranasal drug delivery, their nanosize, coupled with the non-ionic surfactants and bile salts in their structure, provide promising scenarios for utilizing them in nose to brain drug delivery.

To gain the maximum benefit from the developed intranasal bilosomes, the nasal mucociliary transit time should be extended to allow for more residence of the applied dosage form inside the nasal cavity, improving drug absorption. This can be achieved by loading the developed bilosomes into a mucoadhesive in situ gelling system with high viscosity capable of resisting rapid mucociliary clearance [21,22].

Therefore, the objective of this study was to fabricate zolmitriptan-loaded bilosomes by applying 3^3 Box–Behnken design and trying different formulation factors as well as loading the optimal bilosomal formulation into a mucoadhesive in situ gelling system with extended nasal mucociliary transit time. A temperature-induced in situ gelling system which transforms into gel form at body temperature was formulated using poloxamer 407. To boost the nasal residence time of the in situ gelling system, a mucoadhesive polymer (hydroxypropyl methyl cellulose) was added. The influence of formulation variables on entrapment efficiency, particle size and zeta potential, in addition to drug release, were evaluated. Furthermore, biological evaluation for the potential of brain drug delivery was assessed in rats.

2. Materials and Methods

2.1. Materials

Zolmitriptan was kindly supplied and certified by Global Nabi Pharmaceuticals (GNP), 6th of October, Giza, Egypt (Batch number: ZT 18040001). Brij® 35 (polyoxyethylene (23) lauryl ether), Brij® O10 (polyoxylethylene (10) oleyl ether), cholesterol, hydroxypropyl methylcellulose (HPMC) (viscosity 1500–4500 cp at 37 °C), poloxamer 407, sodium deoxycholate, Span® 20 (sorbitan monolaurate), Span® 40 (sorbitan monopalmitate), Span® 60 (sorbitan monostearate), Span® 80 (sorbitan monooleate), Tween® 65 (polyoxyethylene sorbitan tristearate), Tween® 80 (polyoxyethylene sorbitan monooleate) and dialysis tubing cellulose membrane (molecular weight cutoff 14,000 g/mol) were procured from Sigma-Aldrich, St. Louis, MO, USA. Methylene blue was obtained from El-Nasr Pharmaceutical Chemicals Company, Abu-Zaabal, Cairo, Egypt. Normal saline was purchased from Otsuka Pharmaceutical Co., Egypt. Acetonitrile and formic acid (both of HLPC grade) were supplied by Romil Limited, London, UK and E. Merk, D-6100 Darmstadt, Germany, respectively. Torsemide was provided and certified by DELTA Pharma, Cairo, Egypt. The water used was distilled de-ionized water. The other chemicals were of reagent grade and used as provided.

2.2. *Optimization of Bilosomes*

2.2.1. Preparation of Zolmitriptan-Loaded Niosomes

Zolmitriptan-loaded niosomes were formed using the thin film hydration method [23], with minor modifications. In brief, 20 mg of drug were mixed with a 200 mg equimolar mixture of cholesterol and a non-ionic surfactant; all were dissolved in 10 mL chloroform/methanol mixture (3:7 v/v) in a round-bottomed flask. The organic solvent was evaporated at 60 °C under vacuum utilizing a rotary evaporator (Rotavapor, Heidolph VV 2000, Burladingen, Germany) adjusted at 90 rpm for 30 min to confirm complete elimination of the organic solvent. Following this, the formed thin dry film on the flask inner wall was hydrated using 10 mL distilled water. The hydration step was performed under normal pressure in the presence of glass beads for 1 h at 60 °C, utilizing the rotary evaporator which revolved at 90 rpm. Following this, the hydrated film dispersion was sonicated for 2 min using a bath sonicator (Crest ultrasonics corp., Trenton, NJ, USA) to ensure the formation of homogenous dispersion without any aggregates, then kept overnight at 6 °C. Eight non-ionic surfactants having different HLB values were utilized to prepare eight different niosomal formulations. The used surfactants were Span® 20, Span® 40, Span® 60, Span® 80, Tween® 65, Tween® 80, Brij® 35 and Brij® O10.

Evaluation of the Prepared Zolmitriptan-Loaded Niosomes

For each of the prepared niosomal formulations, drug entrapment efficiency (EE), particle size (PS) and polydispersity index (PDI) were evaluated.

Assessment of Entrapment Efficiency (EE)

To assess the EE% of the formed niosomal formulations, 1 mL of niosomal dispersion was mixed with 9 mL ethanol followed by sonication for 5 min using a bath sonicator. Actual drug content was measured spectrophotometrically (model UV-1601 PC; Shimadzu, Kyoto, Japan) by assaying its UV absorbance at a wavelength of 285 nm, after suitable dilution.

Additionally, the same volume (1 mL) of the niosomal formulation was ultra-centrifuged at 15,000 rpm, 4 °C for 90 min by means of a cooling centrifuge (Beckman, Fullerton, Canada). The supernatant was discarded and the residue was dissolved in 10 mL ethanol under sonication for 5 min in a bath sonicator to quantify the amount of entrapped drug [24]. Zolmitriptan content was assayed spectrophotometrically as before. EE% was determined as follows:

$$EE\ \% = (\text{Amount of entrapped drug}/\text{Actual drug content}) \times 100$$

Assessment of Particle Size (PS) and Polydispersity Index (PDI)

Furthermore, the niosomal preparations were assessed for their PS and PDI values. The examined formulations were suitably diluted with distilled water (1:10 v/v) until reaching faint opalescence, followed by analysis via ZetaSizer Nano ZS (Malvern Instruments, Worcestershire, UK). Moreover, particle size distribution was assessed via the determination of PDI. The used cuvettes were quartz, and the refractive index was adjusted at 1.33.

Statistical Analysis

One-way ANOVA followed by the least significance difference (LSD) test was applied to compare the EE% of the prepared zolmitriptan-loaded niosomal formulations using SPSS 17® (SPSS Inc., Chicago, IL, USA). Zolmitriptan-loaded niosomes with the highest EE% were chosen as the optimal drug-loaded niosomal formulation. Data were gathered from two different batches for each preparation. Means and standard deviations were calculated from triplicate test results for every batch.

2.2.2. Preparation of Zolmitriptan-Loaded Bilosomes

The same method utilized to prepare zolmitriptan-loaded niosomes was applied to prepare drug-loaded bilosomes, with bile salt (sodium deoxycholate) added to the chloroform/methanol solvent mixture. The resultant organic solution was treated as in the preparation of drug-loaded niosomes. Fifteen formulations were prepared using different weights of sodium deoxycholate and cholesterol/Span® 40 mixture, as well as different molar ratios of cholesterol: Span® 40 according to the constructed Box-Behnken statistical design.

Optimization of Zolmitriptan-Loaded Bilosomes

A three-factor, three-level Box-Behnken design (3^3) was constructed in order to explore the effects of formulation factors on the main properties of the fabricated bilosomes and optimize their composition, for which Design-Expert® software (Stat-Ease, Inc., Minneapolis, MN, USA) was employed. The independent variables were the amount of sodium deoxycholate (X_1; 5, 10, 15 mg), the amount of cholesterol/Span® 40 mixture (X_2; 100, 200, 300 mg), and the molar ratio of cholesterol: Span® 40 (X_3; 1:1, 1:5, 1:9 *w*/*w*). Entrapment efficiency (Y_1), particle size (Y_2), polydispersity index (Y_3), zeta potential (Y_4), total % of zolmitriptan released after 0.5 h (Q0.5 h; Y_5), and drug release efficiency (Y_6) were chosen to be the dependent variables. Regarding the optimized formulation, responses Y_1, Y_5 and Y_6 were preferred to be maximized, whereas other responses (Y_2, Y_3 and Y_4) were desired to be minimized. According to the designed study, 15 formulations were prepared; 13 of them contained the midpoints of the investigated factors, while the center formulation was formulated three times. Two batches were prepared and results were collected in triplicates for each batch. The Box-Behnken design is presented in Table 1 and the detailed composition of the prepared drug-loaded bilosomal formulations is given in Table 2.

Table 1. Design parameters and experimental conditions for Box–Behnken (3^3) design.

Independent Variable (Factor)	Level		
	Low (−1)	Medium (0)	High (+1)
X_1: Sodium deoxycholate amount (mg)	5	10	15
X_2: Cholesterol/Span® 40 amount (mg)	100	200	300
X_3: Cholesterol: Span® 40 molar ratio (*w*/*w*)	1:1	1:5	1:9
Dependent variable (Response)	**Desirability Constraint**		
Y_1: Entrapment efficiency (%)	Maximize		
Y_2: Particle size (nm)	Minimize		
Y_3: Polydispersity index	Minimize		
Y_4: Zeta potential (mV)	Minimize		
Y_5: Q0.5 h (%)	Maximize		
Y_6: Release efficiency (%)	Maximize		

Abbreviations; Q0.5 h (%), Total percentage of drug released after 0.5 h.

Table 2. Composition of the prepared zolmitriptan-loaded bilosomes.

Formulation Code	Composition		
	Sodium Deoxycholate (mg)	Cholesterol/Span® 40 Mixture (mg)	Cholesterol: Span® 40 Molar Ratio
	Midpoint Formulations		
F1	5	100	1:5
F2	15	100	1:5
F3	5	300	1:5
F4	15	300	1:5
F5	5	200	1:1
F6	15	200	1:1
F7	5	200	1:9
F8	15	200	1:9
F9	10	100	1:1
F10	10	300	1:1
F11	10	100	1:9
F12	10	300	1:9
	Center point formulations		
F13	10	200	1:5
F14	10	200	1:5
F15	10	200	1:5

Drug concentration was kept constant (2 mg/mL) in all formulations.

Characterization of the Prepared Zolmitriptan-Loaded Bilosomes—Assessment of Entrapment Efficiency, Particle Size (PS), Polydispersity Index (PDI) and Zeta Potential (ZP)

The same methods and steps used for assessing the drug-loaded niosomes were followed for the determination of the EE%, PS and PDI of the bilosomes. Additionally, the surface charge of the formulated bilosomes was evaluated by determining the ZP so as to evaluate the physical stability of the examined samples using ZetaSizer Nano ZS.

Characterization of the Prepared Zolmitriptan-Loaded Bilosomes—In Vitro Release Studies

For each investigated formulation, the dialysis bag technique was applied [25], where a certain volume equivalent to 4 mg entrapped drug was transferred in a dialysis bag which was pre-soaked 12 h in distilled water. The filled dialysis bag was properly secured from both ends and then dipped in 100 mL phosphate buffered saline (PBS, pH 7.4) in an amber colored glass bottle to assure the sink conditions. The bottles were then put in a thermostatically controlled shaking water bath (GFL, Gesellschatt laboratories, Berlin, Germany) operating at 100 shakes per min at 37 °C ± 0.5. Three mL samples of the release medium were withdrawn at specified time intervals (0.5, 1, 2, 3, 4, 6 and 8 h) and immediately substituted by an equivalent volume of fresh PBS. Samples were assayed spectrophotometrically for zolmitriptan content at λ_{max} 285 nm. This experiment was repeated for zolmitriptan aqueous dispersion (4 mg/2 mL) to check the appropriateness of the utilized dialysis cellulose membrane. For comparison purposes, the total percentage of drug released after 0.5 h (Q0.5 h), as well as the release efficiency (*RE*), were calculated for each of the investigated formulations. The *RE* parameter was the area under the release curve, expressed as the percentage of the rectangle area represented by 100% release at the same time. The following equation was used for calculation of *RE*% [26]:

$$RE\% = \int_0^t y.dt/y100\ t \times 100$$

where the integral represents the area under the release curve until time t, and y_{100} is the area of the rectangle representing 100% release at equivalent time. The best kinetic model was determined by fitting the obtained release data to the zero-order, Higuchi and Korsmeyer-Peppas models [27,28].

2.3. *Mucoadhesive In Situ Gelling System*

2.3.1. Preparation of Mucoadhesive In Situ Gelling System Containing the Optimal Bilosomes

The mucoadhesive in situ gelling system was fabricated using the cold method [29]. Different gelling systems were prepared using different polymers at different concentrations (Table S1). A 3^3 general factorial design using Design-Expert® software was utilized to investigate the effect of formulation variables. The optimal gelling system was selected based on the desirability function (0.705). The optimal zolmitriptan-loaded bilosomes was dispersed in an aqueous solution of hydroxypropyl methyl cellulose (HPMC, the mucoadhesive polymer). A calculated amount of poloxamer 407 was then added slowly under magnetic stirring (WiseStir, Daihan Scientific Company, Daihan, Chhattisgarh, India) adjusted at 100 rpm at room temperature. The prepared dispersion was preserved in a refrigerator at 6 ± 2 °C for 24 h to equilibrate and form a clear solution. The used concentration of HPMC was 0.5% *w*/*v* and that of poloxamer 407 was 17% *w*/*v*. Batches were prepared in duplicates and the mean± standard deviations were calculated for three measurements for each batch.

2.3.2. Characterization of the Prepared Mucoadhesive In Situ Gelling System

The optimal zolmitriptan-loaded bilosomal formulation in the prepared mucoadhesive in situ gelling system was re-characterized for its EE%, PS, PDI and ZP as was previously done for the free bilosomes prior to incorporation into the gel system. The prepared mucoadhesive in situ gelling system containing the optimal bilosomal formulation was characterized for drug release parameters (Q0.5 h and *RE*%), sol to gel transition temperature, nasal mucociliary transit time and rheological constants (consistency index and flow index).

Assessment of Release Parameters of Zolmitriptan from the Prepared Mucoadhesive In Situ Gelling System

The in vitro release testing was conducted using the dialysis bag diffusion method for the cold in situ gelling system loaded with optimal bilosomes, as previously described under the in vitro release testing of bilosomes and the percentage of total zolmitriptan released after 0.5 h and *RE*% was calculated.

Assessment of Sol to Gel Transition Temperature and Time

To determine the sol to gel transition temperature of the prepared gelling system, the tilting method was used [30]. A test tube containing 2 mL aliquot of the formulated clear solution of the cold mucoadhesive in situ gel was covered with Parafilm® and affixed in a water bath. The temperature of the water bath was elevated gradually, starting from 20 °C, in increments of 0.5 °C every 10 min. The content was visually inspected for gelation by tilting it by 90°. The gelation temperature of the investigated formulation was its sol to gel transition temperature.

The sol to gel transition time was investigated using the test tube inversion method [31]. In brief, 1 mL of the mucoadhesive in situ gelling system (sol) was transferred into a 5 mL stoppered test tube which was placed a thermostatically controlled water bath kept at 37 °C. The transition time was determined by tilting the tube every 10 s till no flow was detected.

Assessment of Rheological Constants

The rheological characteristics of the investigated gelling system were assessed using a cone and plate viscometer (Brookfield viscometer; type DVT-2). The plate was connected to a water bath to keep its temperature at 35 ± 0.1 °C. A half-mL sample of the investigated cold system was transferred to the plate. The shear rate was elevated gradually from

0.5 to 100 min^{-1} and the viscosity reading was recorded [32]. The power law constitutive equation was then applied to the results [33]:

$$\eta = my^{n-1}$$

where η is the viscosity (cp), y is the shear rate (s^{-1}), and m and n are constants representing consistency and flow indices, respectively.

Transmission Electron Microscopy (TEM)

Morphological examination of the optimal zolmitriptan-loaded bilosomal formulation as well as the prepared mucoadhesive in situ gelling system containing it was performed in order to assess aqueous dispersion. TEM (Lecia Image, Wetzlar, Germany) connected to camera model TKC 1380 JVC (Victor Company, Tokyo, Japan) at an accelerating voltage of 80 kV was used. A sample drop was placed on a carbon-coated copper grid surface and left for one minute; any excess was dried by a tip of filter paper.

Differential Scanning Calorimetry (DSC)

DSC was applied to both the optimal zolmitriptan-loaded bilosomes and the mucoadhesive in situ gelling system containing them after lyophilizing both.

Samples were initially frozen at −20 °C then lyophilized for 24 h (Lyophilizer; Novalyphe-NL 500; Savant Instruments Corp., Holbrook, NY, USA) with pressure adjusted at 7×10^{-2} mbar and condenser temperature maintained at −45 °C. The reconstitution time of the lyophilized samples was assessed by adding the same volume of distilled water prior to the lyophilization process to the dried samples. The time recorded till the formation of dispersion free from any aggregates was taken as the reconstitution time [34].

DSC analysis was also performed for zolmitriptan powder, a physical mixture of the individual components of the bilosomes, and the individual components of the gelling system. About 4 mg of each sample was scanned separately in aluminum pans from 30 to 300 °C at a heating rate of 10 °C/min under an inert nitrogen flow of 25 mL/min.

Determination of Nasal Mucociliary Transit Time

The nasal mucociliary transit time was assessed by an in vivo method described by Lale et al. [35], with slight adjustments. Nine rats (weighing 200–250 g) participated in this study. Animal use in this study was in accordance with the National Institutes of Health Guide for The Care and Use of Laboratory Animals (NIH, publication No.85-23, 1996). Rats were divided into three equal groups (n = 3). Animals were anesthetized by intramuscular injection of sodium thiopental (7 mg/kg) at the beginning of the experiment. A volume of 10 µL of the prepared in situ gelling system loaded with the optimal bilosomes and containing methylene blue dye (5 mg/mL) was introduced into the right nostril of the animals of Group 1 using a micropipette. Swabs from the nasopalatine canal and pharynx were done via oral cavity (using a moistened cotton-tipped applicator) each minute post application, for a total period of 60 min. Each swab was visually examined for the blue color of the dye. The time taken for the appearance of the blue dye was recorded as the mucociliary transit time [30]. The experiment was also performed with the optimal bilosomes pre-mixed with methylene blue (Group 2) as well as with methylene blue solution in saline, which was used as a control (Group 3).

2.4. *In Vivo Animal Study*

2.4.1. Study Design and Dose Administration

This study was conducted to compare the pharmacokinetic parameters of zolmitriptan when using three different treatments. The investigated treatments were the optimal zolmitriptan-loaded bilosomes (Treatment A), the mucoadhesive in situ gelling system containing it (Treatment B), and the drug solution (Treatment C). A non-blind, three-treatment, one-period, randomized parallel design was used. Ninety male rats (weighing 200–250 g) participated in this study. The protocol of the study was approved by the institutional review board, Research Ethics Committee, Faculty of Pharmacy, Cairo University (PI 2326). The rats were housed nine per cage at ambient temperature with free access to food and water and a 12 h light/dark cycle. The animals were categorized into three equal groups ($n = 30$). Group 1 received intranasal (IN) Treatment A, Group 2 received IN Treatment B and Group 3 received intravenous (IV) Treatment C (used as a control). The dose of zolmitriptan in all treatments was 5 mg/kg [36]. The study lasted for 12 h and the animals were visually inspected throughout the study period for any behavioral disorder or sign of illness. At time intervals 0 (pre-dose), 0.25, 0.5, 1, 1.5, 2, 4, 6, 8 and 12 h following administration, three rats from each group were mercy sacrificed and plasma and brain samples were collected from them. Blood was collected from the trunk of the sacrificed animals into heparinized tubes and centrifuged (using Centurion Scientific LTD. Centrifuge, West Sussex, UK) at 4000 rpm for 15 min at 25 °C to separate plasma. In addition, the dissected brain was washed with normal saline, cleaned of all attaching tissue/fluid, and then homogenized with saline (three-fold its volume) for 1 min at 24,000 rpm using Pro scientific Homogenizer, (Oxford, UK). Plasma and brain samples were preserved at −20 °C pending analysis.

2.4.2. Chromatographic Conditions

A sensitive, selective and validated LC-MS/MS method for quantitative determination of zolmitriptan in plasma and brain tissues was adopted [37,38]. Torsemide was utilized as an internal standard. The detector was a triple quadrupole MS/MS (Waters Corp., Milford, MA, USA) and positive ionization mode was used for zolmitriptan and torsemide monitoring. Empower™ 2 CDS Software solutions was used for data acquisition and data integration. The used column was a reverse-phase column (C_{18}, 50 × 2.1 mm, Waters Corp., Milford, MA, USA). The mobile phase was a mixture of acetonitrile and 0.1% aqueous solution of formic acid 4:1 (v/v). Isocratic chromatographic separation was done at 40 °C and a flow rate of 0.2 mL/min.

2.4.3. Sample Preparation

A certain volume of plasma or homogenized brain sample (0.5 mL) was mixed with a 50 µL solution of torsemide in acetonitrile (100 ng/mL). The mixture was vortexed for 30 s and then centrifuged at 3000× g for 15 min. The supernatant was withdrawn and filtered through a 0.45 µm Millipore® filter. A centrifugal vacuum concentrator (Vacufuge 5301, Eppendorf, Hamburg, Germany) was utilized to dry the filtrate at 40 °C, which was then reconstituted with 100 µL mobile phase. A volume of 20 µL of the reconstituted sample was injected into the column using the autosampler.

2.4.4. In Vivo Brain and Systemic-Kinetic Studies

The main pharmacokinetic parameters of zolmitriptan from the three treatments were determined in both plasma and homogenized brain tissues. For plasma samples, the mean plasma concentration of the drug was illustrated against time, and the peak plasma concentration (C_{max}) and time taken to reach it (t_{max}) were calculated. The area under the zolmitriptan plasma concentration–time curve ($AUC_{0–12\ h}$) represents the total amount of drug in plasma over 12 h. C_{max}, t_{max}, $AUC_{0–12\ h}$, $AUC_{0–\infty}$, mean residence time (MRT, calculated by the trapezoidal rule), as well as the time for half the initial dose to be eliminated ($t_{1/2}$) and the drug elimination rate constant (k) were calculated by non-compartmental pharmacokinetic models using Kinetica® software (version 5.0, 2017, Thermo Fisher Scientific, Waltham, MA, USA. The values of absolute bioavailability of the drug in plasma from the applied IN Treatments (A and B) were calculated relative to an intravenous aqueous solution of drug in normal saline.

For brain samples, the mean concentration of the drug in the homogenized brain was plotted versus time, and the main pharmacokinetic parameters of the drug in brain tissues (C_{max}, t_{max}, $AUC_{\ 0–12\ h}$, $t_{1/2}$ and k) were determined as was done for the plasma samples. The values of drug bioavailability in the brain from the applied IN Treatments (A and B) compared to IV solution (Treatment C) were also calculated. In addition, two indices were calculated to express zolmitriptan targeting to the brain. These indices were drug targeting efficiency (DTE) [30] and nose to brain direct transport percentage (DTP) [39]. These indices were determined from the respective equations:

$$\text{DTE}(\%) = \left(\frac{\frac{B_{IN}}{P_{IN}}}{\frac{B_{IV}}{P_{IV}}}\right) \times 100$$

$$\text{DTP}(\%) = \left(\frac{B_{IN} - B_x}{B_{IN}}\right) \times 100$$

where B and P are AUC_{0-12} in brain and plasma, respectively, IN and IV stand for intranasal and intravenous application, respectively, and B_x is the brain AUC portion contributed by systemic circulation through the blood–brain barrier (BBB) subsequent IN application. B_x was determined as follows [39]:

$$B_x = \left(\frac{B_{IV} \times P_{IN}}{P_{IV}}\right) \times 100$$

2.4.5. Statistical Analysis

One-way ANOVA was carried out using SPSS 17.0 software followed by LSD test. Differences were significant at $p < 0.05$.

3. Results and Discussion

3.1. Optimization of Bilosomes

3.1.1. Preparation of Zolmitriptan-Loaded Niosomes

As explained before, this study aimed at preparing zolmitriptan-loaded non-ionic surfactant nano-vesicles for brain targeting. Non-ionic surfactant nano-vesicles consist of niosomes and bilosomes; the former is considered a precursor for the latter. In other words, preparing good bilosomes requires starting with good niosomes. A very important variable affecting the quality of the prepared niosomes is the type of non-ionic surfactant used. In order to choose a suitable surfactant for the preparation of zolmitriptan-loaded niosomes, eight non-ionic surfactants with different HLB values were used under fixed conditions to inspect the effect of surfactant type on the EE of the formed vesicles. The investigated surfactants covered an HLB range of 4.3–16.0.

Evaluation of the Prepared Zolmitriptan-Loaded Niosomes

As entrapment of the water-soluble drug (zolmitriptan) in niosomes, which are lipid-rich vesicles, was the main challenge in the preparation of such vesicles, EE% was set as the evaluation criterion for the quality of the prepared niosomes.

Table 3 represents the EE% of zolmitriptan-loaded niosomes prepared using different surfactants. It can be seen that the EE% of vesicles prepared using any of the sorbitan esters was significantly higher than that prepared using any of the Tweens or Brijs as a surfactant. The EE% of niosomes prepared using sorbitan esters ranged from 14.90 $\pm$ 0.70% to 44.70 $\pm$ 1.17%, whereas the highest EE% of niosomes prepared using any of the Tweens or Brijs did not exceed 11.90 $\pm$ 1.65%. Differences in EE% between different surfactant types were found to be significant ($p < 0.05$). This could be ascribed to the different HLB values of the used surfactants and, consequently, the difference in their lipophilicity [40,41]. Values of EE% were found to increase as the HLB value of the used surfactant decreased (i.e., lipophilicity increased). Tweens and Brijs have HLB values > 10, indicating more hydrophilicity, which caused the vesicular membrane to be more permeable and leaky to the drug, leading to lower EE% values compared to vesicles prepared using sorbitan esters (with low HLB values ranging from 4.3–8.6).

Table 3. Entrapment efficiency percent of zolmitriptan-loaded niosomes prepared using different non-ionic surfactants with different HLB values.

Non-Ionic Surfactant		EE%
Name	HLB	
Span® 20	8.6	14.90 ± 0.70
Span® 40	6.7	44.72 ± 1.17
Span® 60	4.7	33.33 ± 1.55
Span® 80	4.3	24.60 ± 1.35
Tween® 65	10.5	11.90 ± 1.65
Tween® 80	15.0	6.50 ± 0.70
Brij® 35	16.0	9.70 ± 0.70
Brij® O10	12.0	8.80 ± 0.83

Results are expressed as mean values ± SD, Abbreviations; EE, Entrapment efficiency.

Among the niosomes prepared using different sorbitan esters as surfactants, it was noticed that of EE% values of niosomes prepared using Span® 40 or Span® 60 (44.42 ± 1.17% and 33.33 ± 1.55%, respectively) were significantly higher ($p < 0.05$) than those prepared using Span® 20 or Span® 80 (14.90 ± 0.7% and 24.60 ± 1.35%, respectively). This could be related to the intrinsic properties of the sorbitan ester type used, especially the phase transition temperature. Span® 40 and Span® 60 are solid at ambient temperature due to their relatively high phase transition temperatures compared to Span® 20 or Span® 80. The stated phase transition temperatures are 48 and 53 °C versus 16 and −12 °C, respectively [40]. This temperature affects the nature of the surfactant bilayer being either in liquid or gel state, with the latter state occurring at higher phase transition temperatures. This gel state is characterized by the ordered arrangement of the surfactant alkyl chain, and hence leads to formation of less leaky bilayers [42].

Finally, by relating the EE% values of the formed niosomes utilizing either Span® 40 or Span® 60, it was evident that Span® 40 excelled significantly ($p < 0.05$). This might be attributed to the relatively higher surface free energy of Span® 40 (associated with higher HLB values) leading to the formation of vesicles of larger particle size with enhanced capability in terms of entrapping water-soluble drugs [43,44].

The relationship between PS and EE% was further confirmed by measuring the PS values of the investigated niosomes. The PS values of the prepared niosomes ranged from 308.31 ± 3.42 to 490.29 ± 6.53 nm, indicating the formation of nanovesicles. By comparing the PS of niosomes prepared with either Span® 40 or Span® 60, it was obvious that the former led to the formation of larger PS values compared to the latter, which could explain the enhanced EE% obtained with Span® 40-based niosomes. The obtained PS values were 434.67 ± 9.75 and 383.56 ± 8.39 nm, respectively. The obtained PDI values of the prepared niosomes were between 0.213 ± 0.014 to 0.411 ± 0.007, indicating·homogenous dispersion with low PDI values [45].

It can be concluded from the previous discussion that Span® 40 was the surfactant that succeeded in enhancing the EE% of the drug. The EE% of niosomes prepared using Span® 40 was quite satisfactory, as it is logical that entrapment of a water soluble drug in lipid niosomes is a great challenge. Accordingly, a niosomal formulation prepared using Span® 40 was chosen to complete this study and prepare bile salt-enriched zolmitriptan-loaded niosomes (i.e., bilosomes) for further investigation.

3.1.2. Investigation of the Effect Process Variables on the Properties of Zolmitriptan-Loaded Bilosomes

Statistical design was needed to correlate the main properties of the prepared drug-loaded bilosomes to the different formulation factors, to study the interaction between the investigated factors, and finally to suggest a formulation with optimized composition. A Box–Behnken (3^3) design was constructed to optimize the composition of the zolmitriptan-loaded bilosomes. The pre-determination of the used surfactant during the preparation of the niosomes reduced the number of investigated formulation factors. In addition, the total number of 15 test runs needed for Box–Behnken design is fewer than that needed for a central composite design with the same number of repeats (17 runs) or that needed for a 3^3 factorial design without repeats (27 runs) [46]. In addition, the used design enables studying of the interactions between different factors. For this reason, a Box–Behnken design was chosen in order to optimize the composition of the prepared bilosomes. The main output data of the applied design indicated good correlation between the predicted and adjusted R^2 values for all responses with differences between them not exceeding 0.2, which confirmed that the applied design was appropriate for predicting response values [47]. Additionally, adequate precision for all the investigated responses exceeded the value of four; which is the desirable value. As adequate precision measures the signal to noise ratio, the results indicated that the applied model can be utilized for navigating the design space [48]. Furthermore, it can be concluded that the statistical model designed to be applied in this study is a valid one (Table S2).

Effect on Entrapment Efficiency (EE)

All the investigated bilosomes had a drug content approximately equal to 100%, as the actual drug content did not show any significant difference from theoretical one (20 mg). This indicated that there was no significant drug loss during preparation.

As revealed in Table 4, the EE% of the investigated zolmitriptan-loaded bilosomes ranged from 33.53 ± 1.59 to 74.33 ± 1.32% for formulations F9 and F12, respectively. ANOVA testing showed a non-significant effect of sodium deoxycholate amount (X_1) on the EE% (Y_1) of bilosomes (p = 0.0815) and significant effects of both the amount (X_2) and molar ratio (X_3) of cholesterol/Span® 40 mixture (p < 0.0001 and = 0.0017, respectively), with a significant interaction between the two effective factors (p = 0.018). The individual effects of the two effective formulation factors on the EE% of the prepared bilosomes, as well as their interaction plot, are demonstrated in Figure 1. From Figure 1a, it is clear that increasing the amount of cholesterol/Span® 40 mixture resulted in a significant increase in the EE% of the formed bilosomes. This finding might be attributed to the fact that the cholesterol/non-ionic surfactant mixture represents the backbone and the main vesicle-forming material of bilosomes; thus, increasing amounts might lead to the construction of a larger number of large-sized vesicles, and thus inclusion of larger drug amounts [49]. In addition, at low cholesterol/Span® 40 mixture amounts, decreasing Span® 40 level might lead to more drug leakage, as decreased Span® 40 amounts are not adequate to stabilize the bilosomal membrane [50].

Table 4. Measured responses of Box–Behnken (3^3) design for the prepared zolmitriptan-loaded bilosomes.

Formulation Code	Responses					
	EE (%)	PS (nm)	PDI	ZP (mV)	Q0.5 h (%)	RE (%)
F1	42.73 ± 1.19	343.33 ± 18.53	0.34 ± 0.03	−41.4 ± 1.15	16.0 ± 0.64	72.0 ± 3.09
F2	37.67 ± 1.33	230.53 ± 12.62	0.49 ± 0.07	−55.0 ± 1.27	22.3 ± 1.00	68.6 ± 2.06
F3	63.40 ± 0.74	448.72 ± 19.32	0.33 ± 0.04	−39.3 ± 0.81	34.8 ± 1.60	76.1 ± 3.04
F4	67.46 ± 0.77	602.20 ± 13.21	0.35 ± 0.04	−54.2 ± 1.50	39.6 ± 1.41	77.3 ± 1.09
F5	51.63 ± 1.22	560.50 ± 20.55	0.26 ± 0.01	−45.0 ± 1.48	38.5 ± 1.24	74.1 ± 1.07
F6	44.97 ± 1.35	527.00 ± 55.27	0.35 ± 0.04	−65.1 ± 2.05	42.4 ± 0.75	70.0 ± 3.08
F7	65.73 ± 1.66	409.27 ± 34.68	0.35 ± 0.04	−44.5 ± 0.50	32.8 ± 1.00	67.8 ± 1.06
F8	51.03 ± 1.59	460.43 ± 48.91	0.28 ± 0.02	−48.8 ± 0.95	38.4 ± 1.22	70.8 ± 2.05
F9	33.53 ± 1.59	531.23 ± 31.97	0.16 ± 0.03	−45.3 ± 0.60	24.5 ± 0.96	46.5 ± 3.02
F10	46.06 ± 1.45	597.96 ± 34.41	0.35 ± 0.04	−51.2 ± 0.70	31.3 ± 0.55	69.2 ± 1.07
F11	37.55 ± 0.83	356.97 ± 42.54	0.16 ± 0.03	−44.8 ± 1.05	18.1 ± 1.00	64.4 ± 3.03
F12	74.33 ± 1.32	352.23 ± 43.37	0.29 ± 0.03	−48.0 ± 0.50	15.5 ± 0.68	63.5 ± 0.14
F13	70.97 ± 1.30	384.40 ± 10.05	0.017 ± 0.00	−45.3 ± 0.64	15.5 ± 0.96	71.9 ± 0.19
F14	71.39 ± 1.30	379.30 ± 10.05	0.019 ± 0.00	−44.3 ± 0.64	16.7 ± 0.96	72.1 ± 0.19
F15	70.83 ± 1.30	398.20 ± 10.05	0.012 ± 0.00	−44.1 ± 0.64	17.4 ± 0.96	71.8 ± 0.19

Abbreviations; EE, Entrapment efficiency; PS, Particle size; PDI, Polydispersity index; ZP, Zeta potential; Q0.5 h, Total percentage of zolmitriptan released after 0.5 h; RE, Release efficiency.

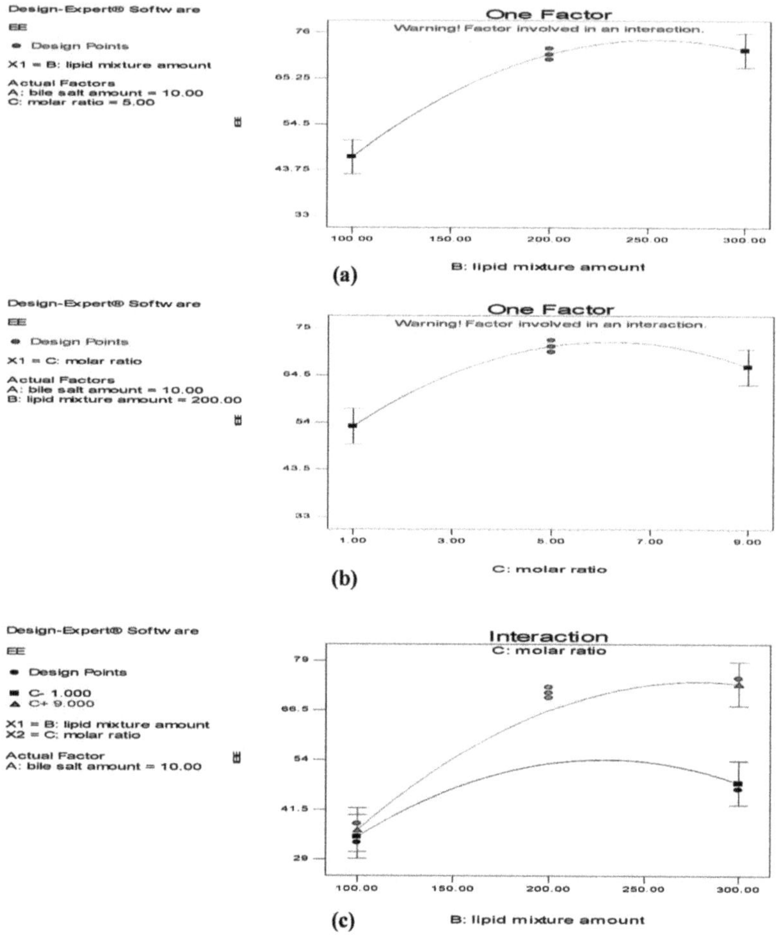

Figure 1. Line plots for the effects of cholesterol/Span® 40 mixture amount (**a**) and cholesterol: Span® 40 molar ratio (**b**), and the interactions between them (**c**) on entrapment efficiency of the prepared zolmitriptan-loaded bilosomes.

Figure 1b reveals that increasing the proportion of cholesterol in the cholesterol/Span® 40 mixture (in other words, moving from cholesterol: Span® 40 molar ratio 1:9 to 1:1) resulted in a significant reduction in their EE%. This is evident as the values of EE% of bilosomes of formulations F7, F8, F11 and F12 (containing a proportion of cholesterol = 10% of its mixture with Span® 40) were significantly larger than those for the corresponding formulations with higher proportions of cholesterol (=50%), which were formulations F5, F6, F9 and F10. This might be attributed to the competition between cholesterol and the drug for the packing space in bilosomes prepared with relatively high proportions of cholesterol, which disrupted the regular bilayer structure and caused drug leakage [51,52]. In addition, the presence of large amount of cholesterol might increase the hydrophobicity of the interfacial region of the bilayers during the bilosomal preparation which disfavored the entrapment of the hydrophilic zolmitriptan [52]. On the other hand, in formulations with smaller proportions of cholesterol in the mixture with Span® 40, the relatively high proportion of non-ionic surfactant increased the solubility of zolmitriptan in the organic phase during bilosomal preparation and decreased their escape to the aqueous phase, leading to enhanced drug entrapment.

The interaction between the two effective formulation factors (X_2 and X_3) on the EE% of the formed bilosomes is provided in Figure 1c. It is clear that at a cholesterol/Span® 40 molar ratio 1:9, increasing the amount of the mixture resulted in increasing the EE%.

Effect on Particle Size (PS)

Table 4 demonstrates the mean PS values of the formed zolmitriptan-loaded bilosomes. The PS values were between 230.53 ± 12.62 nm (formulation F2) and 602.20 ± 13.21 nm (formulation F4). ANOVA testing indicated a non-significant effect ($p > 0.05$) of sodium deoxycholate amount (X_1) on the mean PS as well as significant effects of both the amount of cholesterol/Span® 40 mixture (X_2) and the molar ratio (X_3) between its components ($p = 0.026$ and 0.017, respectively); however, no interaction between the effective factors was indicated. The effects of the investigated formulation factors on PS are presented graphically in Figure 2.

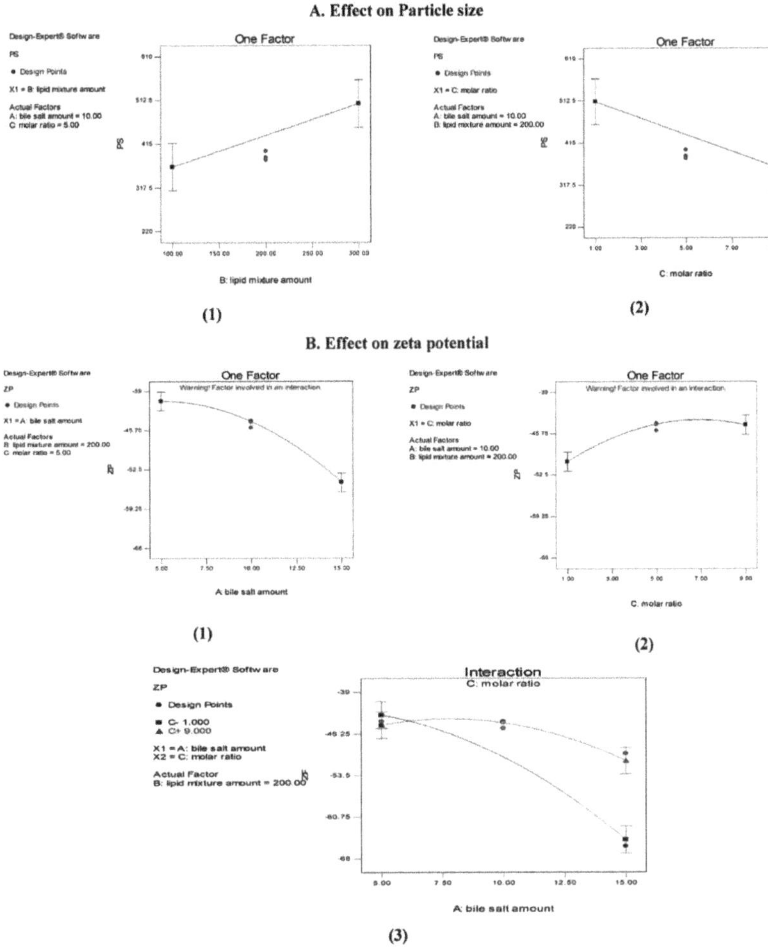

Figure 2. (**A**) Line plots of the effects of cholesterol/Span® 40 mixture amount and (1) cholesterol: Span® 40 molar ratio (2) on particle size. (**B**) Line plots for the effects of sodium deoxycholate amount (1), cholesterol: Span® 40 molar ratio and (2) the interaction between them (3) on zeta potential of the prepared zolmitriptan-loaded bilosomes.

From Figure 2(A1) it is clear that increasing the amount of cholesterol/Span® 40 mixture from 100 mg (in formulations F1, F2, F9 and F11) to 300 mg in the corresponding formulations (F3, F4, F10 and F12) led to a significant increase in the PS of the prepared bilosomes. There are different explanations for this finding. As mentioned before, cholesterol/Span® 40 mixture is the building unit of bilosomes; thus, increasing its amount enhanced the formation of larger number of large-sized vesicles [49,52,53]. Another explanation relates the larger size of the bilosomes prepared using larger amount of cholesterol/Span® 40 mixture to their higher EE%. In addition, as water-soluble drugs like zolmitriptan favor entrapment in the vesicles' aqueous core, this might cause a mutually repulsive interaction between the drug and the polar heads of the surfactant, leading to an increase in PS [43,54].

From Figure 2(A2) it can be seen that increasing the proportion of cholesterol in the cholesterol/Span® 40 mixture resulted in a significant increase in the PS of the produced bilosomes. We believe that this is due to the packing of cholesterol molecules between the surfactant alkyl chain, leading to larger vesicular size [43,55].

Effect on Polydispersity Index (PDI)

PDI is a numerical value ranging from zero to one used to express the homogeneity of particle size distribution. When this index approaches zero, this indicates highly monodispersed particles, whereas, when it approaches one, this suggests highly polydispersed vesicles [56,57]. As presented in Table 4, the PDI of all the formed bilosomes ranged from 0.012 ± 0.00 to 0.49 ± 0.07 (for formulations F15 and F2, respectively) which indicated narrow size distribution of the prepared bilosomes. ANOVA testing indicated that the PDI of the prepared vesicles was not significantly ($p > 0.05$) influenced by the studied factors.

Effect on Zeta Potential (ZP)

The ZP of zolmitriptan-loaded bilosomes was between -65.1 ± 2.05 and -39.3 ± 0.81 mV (for formulations F6 and F3, respectively), confirming that the formed bilosomes had sufficient negative charge to maintain electric repulsion between them and inhibit their aggregation, and hence, better stability [58]. This negative charge in all formulations was mostly due to the use of the anionic bile salt sodium deoxycholate [59]. The results of ANOVA testing demonstrated a non-significant effect ($p > 0.05$) of the amount of cholesterol/Span® 40 mixture (X_2) and significant effects of both sodium deoxycholate amount (X_1) and cholesterol:Span® 40 molar ratio (X_3) ($p < 0.0001$ and $=0.0009$, respectively), with a significant interaction between the latter two effects ($p = 0.0017$). The individual effects of factors X_1 and X_3 on ZP of the prepared bilosomes, in addition to the line plot representing the interaction between them, are illustrated in Figure 2B. From Figure 2(B1), it is clear that increasing the sodium deoxycholate amount from 5 mg (in formulations F1, F3, F5 and F7) to 15 mg in the corresponding formulations (F2, F4, F6 and F8) led to a significant increase in the absolute ZP value of the resultant bilosomes, which may be due to the anionic nature of this bile salt [60].

Figure 2(B2) reveals that increasing Span® 40 proportion in the cholesterol/Span® 40 mixture in the prepared bilosomes resulted in a significantly less negative ZP values. This is evident in the values of ZP for formulations prepared using a cholesterol:Span® 40 molar ratio of 1:1 (F5, F6, F9 and F10) being significantly more negative than the corresponding ones prepared using a molar ratio of 1:9 (namely, F7, F8, F11 and F12). This may be due to the shielding effect of the excess non-ionic surfactant. As the used non-ionic surfactant is hydrophilic in nature, it might reside on the vesicular bilayer surface, leading to a less negative ZP [60,61]. From Figure 2(B3), it is clear that at a low cholesterol/Span® 40 molar ratio, increasing the sodium deoxycholate amount resulted in increasing the negative ZP of the produced bilosomes. This is logical because, as explained before, this bile salt is the main cause of the negative potential of the prepared bilosomes.

Effect on In Vitro Release Studies

The percentages of zolmitriptan released from the investigated bilosomes and drug aqueous dispersion are plotted versus time in Figure 3. The release profile of zolmitriptan from its dispersion revealed fast drug release, with about 99.8% of the drug released in the first 3 h. This assumed the free diffusion of drug through the dialysis membrane, indicating that the membrane used does not hinder drug availability in the release medium. Conversely, drug release from the prepared bilosomes was seen to be slower than that from its aqueous dispersion, which is quite logical.

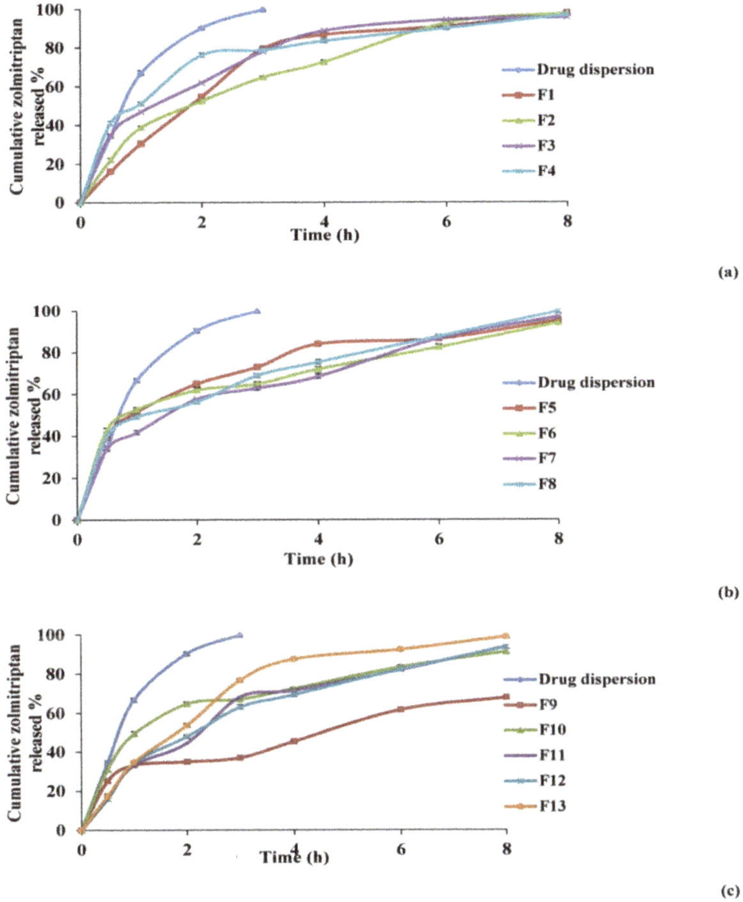

Figure 3. Release profiles of zolmitriptan from the prepared bilosomes compared to aqueous drug dispersion in phosphate buffer saline (pH 7.4); F1–F4 (**a**), F5–F8 (**b**) and F9–F13 (**c**).

Figure 3 also shows that the release of zolmitriptan from the investigated bilosomes was biphasic. An initial flush release of the drug took place within the first 0.5 h, followed by a slower release phase. The initial phase can be attributed to the fast release of adsorbed or surface drug in the release medium, owing to its hydrophilic nature [62], while the second phase of drug release was believed to be regulated by release through the swollen vesicle bilayers [63]. The biphasic release profiles of the drug from all the investigated bilosomes are expected to be of great benefit. Being an anti-migraine drug, the initial amount released would offer rapid onset of pain relief, while the slower subsequent release would keep the patient under prophylaxis from migraine over 8 h.

To compare zolmitriptan release from different drug-loaded bilosomes, two release parameters were applied: Q0.5 h and *RE*% from zero time to 8 h (Table 4). Q0.5 h percentage ranged from 15.5 ± 0.68% to 42.4 ± 0.75% for formulations F12 and F6, respectively. Furthermore, the lowest *RE*% result was recorded for F9 (46.5 ± 3.02%), while the highest was for F4 (77.3 ± 1.09%).

ANOVA analysis of Q0.5 h results showed a non-significant effect ($p > 0.05$) of sodium deoxycholate amount (X_1) and significant effects of both cholesterol/Span® 40 mixture amount (X_2) and the molar ratio (X_3) between components ($p = 0.0109$ and 0.0202, respectively), with no interaction between effective factors. The effect of the investigated formulation variables on Q0.5 h is represented graphically in Figure 4.

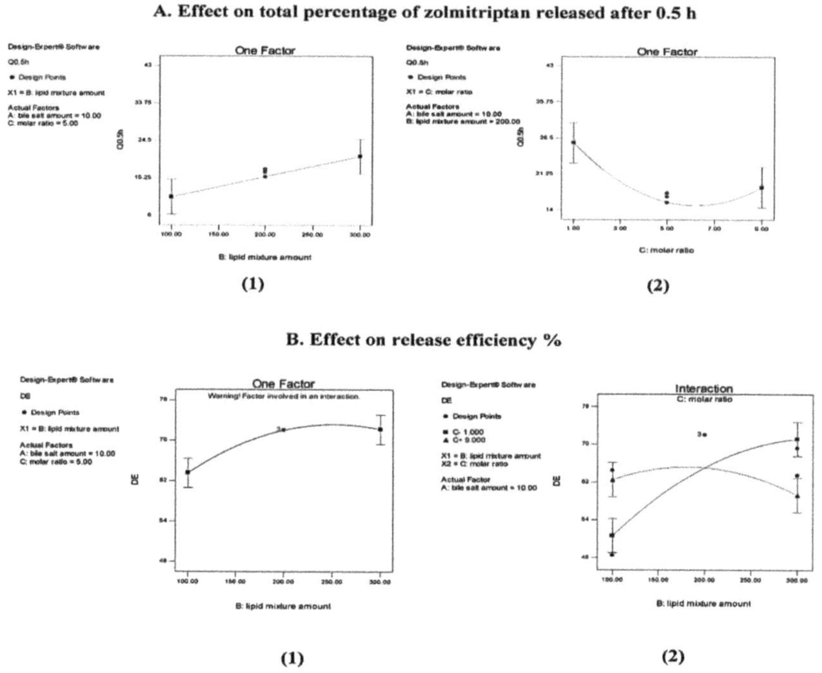

Figure 4. (**A**) Line plots of the effects of cholesterol/Span® 40 mixture amount (1) and cholesterol: Span® 40 molar ratio (2) on total percentage of zolmitriptan released after 0.5 h. (**B**) Line plots for the effect of the amount of cholesterol: Span® 40 mixture (1) and the interaction between it and cholesterol: Span® 40 molar ratio (2) on release efficiency % of the drug up to 8 h.

Regarding the effect of the amount of cholesterol/Span® 40 mixture on Q0.5 h of the prepared bilosomes, it was evident that formulations containing larger amounts of cholesterol/Span® 40 mixture (for example, formulations F3, F4, and F10) possessed higher Q0.5 h values than those for the corresponding formulations containing smaller amounts (F1, F2 and F9), as illustrated in Figure 4(A1). This can be credited to the significant elevation in EE% of the prepared bilosomes by increasing the amount of incorporated cholesterol/Span® 40 mixture (as previously discussed), which was associated with increased driving force for the drug to be released, in line with Fick's first law [64].

Figure 4(A2) shows that increasing cholesterol proportion from 10% to 50% in the cholesterol: Span® 40 molar ratio 1:9 and 1:1 in formulations F7, F8, F11 and F12 compared to the corresponding formulations F5, F6, F9 and F10 led to a significant increase in the Q0.5 h values. This finding might be explained by the ability of cholesterol to disrupt the bilosomal membrane linear structure, as previously discussed [51,52]. This logically led to drug leakage, and hence enhanced drug release and higher Q0.5 h values.

It is obvious that using Q0.5 h as a release parameter involves comparison of single release points in order to evaluate the ability of the investigated formulations to release a fast initial dose of the loaded drug. On the other hand, the concept of *RE*% has some advantages over the single point parameter, the most important being that it can be theoretically related to in vivo data [65].

Concerning *RE*%, ANOVA results showed a non-significant effect ($p > 0.05$) of both the amount of sodium deoxycholate (X_1) and cholesterol/Span® 40 molar ratio (X_3), and a significant effect of the amount of cholesterol/Span® 40 mixture (X_2) ($p = 0.0021$). The effect of the variable X_2 is illustrated in Figure 4B. From Figure 4(B1) and Table 4, it is clear that increasing the amount of cholesterol/Span® 40 mixture from 100 mg to 300 mg caused a statistically significant increase in *RE*%, as revealed by comparing the results obtained from formulations F1, F2 and F9 with those obtained from the corresponding formulations F3, F4 and F10. The increase can be attributed to the enhancement in terms of EE% of these bilosomes (as previously discussed), leading to the increase in drug concentration gradient and consequently to the enhancement of drug release. Statistical analysis also revealed a significant interaction between the amount of cholesterol/Span® 40 mixture and the molar ratio between them ($p = 0.0026$). The line plot of the interaction presented in Figure 4(B2) shows that at a cholesterol: Span® 40 molar ratio of 1:1, when the amount of this mixture was increased from 100 mg to 300 mg, the calculated value of *RE*% increased.

The drug release data presented best fit with the Korsmeyer-Peppas model, with correlation coefficient values (r) above 0.96.

3.1.3. Selection of the Optimized Zolmitriptan-Loaded Bilosomes

The target of the optimization process is to specify the optimum levels of any variable required for the preparation of a pharmaceutical product with high quality. In this work, Design-Expert® software was used to employ a numerical optimization approach, using the desirability function to overcome the multiple and opposing responses [66]. When applied, this numerical analysis developed suggested zolmitriptan-loaded bilosomes with an overall desirability of 0.758. This formulation was suggested to be prepared using 5 mg sodium deoxycholate (X_1) and 255 mg of cholesterol/Span® 40 mixture (X_2) with a cholesterol:Span® 40 molar ratio of 1:7.7 (X_3). To evaluate the optimization capability of the model generated according to the Box–Behnken design, the suggested zolmitriptan-loaded bilosomes were prepared and characterized as was done for the previously prepared bilosomes. For each response, the observed value of the suggested bilosomes was collected with the expected one as well as the residual values which represented the difference between the expected and observed values of each response (Table 5). The residual values of all responses were small (not exceeding 2.1), signifying the reasonability of the optimization process. Thus, the suggested zolmitriptan-loaded bilosomes could be nominated as the optimal one, and it was used for further investigation.

Table 5. Optimal levels of factors of the suggested zolmitriptan-loaded bilosomes with the expected, observed and residual values of each response.

Factor		Optimal Level	
X_1: Sodium deoxycholate amount (mg)		5	
X_2: Cholesterol/Span® 40 amount (mg)		255	
X_3: Cholesterol: Span® 40 molar ratio (w/w)		1:7.7	
Response	**Expected value**	**Observed value**	**Residual value** [a]
Y_1: Entrapment efficiency (%)	71.70	70.34 ± 0.10	1.36
Y_2: Particle size (nm)	399.27	399.80 ± 4.95	−0.53
Y_3: Polydispersity index	0.33	0.33 ± 0.05	−0.004
Y_4: Zeta potential (mv)	−42.50	−41.90 ±0.19	−0.60
Y_5: Q0.5 h (%) [a]	31.87	32.20 ± 1.09	−0.33
Y_6: Release Efficiency (%)	73.86	71.76 ± 0.34	2.10

[a] Residual value = expected value—observed value.

3.2. Mucoadhesive In Situ Gelling System

3.2.1. Characterization of the Prepared Mucoadhesive In Situ Gelling System

The loaded bilosomes in the prepared mucoadhesive in situ gelling system had an EE of 73.63 ± 1.12%, PS of 417.56 ± 16.52 nm, PDI of 0.32 ± 0.01 and ZP of −41.6 ± 0.66. These values were found to be non-significantly different from those previously obtained by free bilosomal dispersion, and p values were calculated to be 0.061, 0.059, 0.072 and 0.081, respectively.

3.2.2. Assessment of Release Parameters of Zolmitriptan from the Prepared Mucoadhesive In Situ Gelling System

The drug release profiles of the prepared in situ gelling system as well as of the free optimal bilosomes are given in Figure 5a. The release best fitted the Korsmeyer–Peppas model, with an r value equal to 0.98. As shown in the figure, drug release from the prepared mucoadhesive in situ gelling system retained the biphasic profile given before from the prepared bilosomes, with an obvious reduction in the initial amount released. The Q0.5 h value of the drug released from the optimal bilosomes loaded in the gelling system decreased by around 50% compared to the free ones ($p = 0.002$). This might be due to the increased viscosity and density of the gelling system compared to free bilosomes, resulting in the slowing of drug diffusion and release [67–69]. Regarding the *RE%*, it was found that the difference between both the gelling system and free bilosomes was statistically non-significant ($p > 0.05$). It is worth to noting that in spite of the significant decrease in Q0.5 h of zolmitriptan from bilosomes when incorporated into the mucoadhesive in situ gelling system, the overall amount of drug released in a defined time (representing drug *RE*) did not display any significant change. In other words, the incorporation of drug-loaded bilosomes in the mucoadhesive in situ gelling system resulted in delayed drug release onset, with no effect on the total amount of drug released.

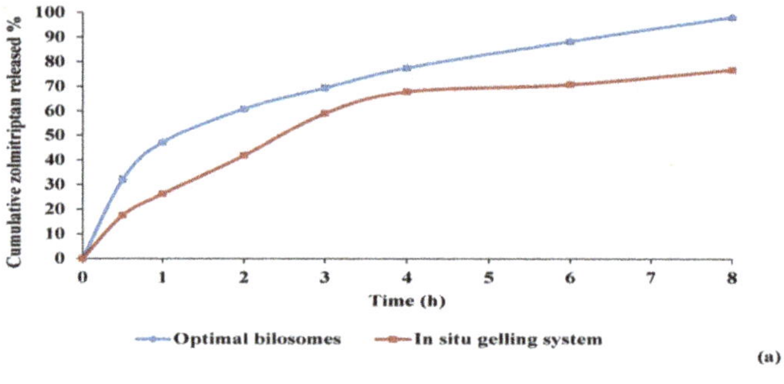

(a)

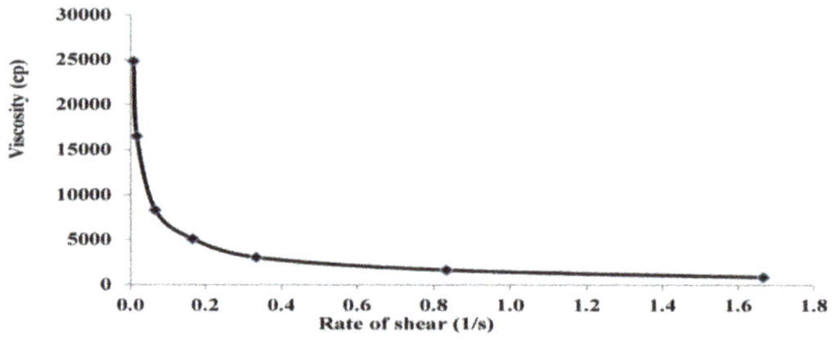

(b)

Figure 5. (**a**) Release profiles of zolmitriptan dispersion from the optimal bilosomes and the prepared mucoadhesive in situ gelling system containing them in phosphate buffer saline, pH 7.4; (**b**) Relation between viscosity and rate of shear for the prepared mucoadhesive in situ gelling system.

3.2.3. Assessment of Sol to Gel Transition Temperature and Time

The sol to gel transition temperature of the prepared mucoadhesive in situ gelling system was 34.03 ± 0.45 °C. This transition temperature is close to the acceptable range for nasal administration, which has been stated by other researchers to be between 25 and 33 °C [30]. The sol to gel transition time was recorded to be 20.00 ± 1.00 s.

3.2.4. Assessment of Rheological Constants

The rheological behavior of the mucoadhesive in situ gelling system loaded with optimal bilosomes was assessed using two indices, consistency and flow. Consistency index (m) represents the consistency or the thickness of the investigated fluid, which is more or less equivalent to the viscosity. On the other hand, flow index (n) represents the flow behavior of the fluid. When the value of n equals unity, this indicates Newtonian flow, while when it is bigger than one, the fluid shows dilatant flow (i.e., shear thickening). Values of n between zero and one indicate that the flow of the fluid is of a pseudo-plastic type, exhibiting shear thinning behavior [70–72].

For the prepared gelling system, the values of its viscosity at different shear rate values were reported at 35 °C, which represents the average temperature of nasal cavity. The calculated values of indices m and n were found to be 17717.40 and 0.39, respectively. The relatively large value of m indicated that the system is somewhat viscous, which could be explained by the plate temperature (35 °C) exceeding the sol to gel transition temperature of the investigated gelling system, leading to system gelation and an increase in its viscosity. As the value of n was less than unity, the investigated system exhibited shear-thinning flow. This flow is confirmed by the relation between viscosity and shear stress (Figure 5b). Such shear thinning behavior can be accredited to the decrease in viscosity by increasing shear rate [58,73]. The externally applied shear rate, responsible for the shear thinning behavior, could be achieved in vivo by the physiological ciliary movement, which is about 1000 beats per min [74]. This shear thinning behavior would allow for gradual release of the drug from the gel over time.

3.2.5. Transmission Electron Microscopy (TEM)

Micrographs of all the examined samples showed that all samples were non-aggregating, almost spherical vesicles with well-defined walls and a smooth surface (Figure S1). This indicated that incorporation of the optimal zolmitriptan-loaded bilosomes in the mucoadhesive in situ gelling system used did not significantly affect their shape.

3.2.6. Differential Scanning Calorimetry (DSC)

The lyophilized samples showed complete dispersion, with a reconstitution time of 16.67 ± 1.52 and 19.00 ± 1.00 s for the optimal bilosomal formulation and mucoadhesive in situ gelling system containing the bilosomal formulation, respectively. The thermal behavior of the pure drug, the lyophilized optimal bilosomes and the physical mixture of its components are demonstrated in Figure S2. A DSC thermogram of zolmitriptan exhibited a characteristic melting endothermic peak at 137.6 °C, signifying its crystalline nature. This peak could be observed in the physical mixture thermogram as well. However, this characteristic peak was not detected in the thermogram of the lyophilized optimal bilosomes, indicating the transformation of zolmitriptan to the amorphous form [75,76]. Additionally, the DSC thermograms of the prepared mucoadhesive in situ gelling system and the physical mixture of its components are presented in Figure S2. The characteristic drug peak can be noticed in the physical mixture thermogram but is not detected in the thermogram of the lyophilized mucoadhesive in situ gelling system, indicating the preservation of the drug-loaded bilosomal structure after being loaded inside the gelling system.

3.2.7. Determination of Nasal Mucociliary Transit Time

Mucociliary clearance is the defense mechanism of the respiratory tract body against inhaled foreign substances. Hence, it is responsible for the quick clearance of nasally administered drugs to the nasopharynx, resulting in a significant decrease in their absorption [77]. In this study, nasal mucociliary transit time was assessed by measuring the time required by the applied system to reach the nasopalatine canal and the pharynx. The measured time expresses the time period during which the system can stay in the nasal cavity and thus available for drug absorption.

To avoid the difficulty of analyzing the drug in swabs taken from the nasopalatine canal and pharynx every minute, a blue dye (methylene blue) was mixed with the investigated samples to act as an indicator of the site it reached. In this study, the control solution (methylene blue in saline) appeared in swabs taken within the first minute of its application to the nasal cavity, indicating the successful administration of the dye solution to the laboratory animals.

The nasal mucociliary transit time of the optimal bilosomes was also determined and compared to results obtained from the prepared mucoadhesive in situ gelling system containing them in order to investigate the effect of incorporation in gelling system on their nasal mucociliary clearance. The nasal mucociliary transit time for dispersion of the optimal bilosomes was found to be 2.5 ± 0.71, versus 22.36 ± 0.41 min for the mucoadhesive in situ gelling system ($p < 0.05$). This is logical, as the prepared system is converted in the nasal cavity to a gel with higher viscosity and less clearance and, in addition, the incorporated mucoadhesive polymers increase the residence time of the prepared in situ gelling system in the nasal cavity by adhering to nasal mucosa [30].

3.3. *In Vivo Animals*

All the participating animals tolerated the drug, the examined preparations and the applied study design well, as they all remained alive and showed normal behavior and vitality until the final last sampling time. The applied LC/MS-MS method showed a lower limit of quantification (LLOQ) of 0.03 ng/mL in both plasma and brain tissues and showed good linearity, from 0.03 to 100 ng/mL (R^2 of the corresponding lines were 0.9993 and 0.9990, respectively).

In Vivo Brain and Systemic–Kinetic Studies

For each of the three applied treatments, zolmitriptan concentration in both plasma and homogenized brain was plotted versus time; the resulting curves are given in Figure 6.

It can be seen that the shapes of the zolmitriptan plasma concentration–time curves (Figure 6a) for bilosomes after IN administration either in the form of free bilosomes (Treatment A) or bilosomes contained in mucoadhesive in situ gel (Treatment B) obviously differed from that obtained for the IV drug solution (Treatment C). The former two treatments showed lower C_{max} values and longer t_{max} values. This indicates a difference in drug bioavailability between the IN treatments and the IV solution. The pharmacokinetic parameters of the drug from the three applied treatments are collected in Table 6. Zolmitriptan reached C_{max} of 535.59 ± 9.04 ng/mL (after 0.25 h) when applied as an IV solution. The values of C_{max} of the drug from the optimal bilosomes and the mucoadhesive in situ gel after IN administration were significantly lower ($p < 0.05$) than that for IV solution, being 108.58 ± 1.94 and 86.66 ± 4.13 ng/mL, respectively (both were reached after 0.5 h). Concerning the $AUC_{0\text{–}12\,h}$ values under the plasma/time curve, it was found that the calculated values for Treatments A and B (361.86 ± 6.89 and 340.64 ± 36.48 ng·h/mL; respectively) were significantly smaller ($p < 0.05$) than that calculated for Treatment C (1579.32 ± 33.48 ng·h/mL). However, the difference in $AUC_{0\text{–}12\,h}$ between Treatments A and B was statistically non-significant ($p = 0.082$). The same effect was obtained when $AUC_{0\text{-}C}$ was calculated, as revealed in Table 6. The obtained values with Treatments A and B might explain the availability of the drug in the brain tissues, which will be indicated by investigating brain kinetics. In addition, statistically non-significant differences ($p > 0.05$) were found between the three treatments concerning the time required to eliminate half the administered dose ($t_{1/2}$) as well as in the elimination rate constant (k). The obtained values of drug $t_{1/2}$ and k ranged from 2.5 to 3 h and from 0.231± 0.006 to 0.277 ±0.003 h^{-1}, respectively. These values were in agreement with those stated for zolmitriptan in the Electronic Medicines Compendium (EMC, Datapharm Ltd.) [78]. Regarding the MRT values, it was found that both Treatments A and B (4.08 and 4.80 h, respectively) possessed significantly larger values ($p < 0.05$) compared to Treatment C (3.33 h). Additionally, no significant difference in *MRT* values was detected between both Treatments A and B ($p > 0.05$). This could be due to the enhanced ability of the lipid nanovesicles like bilosomes to enhance nasal permeation of zolmitriptan through disrupting the mucosal membrane of the nose. Hence, due to the absorption process, the *MRT* of both Treatments A and B was found to be longer than that obtained after IV administration of the drug solution [11,79].

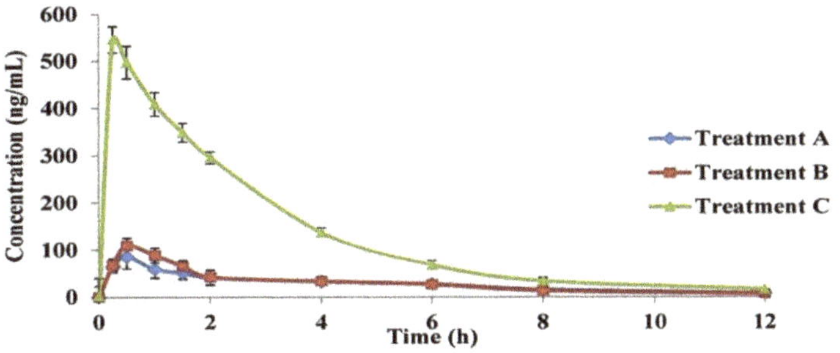

(a)

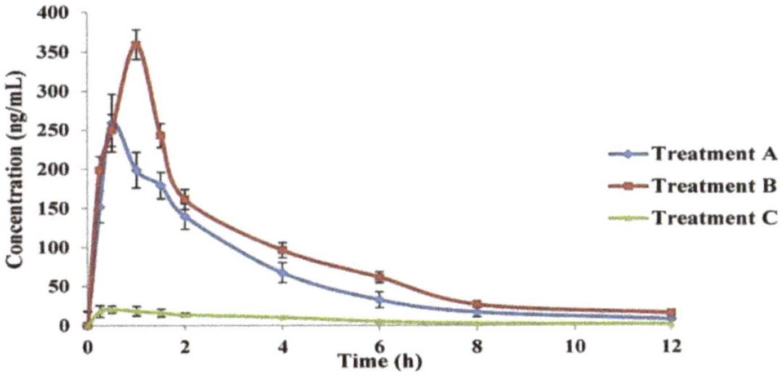

(b)

Figure 6. Zolmitriptan concentration versus time curves for plasma (**a**) and brain tissues (**b**) after administration of intranasal optimal bilosomes (Treatment A), intranasal mucoadhesive in situ gelling system (Treatment B), and intravenous zolmitriptan solution (Treatment C).

As revealed by the above plasma data, the values of absolute bioavailability of zolmitriptan in plasma from the optimal bilosomes (Treatment A) and from the mucoadhesive in situ gelling system (Treatment B) were 23.65 and 22.78%, respectively, with a statistically non-significant difference between them ($p > 0.05$). The small values of absolute bioavailability of the drug in plasma after administration of nasal bilosome treatments might be due to brain targeting of the drug. To confirm the brain targeting potential of the prepared bilosomes when applied IN, and to exclude any other factor that may result in poor plasma bioavailability of the drug, zolmitriptan concentration in homogenized brain tissues was estimated.

Zolmitriptan concentration in the homogenized brain samples was calculated and plotted versus time for the three treatments, as shown in Figure 6b. The curves of the three treatments are obviously different in shape. It is evident that Treatment B (IN mucoadhesive in situ gelling system containing the bilosomal formulation) showed the highest C_{max}, followed by Treatment A (IN free bilosomal formulation), while Treatment C possessed the lowest C_{max}. It is also obvious that the t_{max} from Treatment B is the longest among the applied treatments. Table 6 shows the brain kinetic parameters of the applied treatments; the values of C_{max} were 260.43 ± 6.90, 360.30 ± 7.78 and 21.13 ± 2.09 ng/mL for Treatments A, B and C, respectively, with significant differences between all of them ($p < 0.05$). Treatment B showed the longest t_{max} (1 h) ($p < 0.05$) when compared to Treatments A and C ($t_{max} = 0.5$ h). Table 6 also shows that the largest value of $AUC_{0\text{–}12\,h}$ in brain was obtained by Treatment B (1081.88 ± 43.37 ng·h/mL), followed by Treatment A (768.24 ± 43.69 ng·h/mL), then Treatment C (91.92 ± 12.20 ng·h/mL), with significant differences ($p < 0.05$). The same effect between the three investigated treatments was obtained when comparing $AUC_{0\text{-}C}$ values. The $t_{1/2}$ and k values of zolmitriptan from the three treatments showed non-significant differences (p-values < 0.05). By comparing the MRT values, it was found that the three treatments differed significantly from each other ($p < 0.05$), with Treatment B showing the highest MRT value (3.87 h) and Treatment C giving the least value (3.31 h). This extended MRT obtained with Treatment B compared to Treatment A might be attributed to the extended mucociliary transit time of the gelling system, which led to less clearance and hence better drug delivery to the brain through the olfactory duct [21].

Table 6. Pharmacokinetic parameters of zolmitriptan in plasma and brain after administration of intranasal optimal bilosomes (Treatment A), intranasal mucoadhesive in situ gelling system (Treatment B) and intravenous solution (Treatment C).

	In Plasma		
Parameter	**Treatment A**	**Treatment B**	**Treatment C**
C_{max}**(ng/mL)** [a]	108.58 ± 1.94	86.66 ± 4.13	535.59 ± 9.04
t_{max}**(h)** [b]	0.5	0.5	0.25
$AUC_{0\text{–}12\,h}$**(ng·h/mL)** [c]	361.86 ± 6.89	340.64 ± 36.48	1579.32 ± 33.48
$AUC_{0\text{–}\infty}$**(ng·h/mL)** [d]	388.62 ± 4.77	370.43 ± 31.26	1643.89 ± 35.43
$K(h^{-1})$	0.251 ± 0.010	0.231 ± 0.006	0.277 ± 0.003
$t_{1/2}$**(h)**	2.76 ± 0.15	3.00 ± 0.24	2.5 ± 0.38
MRT [e]	4.08	4.80	3.33
Absolute bioavailability (%) *	23.65	22.78	—
	In Brain		
Parameter	**Treatment A**	**Treatment B**	**Treatment C**
C_{max}**(ng/mL)** [f]	260.43 ± 6.90	360.30 ± 7.78	21.13 ± 2.09
t_{max}**(h)** [g]	0.5	1	0.5
$AUC_{0\text{–}12\,h}$**(ng·h/mL)** [h]	768.24 ± 43.69	1081.88 ± 43.37	91.92 ± 12.20
$AUC_{0\text{–}\infty}$**(ng·h/mL)** [i]	801.15 ± 46.94	1147.08 ± 51.79	97.73 ± 13.86
$K(h^{-1})$	0.275 ± 0.011	0.25 ± 0.003	0.256 ± 0.003
$t_{1/2}$**(h)**	2.52 ± 0.18	2.77 ± 0.16	2.70 ± 0.31
MRT(h) [j]	3.36	3.87	3.31
Brain bioavailability (%) **	819.75	1173.64	—

Results are mean values ± SD, in plasma data and compared to Treatment C; [a] $p < 0.05$ (0.0015 and 0.0012 for Treatments A and B, respectively), [b] $p < 0.05$ (0.0072 for both Treatments A and B), [c] $p < 0.05$ (0.0014 and 0.0011 for Treatments A and B, respectively). No significant difference was detected between Treatments A and B, [d] $p < 0.05$ (0.00138 and 0.00114 for Treatments A and B, respectively). No significant difference was detected between Treatments A and B, [e] $p < 0.05$ (0.0017 and 0.00109 for Treatments A and B, respectively). No significant difference was detected between Treatments A and B. * p < 0. 05 (0.278 between Treatments A and B), In brain data and compared to Treatment C; [f] $p < 0.05$ (0.0021 and 0.0017 for Treatments A and B, respectively), [g] $p < 0.05$ (0.0074 for Treatment B), [h] $p < 0.05$ (0.0023 and 0.0013 for Treatments A and B, respectively). No significant difference was detected between Treatments A and B, [i] $p < 0.05$ (0.0022 and 0.0014 for Treatments A and B, respectively). No significant difference was detected between Treatments A and B, [j] $p < 0.05$ (0.0023 and 0.0014 for Treatments A and B, respectively). No significant difference was detected between Treatments A and B. ** $p < 0.05$ (0.004 between Treatments A and B).

As revealed from the brain data in Table 6, the brain bioavailability of the drug from IN optimal bilosomes (Treatment A) relative to IV solution (Treatment C) is 819.75% and that from IN mucoadhesive in situ gelling system (Treatment B) is 1173.64%. These results indicated that nasal application of the prepared bilosomes (either as dispersion or contained in mucoadhesive in situ gel) resulted in brain targeting of the incorporated zolmitriptan. The relative brain bioavailability of the drug from Treatment B was calculated to be 1.4-fold more than from Treatment A which might be accredited to the relatively long nasal mucociliary transit time of the mucoadhesive in situ gelling system (22.36 $\pm$ 0.41 min) as mentioned before. This long transit time enhanced the residence of the gelling system onto the nasal mucosa offering the time required for the drug to diffuse through the in situ formed viscous gel, hence better drug absorption [22,80]. This finding can explain the delayed t_{max} of the drug in brain on administration of Treatment B.

In addition, the obtained values of $AUC_{0\text{–}12\,h}$ (total drug amount) in both plasma and brain were compared using two parameters, drug targeting efficiency (DTE %) and direct transport percentage (DTP %), which were calculated. DTE expresses the result of dividing the ratio of total drug amount in brain to that in plasma for the IN treatment by the same ratio for the IV one. Thus, a 100% value of DTE represents an equal proportion of drug concentration in the brain for both the IN and IV routes of administration. If the value of the calculated DTE exceeds 100%, this represents preferential brain targeting of the drug from the IN route; if this value is less than 100%, it indicates preferential brain targeting from the IV route [30]. The DTE values for the applied IN Treatments (A and B) were calculated to be 3652.2 % and 5451.8% for Treatments A and B, respectively. Needless to say, the higher value of DTE calculated for Treatment B is due to the nature of its dosage form, as the prepared mucoadhesive in situ gelling system stayed at the site of application for longer time than bilosomal dispersion, leading to a higher $AUC_{0\text{–}12\,h}$ and, consequently, a higher value of DTE. The calculated values of DTE (in addition to the obtained pharmacokinetic parameters) confirmed that the administered Treatments A and B resulted in favored zolmitriptan delivery to the brain compared to Treatment C. In other words, IN administration of the prepared zolmitriptan-loaded bilosomes resulted in boosted brain targeting with higher drug availability in the brain obtained by the prepared bilosome-containing mucoadhesive in situ gel.

To understand the possible pathways that the drug molecules go through to reach the brain, a brief overview of the anatomy of the nose should first be highlighted. The nasal cavity is divided into two main areas, respiratory and olfactory. The former is highly vascularized, while the latter is stimulated by the olfactory nerve [81].

Previous researchers have explained that there are two pathways for a drug to reach the brain when applied IN. The drug may be absorbed from the respiratory area of the nasal cavity into the general circulation through the nasal mucosa; it then permeates through the BBB to reach the brain. In the other pathway, the drug may be transported from the olfactory area of the nasal cavity to the olfactory bulb and then directly to the brain [82]. Although the olfactory epithelium constitutes only about 5% of the total area of the nasal cavity in humans [83], it is of significant interest when delivering drugs directly to the brain (bypassing the BBB) is required [84]. This unique feature of the olfactory epithelium is due to the existence of the olfactory neurons which are the receptors of the olfactory nerve. The olfactory nerve originates from the olfactory bulb, then reaches the olfactory area where olfactory neurons are embedded within its mucosa [85]. Additionally, there are two different mechanisms by which drug molecules can be transported from the olfactory area to olfactory bulb and then finally to different parts of the brain. These mechanisms are the intracellular and extracellular routes. Regarding the intracellular mechanism, the olfactory neurons internalize the drug molecule to be released later by exocytosis from neuron's projection area. In the extracellular pathway, the drug initially crosses the epithelial membrane of the nose to the lamina propria area containing the neurons, located in the olfactory area of the nasal cavity [82].

To assess the relative contribution of the direct nose to brain pathway (i.e., olfactory pathway) in the overall brain delivery of zolmitriptan from the applied IN Treatments, the values of DTP % of the drug from Treatments A and B were calculated. A negative DTP value designates efficient drug delivery to the brain through the BBB, while a positive one designates a major contribution of the direct nose to brain pathway [30]. The calculated values of DTP were found to be 97.2 and 98.1% for Treatments A and B, respectively. The positive values of the calculated DTP indicated predominance of direct olfactory delivery of zolmitriptan to the brain for both bilosome treatments when applied in the nasal cavity. Enhanced DTE values as well as positive DTP values indicated the successful delivery of the drug to the brain tissues. These findings can be credited to the small particle size of the formed bilosomes, along with their elasticity. These properties promote both intracellular and extracellular drug transport to the brain, as previously mentioned. Their small size enabled the zolmitriptan-loaded bilosomes to be engulfed by the neurons of the olfactory nerve (i.e., intracellular drug transport), and the elasticity of the prepared bilosomes enabled them to squeeze and pass through the narrow extracellular route directly to the brain [86]. Enhancement of brain targeting of drugs when incorporated in nanocarriers for IN application has been reported by many researchers [11,87–89]. Moreover, it has been reported elsewhere that the presence of poloxamer 407 in the used in situ gel might lead to entanglement with the glycoprotein chains of the nasal mucosa, hence permitting better residence, absorption and penetration [90,91]. Additionally, the literature includes several examples showing the safety of the used components for intranasal applications, namely, cholesterol, Span® 40 [92], sodium deoxycholate, and poloxamer 407 [93], and HPMC [94].

4. Conclusions

In the present study, zolmitriptan-loaded bilosomes were constructed using the thin film hydration technique, applying a Box–Behnken design after preliminary selection of the best non-ionic surfactant (Span® 40). Sodium deoxycholate amount (5, 10 and 15 mg), cholesterol/Span® 40 mixture amount (100, 200 and 300 mg) and the molar ratio between the mixture components (1:1, 1:5 and 1:9 *w*/*w*) were selected as independent factors. The optimum bilosomal formulation was suggested, after statistical analysis, to be made up of sodium deoxycholate (5 mg) and a cholesterol/Span® 40 mixture of 255 mg at a molar ratio of 1:7.7 *w*/*w*. The selection was based on entrapment efficiency percentage, particle size, zeta potential and in vitro drug release. The optimum bilosomal formulation was loaded into a mucoadhesive in situ gel formed from a mixture of poloxamer 407 and HPMC. The mucoadhesive gel containing the bilosomal formulation possessed a sol–gel temperature of 34.03 °C and prolonged nasal mucociliary transit time of 22.36 min. Higher C_{max} and $AUC_{0-\infty}$ coupled with longer t_{max} values in homogenized brain tissues revealed the superiority of the gel compared to free bilosomal dispersion (both administered intranasally), as well as the IV solution, in rats. Furthermore, the fabricated gelling system revealed successful brain targeting, which was confirmed by higher DTE and positive DTP values.

In conclusion, the developed formulation offered a promising intranasal substitute with boosted therapeutic effect for treating migraine suffering patients.

Supplementary Materials: The following are available online at https://www.mdpi.com/article/10.3390/pharmaceutics13111828/s1, Table S1: Composition and characterization of the mucoadhesive in situ gelling formulations prepared according to 3^3 general factorial design using Design-Expert® software. Table S2: Main output data of the Box–Behnken (3^3) design for the analysis of zolmitriptan-loaded bilosomes F1–F15[a]. Figure S1: Transmission electron micrographs of the optimal zolmitriptan-loaded bilosomes (a) and the mucoadhesive in situ gelling system containing them (b). Figure S2: Differential scanning calorimetry thermograms of zolmitriptan (a), physical mixture of components of optimal zolmitriptan-loaded bilosomes (b), lyophilized powder of the optimal bilosomes (c), physical mixture of components of the prepared mucoadhesive in situ gelling system loaded with optimal bilosomes (d) and lyophilized mucoadhesive in situ gelling system loaded with optimal bilosomes (e). Supplementary Material S1: Effect of storage.

Author Contributions: Conceptualization, M.M.E.T., M.H.A.-E., M.A.K. and N.A.E.; methodology, M.M.E.T., M.H.A.-E. and M.A.K.; software, M.M.E.T.; investigation, M.M.E.T., M.H.A.-E., M.A.K. and N.A.E.; resources, M.M.E.T.; statistical analysis, M.M.E.T.; writing—original draft preparation, M.M.E.T., M.H.A.-E. and N.A.E.; writing—review and editing, M.M.E.T., M.H.A.-E. and N.A.E.;

supervision, M.H.A.-E., M.A.K. and N.A.E. All authors have read and agreed to the published version of the manuscript.

Funding: This research has not received any sort of funding from any organization, in the public or private sectors.

Institutional Review Board Statement: Not applicable.

Informed Consent Statement: Not applicable.

Data Availability Statement: The data presented in this study are available in the article and Supplementary Material.

Conflicts of Interest: The authors report no conflicts of interest in this work.

References

1. Jensen, R.; Stovner, L.J. Epidemiology and Comorbidity of Headache. *Lancet Neurol.* **2008**, *7*, 354–361. [CrossRef]
2. Peterlin, B.L.; Rapoport, A.M. Clinical pharmacology of the serotonin receptor agonist, zolmitriptan. *Expert Opin. Drug Metab. Toxicol.* **2007**, *3*, 899–911. [CrossRef] [PubMed]
3. Feigin, V.L.; Abajobir, A.A.; Abate, K.H.; Abd-Allah, F.; Abdulle, A.M.; Abera, S.F.; Abyu, G.Y.; Ahmed, M.B.; Aichour, A.N.; Aichour, I.; et al. Global, regional, and national burden of neurological disorders during 1990–2015: A systematic analysis for the Global Burden of Disease Study 2015. *Lancet Neurol.* **2017**, *16*, 877–897. [CrossRef]
4. Weatherall, M.W. The diagnosis and treatment of chronic migraine. *Ther. Adv. Chronic Dis.* **2015**, *6*, 115–123. [CrossRef]
5. Russell, M.; Rasmussen, B.K.; Fenger, K.; Olesen, J. Migraine without aura and migraine with aura are distinct clinical entities: A study of four hundred and eighty-four male and female migraineurs from the general population. *Cephalalgia* **1996**, *16*, 239–245. [CrossRef]
6. Kurth, T.; Slomke, M.A.; Kase, C.S.; Cook, N.R.; Lee, I.M.; Gaziano, J.M.; Diener, H.C.; Buring, J.E. Migraine, headache, and the risk of stroke in women: A prospective study. *Neurology* **2005**, *64*, 1020–1026. [CrossRef]
7. Prajapati, S.T.; Patel, M.V.; Patel, C.N. Preparation and evaluation of sublingual tablets of zolmitriptan. *Int. J. Pharm. Investig.* **2014**, *4*, 27–31. [CrossRef]
8. Mahmoud, A.A.; Salah, S. Fast relief from migraine attacks using fast-disintegrating sublingual zolmitriptan tablets. *Drug Dev. Ind. Pharm.* **2012**, *38*, 762–769. [CrossRef]
9. Spencer, C.M.; Gunasekara, N.S.; Hills, C. Zolmitriptan. *Drugs* **1999**, *58*, 347–374. [CrossRef]
10. Gizurarson, S. Anatomical and histological factors affecting intranasal drug and vaccine delivery. *Curr. Drug Deliv.* **2012**, *9*, 566–582. [CrossRef]
11. Abd-Elal, R.M.; Shamma, R.N.; Rashed, H.M.; Bendas, E.R. Trans-nasal zolmitriptan novasomes: In-vitro preparation, optimization and in-vivo evaluation of brain targeting efficiency. *Drug Deliv.* **2016**, *23*, 3374–3386. [CrossRef]
12. Mann, J.F.; Scales, H.E.; Shakir, E.; Alexander, J.; Carter, K.C.; Mullen, A.B.; Ferro, V.A. Oral delivery of tetanus toxoid using vesicles containing bile salts (bilosomes) induces significant systemic and mucosal immunity. *Methods* **2006**, *38*, 90–95. [CrossRef]
13. Aburahma, M.H. Bile salts-containing vesicles: Promising pharmaceutical carriers for oral delivery of poorly water-soluble drugs and peptide/protein-based therapeutics or vaccines. *Drug Deliv.* **2016**, *23*, 1847–1867. [CrossRef]
14. Shukla, A.; Singh, B.; Katare, O. Significant systemic and mucosal immune response induced on oral delivery of diphtheria toxoid using nano-bilosomes. *Br. J. Pharmacol.* **2011**, *164*, 820–827. [CrossRef]
15. Shukla, A.; Khatri, K.; Gupta, P.N.; Goyal, A.K.; Mehta, A.; Vyas, S.P. Oral immunization against hepatitis B using bile salt stabilized vesicles (bilosomes). *J. Pharm. Pharm. Sci.* **2008**, *11*, 59–66. [CrossRef]
16. Duangjit, S.; Opanasopit, P.; Rojanarata, T.; Ngawhirunpat, T. Evaluation of meloxicam-loaded cationic transfersomes as transdermal drug delivery carriers. *Aaps Pharmscitech* **2013**, *14*, 133–140. [CrossRef]
17. Saifi, Z.; Rizwanullah, M.; Mir, S.R.; Amin, S. Bilosomes nanocarriers for improved oral bioavailability of acyclovir: A complete characterization through in vitro, ex-vivo and in vivo assessment. *J. Drug Deliv. Sci. Technol.* **2020**, *57*, 101634. [CrossRef]
18. Pavlović, N.; Goločorbin-Kon, S.; Đanić, M.; Stanimirov, B.; Al-Salami, H.; Stankov, K.; Mikov, M. Bile acids and their derivatives as potential modifiers of drug release and pharmacokinetic profiles. *Front. Pharmacol.* **2018**, *9*, 1283. [CrossRef] [PubMed]
19. Abdelalim, L.R.; Abdallah, O.Y.; Elnaggar, Y.S. High efficacy, rapid onset nanobiolosomes of sildenafil as a topical therapy for erectile dysfunction in aged rats. *Int. J. Pharm.* **2020**, *591*, 119978. [CrossRef]
20. Janga, K.Y.; Tatke, A.; Balguri, S.P.; Lamichanne, S.P.; Ibrahim, M.M.; Maria, D.N.; Jablonski, M.M.; Majumdar, S. Ion-sensitive in situ hydrogels of natamycin bilosomes for enhanced and prolonged ocular pharmacotherapy: In vitro permeability, cytotoxicity and in vivo evaluation. *Artif. Cells Nanomed. Biotechnol. Int. J.* **2018**, *46*, 1039–1050. [CrossRef]
21. Shang, Y.; Inthavong, K.; Qiu, D.; Singh, N.; He, F.; Tu, J. Prediction of nasal spray drug absorption influenced by mucociliary clearance. *PLoS ONE* **2021**, *16*, e0246007. [CrossRef] [PubMed]
22. Aderibigbe, B.A. In situ-based gels for nose to brain delivery for the treatment of neurological diseases. *Pharmaceutics* **2018**, *10*, 40. [CrossRef] [PubMed]

23. Yaghoobian, M.; Haeri, A.; Bolourchian, N.; Shahhosseni, S.; Dadashzadeh, S. The impact of surfactant composition and surface charge of niosomes on the oral absorption of repaglinide as a BCS II model drug. *Int. J. Nanomed.* **2020**, *15*, 8767–8781. [CrossRef] [PubMed]
24. Tawfik, M.A.; Tadros, M.I.; Mohamed, M.I.; El-Helaly, S.N. Low-frequency versus high-frequency ultrasound-mediated transdermal delivery of agomelatine-loaded invasomes: Development, optimization and in-vivo pharmacokinetic assessment. *Int. J. Nanomed.* **2020**, *15*, 8893–8910. [CrossRef]
25. Mahmoud, A.A.; Elkasabgy, N.A.; Abdelkhalek, A.A. Design and characterization of emulsified spray dried alginate microparticles as a carrier for the dually acting drug roflumilast. *Eur. J. Pharm. Sci.* **2018**, *122*, 64–76. [CrossRef]
26. Khan, K.; Ka, K.; CT, R. Effect of compaction pressure on the dissolution efficiency of some direct compression systems. *Pharmaceutica. Acta Helv.* **1972**, *47*, 594–607.
27. Peppas, N. Analysis of Fickian and non-Fickian drug release from polymers. *Pharm. Acta Helv.* **1985**, *60*, 110–111.
28. Korsmeyer, R.; Gurny, R.; Doelker, E.; Buri, P.; Peppas, N.A. Mechanisms of potassium chloride release from compressed, hydrophilic, polymeric matrices: Effect of entrapped air. *J. Pharm. Sci.* **1983**, *72*, 1189–1191. [CrossRef]
29. Zaki, N.M.; Awad, G.A.; Mortada, N.D.; Abd ElHady, S.S. Enhanced bioavailability of metoclopramide HCl by intranasal administration of a mucoadhesive in situ gel with modulated rheological and mucociliary transport properties. *Eur. J. Pharm. Sci.* **2007**, *32*, 296–307. [CrossRef]
30. Fatouh, A.M.; Elshafeey, A.H.; Abdelbary, A. Agomelatine-based in situ gels for brain targeting via the nasal route: Statistical optimization, in vitro, and in vivo evaluation. *Drug Deliv.* **2017**, *24*, 1077–1085. [CrossRef]
31. Liu, L.; Tang, X.; Wang, Y.; Guo, S. Smart gelation of chitosan solution in the presence of NaHCO3 for injectable drug delivery system. *Int. J. Pharm.* **2011**, *414*, 6–15. [CrossRef]
32. Simões, A.; Miranda, M.; Cardoso, C.; Veiga, F.; Vitorino, C. Rheology by design: A regulatory tutorial for analytical method validation. *Pharmaceutics* **2020**, *12*, 820. [CrossRef]
33. Tung, I.-C. Rheological behavior of poloxamer 407 aqueous solutions during sol-gel and dehydration processes. *Int. J. Pharm.* **1994**, *107*, 85–90. [CrossRef]
34. Ohshima, H.; Miyagishima, A.; Kurita, T.; Makino, Y.; Iwao, Y.; Sonobe, T.; Itai, S. Freeze-dried nifedipine-lipid nanoparticles with long-term nano-dispersion stability after reconstitution. *Int. J. Pharm.* **2009**, *377*, 180–184. [CrossRef]
35. Lale, A.; Mason, J.; Jones, N. Mucociliary transport and its assessment: A review. *Clin. Otolaryngol. Allied Sci.* **1998**, *23*, 388–396. [CrossRef]
36. El-Nabarawy, N.A.; Teaima, M.H.; Helal, D.A. Assessment of spanlastic vesicles of zolmitriptan for treating migraine in rats. *Drug Des. Dev. Ther.* **2019**, *13*, 3929–3937. [CrossRef]
37. Dalpiaz, A.; Marchetti, N.; Cavazzini, A.; Pasti, L.; Velaga, S.; Gavini, E.; Beggiato, S.; Ferraro, L. Quantitative determination of zolmitriptan in rat blood and cerebrospinal fluid by reversed phase HPLC–ESI-MS/MS analysis: Application to in vivo preclinical pharmacokinetic study. *J. Chromatogr. B* **2012**, *901*, 72–78. [CrossRef]
38. Chen, X.; Liu, D.; Luan, Y.; Jin, F.; Zhong, D. Determination of zolmitriptan in human plasma by liquid chromatography–tandem mass spectrometry method: Application to a pharmacokinetic study. *J. Chromatogr. B* **2006**, *832*, 30–35. [CrossRef]
39. Vyas, T.K.; Babbar, A.K.; Sharma, R.K.; Misra, A. Intranasal mucoadhesive microemulsions of zolmitriptan: Preliminary studies on brain-targeting. *J. Drug Target.* **2005**, *13*, 317–324. [CrossRef]
40. Mohamed, D.F.; Abdel-Mageed, A.; Abdel-Hamid, F.; Ahmed, M. In-vitro and in-vivo evaluation of niosomal gel containing aceclofenac for sustained drug delivery. *Int. J. Pharm. Sci. Res.* **2014**, *1*, 1.
41. Dinarvand, R.; Moghadam, S.H.; Sheikhi, A.; Atyabi, F. Effect of surfactant HLB and different formulation variables on the properties of poly-D, L-lactide microspheres of naltrexone prepared by double emulsion technique. *J. Microencapsul.* **2005**, *22*, 139–151. [CrossRef]
42. Kazi, K.M.; Mandal, A.S.; Biswas, N.; Guha, A.; Chatterjee, S.; Behera, M.; Kuotsu, K. Niosome: A future of targeted drug delivery systems. *J. Adv. Pharm. Technol. Res.* **2010**, *1*, 374–380.
43. Fouda, N.H.; Abdelrehim, R.T.; Hegazy, D.A.; Habib, B.A. Sustained ocular delivery of Dorzolamide-HCl via proniosomal gel formulation: In-vitro characterization, statistical optimization, and in-vivo pharmacodynamic evaluation in rabbits. *Drug Deliv.* **2018**, *25*, 1340–1349. [CrossRef]
44. Yoshioka, T.; Sternberg, B.; Florence, A.T. Preparation and properties of vesicles (niosomes) of sorbitan monoesters (Span 20, 40, 60 and 80) and a sorbitan triester (Span 85). *Int. J. Pharm.* **1994**, *105*, 1–6. [CrossRef]
45. ElShagea, H.N.; ElKasabgy, N.A.; Fahmy, R.H.; Basalious, E.B. Freeze-dried self-nanoemulsifying self-nanosuspension (snesns): A new approach for the preparation of a highly drug-loaded dosage form. *AAPS PharmSciTech* **2019**, *20*, 258. [CrossRef]
46. Mason, R.L.; Gunst, R.F.; Hess, J.L. *Statistical Design and Analysis of Experiments: With Applications to Engineering and Science*; John Wiley & Sons: Hoboken, NJ, USA, 2003; Volume 474, pp. 24–28.
47. Annadurai, G.; Ling, L.Y.; Lee, J.F. Statistical optimization of medium components and growth conditions by response surface methodology to enhance phenol degradation by Pseudomonas putida. *J. Hazard. Mater.* **2008**, *151*, 171–178. [CrossRef]
48. Chauhan, B.; Gupta, R. Application of statistical experimental design for optimization of alkaline protease production from Bacillus sp. RGR-14. *Process. Biochem.* **2004**, *39*, 2115–2122. [CrossRef]
49. Thomas, L.; Viswanad, V. Formulation and optimization of clotrimazole-loaded proniosomal gel using 32 factorial design. *Sci. Pharm.* **2012**, *80*, 731–748. [CrossRef]

50. Mokhtar, M.; Sammour, O.A.; Hammad, M.A.; Megrab, N.A. Effect of some formulation parameters on flurbiprofen encapsulation and release rates of niosomes prepared from proniosomes. *Int. J. Pharm.* **2008**, *361*, 104–111. [CrossRef]
51. Moribe, K.; Maruyama, K.; Iwatsuru, M. Encapsulation characteristics of nystatin in liposomes: Effects of cholesterol and polyethylene glycol derivatives. *Int. J. Pharm.* **1999**, *188*, 193–202. [CrossRef]
52. Khalil, R.M.; Abdelbary, G.A.; Basha, M.; Awad, G.E.; El-Hashemy, H.A. Enhancement of lomefloxacin Hcl ocular efficacy via niosomal encapsulation: In vitro characterization and in vivo evaluation. *J. Liposome Res.* **2017**, *27*, 312–323. [CrossRef] [PubMed]
53. Adel, I.M.; ElMeligy, M.F.; Abdelrahim, M.E.; Maged, A.; Abdelkhalek, A.A.; Abdelmoteleb, A.M.; Elkasabgy, N.A. Design and Characterization of Spray-Dried Proliposomes for the Pulmonary Delivery of Curcumin. *Int. J. Nanomed.* **2021**, *16*, 2667–2687. [CrossRef] [PubMed]
54. Uchegbu, I.F.; Florence, A.T. Non-ionic surfactant vesicles (niosomes): Physical and pharmaceutical chemistry. *Adv. Colloid Interface Sci.* **1995**, *58*, 1–55. [CrossRef]
55. Abdelkader, H.; Ismail, S.; Kamal, A.; Alany, R.G. Preparation of niosomes as an ocular delivery system for naltrexone hydrochloride: Physicochemical characterization. *Die Pharm. -Int. J. Pharm. Sci.* **2010**, *65*, 811–817.
56. Salama, A.H.; Abdelkhalek, A.A.; Elkasabgy, N.A. Etoricoxib-loaded bio-adhesive hybridized polylactic acid-based nanoparticles as an intra-articular injection for the treatment of osteoarthritis. *Int. J. Pharm.* **2020**, *578*, 119081. [CrossRef]
57. Abd-Elsalam, W.H.; ElKasabgy, N.A. Mucoadhesive olaminosomes: A novel prolonged release nanocarrier of agomelatine for the treatment of ocular hypertension. *Int. J. Pharm.* **2019**, *560*, 235–245. [CrossRef]
58. Kamel, R.; El-Wakil, N.A.; Abdelkhalek, A.A.; Elkasabgy, N.A. Topical cellulose nanocrystals-stabilized nanoemulgel loaded with ciprofloxacin HCl with enhanced antibacterial activity and tissue regenerative properties. *J. Drug Deliv. Sci. Technol.* **2021**, *64*, 102553.
59. Gagliardi, A.; Paolino, D.; Iannone, M.; Palma, E.; Fresta, M.; Cosco, D. Sodium deoxycholate-decorated zein nanoparticles for a stable colloidal drug delivery system. *Int. J. Nanomed.* **2018**, *13*, 601–614. [CrossRef]
60. Lupo, N.; Steinbring, C.; Friedl, J.D.; Le-Vinh, B.; Bernkop-Schnürch, A. Impact of bile salts and a medium chain fatty acid on the physical properties of self-emulsifying drug delivery systems. *Drug Dev. Ind. Pharm.* **2021**, *47*, 22–35. [CrossRef]
61. Huang, Y.-B.; Tsai, M.J.; Wu, P.C.; Tsai, Y.H.; Wu, Y.H.; Fang, J.Y. Elastic liposomes as carriers for oral delivery and the brain distribution of (+)-catechin. *J. Drug Target.* **2011**, *19*, 709–718. [CrossRef]
62. Govender, T.; Stolnik, S.; Garnett, M.C.; Illum, L.; Davis, S.S. PLGA nanoparticles prepared by nanoprecipitation: Drug loading and release studies of a water soluble drug. *J. Control. Release* **1999**, *57*, 171–185. [CrossRef]
63. Pardakhty, A.; Varshosaz, J.; Rouholamini, A. In vitro study of polyoxyethylene alkyl ether niosomes for delivery of insulin. *Int. J. Pharm.* **2007**, *328*, 130–141. [CrossRef]
64. Williams, M. *The Mathematics of Diffusion*; Crank, J., Ed.; Clarendon Press: Oxford, UK, 1975; p. 414.
65. Serra, C.H.d.R.; Chang, K.H.; Dezani, T.M.; Porta, V.; Storpirtis, S. Dissolution efficiency and bioequivalence study using urine data from healthy volunteers: A comparison between two tablet formulations of cephalexin. *Braz. J. Pharm. Sci.* **2015**, *51*, 383–392. [CrossRef]
66. Malakar, J.; Nayak, A.K.; Goswami, S. Use of response surface methodology in the formulation and optimization of bisoprolol fumarate matrix tablets for sustained drug release. *ISRN Pharm.* **2012**, *2012*, 35–38. [CrossRef]
67. Kassem, M.A.; Aboul-Einien, M.H.; El Taweel, M.M. Dry gel containing optimized felodipine-loaded transferosomes: A promising transdermal delivery system to enhance drug bioavailability. *AAPS PharmSciTech* **2018**, *19*, 2155–2173. [CrossRef]
68. Elela, M.M.A.; ElKasabgy, N.A.; Basalious, E.B. Bio-shielding in situ forming gels (BSIFG) loaded with lipospheres for depot injection of quetiapine fumarate: In vitro and in vivo evaluation. *AAPS PharmSciTech* **2017**, *18*, 2999–3010. [CrossRef]
69. Adel, S.; ElKasabgy, N.A. Design of innovated lipid-based floating beads loaded with an antispasmodic drug: In-vitro and in-vivo evaluation. *J. Liposome Res.* **2014**, *24*, 136–149. [CrossRef]
70. Copetti, G.; Grassi, M.; Lapasin, R.; Pricl, S. Synergistic gelation of xanthan gum with locust bean gum: A rheological investigation. *Glycoconj. J.* **1997**, *14*, 951–961. [CrossRef]
71. Owen, D.H.; Peters, J.J.; Katz, D.F. Rheological properties of contraceptive gels. *Contraception* **2000**, *62*, 321–326. [CrossRef]
72. Chang, J.Y.; Oh, Y.K.; Choi, H.G.; Kim, Y.B.; Kim, C.K. Rheological evaluation of thermosensitive and mucoadhesive vaginal gels in physiological conditions. *Int. J. Pharm.* **2002**, *241*, 155–163. [CrossRef]
73. Abdel-Salam, F.S.; Elkheshen, S.A.; Mahmoud, A.A.; Basalious, E.B.; Amer, M.S.; Mostafa, A.A.; Elkasabgy, N.A. In-situ forming chitosan implant-loaded with raloxifene hydrochloride and bioactive glass nanoparticles for treatment of bone injuries: Formulation and biological evaluation in animal model. *Int. J. Pharm.* **2020**, *580*, 119213. [CrossRef]
74. Gizurarson, S. The effect of cilia and the mucociliary clearance on successful drug delivery. *Biol. Pharm. Bull.* **2015**, *38*, 497–506. [CrossRef]
75. El-Mahrouk, G.; Aboul-Einien, M.H.; Elkasabgy, N.A. Formulation and evaluation of meloxicam orally dispersible capsules. *Asian J Pharm Sci.* **2009**, *4*, 8–22.
76. Adel, I.M.; ElMeligy, M.F.; Abdelkhalek, A.A.; Elkasabgy, N.A. Design and characterization of highly porous curcumin loaded freeze-dried wafers for wound healing. *Eur. J. Pharm. Sci.* **2021**, *164*, 105888. [CrossRef]
77. Schipper, N.G.; Verhoef, J.C.; Mercus, F.W. The nasal mucocilliary clearance relevance to nasal drug delivery. *Pharm Res.* **1991**, *8*, 807–814. [CrossRef]

78. EMC. Zomig Tablets 2.5 mg. Available online: https://www.medicines.org.uk/emc/product/1372/smpc#gref (accessed on 20 August 2021).
79. Salama, H.A.; Mahmoud, A.A.; Kamel, A.O.; Abdel Hady, M.; Awad, G.A. Brain delivery of olanzapine by intranasal administration of transfersomal vesicles. *J. Liposome Res.* **2012**, *22*, 336–345. [CrossRef]
80. Fahmy, U.A.; Badr-Eldin, S.M.; Ahmed, O.A.; Aldawsari, H.M.; Tima, S.; Asfour, H.Z.; Al-Rabia, M.W.; Negm, A.A.; Sultan, M.H.; Madkhali, O.A.; et al. Intranasal niosomal in situ gel as a promising approach for enhancing flibanserin bioavailability and brain delivery: In vitro optimization and ex vivo/in vivo evaluation. *Pharmaceutics* **2020**, *12*, 485. [CrossRef]
81. Kapoor, M.; Cloyd, J.C.; Siegel, R.A. A review of intranasal formulations for the treatment of seizure emergencies. *J. Control. Release* **2016**, *237*, 147–159. [CrossRef]
82. Crowe, T.P.; Greenlee, M.H.; Kanthasamy, A.G.; Hsu, W.H. Mechanism of intranasal drug delivery directly to the brain. *Life Sci.* **2018**, *195*, 44–52. [CrossRef]
83. Soane, R.; Hinchcliffe, M.; Davis, S.S.; Illum, L. Clearance characteristics of chitosan based formulations in the sheep nasal cavity. *Int. J. Pharm.* **2001**, *217*, 183–191. [CrossRef]
84. Alsarra, I.A.; Hamed, A.Y.; Alanazi, F.K.; El Maghraby, G.M. *Vesicular Systems for Intranasal Drug Delivery, in Drug Delivery to the Central Nervous System*; Springer: Berlin/Heidelberg, Germany, 2010; pp. 175–203.
85. Shepherd, G. Responses of mitral cells to olfactory nerve volleys in the rabbit. *J. Physiol.* **1963**, *168*, 89100. [CrossRef] [PubMed]
86. Seju, U.; Kumar, A.; Sawant, K.K. Development and evaluation of olanzapine-loaded PLGA nanoparticles for nose-to-brain delivery: In vitro and in vivo studies. *Acta Biomater.* **2011**, *12*, 4169–4176. [CrossRef] [PubMed]
87. Yu, C.; Gu, P.; Zhang, W.; Cai, C.; He, H.; Tang, X. Evaluation of submicron emulsion as vehicles for rapid-onset intranasal delivery and improvement in brain targeting of zolmitriptan. *Drug Deliv.* **2011**, *18*, 578–585. [CrossRef] [PubMed]
88. Yu, C.; Gu, P.; Zhang, W.; Qi, N.; Cai, C.; He, H.; Tang, X. Preparation and evaluation of zolmitriptan submicron emulsion for rapid and effective nasal absorption in beagle dogs. *Drug Dev. Ind. Pharm.* **2011**, *37*, 1509–1516. [CrossRef]
89. Khezri, F.A.N.Z.; Lakshmi, C.S.R.; Bukka, R.; Nidhi, M.; Nargund, S.L. Pharmacokinetic study and brain tissue analysis of Zolmitriptan loaded chitosan nanoparticles in rats by LC-MS method. *Int. J. Biol. Macromol.* **2020**, *142*, 52–62. [CrossRef]
90. Al Khateb, K.; Ozhmukhametova, E.K.; Mussin, M.N.; Seilkhanov, S.K.; Rakhypbekov, T.K.; Lau, W.M.; Khutoryanskiy, V.V. In situ gelling systems based on Pluronic F127/Pluronic F68 formulations for ocular drug delivery. *Int. J. Pharm.* **2016**, *502*, 70–79. [CrossRef]
91. Chatterjee, B.; Amalina, N.; Sengupta, P.; Mandal, U.K. Mucoadhesive polymers and their mode of action: A recent update. *J. Appl. Pharm. Sci.* **2017**, *7*, 195–203.
92. Abou-Taleb, H.A.; Khallaf, R.A.; Abdel-Aleem, J.A. Intranasal niosomes of nefopam with improved bioavailability: Preparation, optimization, and in-vivo evaluation. *Drug Des. Dev. Ther.* **2018**, *12*, 3501–3516. [CrossRef]
93. Salem, H.F.; Kharshoum, R.M.; Abou-Taleb, H.A.; Naguib, D.M. Nanosized transferosome-based intranasal in situ gel for brain targeting of resveratrol: Formulation, optimization, in vitro evaluation, and in vivo pharmacokinetic study. *AAPS PharmSciTech* **2019**, *20*, 1–14. [CrossRef]
94. Sherje, A.P.; Londhe, V. Development and evaluation of pH-responsive cyclodextrin-based in situ gel of paliperidone for intranasal delivery. *AAPS PharmSciTech* **2018**, *19*, 384–394. [CrossRef]

pharmaceutics

Article

[18F]2-Fluoro-2-deoxy-sorbitol PET Imaging for Quantitative Monitoring of Enhanced Blood-Brain Barrier Permeability Induced by Focused Ultrasound

Gaëlle Hugon [1], Sébastien Goutal [1], Ambre Dauba [1], Louise Breuil [1], Benoit Larrat [2], Alexandra Winkeler [1], Anthony Novell [1] and Nicolas Tournier [1,*]

[1] CEA, CNRS, Inserm, BioMaps, Université Paris-Saclay, 91401 Orsay, France; gaelle.hugon@universite-paris-saclay.fr (G.H.); sebastien.goutal@universite-paris-saclay.fr (S.G.); ambre.dauba@universite-paris-saclay.fr (A.D.); louise.breuil@universite-paris-saclay.fr (L.B.); alexandra.winkeler@universite-paris-saclay.fr (A.W.); anthony.novell@universite-paris-saclay.fr (A.N.)

[2] CNRS, CEA, DRF/JOLIOT/NEUROSPIN/BAOBAB, Université Paris-Saclay, 91191 Gif-sur-Yvette, France; benoit.larrat@cea.fr

* Correspondence: n.tournier@universite-paris-saclay.fr

Abstract: Focused ultrasound in combination with microbubbles (FUS) provides an effective means to locally enhance the delivery of therapeutics to the brain. Translational and quantitative imaging techniques are needed to noninvasively monitor and optimize the impact of FUS on blood-brain barrier (BBB) permeability in vivo. Positron-emission tomography (PET) imaging using [18F]2-fluoro-2-deoxy-sorbitol ([18F]FDS) was evaluated as a small-molecule (paracellular) marker of blood-brain barrier (BBB) integrity. [18F]FDS was straightforwardly produced from chemical reduction of commercial [18F]2-deoxy-2-fluoro-D-glucose. [18F]FDS and the invasive BBB integrity marker Evan's blue (EB) were i.v. injected in mice after an optimized FUS protocol designed to generate controlled hemispheric BBB disruption. Quantitative determination of the impact of FUS on the BBB permeability was determined using kinetic modeling. A 2.2 ± 0.5-fold higher PET signal (n = 5; $p < 0.01$) was obtained in the sonicated hemisphere and colocalized with EB staining observed post mortem. FUS significantly increased the blood-to-brain distribution of [18F]FDS by 2.4 ± 0.8-fold (V_T; $p < 0.01$). Low variability (=10.1%) of V_T values in the sonicated hemisphere suggests reproducibility of the estimation of BBB permeability and FUS method. [18F]FDS PET provides a readily available, sensitive and reproducible marker of BBB permeability to noninvasively monitor the extent of BBB disruption induced by FUS in vivo.

Keywords: blood-brain barrier; integrity marker; sorbitol; positron emission tomography; focused ultrasound

Citation: Hugon, G.; Goutal, S.; Dauba, A.; Breuil, L.; Larrat, B.; Winkeler, A.; Novell, A.; Tournier, N. [18F]2-Fluoro-2-deoxy-sorbitol PET Imaging for Quantitative Monitoring of Enhanced Blood-Brain Barrier Permeability Induced by Focused Ultrasound. *Pharmaceutics* **2021**, *13*, 1752. https://doi.org/10.3390/pharmaceutics13111752

Academic Editors: Vibhuti Agrahari and Prashant Kumar

Received: 17 September 2021
Accepted: 14 October 2021
Published: 20 October 2021

Publisher's Note: MDPI stays neutral with regard to jurisdictional claims in published maps and institutional affiliations.

1. Introduction

The blood-brain barrier (BBB) plays a critical role in protecting the brain from potentially harmful substances of the circulation while controlling brain homeostasis [1]. Integrity of the BBB is mainly carried out by tight junctions between adjacent endothelial cells forming the brain microvasculature [2]. This considerably limits the paracellular (i.e., between cells) passage of solutes across the BBB which contributes to the sanctuary site property of the brain [2,3]. Many drug molecules and therapeutics cannot naturally permeate the intact BBB into the brain parenchyma. As a consequence, the BBB is a bottleneck in the development of central nervous system (CNS)-targeting therapeutics, which complicates the treatment of brain diseases, notably cerebral malignancies [4].

Numerous strategies and technologies have been proposed to overcome the BBB and achieve sufficient brain delivery of therapeutics [5]. Among these strategies, focused ultrasound in combination with microbubbles (FUS) is emerging as an effective means to locally and temporarily enhance BBB permeability, mainly through the "opening" of the paracellular route by disruption of the tight junctions [6]. A large body of preclinical research has convincingly shown that FUS enhanced the brain exposure of small molecules, biologics or gene therapy [7–11]. More than 30 clinical trials using FUS-induced BBB disruption are ongoing and assessed the translational potential and clinical safety of the technique [12–17].

The development of FUS is tightly linked to the availability of markers of BBB integrity, with the aim to quantitatively assess the impact of various FUS conditions in enhancing BBB permeability [18]. In the literature, many different BBB integrity markers have been described for nonclinical in vitro and ex vivo (terminal) experiments [19]. Low molecular weight (MW, g/mol) hydrophilic molecules such as fluorescein (MW = 332, fluorescent detection), (radio)labeled analogues of sucrose (MW = 342) or mannitol (MW = 182) (Figure 1A) are usually preferred as quantitative "paracellular" markers of membrane integrity (Figure 1) [1,20]. Low MW is associated with enhanced sensitivity to subtle change in barrier permeability compared with higher MW compounds such as Evan's blue (EB, MW = 961, highly bound to plasma proteins), radiolabeled proteins (albumin MW = 65,000), dextrans (MW = 1500–70,000) or inulin (MW = 6179) [1,21].

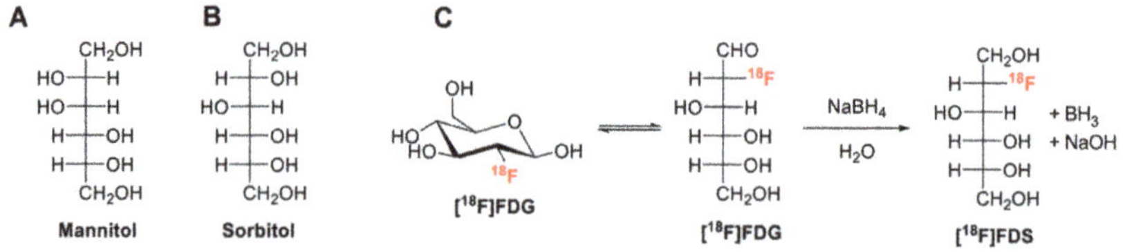

Figure 1. Chemical structures of mannitol (**A**), sorbitol (**B**). Chemical reduction of [^{18}F]2-fluoro-2-deoxy-glucose ([^{18}F]FDG) to [^{18}F]2-fluoro-2-deoxy-sorbitol ([^{18}F]FDS) using sodium borohydride ($NaBH_4$) is shown in (**C**).

Translational imaging techniques such as magnetic resonance imaging (MRI), single-photon emitting computed tomography (SPECT) or positron emission tomography imaging (PET) are increasingly regarded as methods to noninvasively monitor the impact of FUS on BBB permeability [18]. So far, dynamic contrast-enhanced (DCE), T1 relaxometry and dynamic susceptibility contrast MRI using gadolinium (Gd)-based contrast agents such as gadoterate (MW = 558), Gd-DTPA (Gd-diethylene triamine pentaacetic acid, MW = 546) [22,23] or large iron nanoparticles [24] have been used to detect BBB disruption in vivo. Brain SPECT using [^{99m}Tc]DTPA (MW = 487) is also widely used as a BBB integrity marker [25]. The predominant use of MRI and SPECT to investigate BBB integrity is likely due to the wide availability of corresponding imaging probes [26]. In humans, the clinical proof-of-concept of FUS-induced BBB disruption has been achieved using DCE-MRI to assess and localize BBB disruption in vivo [12]. However, accurate and absolute quantification of the brain penetration of contrast agent using MRI is very challenging [22]. More quantitative neuroimaging techniques are needed to accurately estimate the impact of FUS on BBB integrity.

Compared with MRI or SPECT, PET imaging benefits from absolute quantitative performances and high sensitivity so that quantitative determination of the concentration of microdose radiolabeled compounds in the brain is possible. Furthermore, high frame rate allows for kinetic modeling and estimation of transfer rate across the BBB [18]. For most imaging centers, the main limitation of PET is the limited availability of compounds other than commercial and daily produced radiopharmaceuticals such as [^{18}F]2-fluoro-2-deoxy-D-glucose ([^{18}F]FDG, Figure 1). Consistently, PET using radiolabeled low- or high-MW makers of BBB integrity such as [^{18}F]1-fluoro-1-deoxy-D-mannitol (MW = 183) [27] or [^{11}C]inulin (MW = 6179) [28], which synthesis requires production of radioisotope by a cyclotron and dedicated radiochemistry facilities, did not reach mainstream use.

Sorbitol (Figure 1B), a stereoisomer of mannitol, is a non-transported hydrophilic small molecule (MW = 182) that is poorly metabolized in mammals. The fluorinated derivative

[^{18}F]2-fluoro-2-deoxy-sorbitol ([^{18}F]FDS, MW = 183, Figure 1C) can be virtually obtained in all nuclear medicine departments and molecular imaging laboratory from simple chemical reduction of commercial [^{18}F]FDG [29]. [^{18}F]FDS shows nonsignificant brain uptake in healthy rodents and humans [30] and benefits from favorable pharmacokinetic properties for quantitative PET imaging in vivo [31].

This study aimed at evaluating [^{18}F]FDS PET for quantitative monitoring of enhanced BBB permeability induced by FUS in vivo. To this end, transcranial FUS conditions were optimized to induce hemispheric BBB disruption in mice. The kinetics of [^{18}F]FDS across the BBB were compared in the sonicated and nonsonicated hemispheres.

2. Materials and Methods

2.1. Production of [^{18}F]FDS

Synthesis of [^{18}F]2-fluoro-2-deoxy-sorbitol ([^{18}F]FDS) from commercial [^{18}F]FDG (Figure 1C) and quality control was described by Li et al. [29]. Briefly, $NaBH_4$ (2 mg) was added to 4 mL [^{18}F]FDG (180–200 MBq, Curium, Saclay, France). After 15 min reaction at room temperature, 10 µL acetic acid (0.15 mmol) was added. The mixture was passed through a Sep-Pak Alumina-N-Plus-Long cartridge (Waters, Guyancourt, France). Radiochemical purity was checked using radio-thin-layer chromatography (TLC) using silica gel-coated alumina plates (Merck, Guyancourt, France). The mobile phase consisted in acetonitrile/water (80/20, *v/v*).

2.2. Focused Ultrasound

The method for spatially controlled BBB disruption was optimized from previous work [10] to induce reproducible BBB disruption in the right brain hemisphere only. Experiments were performed using female NMRI nu/nu mice. Seven-week-old mice were anesthetized with 1.5% isoflurane in O_2/air (50/50, *v/v*). A catheter was inserted in the tail vein and the animal was transferred to the sonication system. As NMRI nu/nu mice lack body hairs shaving of the head could be omitted. Microbubbles (50 µL, SonoVue®, Bracco, Italy) were intravenously administrated in the tail vein before the beginning of the FUS (n = 5) or sham (no FUS, n = 3) session.

FUS were delivered by a spherically focused transducer (active diameter 25 mm, focal depth 20 mm, axial resolution 5 mm, lateral resolution 1 mm, Imasonic, Voray sur l'Ognon, France) centered at 1.5 MHz. The transducer was connected to a single-channel programmable generator (Image Guided Therapy, Pessac, France), mounted on a motorized *XYZ*-axis stage, and positioned above the mouse head maintained under anesthesia. The device was coupled to the mouse head using a latex balloon (filled with deionized and degassed water) and coupling gel. The distance between the transducer and the skull was adjusted by the displacement of the motorized axis (Z) and the filling of the balloon in order to target the center of the right brain hemisphere, at the focal distance (i.e., 20 mm). The FUS sequence used a peak negative pressure of 525 kPa (calibrated in deionized water). Therefore, the transmitted in situ pressure in the mouse brain was previously estimated to be 420 kPa considering a transmission loss through the skull of 20% at 1.5 MHz [32]. A mechanical scan (*XY*-axis) was synchronized to the generator output in order to induce a hemispheric brain BBB opening of 6 mm (anterior-posterior) × 3.6 mm (lateral right hemisphere). This 3.5 s sequence was repeated 36 times for a total exposure of 126.4 s with a global ultrasound duty of 71%.

2.3. Evan's Blue Extravasation Test

Evan's blue (EB) extravasation test was used as a positive control to visually check and localize BBB disruption induced by the FUS protocol. Solution of EB (obtained from Sigma-Aldrich, Saint-Quentin Fallavier, France) was freshly prepared at 4% in NaCl 0.9% as previously described [33]. Mice received 100 µL EB i.v., immediately after FUS. One hour after injection, i.e., at the end of PET acquisition, animals were euthanized and brains were removed to visually assess EB extravasation. Due to circulating radioactivity in

[^{18}F]FDS-injected animals, no perfusion washout was performed to remove blood and EB from the brain vasculature. Coregistration of the brain distribution of EB and the [^{18}F]FDS PET signal in the brain obtained in an animal of the FUS group was performed. The frozen brain was sectioned with a cryostat (Leica CM3050 S, Leica, Wetzlar, Germany). Brain sections were scanned with a 20× lens, using an AxiObserver Z1 microscope (Zeiss, Jena, Germany) to observe distribution of EB-associated fluorescence in coronal slices. Then, representative EB brain slice and corresponding PET images obtained in the same animal were coregistered on MRI template to compare the PET signal in vivo with EB fluorescence ex vivo.

2.4. [^{18}F]FDS PET Imaging

Immediately after EB injection (<60 s), anesthetized mice were transferred to the microPET scanner (Inveon, microPET, Siemens Healthcare, Knoxville, TN, USA). [^{18}F]FDS was administered intravenously (4.2 ± 0.76 MBq) using a microinjection pump at the rate of 0.2 mL·min^{-1} during 60 s (n = 5 FUS; n = 3 sham). Dynamic PET acquisition (60 min) started with [^{18}F]FDS injection.

PET images were reconstructed using the three-dimensional ordered subset expectation maximization with maximum a posteriori algorithm (3D OSEM/MAP) and corrected for attenuation, random coincidences and scattering. Volumes of interests (VOI$_s$) were manually delineated using Pmod software (version 3.8, PMOD Technologies Ltd., Zurich, Switzerland). In the FUS group, extravasation of ^{18}F-FDS was obvious in the sonicated area on late PET images. The region with disrupted BBB was delineated and mirrored to the contralateral hemisphere. In sham animals, VOI$_s$ were drawn in each brain hemisphere. Another VOI was drawn on the aorta (blood-pool), obvious on early time-frames, to generate an image derived input function (IDIF).

Time activity curves (TACs) were corrected for radioactive decay, injected dose and animal weight and reported as standardized uptake value (SUV) vs. time. Area under the TAC (AUC) was calculated from either 0 to 15, 30 or 60 min (AUC$_{brain}$) as well as corresponding AUC$_{brain}$/AUC$_{blood}$. Kinetic modeling of the 60 min PET data was performed using either the Logan graphical method [34] and a 1-tissue compartment (1-TC) model using IDIF to estimate the total volume of distribution (V_T, mL·cm^{-3}) of [^{18}F]FDS and describe its transport across the BBB. Parametric images were generated to visualize the distribution of V_T (1-TC model) of [^{18}F]FDS in the brain and peripheral tissues.

2.5. Statistics

Data are presented as mean ± S.D. Statistical analysis was performed using GraphPad Prism software version 9.1, La Jolla, CA, USA. Outcome parameters of kinetic modeling were compared using a two-way ANOVA with "hemisphere" and "group" as factors followed by Tukey's multiple comparison test. Ratio of radioactivity measured in the right to the left hemisphere, as well as blood data obtained in the FUS and the sham group were compared using the Mann–Whitney U test. The Pearson's test was used to test the correlation between different kinetic parameters obtained in the same brain regions. Statistical significance was set a $p < 0.05$. Intragroup variability of outcome parameters was estimated by the coefficient of variation (CV = 100 × S.D./mean).

3. Results

Chemical transformation of [^{18}F]FDG into [^{18}F]FDS was very effective (Figure 1). Radio-TLC analysis of the preparation revealed a single peak with retardation factor (Rf) = 0.6, consistent with the presence of [^{18}F]FDS [29]. The Rf of untransformed [^{18}F]FDG, tested using the same TLC conditions, was 0.9 (data not shown). No [^{18}F]FDG could be detected using this method in the final preparation of [^{18}F]FDS.

In FUS animals, strong EB staining was observed in the posterior part of the sonicated (right) hemisphere only (Figure 2A). This contrasted with the low EB staining still observed in brain vessels of the contralateral hemisphere, as well as in sham animals, because no washing out was performed to remove the circulating blood from the resected brain tissue. This confirmed that enhanced EB staining could be used as a positive control for effective BBB disruption.

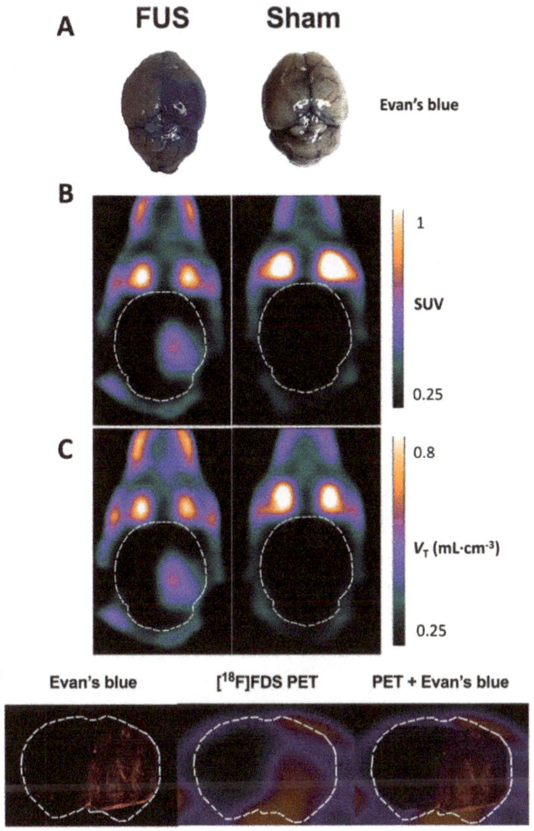

Figure 2. Impact of focused ultrasound (FUS) on blood-brain barrier (BBB) integrity assessed using Evan's blue extravasation and positron emission tomography (PET) using [^{18}F]2-fluoro-2-deoxy-sorbitol ([^{18}F]FDS). Extravasation of Evan's blue was obvious in the right brain hemisphere of animals of the FUS group (**A**). Standardized uptake value (SUV)-normalized brain PET images (sum 30–60 min) of [^{18}F]FDS uptake after hemispheric BBB disruption induced by focused ultrasound (FUS) or without (sham) are shown in (**B**). Corresponding parametric images describing the total volume of distribution (V_T), estimated using the one-tissue compartment model from 0 to 60 min are shown in (**C**). In (**D**), the distribution of the fluorescence of the Evan's blue dye in a coronal slice of mouse brain after FUS protocol obtained ex vivo was overlaid to the corresponding slice of [^{18}F]FDS PET image obtained in vivo in the same animal.

Similarly, no washing out of circulating blood radioactivity was performed to interpret in vivo PET images. PET images in sham animals confirmed the negligible baseline brain uptake of brain [^{18}F]FDS across the intact BBB (Figure 2B), whereas a strong PET signal could be monitored in the sonicated brain hemisphere of FUS animals. Parametric PET images, expressed in $V_{T\text{-}1TC;60min}$ closely resembled the PET images in SUV units (Figure 2C). Images revealed a region with obvious increase in [^{18}F]FDS uptake that was strictly localized in the right hemisphere, with very limited impact on the left hemisphere. Brain distribution of [^{18}F]FDS PET signal was consistent with EB extravasation observed in the whole brain (Figure 2A).

Moreover, brain distribution of the fluorescent signal of EB observed ex vivo in the right brain hemisphere with higher spatial resolution was similar to the [^{18}F]FDS PET signal obtained in the same animal of the FUS group (Figure 2D). It should be noted that although no washout was performed, no fluorescent signal was observed in the contralateral brain hemisphere underlining specific leakage of EB into the brain parenchyma. Interestingly, mapping of [^{18}F]FDS brain distribution within the sonicated area displayed a gradient from the center to the periphery which was not observed using EB as a BBB integrity marker.

In hemispheres with intact BBB (sham animals or contralateral hemisphere), brain PET signal increased rapidly with maximal uptake at T_{max} = 4 min, followed by slow decrease of the radioactivity. FUS selectively enhanced the brain PET signal and T_{max} was achieved later at ~13.5 min, followed by a plateau (Figure 3A,B). SUV values in the sonicated (right) hemisphere at 15, 30 and 60 min were significantly higher than in the nonsonicated (left) hemisphere ($p < 0.01$, Figure 3A). Brain exposure ($AUC_{0\text{–}60min}$) of [^{18}F]FDS in the sonicated volume was 2.2 ± 0.5-fold higher compared with the contralateral volume ($p < 0.01$) and 1.8 ± 0.4-fold higher than the mean $AUC_{0\text{–}60min}$ measured in the corresponding (right) hemisphere of the sham group ($p < 0.05$, Figure 4A). The ratio of the PET signal in the sonicated volume to the contralateral region increased from 0 to 15 min to reach a plateau (Figure 3C). FUS did not impact the kinetics [^{18}F]FDS in the blood-pool with significant difference in neither SUV values nor AUC_{blood} between the FUS and the sham group ($p > 0.05$, Figure 3D).

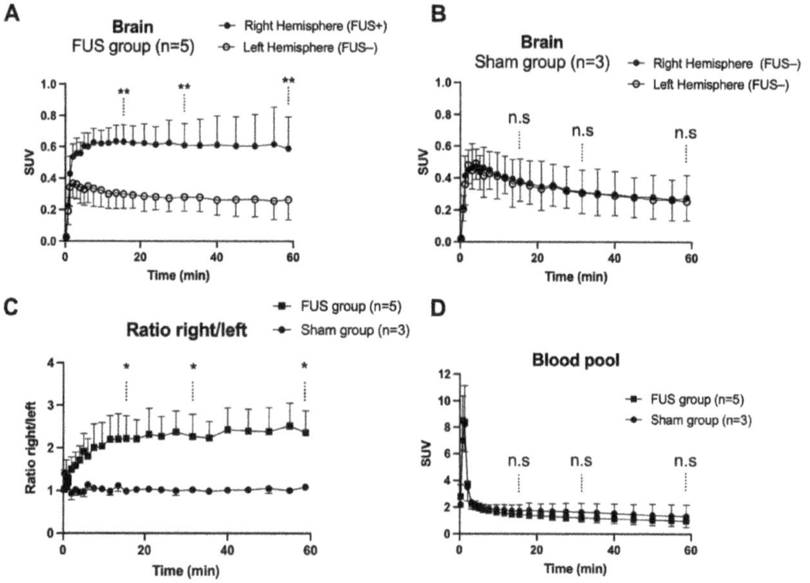

Figure 3. Brain kinetics of [^{18}F]2-fluoro-2-deoxy-sorbitol ([^{18}F]FDS). BBB disruption was obtained in the right brain hemisphere using focused ultrasound (FUS group, n = 5, in (**A**), but not in the sham group (n = 3, in (**B**)). The time course of the right/left ratio of the PET signal in FUS and sham animals is shown in (**C**). Corresponding image-derived input functions are shown in (**D**). Data are mean ± S.D Statistical comparison of values obtained at 15, 30 and 60 min after injection of [^{18}F]FDS is reported with * $p < 0.05$, ** $p < 0.01$, n.s = nonsignificant.

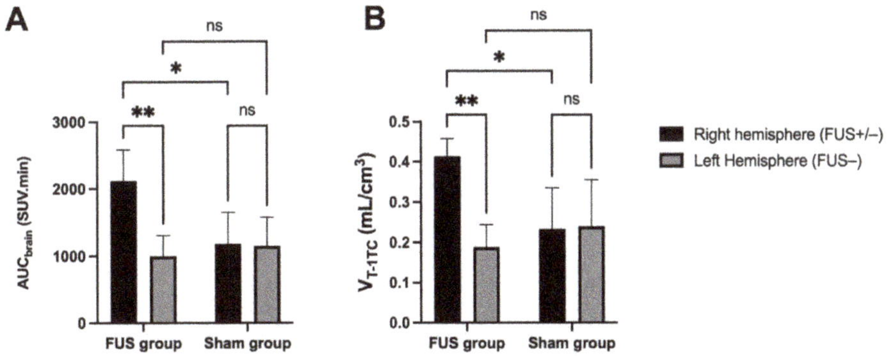

Figure 4. Comparison of [^{18}F]FDS brain PET data. Ultrasound-induced BBB disruption (FUS+) was obtained in the right brain hemisphere of the FUS group (n = 5) while BBB in the contralateral brain hemisphere was intact (FUS−). The brain exposure of [^{18}F]FDS was estimated by the area under the time-activity curve (AUC_{brain}, in (**A**). Brain distribution was estimated by $V_{T\text{-}1TC}$ (1-tissue compartment model, in (**B**) using an image-derived input function. Data were also compared with a sham group (no FUS, n = 3). Data are reported as mean ± S.D with * $p < 0.05$ and ** $p < 0.01$.

Brain TACs of [^{18}F]FDS were accurately described with acceptable fit (error < 3%) by V_T estimated using the 1-TC model (Figure 4B). The Logan graphical method provided similar estimation of brain V_T (correlation $p < 0.001$, R^2 = 0.99, Figure 5). A significant increase in the $V_{T\text{-}1TC}$ of [^{18}F]FDS was observed in the sonicated region compared with the contralateral region (2.43 ± 0.8-fold increase, $p < 0.01$) or the brain of sham animals (1.9 ± 0.2-fold increase, $p < 0.05$) (Figure 4). In the FUS group, the variability of $V_{T\text{-}1TC}$ values was lower in the sonicated brain (CV = 10.1%) compared with the nonsonicated brain (CV = 29.7%). The influx and efflux transfer rates K_1 and k_2 were estimated with acceptable fit (error < 7%). However, K_1 values were associated with a high intragroup variability in the nonsonicated brain (CV = 37.6%) compared with the sonicated brain (CV = 18.5%), which questions the relevance of K_1 and k_2 to describe the extremely low BBB penetration of [^{18}F]FDS across the intact BBB. $V_{T\text{-}1TC}$ was therefore retained as the gold-standard parameter to describe the brain distribution of [^{18}F]FDS in all tested conditions.

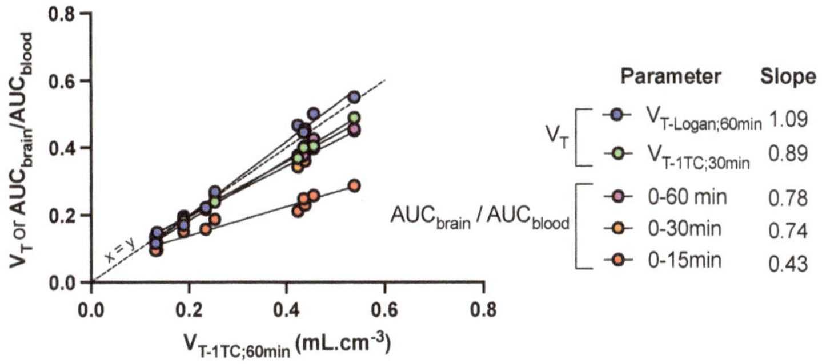

Figure 5. Sensitivity of kinetic parameters to describe the impact of FUS on the brain distribution of [^{18}F]FDS in mice. Mice (n = 5) underwent blood-brain barrier disruption induced by focused ultrasound in the right hemisphere only. Kinetic modeling was performed to estimate the total brain distribution (V_T) using the one-tissue compartment model ($V_{T\text{-}1TC}$) estimated from 0 to 60 min after injection of [^{18}F]FDS. $V_{T\text{-}1TC;0\text{–}60min}$ values were correlated with $V_{T\text{-}1TC}$ estimated from 0 to 30 min ($V_{T\text{-}1TC;0\text{–}30min}$), V_T estimated using the Logan graphical method from 0 to 60 min ($V_{T\text{-}Logan;60min}$) or the ratio of the time-activity curves (AUC) measured in brain regions and blood (AUC_{brain}/AUC_{blood}) from 0 to 15, 30 or 60 min. The slope of the linear correlation is reported.

Other quantification methods were tested to either reduce the length of PET acquisition or simplify analysis of the PET data. $V_{T\text{-}1TC}$ values estimated from 0 to 30 min ($V_{T\text{-}1TC;30min}$), as well as AUC_{brain}/AUC_{blood} measured from either 0 to either 30 or 60 min, was significantly correlated with $V_{T\text{-}1TC;60min}$ ($p < 0.001$, $R^2 = 0.99$) with limited loss in the sensitivity to detect enhanced brain distribution of [^{18}F]FDS induced by FUS (Figure 5). However, further reduction of the length of PET frame tended to underestimate the brain distribution of [^{18}F]FDS, especially in in the sonicated hemisphere. Nevertheless, AUC_{brain}/AUC_{blood} from 0 to 15 min was still significantly correlated with $V_{T\text{-}1TC}$ values ($p < 0.001$, $R^2 = 0.94$) but the slope of the linear regression was <0.5. (Figure 5)

4. Discussion

In the present study, [^{18}F]FDS PET imaging was validated for the first time as a translational and quantitative marker of BBB permeability to estimate the impact of spatially-controlled FUS on BBB integrity in mice.

Unlike [^{18}F]FDG, [^{18}F]FDS is poorly taken up by mammalian cells because it lacks transporters and/or enzymes for specific cell uptake and retention [29]. [^{18}F]FDS PET has been previously validated in animals and humans to study renal function [35] or detect/estimate bacterial burden in tissues because sorbitol is a specific metabolic substrate of some strains of Gram-negative bacteria [36]. [^{18}F]FDS therefore benefits from extensive clinical pharmacology and safety data as an experimental radiopharmaceutical drug [30]. However, to our knowledge, the impact of BBB integrity on the brain kinetics of [^{18}F]FDS has never been evaluated so far.

[^{18}F]FDS benefits from the characteristics of an "ideal" marker of BBB integrity [21]. This includes, metabolic stability, low binding to plasma proteins (<0.1%) and low baseline brain uptake when the BBB is intact [30,31]. Interestingly, Li et al. reported that [^{18}F]FDS visually accumulated in orthotopic brain tumor xenografts in mice, despite negligible uptake by implanted glioma cells in vitro [29]. Given the substantial sensitivity of [^{18}F]FDS to the integrity of the BBB, it can be hypothesized that the local BBB leakage in the tumor environment, rather than uptake by cancer cells, may explain the enhanced [^{18}F]FDS PET signal observed by Li and colleagues in the tumor area [29]. Further experiments are however needed to validate the use of [^{18}F]FDS to quantitatively monitor the permeability of the blood-tumor barrier. Similarly, we advocate that the high sensitivity of [^{18}F]FDS to BBB integrity may be considered for correct estimation of bacterial burden in brain lesions using [^{18}F]FDS PET [37].

Pharmacokinetic modeling of brain [^{18}F]FDS PET data is relatively simple. Estimation of brain V_T, using either the graphical method (Logan plot) or compartmental modeling (1-TC) provided similar outcome parameters to describe the distribution of [^{18}F]FDS in both the sonicated and the non-sonicated brain, with low intragroup variability. In the FUS group, variability was strikingly lower (CV ~10%) in the sonicated brain regions compared with regions with the intact BBB (CV ~30%). This may be explained by the lower PET signal in the brain with intact BBB, associated with higher signal-to-noise ratio compared with the sonicated brain in which the PET signal is higher. Altogether, this suggests that V_T, which takes any change in the plasma kinetics of [^{18}F]FDS into account, provides a reliable and sensitive outcome parameter to describe the BBB permeation of [^{18}F]FDS across the BBB. Estimation of $V_{T\text{-}1TC}$ from 30 min PET data offers a compromise to observe and delineate the blood pool in aorta at early time-frames and allow for correct estimation of the brain distribution of [^{18}F]FDS while reducing the total length of PET acquisition (Figure 5).

Simplified parameters were tested to quantitatively estimate the impact of FUS on the brain uptake of [^{18}F]FDS. AUC_{brain}/AUC_{blood} measured from 0 to 30 or 60 min after injection accurately predicted V_T and can be used as a surrogate parameter to estimate BBB permeation with limited impact on the sensitivity of the method compared with 60 min scan (Figure 5). V_T or AUC_{brain}/AUC_{blood} should be used, rather than AUC_{brain}, in situations where change in the blood kinetics of [^{18}F]FDS is expected, such as renal disorders to correctly estimate the blood to brain distribution of [^{18}F]FDS [38].

The FUS method reported in this project allows for localized BBB disruption in the right hemisphere while keeping the contralateral hemisphere intact, as confirmed using the post mortem EB extravasation test. In this situation, the contralateral hemisphere can serve as a convenient reference region to accurately estimate the impact of FUS on enhanced [^{18}F]FDS brain uptake (AUC_{brain}, Figure 3C). However, in many situations, BBB disruption induced by FUS or other methods may affect the whole brain or cannot be localized a priori [39]. In the absence of such reference region, increase in BBB permeability can be quantified by comparing [^{18}F]FDS V_T or AUC_{brain}/AUC_{blood} obtained in a control (sham) group or in the same animals before any intervention, following a longitudinal design. This illustrates the added value of absolute quantitative PET compared with other neuroimaging techniques for noninvasive determination of different levels of BBB permeation in various situations [26].

Mapping of enhanced [^{18}F]FDS PET signal induced by FUS in the brain was consistent with EB extravasation observed ex vivo and in vitro, although exact co-registration of PET images with brain slices is very challenging. This suggests a limited diffusion of [^{18}F]FDS from the sonicated to the nonsonicated brain with intact BBB. Interestingly, brain distribution within the sonicated area displayed a gradient from the center to the periphery (Figure 2). It may be hypothesized that heterogeneity in intensity of delivered ultrasound may occur within the sonicated area as a consequence of loss of ultrasound transmission relative to the transducer angulation at the skull surface. Interestingly, such a phenomenon could not be detected using high-MW markers of BBB integrity such as gadoterate or using EB extravasation in the same animals (Figure 2).

Several recent examples illustrate the added value of PET imaging to investigate the impact of FUS on BBB structure and function in vivo [18]. First, brain uptake of [^{18}F]FDG, which is actively transported by glucose transporter 1 (GLUT1), was shown to be lower during FUS-induced BBB disruption, consistent with the local decrease in GLUT1 expression in the sonicated brain. Baseline [^{18}F]FDG uptake and GLUT1 expression were fully restored 24 h after FUS [40]. P-glycoprotein (P-gp) and breast cancer resistance protein (BCRP) are the main efflux transporters expressed at the BBB [2]. We have shown that FUS-induced BBB disruption did not significantly impact the efflux transport of the P-gp substrate [^{11}C]*N*-desmethyl-loperamide and the dual P-gp/BCRP substrate [^{11}C]erlotinib in rats [33]. These particular PET probes may however lack the sensitivity to detect subtle changes in transporter function [41]. Decrease in P-gp expression has been reported 24–48 h after FUS [42,43]. However, long-term impact on efflux transport function at the BBB remains to be investigated in details. In this framework, [^{18}F]FDS may offer a quantitative tool to estimate the dynamics of BBB disruption and restoration after FUS with suitable temporal resolution [24]. Altogether, this suggests that [^{18}F]FDS enriches the PET imaging toolbox to investigate the short- and long-term impact of FUS on BBB permeability with respect to its molecular environment, including regulation of tight junction expression [18].

Simple production of [^{18}F]FDS from commercial [^{18}F]FDG makes it an appealing radiopharmaceutical candidate for determination of BBB permeability using quantitative PET. [^{18}F]FDS is not a "ready-to-inject" preparation compared with [^{18}F]FDG, although radiopharmaceutical production and shipment could theoretically be ensured by an external manufacturer. However, most radiopharmaceuticals used in nuclear medicine and molecular imaging departments require handling by a radiopharmacy team, chemical reaction and quality control [44]. Efforts are moreover being made to develop kit formulation for radiosynthesis of [^{18}F]FDS to simplify the production of this radiopharmaceutical [45]. Radiosynthesis of [^{18}F]FDS for animal or clinical use can therefore be achieved in most molecular imaging departments, including those not equipped with radiochemistry facilities [37]. From a clinical perspective, the radiation dosimetry of this radiopharmaceutical was shown suitable for human use, although radiation exposure can be a limitation for the repeated use of [^{18}F]FDS PET in humans [30].

This study has some limitations. The evaluation of the impact of FUS using [^{18}F]FDS PET was evaluated in healthy animals only. As a consequence, FUS induced a large increase in the BBB penetration of [^{18}F]FDS, starting from a low baseline brain uptake. In this situation, statistical significance was reached using a small number of individuals. However, a large body of translational research supports that BBB integrity is compromised in many CNS pathological conditions including multiple sclerosis, hypoxic/ischemic insult, traumatic injury, Parkinson's and Alzheimer's diseases, epilepsy and brain tumors [1]. Different non-clinical models have shown that BBB leakage is a common feature of the neuroinflammatory cascade and contributes to disease-associated brain damage [3,46]. PET imaging is expected to offer more quantitative insight into BBB permeability in such pathophysiological conditions [27,47–49]. Nevertheless, further experiments are needed, probably in a larger number of animals, to test whether [^{18}F]FDS has the sensitivity and appropriate test-retest variability to be useful as permeability marker to investigate the dynamics of disease-associated changes in BBB integrity in longitudinal studies. NMRI nu/nu mice are widely used as a model for cancer treatment, including orthotopic brain tumors, which will be the logical next step for the evaluation of the impact of FUS using [^{18}F]FDS PET imaging [50]. We assume that the use of female individuals of this immunodeficient mouse strain in the present study is not likely to bias the immediate impact of FUS-induced BBB disruption compared with male and/or immunocompetent mouse strains. Nevertheless, immunodeficiency was shown to improve the long-term integrity of the BBB in a model of intracerebral hemorrhage [51]. Longitudinal studies using quantitative [^{18}F]FDS PET imaging may be useful to further investigate the time-dependent cross-talk between the immune system and BBB permeability in pathophysiological situations [46].

Restoration of BBB structure and function is increasingly the subject of investigations as a therapeutic target to prevent or limit the outcome of neurological disorders [52]. Conversely, temporary FUS-induced BBB disruption is also regarded as a potential therapeutic strategy in various CNS diseases. FUS alone was shown to achieve promising results at reducing the amyloid load in Alzheimer's disease or at inducing neurogenesis [53,54]. This questions the long-term impact of the temporary FUS-induced BBB disruption in a situation where BBB integrity and function are already compromised [3]. This complex situation illustrates the crucial need for quantitative PET imaging techniques to untangle the impact of FUS on BBB permeability in relation to brain function in animal models and patients [18].

5. Conclusions

[^{18}F]FDS PET imaging presents essential properties to become an effective and quantitative marker of BBB permeability, which include availability, safety, low MW, low distribution across the intact BBB and low diffusion from the sonicated volume to the non-sonicated brain with intact BBB. This is demonstrated here for the first time using local induction of BBB permeability by FUS. [^{18}F]FDS PET offers a very instrumental imaging marker to finely and dynamically measure BBB permeability variations over time scales of minutes.

Author Contributions: Conceptualization, G.H., A.N. and N.T.; methodology, S.G., L.B., B.L., A.W. and N.T.; software, G.H., S.G. and B.L.; validation, L.B., A.W., A.N. and N.T.; formal analysis, G.H., and A.D.; investigation, G.H., S.G., A.D., A.W. and A.N.; resources, A.N., B.L. and N.T.; data curation, N.T.; writing—original draft preparation, G.H. and N.T.; writing—review and editing, G.H, S.G., A.W., B.L., A.N. and N.T.; visualization, S.G., A.D. and L.B.; supervision, N.T. and A.N.; funding acquisition, A.N., A.W. and N.T. All authors have read and agreed to the published version of the manuscript.

Funding: Ambre Daubat received grant from Agence Nationale de la Recherche (grant DROPMUT, ANR-19-CE19-0011). Gaëlle Hugon received a PhD grant from the CEA (French Atomic and Alternative Energy commission) and the DGA (Direction Générale des Armées). Louise Breuil received a grant from CEA/AP-HP. This work was performed on a platform member of France Life Imaging network (grant ANR-11-INBS-0006).

Institutional Review Board Statement: All animal experiments were performed in accordance with the recommendations of the European Community (2010/63/UE) and the French National Committees (law 2013-118) for the care and use of laboratory animals. The experimental protocol was approved by a local ethics committee for animal use (Comité d'éthique pour expérimentation animale Ile-de-France n° 44) and by the French ministry of agriculture (APAFIS 16292-2018072609593031 v7, accepted the 1 June 2017).

Informed Consent Statement: Not applicable.

Data Availability Statement: Data is contained within the article or Appendix A.

Acknowledgments: We thank Maud Goislard and Philippe Gervais for helpful technical assistance.

Conflicts of Interest: The authors declare no conflict of interest.

Appendix A

Individual time-activity curves (SUV) units in the brain and arterial blood-pool of mice in the FUS group (n = 5) and the sham group (n = 3).

Table A1. SUV values—right hemisphere.

	FUS Group (FUS+)					Sham Group (FUS−)		
Time (min)	Mouse 1	Mouse 2	Mouse 3	Mouse 4	Mouse 5	Mouse 1	Mouse 2	Mouse 3
0.25	0.016	0.024	0.032	0.026	0.017	0.033	0.033	0.010
0.75	0.195	0.216	0.312	0.222	0.178	0.232	0.278	0.135
1.25	0.433	0.382	0.614	0.378	0.330	0.403	0.542	0.295
2	0.566	0.581	0.603	0.396	0.527	0.325	0.580	0.437
3	0.633	0.530	0.664	0.420	0.534	0.324	0.624	0.441
4	0.565	0.550	0.642	0.452	0.580	0.396	0.596	0.421
5	0.605	0.579	0.698	0.479	0.657	0.338	0.543	0.430
6	0.591	0.587	0.711	0.478	0.635	0.370	0.610	0.409
7.5	0.589	0.636	0.680	0.498	0.730	0.377	0.582	0.394
9.5	0.585	0.624	0.650	0.506	0.733	0.320	0.578	0.372
11.5	0.574	0.626	0.639	0.506	0.768	0.299	0.555	0.346
13.5	0.600	0.620	0.648	0.505	0.794	0.292	0.529	0.362
15.5	0.582	0.645	0.612	0.508	0.807	0.262	0.538	0.327
18	0.569	0.613	0.621	0.512	0.804	0.246	0.521	0.333
21	0.561	0.592	0.600	0.520	0.840	0.220	0.525	0.295
24	0.555	0.607	0.564	0.531	0.813	0.254	0.502	0.310
27.5	0.525	0.615	0.550	0.553	0.879	0.209	0.489	0.280
31.5	0.511	0.595	0.534	0.547	0.856	0.204	0.465	0.271
35.5	0.495	0.561	0.516	0.560	0.907	0.167	0.471	0.270
40	0.497	0.559	0.494	0.568	0.940	0.176	0.457	0.262
45	0.470	0.555	0.489	0.579	0.932	0.185	0.416	0.246
50	0.462	0.559	0.457	0.592	0.953	0.165	0.433	0.244
55	0.448	0.538	0.461	0.604	1.029	0.163	0.405	0.224
58.75	0.418	0.528	0.455	0.609	0.929	0.163	0.435	0.231

Table A2. SUV values—left hemisphere.

	FUS Group (FUS−)					Sham Group (FUS−)		
Time (min)	Mouse 1	Mouse 2	Mouse 3	Mouse 4	Mouse 5	Mouse 1	Mouse 2	Mouse 3
0.25	0.019	0.039	0.031	0.032	0.009	0.019	0.032	0.007
0.75	0.194	0.117	0.323	0.213	0.108	0.206	0.277	0.131
1.25	0.330	0.264	0.547	0.337	0.236	0.304	0.511	0.269
2	0.389	0.301	0.520	0.295	0.331	0.420	0.613	0.409
3	0.326	0.278	0.515	0.309	0.375	0.369	0.584	0.393
4	0.282	0.264	0.510	0.292	0.351	0.405	0.599	0.466
5	0.257	0.250	0.499	0.294	0.350	0.372	0.604	0.390

Table A2. *Cont.*

	FUS Group (FUS+)					Sham Group (FUS−)		
Time (min)	Mouse 1	Mouse 2	Mouse 3	Mouse 4	Mouse 5	Mouse 1	Mouse 2	Mouse 3
6	0.270	0.256	0.508	0.309	0.401	0.292	0.558	0.390
7.5	0.242	0.233	0.489	0.287	0.420	0.346	0.536	0.403
9.5	0.240	0.227	0.474	0.285	0.394	0.289	0.569	0.377
11.5	0.211	0.226	0.432	0.278	0.352	0.329	0.515	0.361
13.5	0.218	0.213	0.405	0.276	0.419	0.230	0.521	0.341
15.5	0.213	0.235	0.415	0.254	0.379	0.289	0.517	0.325
18	0.216	0.226	0.374	0.259	0.391	0.257	0.482	0.320
21	0.194	0.196	0.360	0.270	0.406	0.209	0.474	0.310
24	0.203	0.223	0.341	0.249	0.389	0.255	0.488	0.301
27.5	0.197	0.204	0.324	0.245	0.395	0.225	0.440	0.297
31.5	0.201	0.198	0.328	0.267	0.406	0.198	0.451	0.273
35.5	0.203	0.205	0.302	0.261	0.421	0.183	0.446	0.273
40	0.179	0.182	0.279	0.257	0.409	0.188	0.427	0.255
45	0.173	0.178	0.262	0.271	0.435	0.177	0.420	0.241
50	0.168	0.178	0.265	0.276	0.444	0.178	0.398	0.215
55	0.153	0.167	0.245	0.266	0.449	0.159	0.409	0.225
58.75	0.160	0.169	0.238	0.278	0.476	0.147	0.380	0.231

Table A3. SUV values—Blood (aorta).

	FUS Group (FUS+/−)					Sham Group (FUS−)		
Time (min)	Mouse 1	Mouse 2	Mouse 3	Mouse 4	Mouse 5	Mouse 1	Mouse 2	Mouse 3
0.25	3.340	2.733	3.691	2.713	1.559	3.811	3.009	0.864
0.75	10.454	7.641	10.710	8.422	5.261	10.480	9.161	3.796
1.25	11.205	9.700	8.331	5.437	7.183	11.001	10.762	5.115
2	4.676	5.277	3.446	1.990	3.324	3.175	3.246	3.890
3	2.352	2.419	2.611	1.615	2.241	2.337	2.027	2.214
4	2.276	2.155	2.378	1.583	2.056	2.272	1.689	1.888
5	2.046	1.923	2.146	1.524	1.953	2.056	1.684	1.797
6	2.002	1.942	1.881	1.418	1.948	2.021	1.547	1.720
7.5	1.870	1.789	1.803	1.441	1.890	1.861	1.486	1.586
9.5	1.691	1.579	1.581	1.382	1.821	1.771	1.355	1.539
11.5	1.497	1.610	1.519	1.337	1.809	1.607	1.263	1.517
13.5	1.501	1.481	1.371	1.314	1.733	1.516	1.241	1.446
15.5	1.426	1.491	1.359	1.320	1.731	1.466	1.194	1.454
18	1.309	1.446	1.206	1.283	1.736	1.383	1.276	1.540
21	1.238	1.409	1.154	1.290	1.730	1.304	1.303	1.512
24	1.118	1.348	1.045	1.260	1.740	1.219	1.154	1.539
27.5	1.060	1.288	0.979	1.291	1.686	1.144	1.179	1.532
31.5	0.959	1.235	0.935	1.262	1.660	1.095	1.206	1.448
35.5	0.924	1.175	0.869	1.274	1.684	1.022	1.154	1.446
40	0.835	1.100	0.814	1.249	1.669	0.941	1.114	1.378
45	0.785	1.021	0.737	1.255	1.666	0.863	1.062	1.269
50	0.705	0.961	0.703	1.251	1.669	0.829	1.092	1.072
55	0.650	0.896	0.657	1.223	1.650	0.760	1.039	0.985
58.75	0.577	0.906	0.573	1.195	1.633	0.748	1.099	0.922

References

1. Kadry, H.; Noorani, B.; Cucullo, L. A blood-brain barrier overview on structure, function, impairment, and biomarkers of integrity. *Fluids Barriers CNS* **2020**, *17*, 69. [CrossRef] [PubMed]
2. Abbott, N.J.; Patabendige, A.; Dolman, D.E.; Yusof, S.R.; Begley, D.J. Structure and function of the blood-brain barrier. *Neurobiol. Dis.* **2010**, *37*, 13–25. [CrossRef] [PubMed]
3. Al Rihani, S.; Darakjian, L.; Deodhar, M.; Dow, P.; Turgeon, J.; Michaud, V. Disease-Induced Modulation of Drug Transporters at the Blood-Brain Barrier Level. *Int. J. Mol. Sci.* **2021**, *22*, 3742. [CrossRef]

4. Pardridge, W.M. The Blood-Brain Barrier: Bottleneck in Brain Drug Development. *NeuroRx* **2005**, *2*, 3–14. [CrossRef] [PubMed]
5. Terstappen, G.C.; Meyer, A.H.; Bell, R.D.; Zhang, W. Strategies for delivering therapeutics across the blood-brain barrier. *Nat. Rev. Drug Discov.* **2021**, *20*, 362–383. [CrossRef]
6. Chen, K.-T.; Wei, K.-C.; Liu, H.-L. Theranostic Strategy of Focused Ultrasound Induced Blood-Brain Barrier Opening for CNS Disease Treatment. *Front. Pharmacol.* **2019**, *10*, 86. [CrossRef]
7. Liu, H.-L.; Fan, C.-H.; Ting, C.-Y.; Yeh, C.-K. Combining Microbubbles and Ultrasound for Drug Delivery to Brain Tumors: Current Progress and Overview. *Theranostics* **2014**, *4*, 432–444. [CrossRef] [PubMed]
8. Couture, O.; Foley, J.; Kassell, N.F.; Larrat, B.; Aubry, J.-F. Review of Ultrasound Mediated Drug Delivery for Cancer Treatment: Updates from Pre-Clinical Studies. *Transl. Cancer Res.* **2014**, *3*, 494–511. [CrossRef]
9. Hynynen, K.; McDannold, N.; Vykhodtseva, N.; Jolesz, F.A. Noninvasive MR Imaging–guided Focal Opening of the Blood-Brain Barrier in Rabbits. *Radiology* **2001**, *220*, 640–646. [CrossRef]
10. Tran, V.L.; Novell, A.; Tournier, N.; Gerstenmayer, M.; Schweitzer-Chaput, A.; Mateos, C.; Jego, B.; Bouleau, A.; Nozach, H.; Winkeler, A.; et al. Impact of blood-brain barrier permeabilization induced by ultrasound associated to microbubbles on the brain delivery and kinetics of cetuximab: An immunoPET study using 89Zr-cetuximab. *J. Control. Release* **2020**, *328*, 304–312. [CrossRef]
11. Alli, S.; Figueiredo, C.A.; Golbourn, B.; Sabha, N.; Wu, M.Y.; Bondoc, A.; Luck, A.; Coluccia, D.; Maslink, C.; Smith, C.; et al. Brainstem blood brain barrier disruption using focused ultrasound: A demonstration of feasibility and enhanced doxorubicin delivery. *J. Control. Release* **2018**, *281*, 29–41. [CrossRef] [PubMed]
12. Carpentier, A.; Canney, M.; Vignot, A.; Reina, V.; Beccaria, K.; Horodyckid, C.; Karachi, C.; Leclercq, D.; Lafon, C.; Chapelon, J.-Y.; et al. Clinical trial of blood-brain barrier disruption by pulsed ultrasound. *Sci. Transl. Med.* **2016**, *8*, 343re2. [CrossRef]
13. Abrahao, A.; Meng, Y.; Llinas, M.; Huang, Y.; Hamani, C.; Mainprize, T.; Aubert, I.; Heyn, C.; Black, S.E.; Hynynen, K.; et al. First-in-human trial of blood-brain barrier opening in amyotrophic lateral sclerosis using MR-guided focused ultrasound. *Nat. Commun.* **2019**, *10*, 4373. [CrossRef] [PubMed]
14. Lipsman, N.; Meng, Y.; Bethune, A.J.; Huang, Y.; Lam, B.; Masellis, M.; Herrmann, N.; Heyn, C.; Aubert, I.; Boutet, A.; et al. Blood-brain barrier opening in Alzheimer's disease using MR-guided focused ultrasound. *Nat. Commun.* **2018**, *9*, 2336. [CrossRef] [PubMed]
15. Mainprize, T.; Lipsman, N.; Huang, Y.; Meng, Y.; Bethune, A.; Ironside, S.; Heyn, C.; Alkins, R.; Trudeau, M.; Sahgal, A.; et al. Blood-Brain Barrier Opening in Primary Brain Tumors with Non-invasive MR-Guided Focused Ultrasound: A Clinical Safety and Feasibility Study. *Sci. Rep.* **2019**, *9*, 321. [CrossRef] [PubMed]
16. Idbaih, A.; Canney, M.; Belin, L.; Desseaux, C.; Vignot, A.; Bouchoux, G.; Asquier, N.; Law-Ye, B.; Leclercq, D.; Bissery, A.; et al. Safety and Feasibility of Repeated and Transient Blood-Brain Barrier Disruption by Pulsed Ultrasound in Patients with Recurrent Glioblastoma. *Clin. Cancer Res.* **2019**, *25*, 3793–3801. [CrossRef]
17. Chen, K.-T.; Lin, Y.-J.; Chai, W.-Y.; Lin, C.-J.; Chen, P.-Y.; Huang, C.-Y.; Kuo, J.S.; Liu, H.-L.; Wei, K.-C. Neuronavigation-guided focused ultrasound (NaviFUS) for transcranial blood-brain barrier opening in recurrent glioblastoma patients: Clinical trial protocol. *Ann. Transl. Med.* **2020**, *8*, 673. [CrossRef]
18. Arif, W.M.; Elsinga, P.H.; Gasca-Salas, C.; Versluis, M.; Martínez-Fernández, R.; Dierckx, R.A.; Borra, R.J.; Luurtsema, G. Focused ultrasound for opening blood-brain barrier and drug delivery monitored with positron emission tomography. *J. Control. Release* **2020**, *324*, 303–316. [CrossRef]
19. Sun, H.; Hu, H.; Liu, C.; Sun, N.; Duan, C. Methods used for the measurement of blood-brain barrier integrity. *Metab. Brain Dis.* **2021**, *36*, 723–735. [CrossRef]
20. Noorani, B.; Chowdhury, E.A.; Alqahtani, F.; Ahn, Y.; Patel, D.; Al-Ahmad, A.; Mehvar, R.; Bickel, U. LC–MS/MS-based in vitro and in vivo investigation of blood-brain barrier integrity by simultaneous quantitation of mannitol and sucrose. *Fluids Barriers CNS* **2020**, *17*, 61. [CrossRef]
21. Saunders, N.R.; Dziegielewska, K.M.; Emøllgård, K.; Habgood, M.D. Markers for blood-brain barrier integrity: How appropriate is Evans blue in the twenty-first century and what are the alternatives? *Front. Neurosci.* **2015**, *9*, 385. [CrossRef]
22. Bernal, J.; Valdés-Hernández, M.D.; Escudero, J.; Heye, A.K.; Sakka, E.; Armitage, P.A.; Makin, S.; Touyz, R.M.; Wardlaw, J.M.; Thrippleton, M.J. A four-dimensional computational model of dynamic contrast-enhanced magnetic resonance imaging measurement of subtle blood-brain barrier leakage. *NeuroImage* **2021**, *230*, 117786. [CrossRef] [PubMed]
23. Elschot, E.P.; Backes, W.H.; Postma, A.A.; Van Oostenbrugge, R.J.; Staals, J.; Rouhl, R.P.; Jansen, J.F. A Comprehensive View on MRI Techniques for Imaging Blood-Brain Barrier Integrity. *Investig. Radiol.* **2021**, *56*, 10–19. [CrossRef]
24. Marty, B.; Larrat, B.; Van Landeghem, M.; Robic, C.; Robert, P.; Port, M.; Le Bihan, D.; Pernot, M.; Tanter, M.; Lethimonnier, F.; et al. Dynamic Study of Blood-Brain Barrier Closure after its Disruption using Ultrasound: A Quantitative Analysis. *J. Cereb. Blood Flow Metab.* **2012**, *32*, 1948–1958. [CrossRef]
25. Yang, F.-Y.; Wang, H.-E.; Lin, G.-L.; Teng, M.-C.; Lin, H.-H.; Wong, T.-T.; Liu, R.-S. Micro-SPECT/CT–Based Pharmacokinetic Analysis of 99mTc-Diethylenetriaminepentaacetic Acid in Rats with Blood-Brain Barrier Disruption Induced by Focused Ultrasound. *J. Nucl. Med.* **2011**, *52*, 478–484. [CrossRef]
26. Tournier, N.; Comtat, C.; Lebon, V.; Gennisson, J.-L. Challenges and Perspectives of the Hybridization of PET with Functional MRI or Ultrasound for Neuroimaging. *Neuroscience* **2020**, *474*, 80–93. [CrossRef]

27. Elmaleh, D.; Shoup, T.; Bonab, A.; Takahashi, K.; Fischman, A. Evaluation of 1-Deoxy-1-[18F]Fluoro-D-Mannitol as a Brain Imaging Tracer for Measuring Osmotic Disruption Following Cancer Therapy. *J. Nucl. Med.* **2014**, *55*, 1123.
28. Hara, T.; Iio, M.; Tsukiyama, T.; Yokoi, F. Measurement of human blood brain barrier integrity using 11C-inulin and positron emission tomography. *Eur. J. Nucl. Med.* **1988**, *14*, 173–176. [CrossRef]
29. Li, Z.; Wu, Z.; Cao, Q.; Dick, D.; Tseng, J.R.; Gambhir, S.S.; Chen, X. The Synthesis of 18F-FDS and Its Potential Application in Molecular Imaging. *Mol. Imaging Biol.* **2008**, *10*, 92–98. [CrossRef] [PubMed]
30. Zhu, W.; Yao, S.; Xing, H.; Zhang, H.; Tai, Y.-C.; Zhang, Y.; Liu, Y.; Ma, Y.; Wu, C.; Wang, H.; et al. Biodistribution and Radiation Dosimetry of the Enterobacteriaceae-Specific Imaging Probe [18F]Fluorodeoxysorbitol Determined by PET/CT in Healthy Human Volunteers. *Mol. Imaging Biol.* **2016**, *18*, 782–787. [CrossRef] [PubMed]
31. Yao, S.; Xing, H.; Zhu, W.; Wu, Z.; Zhang, Y.; Ma, Y.; Liu, Y.; Huo, L.; Zhu, Z.; Li, Z.; et al. Infection Imaging With 18F-FDS and First-in-Human Evaluation. *Nucl. Med. Biol.* **2016**, *43*, 206–214. [CrossRef] [PubMed]
32. Felix, M.-S.; Borloz, E.; Metwally, K.; Dauba, A.; Larrat, B.; Matagne, V.; Ehinger, Y.; Villard, L.; Novell, A.; Mensah, S.; et al. Ultrasound-Mediated Blood-Brain Barrier Opening Improves Whole Brain Gene Delivery in Mice. *Pharmaceutics* **2021**, *13*, 1245. [CrossRef] [PubMed]
33. Goutal, S.; Gerstenmayer, M.; Auvity, S.; Caillé, F.; Mériaux, S.; Buvat, I.; Larrat, B.; Tournier, N. Physical blood-brain barrier disruption induced by focused ultrasound does not overcome the transporter-mediated efflux of erlotinib. *J. Control. Release* **2018**, *292*, 210–220. [CrossRef]
34. Logan, J.; Fowler, J.S.; Volkow, N.D.; Wolf, A.P.; Dewey, S.L.; Schlyer, D.J.; MacGregor, R.R.; Hitzemann, R.; Bendriem, B.; Gatley, S.J.; et al. Graphical Analysis of Reversible Radioligand Binding from Time—Activity Measurements Applied to [N-11C-Methyl]-(−)-Cocaine PET Studies in Human Subjects. *J. Cereb. Blood Flow Metab.* **1990**, *10*, 740–747. [CrossRef] [PubMed]
35. Werner, R.A.; Ordonez, A.; Sanchez-Bautista, J.; Marcus, C.; Lapa, C.; Rowe, S.P.; Pomper, M.G.; Leal, J.P.; Lodge, M.A.; Javadi, M.S.; et al. Novel Functional Renal PET Imaging With 18F-FDS in Human Subjects. *Clin. Nucl. Med.* **2019**, *44*, 410–411. [CrossRef] [PubMed]
36. Weinstein, E.A.; Ordonez, A.A.; DeMarco, V.P.; Murawski, A.M.; Pokkali, S.; MacDonald, E.M.; Klunk, M.; Mease, R.C.; Pomper, M.G.; Jain, S.K. Imaging Enterobacteriaceae infection in vivo with 18F-fluorodeoxysorbitol positron emission tomography. *Sci. Transl. Med.* **2014**, *6*, 259ra146. [CrossRef]
37. Ordonez, A.A.; Wintaco, L.M.; Mota, F.; Restrepo, A.F.; Ruiz-Bedoya, C.A.; Reyes, C.F.; Uribe, L.G.; Abhishek, S.; D'Alessio, F.R.; Holt, D.P.; et al. Imaging Enterobacterales infections in patients using pathogen-specific positron emission tomography. *Sci. Transl. Med.* **2021**, *13*, eabe9805. [CrossRef]
38. Werner, R.A.; Wakabayashi, H.; Chen, X.; Hirano, M.; Shinaji, T.; Lapa, C.; Rowe, S.P.; Javadi, M.S.; Higuchi, T. Functional Renal Imaging with 2-Deoxy-2-18F-Fluorosorbitol PET in Rat Models of Renal Disorders. *J. Nucl. Med.* **2018**, *59*, 828–832. [CrossRef]
39. Fortin, D. Drug Delivery Technology to the CNS in the Treatment of Brain Tumors: The Sherbrooke Experience. *Pharmaceutics* **2019**, *11*, 248. [CrossRef]
40. Yang, F.-Y.; Chang, W.-Y.; Chen, J.-C.; Lee, L.-C.; Hung, Y.-S. Quantitative assessment of cerebral glucose metabolic rates after blood-brain barrier disruption induced by focused ultrasound using FDG-MicroPET. *NeuroImage* **2014**, *90*, 93–98. [CrossRef]
41. Breuil, L.; Marie, S.; Goutal, S.; Auvity, S.; Truillet, C.; Saba, W.; Langer, O.; Caillé, F.; Tournier, N. Comparative vulnerability of PET radioligands to partial inhibition of P-glycoprotein at the blood-brain barrier: A criterion of choice? *J. Cereb. Blood Flow Metab.* **2021**. [CrossRef]
42. Aryal, M.; Fischer, K.; Gentile, C.; Gitto, S.; Zhang, Y.-Z.; McDannold, N. Effects on P-Glycoprotein Expression after Blood-Brain Barrier Disruption Using Focused Ultrasound and Microbubbles. *PLoS ONE* **2017**, *12*, e0166061. [CrossRef]
43. Cho, H.; Lee, H.-Y.; Han, M.; Choi, J.-R.; Ahn, S.; Lee, T.; Chang, Y.; Park, J. Localized Down-regulation of P-glycoprotein by Focused Ultrasound and Microbubbles induced Blood-Brain Barrier Disruption in Rat Brain. *Sci. Rep.* **2016**, *6*, 31201. [CrossRef]
44. Drozdovitch, V.; Brill, A.B.; Callahan, R.J.; Clanton, J.A.; DePietro, A.; Goldsmith, S.J.; Greenspan, B.S.; Gross, M.D.; Hays, M.T.; Moore, S.C.; et al. Use of Radiopharmaceuticals in Diagnostic Nuclear Medicine in the United States: 1960–2010. *Heal. Phys.* **2015**, *108*, 520–537. [CrossRef]
45. Hasegawa, K.; Koshino, K.; Higuchi, T. Facile synthesis of 2-deoxy-2-[18F]fluorosorbitol using sodium borohydride on aluminum oxide. *J. Label. Compd. Radiopharm.* **2021**, *64*, 40–46. [CrossRef]
46. Obermeier, B.; Daneman, R.; Ransohoff, R.M. Development, maintenance and disruption of the blood-brain barrier. *Nat. Med.* **2013**, *19*, 1584–1596. [CrossRef]
47. Okada, M.; Kikuchi, T.; Okamura, T.; Ikoma, Y.; Tsuji, A.B.; Wakizaka, H.; Kamakura, T.; Aoki, I.; Zhang, M.-R.; Kato, K. In-vivo imaging of blood-brain barrier permeability using positron emission tomography with 2-amino-[3-11C]isobutyric acid. *Nucl. Med. Commun.* **2015**, *36*, 1239–1248. [CrossRef] [PubMed]
48. Iannotti, F.; Fieschi, C.; Alfano, B.; Picozzi, P.; Mansi, L.; Pozzilli, C.; Punzo, A.; Del Vecchio, G.; Lenzi, G.L.; Salvatore, M.; et al. Simplified, Noninvasive PET Measurement of Blood-Brain Barrier Permeability. *J. Comput. Assist. Tomogr.* **1987**, *11*, 390–397. [CrossRef] [PubMed]
49. Jones, T.; Rabiner, E.A. PET Research Advisory Company the Development, Past Achievements, and Future Directions of Brain PET. *J. Cereb. Blood Flow Metab.* **2012**, *32*, 1426–1454. [CrossRef] [PubMed]
50. Szadvari, I.; Krizanova, O.; Babula, P. Athymic Nude Mice as an Experimental Model for Cancer Treatment. *Physiol. Res.* **2016**, S441–S453. [CrossRef] [PubMed]

51. Zhang, X.; Liu, W.; Yuan, J.; Zhu, H.; Yang, Y.; Wen, Z.; Chen, Y.; Li, L.; Lin, J.; Feng, H. T lymphocytes infiltration promotes blood-brain barrier injury after experimental intracerebral hemorrhage. *Brain Res.* **2017**, *1670*, 96–105. [CrossRef]
52. Li, J.; Zheng, M.; Shimoni, O.; Banks, W.A.; Bush, A.I.; Gamble, J.R.; Shi, B. Development of Novel Therapeutics Targeting the Blood-Brain Barrier: From Barrier to Carrier. *Adv. Sci.* **2021**, *8*, 2101090. [CrossRef] [PubMed]
53. Burgess, A.; Dubey, S.; Yeung, S.; Hough, O.; Eterman, N.; Aubert, I.; Hynynen, K. Alzheimer Disease in a Mouse Model: MR Imaging–guided Focused Ultrasound Targeted to the Hippocampus Opens the Blood-Brain Barrier and Improves Pathologic Abnormalities and Behavior. *Radiology* **2014**, *273*, 736–745. [CrossRef] [PubMed]
54. Mooney, S.J.; Shah, K.; Yeung, S.; Burgess, A.; Aubert, I.; Hynynen, K. Focused Ultrasound-Induced Neurogenesis Requires an Increase in Blood-Brain Barrier Permeability. *PLoS ONE* **2016**, *11*, e0159892. [CrossRef] [PubMed]

MDPI
St. Alban-Anlage 66
4052 Basel
Switzerland
Tel. +41 61 683 77 34
Fax +41 61 302 89 18
www.mdpi.com

Pharmaceutics Editorial Office
E-mail: pharmaceutics@mdpi.com
www.mdpi.com/journal/pharmaceutics

www.ingramcontent.com/pod-product-compliance
Lightning Source LLC
LaVergne TN
LVHW070503100526
838202LV00014B/1780